Cardiovascular and Metabolic Disease: New Treatment and Future Directions 2.0

Cardiovascular and Metabolic Disease: New Treatment and Future Directions 2.0

Editor

Alfredo Caturano

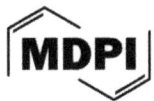

Basel • Beijing • Wuhan • Barcelona • Belgrade • Novi Sad • Cluj • Manchester

Editor
Alfredo Caturano
University of Campania
"Luigi Vanvitelli"
Naples
Italy

Editorial Office
MDPI AG
Grosspeteranlage 5
4052 Basel, Switzerland

This is a reprint of articles from the Special Issue published online in the open access journal *Biomedicines* (ISSN 2227-9059) (available at: https://www.mdpi.com/journal/biomedicines/special_issues/UC4DR3PU81).

For citation purposes, cite each article independently as indicated on the article page online and as indicated below:

Lastname, A.A.; Lastname, B.B. Article Title. *Journal Name* **Year**, *Volume Number*, Page Range.

ISBN 978-3-7258-1667-5 (Hbk)
ISBN 978-3-7258-1668-2 (PDF)
doi.org/10.3390/books978-3-7258-1668-2

© 2024 by the authors. Articles in this book are Open Access and distributed under the Creative Commons Attribution (CC BY) license. The book as a whole is distributed by MDPI under the terms and conditions of the Creative Commons Attribution-NonCommercial-NoDerivs (CC BY-NC-ND) license.

Contents

About the Editor ix

Alfredo Caturano
Cardiovascular and Metabolic Disease: New Treatments and Future Directions 2.0
Reprinted from: *Biomedicines* 2024, 12, 1356, doi:10.3390/biomedicines12061356 1

Seung Eun Jung, Sang Woo Kim and Jung-Won Choi
Exploring Cardiac Exosomal RNAs of Acute Myocardial Infarction
Reprinted from: *Biomedicines* 2024, 12, 430, doi:10.3390/biomedicines12020430 7

Federica Fogacci, Serra İlayda Yerlitaş, Marina Giovannini, Gökmen Zararsız, Paolo Lido, Claudio Borghi, et al.
Sex X Time Interactions in Lp(a) and LDL-C Response to Evolocumab
Reprinted from: *Biomedicines* 2023, 11, 3271, doi:10.3390/biomedicines11123271 24

Alfredo Caturano, Gaetana Albanese, Anna Di Martino, Carmine Coppola, Vincenzo Russo, Raffaele Galiero, et al.
Predictive Value of Fatty Liver Index for Long-Term Cardiovascular Events in Patients Receiving Liver Transplantation: The COLT Study
Reprinted from: *Biomedicines* 2023, 11, 2866, doi:10.3390/biomedicines11102866 35

Irina Tarasova, Olga Trubnikova, Irina Kukhareva, Irina Syrova, Anastasia Sosnina, Darya Kupriyanova, et al.
A Comparison of Two Multi-Tasking Approaches to Cognitive Training in Cardiac Surgery Patients
Reprinted from: *Biomedicines* 2023, 11, 2823, doi:10.3390/biomedicines11102823 50

Teodor Salmen, Ali Abbas Rizvi, Manfredi Rizzo, Valeria-Anca Pietrosel, Ioana-Cristina Bica, Cosmina Theodora Diaconu, et al.
Antidiabetic Molecule Efficacy in Patients with Type 2 Diabetes Mellitus—A Real-Life Clinical Practice Study
Reprinted from: *Biomedicines* 2023, 11, 2455, doi:10.3390/biomedicines11092455 64

Juan Carlos Sánchez-Delgado, Daniel D. Cohen, Paul A. Camacho-López, Javier Carreño-Robayo, Alvaro Castañeda-Hernández, Daniel García-González, et al.
Handgrip Strength Is Associated with Specific Aspects of Vascular Function in Individuals with Metabolic Syndrome
Reprinted from: *Biomedicines* 2023, 11, 2435, doi:10.3390/biomedicines11092435 77

Maria Kercheva, Vyacheslav Ryabov, Aleksandra Gombozhapova, Ivan Stepanov and Julia Kzhyshkowska
Macrophages of the Cardiorenal Axis and Myocardial Infarction
Reprinted from: *Biomedicines* 2023, 11, 1843, doi:10.3390/biomedicines11071843 90

Anna Kurpas, Karolina Supel, Paulina Wieczorkiewicz, Joanna Bodalska Duleba and Marzenna Zielinska
Fibroblast Growth Factor 23: Potential Marker of Invisible Heart Damage in Diabetic Population
Reprinted from: *Biomedicines* 2023, 11, 1523, doi:10.3390/biomedicines11061523 98

Natalia Beloborodova, Alisa Pautova, Marina Grekova, Mikhail Yadgarov, Oksana Grin, Alexander Eremenko, et al.
Microbiota Metabolism Failure as a Risk Factor for Postoperative Complications after Aortic Prosthetics
Reprinted from: *Biomedicines* **2023**, *11*, 1335, doi:10.3390/biomedicines11051335 114

Ioan Alexandru Balmos, Emőke Horváth, Klara Brinzaniuc, Adrian Vasile Muresan, Peter Olah, Gyopár Beáta Molnár, et al.
Inflammation, Microcalcification, and Increased Expression of Osteopontin Are Histological Hallmarks of Plaque Vulnerability in Patients with Advanced Carotid Artery Stenosis
Reprinted from: *Biomedicines* **2023**, *11*, 881, doi:10.3390/biomedicines11030881 126

Moustapha Agossou, Bérénice Awanou, Jocelyn Inamo, Mickael Rejaudry-Lacavalerie, Jean-Michel Arnal and Moustapha Dramé
Impact of Previous Continuous Positive Airway Pressure Use on Noninvasive Ventilation Adherence and Quality in Obesity Hypoventilation Syndrome: A Pragmatic Single-Center Cross-Sectional Study in Martinique
Reprinted from: *Biomedicines* **2023**, *11*, 2753, doi:10.3390/biomedicines11102753 144

Giovanni Cimmino, Francesco Natale, Roberta Alfieri, Luigi Cante, Simona Covino, Rosa Franzese, et al.
Non-Conventional Risk Factors: "Fact" or "Fake" in Cardiovascular Disease Prevention?
Reprinted from: *Biomedicines* **2023**, *11*, 2353, doi:10.3390/biomedicines11092353 152

Weronika Frąk, Joanna Hajdys, Ewa Radzioch, Magdalena Szlagor, Ewelina Młynarska, Jacek Rysz, et al.
Cardiovascular Diseases: Therapeutic Potential of SGLT-2 Inhibitors
Reprinted from: *Biomedicines* **2023**, *11*, 2085, doi:10.3390/biomedicines11072085 186

Silvia Preda, Lucian Câlmâc, Claudia Nica, Mihai Cacoveanu, Robert Țigănașu, Aida Badea, et al.
TAVI in a Heart Transplant Recipient—Rare Case Report and Review of the Literature
Reprinted from: *Biomedicines* **2023**, *11*, 2634, doi:10.3390/biomedicines11102634 204

Ayodeji A. Olabiyi and Lisandra E. de Castro Brás
Cardiovascular Remodeling Post-Ischemia: Herbs, Diet, and Drug Interventions
Reprinted from: *Biomedicines* **2023**, *11*, 1697, doi:10.3390/biomedicines11061697 220

Simonetta Genovesi, Marco Giussani, Giulia Lieti, Antonina Orlando, Ilenia Patti and Gianfranco Parati
Evidence and Uncertainties on Lipoprotein(a) as a Marker of Cardiovascular Health Risk in Children and Adolescents
Reprinted from: *Biomedicines* **2023**, *11*, 1661, doi:10.3390/biomedicines11061661 238

Ozan Demirel, Alexander E. Berezin, Moritz Mirna, Elke Boxhammer, Sarah X. Gharibeh, Uta C. Hoppe, et al.
Biomarkers of Atrial Fibrillation Recurrence in Patients with Paroxysmal or Persistent Atrial Fibrillation Following External Direct Current Electrical Cardioversion
Reprinted from: *Biomedicines* **2023**, *11*, 1452, doi:10.3390/biomedicines11051452 252

Polyxeni Mantzouratou, Eleftheria Malaxianaki, Domenico Cerullo, Angelo Michele Lavecchia, Constantinos Pantos, Christodoulos Xinaris, et al.
Thyroid Hormone and Heart Failure: Charting Known Pathways for Cardiac Repair/Regeneration
Reprinted from: *Biomedicines* **2023**, *11*, 975, doi:10.3390/biomedicines11030975 279

Preeti Kumari Chaudhary, Sachin Upadhayaya, Sanggu Kim and Soochong Kim
The Perspectives of Platelet Proteomics in Health and Disease
Reprinted from: *Biomedicines* **2024**, *12*, 585, doi:10.3390/biomedicines12030585 . . . . **292**

Esther Solano-Pérez, Carlota Coso, Sofía Romero-Peralta, María Castillo-García, Sonia López-Monzoni, Alfonso Ortigado, et al.
New Approaches to the Management of Cardiovascular Risk Associated with Sleep Respiratory Disorders in Pediatric Patients
Reprinted from: *Biomedicines* **2024**, *12*, 411, doi:10.3390/biomedicines12020411 . . . . **314**

About the Editor

Alfredo Caturano

Alfredo Caturano, MD, graduated in Medicine and Surgery from the Second University of Naples (SUN) in 2016. He achieved a Specialization Degree in Internal Medicine in 2021 at the University of Campania "Luigi Vanvitelli". His specialization thesis, concerning the impact of glycemic control on cardiovascular outcomes and mortality in a cohort of patients with type 2 diabetes mellitus in a multifactorial randomized controlled trial, was awarded the 2021 Annapaola Braggio prize by the Italian Society of Diabetology as the best specialization thesis on topics related to insulin resistance. He presently serves as a PhD attendant at the University of Campania "Luigi Vanvitelli" and has been awarded multiple grants from both Italian and European scientific societies.

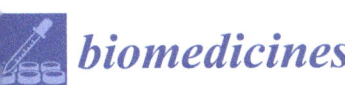 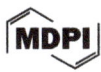

Editorial

Cardiovascular and Metabolic Disease: New Treatments and Future Directions 2.0

Alfredo Caturano [1,2]

[1] Department of Advanced Medical and Surgical Sciences, University of Campania Luigi Vanvitelli, I-80138 Naples, Italy; alfredo.caturano@unicampania.it; Tel.: +39-3338616985
[2] Department of Experimental Medicine, University of Campania Luigi Vanvitelli, I-80138 Naples, Italy

1. Introduction

Over recent decades, cardiovascular diseases (CVDs) and metabolic disorders have emerged as major global health challenges, exacting a heavy toll on human lives and burdening healthcare systems worldwide. Despite advancements in medical science and technology, these conditions persist as leading causes of morbidity and mortality, prompting a critical need for innovative approaches to prevention, diagnosis, and treatment [1,2].

The intersection of cardiovascular diseases and metabolic disorders is complex and multifaceted. The epidemiological landscape reveals a stark reality: a significant proportion of CVD-related deaths are intricately linked to the coexistence of metabolic ailments, particularly diabetes. This nexus demands comprehensive understanding and targeted interventions to mitigate the intertwined risks and complexities inherent in these conditions [3,4].

In the year 2019 alone, an alarming 17.9 million lives were lost to cardiovascular diseases, constituting a staggering 32% of all global deaths [5]. Heart attacks and strokes accounted for a substantial portion of these fatalities, underscoring the urgent need for effective preventive strategies and therapeutic interventions. Moreover, the burden of metabolic diseases, exemplified by the pervasive prevalence of diabetes, adds to the gravity of the situation. In 2019, global diabetes prevalence stood at 9.3%, affecting approximately 463 million individuals worldwide. Projections indicate a steady rise in prevalence, with estimates indicating a rise to 10.2% (578 million) by 2030 and 10.9% (700 million) by 2045 [6]. Alarmingly, 1.5 million deaths are directly attributed to diabetes annually, accentuating the imperative for the early detection and comprehensive management of these interrelated conditions [7].

Behavioral risk factors such as tobacco use, unhealthy dietary patterns, sedentary lifestyles, and excessive alcohol consumption exacerbate the susceptibility to both cardiovascular diseases and metabolic disorders. Therefore, addressing these modifiable risk factors assumes paramount importance in the overarching strategy for disease prevention and control [8–10].

In the realm of therapeutics, recent years have witnessed significant strides in the management of cardiovascular and metabolic diseases. From pharmacological innovations, including the advent of sodium glucose cotransporter 2 inhibitors heralding promising outcomes in heart failure and diabetes management, to advancements in interventional techniques such as immediate revascularization for acute myocardial infarction and cerebral infarction, the landscape of cardiovascular care continues to evolve rapidly [11,12]. Additionally, emerging modalities like mechanical cardiac support and multiorgan transplantation offer novel avenues for managing the most complex manifestations of heart failure, underscoring the transformative potential of cutting-edge interventions [11,13].

This Special Issue has captured the diversity of the studies that focus on the latest scientific insights and technological innovations in the realm of cardiovascular and metabolic disease management.

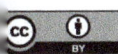

2. Overview of Published Articles

These articles provide a diverse range of insights into cardiovascular and metabolic diseases, reflecting the multifaceted nature of these conditions and the ongoing efforts to better understand and treat them.

Seung Eun Jung et al. (contribution 1) investigated the role of exosomal RNAs, particularly microRNAs, in animal models of acute myocardial infarction (AMI). By identifying differentially expressed miRNAs and validating their functions in vitro, the research enhances our understanding of post-AMI molecular changes and explores the potential of exoRNAs as biomarkers or therapeutic targets.

Federica Fogacci et al. (contribution 2) focused on the effects of Evolocumab, a PCSK9 inhibitor. In this study, the researchers examined how lipoprotein(a) and low-density lipoprotein cholesterol respond to treatment over time, particularly considering sex-related differences. The understanding of these dynamics could contribute to personalized treatment strategies for cardiovascular disease.

Alfredo Caturano et al. (contribution 3) investigated the association between the fatty liver index (FLI) and cardiovascular events in liver transplant recipients; this study underscores the importance of monitoring metabolic parameters and liver health in this unique cohort of patients for cardiovascular disease prevention, suggesting FLI as a potential predictive marker.

Irina Tarasova et al. (contribution 4) evaluated different cognitive training approaches in cardiac surgery patients, highlighting the potential benefits of multi-tasking training for cognitive rehabilitation in the postoperative period.

Teodor Salmen et al. (contribution 5) assessed the efficacy of antidiabetic medications, particularly SGLT-2 inhibitors and GLP-1 receptor agonists, in real-life clinical practice. This study provides valuable insights into their effectiveness in managing type 2 diabetes mellitus, especially when used in conjunction with other medications.

Juan Carlos Sánchez-Delgado et al. (contribution 6) investigated the association between handgrip strength and vascular function in individuals with metabolic syndrome. This study highlights the potential role of muscle strength in mitigating vascular dysfunction, particularly in older adults.

Maria Kercheva et al. (contribution 7) found that kidneys of patients with fatal myocardial infarction (MI) showed a predominance of CD163+ macrophages, while controls without cardiovascular diseases (CVD) had a higher presence of CD163+, CD206+, and CD68+ macrophages. In MI patients, CD80+ and CD206+ macrophages exhibited a biphasic response, decreasing over time post-MI.

Anna Kurpas et al. (contribution 8) found that epicardial global circumferential strain measured using 2D speckle-tracking echocardiography significantly correlated with serum FGF23 levels in patients with type 2 diabetes mellitus, suggesting FGF23 as a potential early marker of myocardial damage in these patients. Additionally, patients with left ventricular diastolic dysfunction had lower estimated glomerular filtration rates and higher hemoglobin A1c levels.

Natalia Beloborodova et al. (contribution 9) found that higher levels of sepsis-associated aromatic microbial metabolites in the blood before and shortly after surgery were linked to postoperative complications in patients with aortic aneurysm. This suggests that an impaired microbiota metabolism plays a significant role in postoperative outcomes, indicating a potential target for new prevention strategies.

Ioan Alexandru Balmos et al. (contribution 10) found that inflammation, microcalcification, and high-grade osteopontin expression are significantly associated with plaque ulceration and atherothrombosis in patients with carotid artery stenosis, indicating their critical roles in plaque formation and destabilization. Higher osteopontin expression was also linked to the presence of a lipid core, suggesting its importance in plaque progression.

Moustapha Agossou et al. (contribution 11) showed the results of a brief report assessing the impact of previous continuous positive airway pressure (CPAP) use on the quality of noninvasive ventilation (NIV) in patients with obesity hypoventilation syndrome.

They found no significant difference in NIV quality between patients with and without prior CPAP use.

Preeti Kumari Chaudhary et al. (contribution 12) reviewed the literature exploring how platelet proteomics can advance the diagnosis and treatment of cardiovascular thromboembolic diseases and cancer. By analyzing peptides and proteins in platelets, researchers can identify disease-specific biomarkers for personalized medicine.

Esther Solano-Pérez et al. (contribution 13) discuss how obstructive sleep apnea (OSA) in children can increase cardiovascular risk. Their review proposes using echocardiography alongside polysomnography to assess cardiac function and structure in OSA patients for better risk management.

Silvia Preda et al. (contribution 14) presented a case study of transcatheter aortic valve implantation (TAVI) in a patient who had previously undergone a heart transplant. It highlights the challenges and potential benefits of using TAVI in heart transplant recipients.

Giovanni Cimmino et al. (contribution 15) focused on analyzing literature data with the aim of exploring emerging non-traditional risk factors for cardiovascular disease and their potential impact on disease development. They discuss how these factors may influence current cardiovascular risk assessment models.

Weronika Frąk et al. (contribution 16) discuss the therapeutic potential of sodium/glucose cotransporter 2 inhibitors in treating cardiovascular diseases. They report the available data on the efficacy of these medications in improving cardiovascular outcomes.

Ayodeji A. Olabiyi et al. (contribution 17) focus their review article on examining the use of dietary interventions and medicinal herbs in treating cardiovascular disease. They propose combining these approaches with pharmaceutical drugs for more effective treatment strategies.

Simonetta Genovesi et al. (contribution 18) dealt with lipoprotein(a) (Lp(a)) as a marker of cardiovascular health risk in young populations. They explore the evidence surrounding Lp(a) and its potential role in assessing cardiovascular risk in children and adolescents.

Ozan Demirel et al. (contribution 19) examined different serum biomarkers for predicting atrial fibrillation recurrence after electrical cardioversion in their review article. They discussed the potential of these biomarkers in improving patient outcomes.

Polyxeni Mantzouratou et al. (contribution 20) performed a literature review on the role of thyroid hormone signaling in cardiac repair and regeneration, reporting that thyroid hormone therapy may benefit heart failure patients.

3. Future Directions

Looking ahead, the landscape of cardiovascular and metabolic disease research holds immense promise for transformative advancements and innovative interventions. As we navigate the complexities of these interconnected conditions, several key avenues emerge as focal points for future exploration and inquiry.

First and foremost, the imperative for personalized medicine in cardiovascular and metabolic disease management is looming large on the horizon [14]. With the advent of precision medicine and genomic technologies, there exists unprecedented potential to tailor interventions to the individual characteristics and needs of patients, thereby optimizing therapeutic outcomes and minimizing adverse effects. Harnessing the power of big data analytics and artificial intelligence, researchers can glean valuable insights into the intricate interplay of genetic, environmental, and lifestyle factors influencing disease susceptibility and progression, paving the way for more targeted and effective treatment strategies [15].

Furthermore, the pursuit of novel therapeutic targets and modalities represents a frontier ripe for exploration. From elucidating the molecular mechanisms underlying disease pathogenesis to identifying druggable targets and developing innovative therapeutics, ongoing research efforts hold promise for revolutionizing the treatment landscape for cardiovascular and metabolic disorders. Emerging areas such as gene editing, stem cell therapy, and regenerative medicine offer tantalizing prospects for disease modification and regeneration, offering new hope for patients with refractory conditions and advanced disease states [16,17].

In parallel, efforts to address the social determinants of health and reduce health disparities remain paramount [18]. Recognizing the profound impact of socioeconomic factors, access to care, and healthcare disparities on disease outcomes, future initiatives must prioritize equitable access to preventive services, early detection, and evidence-based interventions for all segments of the population. By addressing structural barriers and fostering community engagement, healthcare stakeholders can empower individuals to make informed choices and adopt healthy behaviors, thereby mitigating the burden of cardiovascular and metabolic diseases on vulnerable populations. Moreover, the integration of digital health technologies and telemedicine holds immense potential for enhancing disease management and improving patient outcomes. From remote monitoring and teleconsultation to wearable devices and mobile health applications, digital innovations offer unprecedented opportunities to empower patients, enhance care coordination, and facilitate real-time data-driven decision-making. By harnessing the power of technology to bridge geographical barriers, streamline healthcare delivery, and empower patients to actively participate in their own care, we can unlock new frontiers in the prevention and management of cardiovascular and metabolic diseases [19].

In conclusion, the future of cardiovascular and metabolic disease research is characterized by boundless possibilities and transformative potential. By embracing a multidisciplinary approach, leveraging cutting-edge technologies, and prioritizing patient-centered care, we can chart a course towards a future where the burden of these devastating conditions is alleviated, and the promise of improved health and well-being becomes a tangible reality for individuals and communities worldwide.

Funding: This research received no external funding.

Institutional Review Board Statement: The author reviewed literature data and reported results from studies approved by local ethics committees.

Informed Consent Statement: Not applicable.

Data Availability Statement: No dataset was generated for the publication of this article.

Conflicts of Interest: The author declares no conflicts of interest.

List of Contributions

1. Jung, S.E.; Kim, S.W.; Choi, J.-W. Exploring Cardiac Exosomal RNAs of Acute Myocardial Infarction. *Biomedicines* **2024**, *12*, 430.
2. Fogacci, F.; Yerlitaş, S.İ.; Giovannini, M.; Zararsız, G.; Lido, P.; Borghi, C.; Cicero, A.F.G. Sex X Time Interactions in Lp(a) and LDL-C Response to Evolocumab. *Biomedicines* **2023**, *11*, 3271.
3. Caturano, A.; Albanese, G.; Di Martino, A.; Coppola, C.; Russo, V.; Galiero, R.; Rinaldi, L.; Monda, M.; Marfella, R.; Sasso, F.C.; et al. Predictive Value of Fatty Liver Index for Long-Term Cardiovascular Events in Patients Receiving Liver Transplantation: The COLT Study. *Biomedicines* **2023**, *11*, 2866.
4. Tarasova, I.; Trubnikova, O.; Kukhareva, I.; Syrova, I.; Sosnina, A.; Kupriyanova, D.; Barbarash, O. A Comparison of Two Multi-Tasking Approaches to Cognitive Training in Cardiac Surgery Patients. *Biomedicines* **2023**, *11*, 2823.
5. Salmen, T.; Rizvi, A.A.; Rizzo, M.; Pietrosel, V.-A.; Bica, I.-C.; Diaconu, C.T.; Potcovaru, C.G.; Salmen, B.-M.; Coman, O.A.; Bobircă, A.; et al. Antidiabetic Molecule Efficacy in Patients with Type 2 Diabetes Mellitus—A Real-Life Clinical Practice Study. *Biomedicines* **2023**, *11*, 2455.
6. Sánchez-Delgado, J.C.; Cohen, D.D.; Camacho-López, P.A.; Carreño-Robayo, J.; Castañeda-Hernández, A.; García-González, D.; Martínez-Bello, D.; Aroca-Martinez, G.; Parati, G.; Lopez-Jaramillo, P. Handgrip Strength Is Associated with Specific Aspects of Vascular Function in Individuals with Metabolic Syndrome. *Biomedicines* **2023**, *11*, 2435.
7. Kercheva, M.; Ryabov, V.; Gombozhapova, A.; Stepanov, I.; Kzhyshkowska, J. Macrophages of the Cardiorenal Axis and Myocardial Infarction. *Biomedicines* **2023**, *11*, 1843.

8. Kurpas, A.; Supel, K.; Wieczorkiewicz, P.; Bodalska Duleba, J.; Zielinska, M. Fibroblast Growth Factor 23: Potential Marker of Invisible Heart Damage in Diabetic Population. *Biomedicines* **2023**, *11*, 1523.
9. Beloborodova, N.; Pautova, A.; Grekova, M.; Yadgarov, M.; Grin, O.; Eremenko, A.; Babaev, M. Microbiota Metabolism Failure as a Risk Factor for Postoperative Complications after Aortic Prosthetics. *Biomedicines* **2023**, *11*, 1335.
10. Balmos, I.A.; Horváth, E.; Brinzaniuc, K.; Muresan, A.V.; Olah, P.; Molnár, G.B.; Nagy, E.E. Inflammation, Microcalcification, and Increased Expression of Osteopontin Are Histological Hallmarks of Plaque Vulnerability in Patients with Advanced Carotid Artery Stenosis. *Biomedicines* **2023**, *11*, 881.
11. Agossou, M.; Awanou, B.; Inamo, J.; Rejaudry-Lacavalerie, M.; Arnal, J.-M.; Dramé, M. Impact of Previous Continuous Positive Airway Pressure Use on Noninvasive Ventilation Adherence and Quality in Obesity Hypoventilation Syndrome: A Pragmatic Single-Center Cross-Sectional Study in Martinique. *Biomedicines* **2023**, *11*, 2753.
12. Chaudhary, P.K.; Upadhayaya, S.; Kim, S.; Kim, S. The Perspectives of Platelet Proteomics in Health and Disease. *Biomedicines* **2024**, *12*, 585.
13. Solano-Pérez, E.; Coso, C.; Romero-Peralta, S.; Castillo-García, M.; López-Monzoni, S.; Ortigado, A.; Mediano, O. New Approaches to the Management of Cardiovascular Risk Associated with Sleep Respiratory Disorders in Pediatric Patients. *Biomedicines* **2024**, *12*, 411.
14. Preda, S.; Câlmâc, L.; Nica, C.; Cacoveanu, M.; Țigănașu, R.; Badea, A.; Zăman, A.; Ciomag, R.; Nistor, C.; Gașpar, B.S.; et al. TAVI in a Heart Transplant Recipient—Rare Case Report and Review of the Literature. *Biomedicines* **2023**, *11*, 2634.
15. Cimmino, G.; Natale, F.; Alfieri, R.; Cante, L.; Covino, S.; Franzese, R.; Limatola, M.; Marotta, L.; Molinari, R.; Mollo, N.; et al. Non-Conventional Risk Factors: "Fact" or "Fake" in Cardiovascular Disease Prevention? *Biomedicines* **2023**, *11*, 2353.
16. Frąk, W.; Hajdys, J.; Radzioch, E.; Szlagor, M.; Młynarska, E.; Rysz, J.; Franczyk, B. Cardiovascular Diseases: Therapeutic Potential of SGLT-2 Inhibitors. *Biomedicines* **2023**, *11*, 2085.
17. Olabiyi, A.A.; de Castro Brás, L.E. Cardiovascular Remodeling Post-Ischemia: Herbs, Diet, and Drug Interventions. *Biomedicines* **2023**, *11*, 1697.
18. Genovesi, S.; Giussani, M.; Lieti, G.; Orlando, A.; Patti, I.; Parati, G. Evidence and Uncertainties on Lipoprotein(a) as a Marker of Cardiovascular Health Risk in Children and Adolescents. *Biomedicines* **2023**, *11*, 1661.
19. Demirel, O.; Berezin, A.E.; Mirna, M.; Boxhammer, E.; Gharibeh, S.X.; Hoppe, U.C.; Lichtenauer, M. Biomarkers of Atrial Fibrillation Recurrence in Patients with Paroxysmal or Persistent Atrial Fibrillation Following External Direct Current Electrical Cardioversion. *Biomedicines* **2023**, *11*, 1452.
20. Mantzouratou, P.; Malaxianaki, E.; Cerullo, D.; Lavecchia, A.M.; Pantos, C.; Xinaris, C.; Mourouzis, I. Thyroid Hormone and Heart Failure: Charting Known Pathways for Cardiac Repair/Regeneration. *Biomedicines* **2023**, *11*, 975.

References

- Chew, N.W.S.; Ng, C.H.; Tan, D.J.H.; Kong, G.; Lin, C.; Chin, Y.H.; Lim, W.H.; Huang, D.Q.; Quek, J.; Fu, C.E.; et al. The global burden of metabolic disease: Data from 2000 to 2019. *Cell Metab.* **2023**, *35*, 414–428.e3. [CrossRef] [PubMed]
- Cozzolino, D.; Sessa, G.; Salvatore, T.; Sasso, F.C.; Giugliano, D.; Lefebvre, P.J.; Torella, R. The involvement of the opioid system in human obesity: A study in normal weight relatives of obese people. *J. Clin. Endocrinol. Metab.* **1996**, *81*, 713–718. [PubMed]
- Greenfield, D.M.; Snowden, J.A. Cardiovascular Diseases and Metabolic Syndrome. In *The EBMT Handbook: Hematopoietic Stem Cell Transplantation and Cellular Therapies*, 7th ed.; Carreras, E., Dufour, C., Mohty, M., Kröger, N., Eds.; Springer: Cham, Switzerland, 2019; Chapter 55.
- Šiklová, M.; Šrámková, V.; Koc, M.; Krauzová, E.; Čížková, T.; Ondrůjová, B.; Wilhelm, M.; Varaliová, Z.; Kuda, O.; Neubert, J.; et al. The role of adipogenic capacity and dysfunctional subcutaneous adipose tissue in the inheritance of type 2 diabetes mellitus: Cross-sectional study. *Obesity* **2024**, *32*, 547–559. [CrossRef] [PubMed]
- World Health Organization. Cardiovascular Diseases (CVDs). Available online: https://www.who.int/news-room/fact-sheets/detail/cardiovascular-diseases-(cvds) (accessed on 3 May 2024).
- Saeedi, P.; Petersohn, I.; Salpea, P.; Malanda, B.; Karuranga, S.; Unwin, N.; Colagiuri, S.; Guariguata, L.; Motala, A.A.; Ogurtsova, K.; et al. Global and regional diabetes prevalence estimates for 2019 and projections for 2030 and 2045: Results from the International Diabetes Federation Diabetes Atlas, 9th edition. *Diabetes Res. Clin. Pract.* **2019**, *157*, 107843. [CrossRef] [PubMed]
- World Health Organization. Diabetes. Available online: https://www.who.int/health-topics/diabetes#tab=tab_1 (accessed on 3 May 2024).

8. Anděl, M.; Brunerová, L.; Dlouhý, P.; Polák, J.; Gojda, J.; Kraml, P. Posuny v nutričních doporučeních pro zdravé obyvatelstvo a jejich dopad pro diabetickou dietu [Changes in nutritional recommendations for a healthy population and their influence on a diabetic diet]. *Vnitr. Lek.* **2016**, *62*, 539–546. (In Czech) [PubMed]
9. Čížková, T.; Štěpán, M.; Daďová, K.; Ondrůjová, B.; Sontáková, L.; Krauzová, E.; Matouš, M.; Koc, M.; Gojda, J.; Kračmerová, J.; et al. Exercise Training Reduces Inflammation of Adipose Tissue in the Elderly: Cross-Sectional and Randomized Interventional Trial. *J. Clin. Endocrinol. Metab.* **2020**, *105*, dgaa630. [CrossRef] [PubMed]
10. Rodriguez-Araujo, G.; Nakagami, H. Pathophysiology of cardiovascular disease in diabetes mellitus. *Cardiovasc. Endocrinol. Metab.* **2018**, *7*, 4–9. [CrossRef] [PubMed]
11. Schmidt, A.M. Diabetes Mellitus and Cardiovascular Disease. *Arterioscler. Thromb. Vasc. Biol.* **2019**, *39*, 558–568. [CrossRef] [PubMed]
12. Di Francia, R.; Rinaldi, L.; Cillo, M.; Varriale, E.; Facchini, G.; D'Aniello, C.; Marotta, G.; Berretta, M. Antioxidant diet and genotyping as tools for the prevention of liver disease. *Eur. Rev. Med. Pharmacol. Sci.* **2016**, *20*, 5155–5163. [PubMed]
13. Atti, V.; Narayanan, M.A.; Patel, B.; Balla, S.; Siddique, A.; Lundgren, S.; Velagapudi, P. A Comprehensive Review of Mechanical Circulatory Support Devices. *Heart Int.* **2022**, *16*, 37–48. [CrossRef] [PubMed]
14. Kleinberger, J.W.; Pollin, T.I. Personalized medicine in diabetes mellitus: Current opportunities and future prospects. *Ann. N. Y. Acad. Sci.* **2015**, *1346*, 45–56. [CrossRef] [PubMed]
15. Wu, H.; Norton, V.; Cui, K.; Zhu, B.; Bhattacharjee, S.; Lu, Y.W.; Wang, B.; Shan, D.; Wong, S.; Dong, Y.; et al. Diabetes and Its Cardiovascular Complications: Comprehensive Network and Systematic Analyses. *Front. Cardiovasc. Med.* **2022**, *9*, 841928. [CrossRef] [PubMed]
16. Hoang, D.M.; Pham, P.T.; Bach, T.Q.; Ngo, A.T.; Nguyen, Q.T.; Phan, T.T.; Nguyen, G.H.; Le, P.T.T.; Hoang, V.T.; Forsyth, N.R.; et al. Stem cell-based therapy for human diseases. *Signal Transduct. Target. Ther.* **2022**, *7*, 272. [CrossRef] [PubMed]
17. Chancellor, D.; Barrett, D.; Nguyen-Jatkoe, L.; Millington, S.; Eckhardt, F. The state of cell and gene therapy in 2023. *Mol. Ther.* **2023**, *31*, 3376–3388. [CrossRef] [PubMed]
18. Richards, S.E.; Wijeweera, C.; Wijeweera, A. Lifestyle and socioeconomic determinants of diabetes: Evidence from country-level data. *PLoS ONE* **2022**, *17*, e0270476. [CrossRef] [PubMed]
19. Kuan, P.X.; Chan, W.K.; Fern Ying, D.K.; Rahman, M.A.A.; Peariasamy, K.M.; Lai, N.M.; Mills, N.L.; Anand, A. Efficacy of telemedicine for the management of cardiovascular disease: A systematic review and meta-analysis. *Lancet Digit. Health* **2022**, *4*, e676–e691. [CrossRef] [PubMed]

Disclaimer/Publisher's Note: The statements, opinions and data contained in all publications are solely those of the individual author(s) and contributor(s) and not of MDPI and/or the editor(s). MDPI and/or the editor(s) disclaim responsibility for any injury to people or property resulting from any ideas, methods, instructions or products referred to in the content.

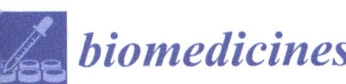 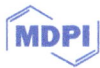

Article

Exploring Cardiac Exosomal RNAs of Acute Myocardial Infarction

Seung Eun Jung [1,†], Sang Woo Kim [2,3,†] and Jung-Won Choi [1,*]

1. Medical Science Research Institute, College of Medicine, Catholic Kwandong University, Gangneung-si 25601, Republic of Korea; top98@naver.com
2. International St. Mary's Hospital, Incheon 22711, Republic of Korea; ksw74@cku.ac.kr
3. Department of Convergence Science, College of Medicine, Catholic Kwandong University, Gangneung-si 25601, Republic of Korea
* Correspondence: gardinia@hanmail.net; Tel.: +82-32-290-2767
† These authors contributed equally to this work.

Abstract: Background: Myocardial infarction (MI), often a frequent symptom of coronary artery disease (CAD), is a leading cause of death and disability worldwide. Acute myocardial infarction (AMI), a major form of cardiovascular disease, necessitates a deep understanding of its complex pathophysiology to develop innovative therapeutic strategies. Exosomal RNAs (exoRNA), particularly microRNAs (miRNAs) within cardiac tissues, play a critical role in intercellular communication and pathophysiological processes of AMI. Methods: This study aimed to delineate the exoRNA landscape, focusing especially on miRNAs in animal models using high-throughput sequencing. The approach included sequencing analysis to identify significant miRNAs in AMI, followed by validation of the functions of selected miRNAs through in vitro studies involving primary cardiomyocytes and fibroblasts. Results: Numerous differentially expressed miRNAs in AMI were identified using five mice per group. The functions of 20 selected miRNAs were validated through in vitro studies with primary cardiomyocytes and fibroblasts. Conclusions: This research enhances understanding of post-AMI molecular changes in cardiac tissues and investigates the potential of exoRNAs as biomarkers or therapeutic targets. These findings offer new insights into the molecular mechanisms of AMIs, paving the way for RNA-based diagnostics and therapeutics and therapies and contributing to the advancement of cardiovascular medicine.

Keywords: exosomal RNA sequencing; exosome; acute myocardial infarction; microRNA; cardiac tissue

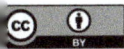

1. Introduction

Myocardial infarction (MI), frequently the initial symptom of coronary artery disease (CAD), is a major contributor to global mortality and disability [1]. Defined as myocardial cell death due to ischemia, MI typically results from thrombosis triggered by rupture or erosion of atherosclerotic plaque in the coronary artery [2]. Onset is rapid, occurring within 20 min of blood supply interruption, leading to irreversible cell death within a few hours [3]. Distinguishing between acute and chronic myocardial injury is essential for early MI detection and mortality reduction [4]. Acute myocardial infarction (AMI), a prominent cardiovascular disease, poses a significant global health challenge [5–7]. Understanding the complex pathophysiology of AMI is vital for developing novel therapeutic strategies [8]. In this complex milieu, exosomal RNAs (exoRNAs) within cardiac tissues play a pivotal role in intercellular communication and the pathophysiological process of AMI [9].

Exosomes, small extracellular vesicles (EV), have garnered significant attention in the scientific community for their role in mediating intercellular communication [10]. These vesicles are known for transporting a diverse array of biomolecules, notably RNAs, among cells, reflecting the physiological and pathological state of their source cells [11,12]. As such, they are increasingly recognized for their potential as biomarkers in disease diagnosis and prognosis. In the specific context of AMI, exoRNAs provide a window into the molecular upheavals occurring within cardiac tissues during the disease's acute phase [13]. Recent research has expanded the understanding of EVs, particularly exosomes and microRNAs (miRNAs or miRs), in the realm of cardiovascular health. These entities are being explored for their therapeutic potential not only in cardiovascular diseases but also cancer and neurological disorders [14,15]. For instance, miR-134 has been identified as a regulator of STAT5B function, making it a promising biomarker and therapeutic agent for breast cancer [16]. Similarly, exosome-derived miR-126 from ADSCs shows potential in reducing cardiac fibrosis and inflammation, thereby mitigating myocardial injury [17]. Moreover, miR-217-containing exosomes have emerged as significant markers in chronic heart failure by modulating cardiac fibrosis and dysfunction. Additionally, exosome-derived miR-21-3p has been identified as a key mediator in cardiac hypertrophy through its regulatory impact on sorbin and SH3 domain containing 2 (*SORBS2*) and PDZ and LIM domain 5 (*PDLIM5*) [18].

The role of miRNAs extends beyond just biomarkers; these small noncoding RNAs are pivotal in controlling gene expression and cellular process, impacting the pathophysiological pathways of MI both directly and indirectly [19,20]. Certain miRNAs have been implicated in inducing cardiomyocyte death through mechanisms including apoptosis, autophagy, and necroptosis, while others play a role in cardiomyocyte proliferation, repair, and intercellular interaction [20]. These insights not only enhance the understanding of MI mechanisms but also underscore the potential of miRNAs as diagnostic biomarkers for this condition.

This study delves into the comprehensive profiling of exoRNAs isolated from cardiac tissues in MI animal models. Employing high-throughput sequencing techniques, it aimed to map the exoRNA landscape in AMI, focusing on the differentially expressed miRNAs This approach included sequencing analysis to identify significant miRNAs in AMI, followed by validation of functions of selected miRNAs through in vitro studies involving primary cardiomyocytes and fibroblasts. This research endeavors to provide a deeper understanding of molecular alterations in cardiac tissues following AMI and explores the potential of exoRNAs as biomarkers and therapeutic targets. The findings of this study make a significant contribution to cardiovascular medicine, offering novel insights into the molecular underpinnings of AMI. This research not only enriches existing knowledge but also paves the way for the development of innovative RNA-based diagnostics and therapeutic strategies, inspiring future research in this critical area of healthcare.

2. Materials and Methods

2.1. Animals

To establish an MI mouse model, 12-week-old male C57BL/6 mice (23 ± 4 g; KOATECH, Pyeongtaek, Republic of Korea) were used. Following anesthesia via zoletil (30 mg/kg Virbac, France) and xylazine (10 mg/kg; Bayer Korea, Ansan, Republic of Korea), the mice were airway ventilated using a ventilator (Harvard Instruments, Holliston, MA, USA). The left anterior descending (LAD) artery was ligated with 6-0 prolene suture (Ethicon, Diegem, Belgium). Subsequently, muscle and skin closure were performed with 4-0 prolene suture (Ethicon) [21]. The mice were divided into three groups: sham, MI-1day, and MI-3day, based on the duration of left anterior descending LAD artery ligation, followed by suture closure [22]. The mice were sacrificed on the designated day to procure heart tissue for analysis, ensuring simultaneous tissue collection across all groups. Ten mice were selected for each group to establish an MI animal model, and finally, five mice were randomly selected per group for further experiments.

2.2. Triphenyltetrazolium Chloride (TTC) Staining

Before TTC staining, the isolated heart tissue was perfused with 1X phosphate-buffer saline (PBS; Biosesang, Seongnam, Republic of Korea) several times. Heart tissues from each experimental group were subjected to TTC staining. For this, tissues were incubated in the 1% TTC (Sigma-Aldrich, St. Louis, MO, USA) solution, which was prepared by dissolving TTC in 1X PBS. The incubation was carried out at 37 °C for 1 h in a state shielded from light to prevent photo-degradation [23,24]. Post-incubation, the tissues were fixed in a 4% paraformaldehyde solution (Biosesang, Seongnam, Republic of Korea) at 4 °C for 4 h. This was followed by sectioning the tissues into 1 mm thick cross-sections for detailed examination. The stained and sectioned heart tissues were then photographed using a digital camera (DIMIS M model, Anyang, Republic of Korea) to document the results of the TTC staining process. The infarcted tissue appears white, while the viable tissue is red. This photographic evidence is crucial for visualizing and analyzing the extent of infarction in heart tissues.

2.3. Exosome Isolation

Heart tissues isolated from each group were dissected into 1 mm^3 pieces using a razor. These tissue fragments were then gently rinsed with cold 1X PBS in a cell strainer fitted with a 70 μm nylon mesh (SPL, Pocheon, Republic of Korea). Five heart tissue fragments from the same group were pooled together in a 50 mL tube. The pooled heart tissues in each tube were incubated in serum-free medium supplemented with 20 mM N-2-hydroxyethylpiperazine-N-2-ethane sulfonic acid (HEPES; Thermo Fisher Scientific, Grand Island, NY, USA), at 37 °C with gentle shaking (200 rpm) for 45 min [25]. This step facilitates the release of exosomes into the medium. Following incubation, the tube was centrifuged at $3000 \times g$ for 15 min at 4 °C. This centrifugation step aimed to pellet intact cells and cellular debris, leaving the supernatant enriched with exosomes. Exosomes were then isolated from the supernatants using an Exo2D EV isolation kit for RNA analysis (EXOSOMEplus, Seoul, Republic of Korea), following the manufacturer's instructions. Briefly, Exo2D reagents were added to the supernatants in a 1:5 ratio, and the mixture was incubated at 4 °C for 1 h. Subsequently, the mixture was centrifuged at $3000 \times g$ for 30 min at 4 °C. The resultant white pellets containing the exosomes were resuspended in 1X PBS and stored at −80 °C for future use. Total RNA was extracted from the purified exosomes using TRIzol reagent (Thermo Fisher Scientific, Rockford, IL, USA), as per the standard protocol. This RNA served as the basis for subsequent RNA analysis and sequencing.

2.4. SmRNA Library Construction and miRNA Sequencing

The smRNA sequencing library was prepared using a TruSeq RNA Sample preparation Kit (Illumina, San Diego, CA, USA), adhering to Illumina's standard procedure. This preparation involved selecting RNA fractions, ligating adapters, and amplifying the sample to construct the library suitable for high-throughput sequencing. The constructed smRNA library was subsequently sequenced on an Illumina Hiseq 2500 Genome Analyzer platform [26]. The sequencing parameters were set to achieve a read length of 50 base pairs (bp) using single-end sequencing. This approach was chosen to optimize the detection and analysis of smRNA species, particularly miRNAs. The size range of the library was determined to be between 145 bp and 160 bp, which is indicative of successful library preparation and suitable for effective miRNA sequencing. All processes related to the smRNA library construction and sequencing were performed externally by MACROGEN Inc. (Seoul, Republic of Korea), ensuring high-quality and reliable sequencing data.

2.5. Data Analysis of miRNA Sequencing

Following smRNA sequencing, the raw sequence data underwent an initial filtering process. This step involved quality-based filtering to separate high-quality reads from the dataset. The processed reads were then further refined by trimming adapter sequences and removing any reads aligned to rRNA sequences. This refinement ensured that the dataset for analysis comprised only relevant and high-quality miRNA sequences. The resulting high-quality, processed reads were then subjected to classification and analysis. Known miRNAs were identified using miRbase v22.1, a comprehensive miRNA sequence database. Other types of RNA sequences were classified using RNAcentral 14.0, a non-coding RNA sequence database. Additionally, the prediction of novel miRNAs was performed using miRDeep2, a tool specifically designed for novel miRNA discovery. The identification of differentially expressed miRNAs was a critical step in this analysis. Statistical methods, including fold change calculation and the exactTest function from the edgeR (version 3.9), were employed. Hierarchical clustering was also utilized to understand the patterns of miRNA expression under different conditions. GO and the KEGG databases were instrumental in analyzing the functions and pathways of the target genes identified in the DE miRNA analysis. These analyses provided insights into the biological implications of the miRNA expression patterns observed. All processes related to the data analysis of miRNA sequencing were conducted by MACROGEN Inc., Seoul, Republic of Korea, ensuring a professional and thorough analysis of the sequencing data.

2.6. Transmission Electron Microscopy (TEM) Analysis

The exosomes extracted from heart tissues were first prepared for TEM analysis by fixing them with a 0.1% paraformaldehyde solution (Biosesang, Seongnam, Republic of Korea) for 30 min. This step is critical in preserving the structural integrity of the exosomes during the subsequent analysis steps. A 10 µL aliquot of each exosome sample was placed on a piece of Parafilm. A formvar/carbon-supported copper grid (200 mesh; Electron Microscopy Sciences, Hatfield, PA, USA) was then floated on top of each sample drop for 7 min [27]. This method allowed the exosomes to adhere to the grid while being sufficiently supported for detailed TEM examination. The grid with adhered exosomes underwent a washing procedure, alternating with three drops of ultrapure water, each wash lasting for a 2 min duration. This step ensured the removal of any residual fixing agent. Subsequently, the grid was stained with a 2% solution of phosphotungstic acid (pH 7.0; Sigma-Aldrich, St. Louis, MO, USA) for 30 s, which provided the contrast necessary to visualize the exosomes under TEM. After staining, the grid was air-dried overnight in a dark environment to prevent any light-induced alterations. Once dried, the exosomes were ready for visualization. The prepared samples were examined under a transmission electron microscope (JEM-F200; JEOL, Tokyo, Japan).

2.7. Immunoblot Analysis

Cells were lysed using RIPA buffer (Thermo Fisher Scientific, Rockford, IR, USA), which was supplemented with 1% phosphatase inhibitor (Sigma-Aldrich, St. Louis, MO, USA) and 1% protease inhibitor (Sigma-Aldrich, St. Louis, MO, USA), to ensure effective breakdown of cell components while preserving protein integrity. The protein concentration in the lysates was quantified using the Pierce BCA Protein Assay Kit (Thermo Fisher Scientific, Rockford, IL, USA), enabling accurate determination of protein amounts for uniform loading in gel electrophoresis. The proteins were then separated by electrophoresis on SDS-PAGE under reducing conditions. Following electrophoresis, the proteins were transferred onto a polyvinylidene difluoride (PVDF; Sigma-Aldrich, St. Louis, MO, USA) membrane to prepare for immunoblotting. To prevent non-specific binding, the membrane was blocked for 1 h with 5% skim milk (BD Difco; Sparks, MD, USA) in TBS-T buffer (10 mM Tris-HCl (Sigma-Aldrich, St. Louis, MO, USA), 150 mM NaCl (Sigma-Aldrich, St. Louis, MO, USA), and 0.1% Tween 20 (Sigma-Aldrich, St. Louis, MO, USA)). It was then incubated overnight at 4 °C with primary antibodies (Santa Cruz Biotechnology, Dallas, TX, USA) at a dilution of 1:1000. Following primary antibody incubation, the membrane was washed three times and then incubated with HRP-conjugated anti-mouse IgG (1:1000; Santa Cruz Biotechnology, Dallas, TX, USA) for 2 h in blocking buffer. After three more washes to remove excess secondary antibody, the membrane was prepared for detection [28,29]. Protein bands were visualized using an ECL kit (Western Blotting Detection Kit; GE Healthcare, Buckinghamshire, UK). The band intensities were quantified using ImageJ software (NIH; version 1.54h), providing a quantitative analysis of protein expression.

2.8. Isolation of Primary Cardiomyocytes and Fibroblasts from Neonatal Mouse Heart

Primary cardiomyocytes and fibroblasts were isolated from 1-day-old C57BL/6 mice (KOATECH, Pyeongtaek, Republic of Korea) using the Primary Cardiomyocyte Isolation Kit (Thermo Fisher Scientific, Rockford, IL, USA) and Primary Fibroblast Isolation Kit (Thermo Fisher Scientific, Rockford, IL, USA), respectively, following the manufacturer's protocols. Neonatal hearts were dissected into 1–3 mm^3 pieces and initially placed separately in chilled Hank's Balanced Salt Solution (HBSS; Thermo Fisher Scientific, Grand Island, NY, USA). After two washes with 0.5 mL of cold HBSS, the heart pieces were subjected to enzymatic digestion. For primary cardiomyocyte isolation, each heart in a tube was treated with 0.5 mL of Enzyme 1 (containing papain) and 0.01 mL of Cardiomyocyte Isolation Enzyme 2 (containing thermolysin), and incubated at 37 °C for 30 min. For primary fibroblast isolation, each heart was treated with 0.2 mL of reconstituted MEF Isolation Enzyme (containing papain) and incubated at 37 °C for 25 min. Following enzymatic digestion, the heart tissues were washed twice with 0.5 mL of cold HBSS. The tissues were then mechanically disrupted by pipetting up and down 25 times for primary cardiomyocytes or 20 times for primary fibroblasts in 0.5 mL of complete DMEM (Thermo Fisher Scientific, Grand Island, NY, USA) containing 10% fetal bovine serum (FBS; HyClone, Logan, UT, USA) and 1% penicillin/streptomycin (Thermo Fisher Scientific, Grand Island, NY, USA). The resultant cell suspensions were combined, and cell concentration and viability were determined. The cells were then seeded at a density of 4×10^4 cells/well in a 96-well plate (SPL, Pocheon, Republic of Korea) for transfection with miRNA mimics. For immunofluorescence analysis, cells were seeded at 2×10^5 cells/well in a 4-well cell culture slide (SPL, Pocheon, Republic of Korea).

2.9. Transfection with miRNA Mimics

Primary cardiomyocytes and fibroblasts were seeded in 96-well plates in preparation for transfection. On the following day, each well was transfected with 20 different miRNA mimics at a concentration of 1 pmol/well using Lipofectamine RNAiMAX (Thermo Fisher Scientific, Rockford, IL, USA) according to the manufacturer's guidelines. A miRNA mimic negative control was utilized for comparison [30]. All miRNA mimics used in this study were sourced from Genolution Pharmaceuticals (Seoul, Republic of Korea), with their specific details provided in Table 1. For control 24 h post-transfection, the cells were shifted to serum-free medium (SFM) and subjected to either normoxic or hypoxic conditions for an additional 24 h. This setup was designed to simulate an in vitro environment analogous to MI. For hypoxic treatment, cells were maintained at 37 °C in 5% CO_2, 5% H_2, and 0.5% O_2, facilitated by an anaerobic atmosphere system (Technomart, Seoul, Republic of Korea).

Table 1. Information about miRNA mimics used for transfection assay.

No.	Target Name	Accession#	Sequence (5′–3′)
1	mmu-miR-30c-1-3p	MIMAT0004616	CUGGGAGAGGGUUGUUUACUCC
2	mmu-miR-149-3p	MIMAT0016990	GAGGGAGGGACGGGGGCGGUGC
3	mmu-miR-206-3p	MIMAT0000239	UGGAAUGUAAGGAAGUGUGUGG
4	mmu-miR-486a-3p	MIMAT0017206	CGGGGCAGCUCAGUACAGGAU
5	mmu-miR-673-3p	MIMAT0004824	UCCGGGGCUGAGUUCUGUGCACC
6	mmu-miR-690	MIMAT0003469	AAAGGCUAGGCUCACAACCAAA
7	mmu-miR-700-5p	MIMAT0017256	UAAGGCUCCUUCCUGUGCUUGC
8	mmu-miR-706	MIMAT0003496	AGAGAAACCCUGUCUCAAAAAA
9	mmu-miR-744-5p	MIMAT0004187	UGCGGGGCUAGGGCUAACAGCA
10	mmu-miR-871-3p	MIMAT0017265	UGACUGGCACCAUUCUGGAUAAU
11	mmu-miR-874-5p	MIMAT0017268	CGGCCCCACGCACCAGGGUAAG
12	mmu-miR-1247-5p	MIMAT0014800	ACCCGUCCCGUUCGUCCCCGGA
13	mmu-miR-1306-3p	MIMAT0009411	ACGUUGGCUCUGGUGGUGAUG
14	mmu-miR-3057-3p	MIMAT0014823	UCCCACAGGCCCAGCUCAUAGC
15	mmu-miR-3086-5p	MIMAT0014880	UAGAUUGUAGGCCCAUUGGA

Table 1. Cont.

No.	Target Name	Accession#	Sequence (5′–3′)
16	mmu-miR-3470a	MIMAT0015640	UCACUUUGUAGACCAGGCUGG
17	mmu-miR-3470b	MIMAT0015641	UCACUCUGUAGACCAGGCUGG
18	mmu-miR-3968	MIMAT0019352	CGAAUCCCACUCCAGACACCA
19	mmu-miR-5107-5p	MIMAT0020615	UGGGCAGAGGAGGCAGGGACA
20	mmu-miR-7225-5p	MIMAT0028418	ACGUAGACUGUGUAGAAGCC

2.10. Cytotoxicity Assay

In evaluating cytotoxicity in the cell cultures, the ToxiLight BioAssay Kit (Lonza, Walkersville, MD, USA) was employed. This kit is a non-destructive cytolysis assay, specifically designed to measure the release of adenylate kinase (AK) from damaged cells. The assay utilizes bioluminescent reaction that correlates with the amount of AK released from lysed cells. For the assay, 0.02 mL of cell culture supernatant was transferred to a new 96-well plate. To this, 0.1 mL of AK test reagent, dissolved in assay buffer, was added. This mixture was then incubated at room temperature for 5 min to allow for the development of the bioluminescent reaction [31,32]. Following the incubation, the bioluminescence intensity was measured using a GloMax Discover Microplate Reader (Promega, Madison, WI, USA).

2.11. Immunofluorescence Analysis

The cell culture slides containing primary cardiomyocytes and fibroblasts were fixed in 4% paraformaldehyde solution (Biosesang, Seongnam, Republic of Korea) overnight at 4 °C. Following fixation, antigen retrieval was performed using a sodium citrate buffer (0.1 M; CureBio, Seoul, Republic of Korea) for 10 minutes at 95 °C. The slides were then permeabilized in 0.2% Triton X-100 (Sigma-Aldrich, St. Louis, MO, USA) for 10 minutes, allowing antibody access to intracellular structures. Subsequently, the slides were blocked with 2.5% normal horse serum (Vector Laboratories, Newark, CA, USA) for 1 h to minimize non-specific binding of the antibodies. After blocking, the slides were incubated with primary antibodies: either anti-cardiac troponin T antibodies (1:200 dilution; Abcam, Cambridge, UK) for cardiomyocytes or anti-vimentin antibodies (1:200 dilution; Abcam, Cambridge, UK) for fibroblasts, overnight at 4 °C. Post-primary antibody incubation, the slides were washed and incubated with appropriate secondary antibodies: either fluorescein isothiocyanate (FITC)-conjugated secondary antibodies (1:500 dilution; Jackson Immunoresearch, West Grove, PA, USA) or rhodamin-conjugated secondary antibodies (1:500 dilution; Millipore, Bedford, MA, USA). Nuclei were stained with 4′,6-diamidino-2-phenylindole (DAPI; 1:5000 dilution; Thermo Fisher Scientific, Rockford, IL, USA) to facilitate the identification of cell structures [30,33]. Finally, the slides were examined under an Olympus IX83 microscope (Evident, Tokyo, Japan) for detailed visualization of the immunofluorescence staining.

2.12. Statistical Analysis

The data were analyzed through two-sample t-test using Statistical Package for the Social Sciences (SPSS, version 14.0K) software and results are expressed as the means ± standard error of the means (SEMs). When the t-test indicated a significant overall treatment effect ($p < 0.05$), differences between groups were assessed using the least-significant difference (LSD) test, with significance set at $p < 0.05$. The p value from the RNA sequencing analysis was automatically extracted by a comparative analysis algorithm called edgeR.

3. Results

3.1. Establishment of MI Animal Models and Isolation of Exosomes from Heart Tissues

ExoRNA sequencing was conducted on exosomes extracted from heart tissues of an established MI mouse model using C57BL/6 mice (Figure 1A). Five mice per group were used for sequencing analysis. To verify MI induction in these models, the heart morphology of the MI models was compared with that of the sham group. Infarction sites were evident in the heart of MI models (Figure 1B). Additionally, the infarcted areas of hearts were compared using TTC staining. This is because TTC staining reacts with mitochondrial enzymes in living cells to form a red compound. Uniform staining was observed in the sham group hearts, while the MI groups exhibited TTC-negative areas at the infarction site (Figure 1B). Exosome size extracted from heart tissues was confirmed using TEM analysis (Figure 1C). Immunoblotting was employed to verify the presence of exosome markers including CD9, CD64, and CD81, with β-actin, α-tubulin, and GAPDH serving as internal controls (Figure 1D).

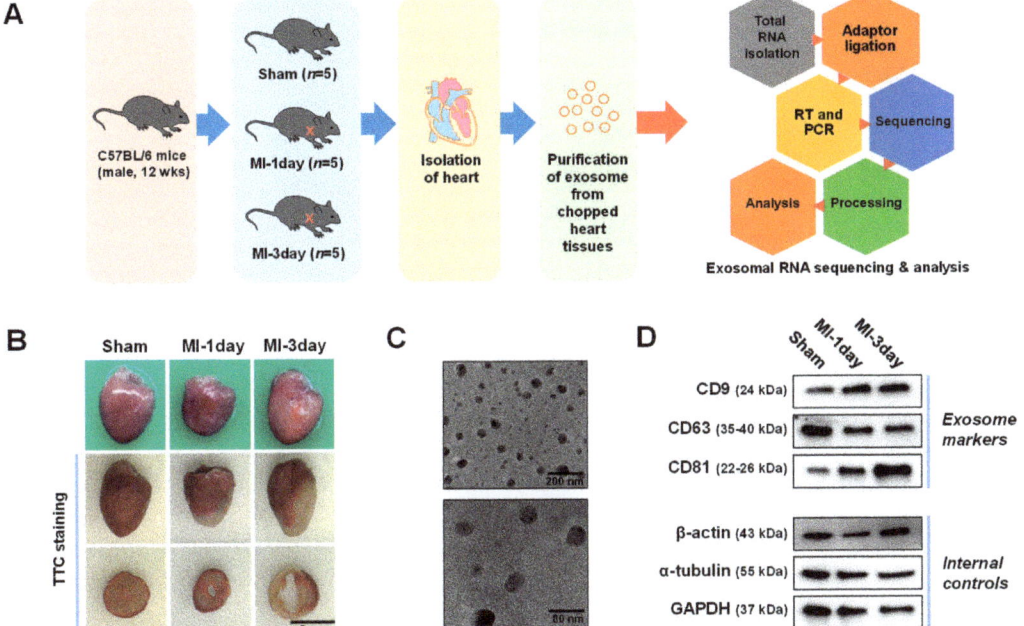

Figure 1. Experimental overview and exosome characterization of extracted from heart tissues. (**A**) Schematic representation of the experimental procedure employed in the current study. (**B**) Group-specific heart images from the myocardial infarction (MI) mouse models, both with and without triphenyltetrazolium chloride (TTC) staining, illustrating the morphological differences among the groups. (**C**) Transmission electron microscopy (TEM) images of isolated exosome stained with phosphotungstic acid, showcasing their structural features. (**D**) Immunoblotting analysis of the isolated exosomes using exosomal markers, including CD9, CD63, and CD81, alongside internal controls. Group designations: sham, control group; MI-1day, MI induced for 1 day; MI-3day, MI induced for 3 days.

3.2. ExoRNA Sequencing and Data Processing

ExoRNA sequencing was conducted on exosomes extracted from the heart tissues of C57BL/6 mice in an MI model. Sequencing adapters were ligated to the exoRNA from heart tissue, followed by reverse transcription (RT) and PCR to amplify cDNA pools (Figure 2A). These cDNA fragments underwent sequencing on an Illumina platform. Data processing involved organizing sequenced reads into categories: trimmed reads (with adapter sequences removed), nonadapter reads (without adapter sequences), short reads (less than 17 bp post-adapter trimming), and low-quality reads (with one or more bases in the trimmed or non-adapter reads). Read counts of each group are presented in Figure 2A. Ribosomal RNA (rRNA) removal was performed to mitigate its abundance effect, with the remaining read counts shown in Figure 2B. Read length distribution across each group is depicted in Figure 2C. Generally, transfer RNA (tRNA) was 70–90 nucleotide (nt), small nucleolar RNA (snoRNA) was about 90 nt, small nuclear RNA (snRNA) was between 100 and 300 nt, miRNA was about 22 nt and PIWI-interacting RNA (piRNA) was about 27 nt in length. The small RNA (smRNA) composition of each sample, indicating the ratio of smRNA types (such as known miRNA, candidate miRNA, rRNA, tRNA, snRNA, snoRNA, etc.), is illustrated in Figure 2D.

A. Read Processing

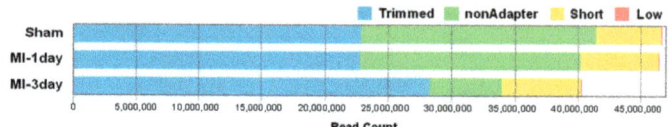

B. Read Filtering

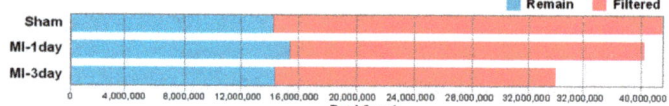

C. Read Length Distribution

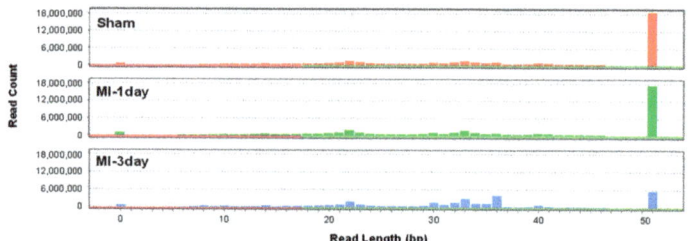

D. RNA Composition

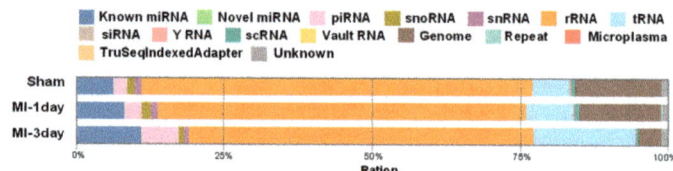

Figure 2. Comprehensive analysis of exosomal RNA (exoRNA) sequencing data. (**A**) Depicts the count distribution of various read types for each group, including trimmed reads, nonadapter reads, short reads and low-quality reads. (**B**) Shows the remaining reads (blue) after the removal of ribosomal RNA (rRNA; red). (**C**) Illustrates the distribution of read lengths across each sample (**D**) Provides a breakdown of the smRNA composition within each sample, categorizing them into various types: miRNA (microRNA), piRNA (PIWI-interacting RNA), snoRNA (small nucleolar RNA), snRNA (small nuclear RNA), rRNA (ribosomal RNA), tRNA (transfer RNA), siRNA (small interfering RNA), Y RNA, scRNA (single-cell RNA).

3.3. Differential Expressed (DE) miRNA Analysis

To assess the similarity between samples, correlation analysis and hierarchical clustering analysis were performed. In the correlation analysis, a value closer to 1 indicates greater similarity. The highest similarity was observed between the sham group and the MI-1day group, followed by the MI-1day and MI-3day groups. The lowest similarity was noted between the sham group and the MI-3day group (Figure 3A). Hierarchical clustering analysis further supported these findings, showing a high similarity between the sham and MI-1day groups and a lower similarity between the combined sham/MI-1day group and the MI-3day group (Figure 3B, left). A heat map, utilizing the Euclidean method and complete linkage in the hierarchical clustering analysis, clustered the mature miRNAs and samples based on their expression levels (normalized value). This clustering highlighted significant differences between at least one pair of total comparison groups (Figure 3B, right). A total of 174 mature miRNAs, which met the criteria of a fold change ($|FC| > 2$) and p-value ($p < 0.05$), were categorized according to differential expression between groups (Figure 3C). These findings were visually represented in smear plots of the average logCPM (X-axis) and log2 fold change (Y-axis), to examine transcripts showing notable expression differences (Figure 3D).

A. Correlation analysis

B. Hierarchical clustering analysis

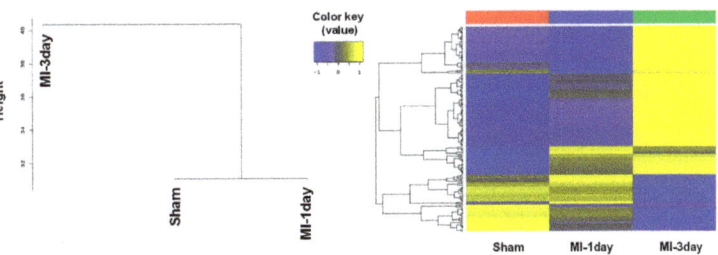

C. Up, down regulated count

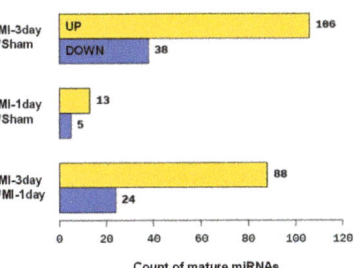

D. Expression level

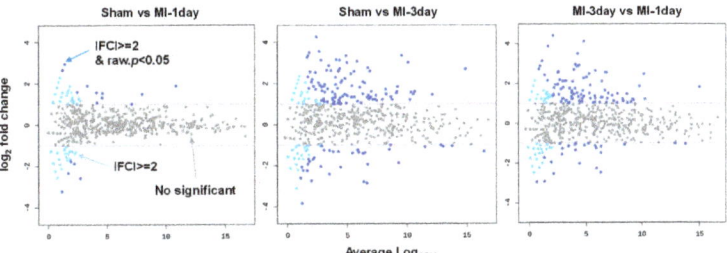

Figure 3. Differential Expression (DE) miRNA analysis from exosomal RNA (exoRNA) sequencing. (**A**) Correlation matrix: This panel presents the correlation matrix of all samples, calculated using Pearson's coefficient based on normalized values. The correlation coefficient (r) ranges from −1 to 1, where values closer to 1 indicate a higher similarity between samples. (**B**) Hierarchical clustering: The left part of this panel shows the hierarchical clustering of samples based on their normalized expression normalized value, where samples with higher expression similarities are grouped together (distance metric = Euclidean distance, linkage method = complete linkage) (left). The right part features a heat map of the two-way hierarchical clustering, utilizing Z-scores of Log2-transformed normalized values for visualization. (**C**) Quantitative analysis of microRNAs (miRNAs): This section displays the number of mature miRNAs that are either up-regulated or down-regulated based on a fold change ($|FC| > 2$) and p-value ($p < 0.05$) for each comparison pair. (**D**) Smear plots: This panel illustrates smear plots representing the expression level of miRNAs. The plots are designed to visually represent the distribution and variance of miRNA expression across samples.

To elucidate the function of exoRNAs from heart tissues in the MI animal model and identify enriched functional terms, gene ontology (GO) and Kyoto Encyclopedia of Genes and Genomes (KEGG) pathway analyses were conducted on the differentially expressed mRNAs of dysregulated miRNAs. These analyses were performed separately for miRNAs showing increased and decreased expressions between MI-1day and sham/MI-3day and sham groups (Figure 4). The GO analysis encompassed three categories: biological process, cellular component, and molecular function. The top seven results from the GO enrichment analysis are presented in Figure 4A. In the MI-1day group, the most enriched biological process terms included organelle organization, regulation of molecular function, and nervous system development. Conversely, in MI-3day group, the terms focused on cell development, protein localization, and cellular catabolic process. The primary cellular component terms for the MI-1day group were cell projection, neuron projection, and vesicle, while for MI-3day group, they were neuron, golgi apparatus, and endomembrane system. The molecular function terms common to both MI-1day and MI-3day groups were ion binding, cation binding, and transition metal ion binding. These findings suggest the involvement of certain miRNAs in the fundamental biological regulation of MI. Additionally, the KEGG pathway analysis highlighted key pathways showing significant differences between MI and sham groups, including endocytosis, the mitogen-activated protein kinase (*MAPK*) signaling pathway, cyclic adenosine monophosphate (*cAMP*) signaling pathway, phosphoinositide 3-kinase (*PI3K*)-*Akt* signaling pathway, and *Ras* signaling pathway (Figure 4B).

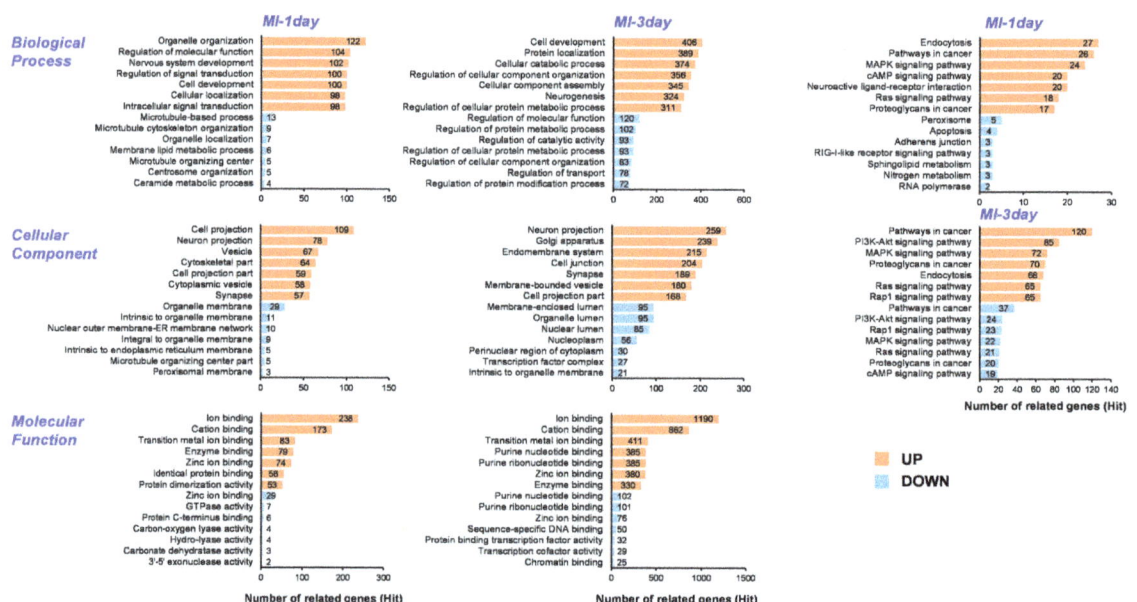

Figure 4. Comprehensive functional enrichment analysis of differentially expressed miRNAs. (**A**) Depicts the top seven gene ontology (GO) terms, providing insights into the biological processes, cellular components, and molecular functions most affected by the dysregulated miRNAs. (**B**) Illustrates the top seven pathways identified in the Kyoto Encyclopedia of Genes and Genomes (KEGG) pathway analysis, highlighting critical pathways impacted by the altered expression of mRNAs across different groups.

3.4. Selection of Differentially Expressed miRNAs

To determine which miRNAs to investigate in vitro from those differentially expressed miRNAs among the groups, a diagram was initially used to chart both increased and decreased miRNAs (Figure 5A). The primary focus of this study was on miRNAs that showed reduced expression in the MI group, as this approach allowed for covering a broader range of miRNAs in the in vitro studies. Subsequently, miRNAs already known to be associated with MI and those exhibiting very low expression levels were excluded to refine the selection of candidate miRNAs for in vitro analysis. Consequently, out of the 49 miRNAs that demonstrated decreased expression in MI groups, 20 were selected for the in vitro functional study (Figure 5B).

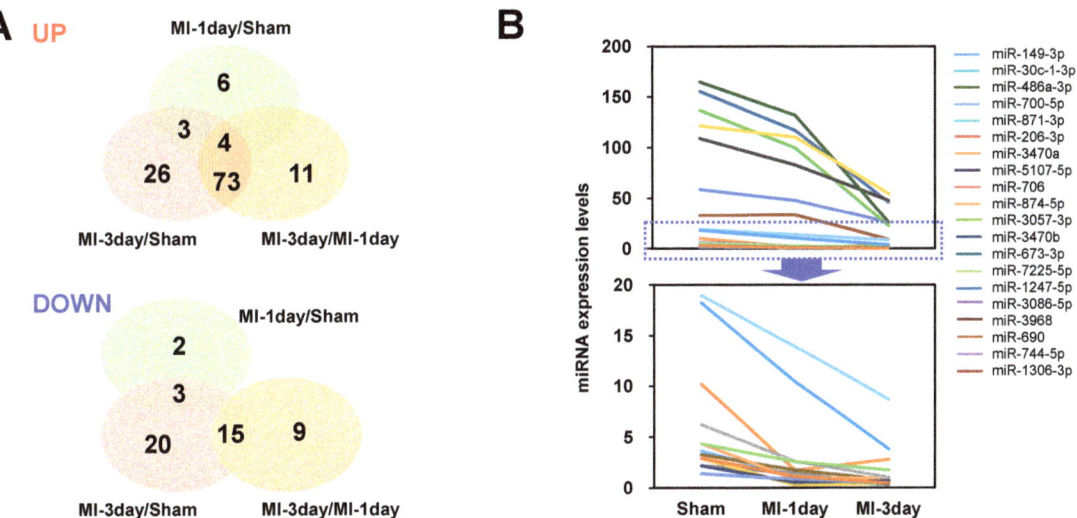

Figure 5. Identification and selection of key candidate microRNAs (miRNAs). (**A**) A diagrammatic representation of the number of miRNAs exhibiting increased (up) or decreased (down) expression upon comparative analysis between groups. This visualization aids in understanding the overall distribution and directional trends of miRNA expression changes. (**B**) A broken line graph displaying the expression profiles of the 20 selectively chosen miRNAs across the groups, enabling a comparative and detailed view of their expression dynamics.

3.5. Effects of Selected miRNAs on Hypoxic Stress-Induced Cell Death

To simulate MI conditions in vitro, primary cardiomyocytes and fibroblasts were isolated from neonatal mouse hearts and subjected to hypoxic stress. These cell types were chosen because they are the most abundant in heart tissue. Following isolation, the cells were characterized using specific cell markers: troponin-T for cardiomyocytes, and vimentin for fibroblasts (Figure 6, left). The cells were then transfected with mimics of 20 selected miRNAs and exposed under hypoxic condition to assess the effects on cell viability. These observations revealed that 19 of the selected miRNAs, with the exception of miR-1247-5p, significantly reduced hypoxic stress-induced cell death in primary cardiomyocytes. In primary fibroblasts, 12 miRNAs (miR-30c-1-3p, miR-149-3p, miR-206-3p, miR-486a-3p, miR-673-3p, miR-690-3p, miR-700-5p, miR-706, miR-744-5p, miR-871-3p, miR-874-5p, and miR-1247-5p) effectively attenuated cytotoxicity under low oxygen conditions (Figure 6, right).

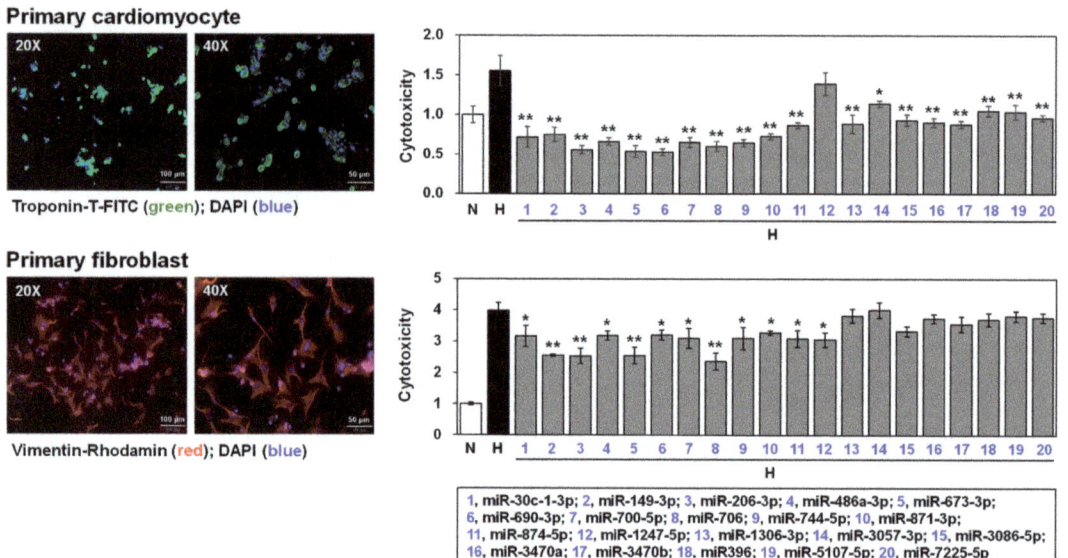

Figure 6. Analysis of cytotoxicity using selected miRNA mimics in primary cardiomyocytes and fibroblasts. On the left, immunofluorescence analysis confirms the presence of specific markers in isolated cells: troponin-T in primary cardiomyocytes and vimentin in primary fibroblasts. The right side of the figure investigates the impact of miRNA mimic treatment on cell survival under hypoxic conditions. In the accompanying bar graph, white and black bars represent the control (miRNA mimic negative control-treated) group, while gray bars denote groups treated with miRNA mimics. Statistical significance between the control and treated groups was assessed using ANOVA. p value annotations indicate levels of significance: * $p < 0.05$ and ** $p < 0.01$, highlight key differences in cytotoxicity responses. The error bar represents the standard deviation between the five wells of the 96-well plates used in the cytotoxicity assay. N, normoxic condition; H, hypoxic condition; FITC, fluorescein isothiocyanate; DAPI, 4′,6-diamidino-2-phenylindole; miR, microRNA.

4. Discussion

4.1. Establishment of MI Model

This study provided a comprehensive profile of exoRNAs, particularly miRNAs, in an MI mouse model established using RNA sequencing techniques. Additionally, the effects of differentially expressed miRNAs in an MI group on hypoxic-induced cell death were also examined in primary cardiomyocytes and fibroblasts. A key achievement of this study was the successfully establishment of an MI animal model using C57BL/6 mice. The occurrence of left ventricular dysfunction and heart failure in rats is an acute renal muscle infarction model, and is primarily used to study the function of MI [34]. Mouse models of MI based on C57BL/6 mice have also been widely used in the study of MI and heart failure [35,36]. Morphological changes in the MI model, confirmed by TTC staining, clearly distinguished between infarcted and non-infarcted areas, validating the model's efficacy (Figure 1B). MI is typically characterized by three phases: the inflammatory phase, proliferative phase, and the maturation phase [37]. During the inflammatory phase, cardiomyocyte death, proinflammatory cytokines secretion, and neutrophil infiltration occur. The proliferative phase is marked by macrophage polarization, myofibroblast proliferation, and collagen deposition. Finally, the maturation phase involves extracellular matrix cross-linking, myofibroblast quiescence, and heart failure. In the present study, the MI mouse model during the acute inflammatory phase of MI was utilized to identify potential biomarkers that could be useful for early-stage MI detection and intervention.

4.2. Exosome Analysis

Furthermore, exosomes were isolated from cardiac tissues and their identity through TEM and immunoblotting analyses was confirmed (Figure 1C,D). Exosomes are heterogeneous populations of 50–250 nm membrane-bound vesicles that contain proteins, lipids, and nucleic acids, playing crucial roles in various disease processes [38]. While exosomes are abundantly present in blood vessels, they are also found in the interstitial spaces of cellular tissues [39]. The exosome analyzed in this study were specifically derived from cells within the heart tissues affected by MI, focusing on those newly released by cells post-MI, rather than those of unclear origin circulating in the blood.

4.3. RNA Sequencing and Analysis

In this study, comprehensive RNA sequencing and data processing of exoRNAs from MI models revealed a diverse spectrum of RNA species. This spectrum included microRNAs (miRNAs), transfer RNAs (tRNAs), small nuclear RNAs (snRNAs), small nucleolar RNAs (snoRNAs), and PIWI-interacting RNAs (piRNAs). The analysis of read length distribution and smRNA composition in this study offers an extensive overview of the exoRNA profile in MI (Figure 2). Such detailed information is vital for deciphering the molecular mechanisms at play in MI, suggesting these RNAs' potential roles in intercellular communication and the cardiac injury response. The DE analysis of miRNAs underlines significant changes in miRNA expression in response to MI (Figure 3). Correlation and hierarchical clustering analyses (Figure 3) indicate that the longer the ligation duration of the left anterior descending (LAD) artery, the more pronounced the differences in miRNA expression between the sham and MI groups. These insights are pivotal for understanding the time-dependent regulation of gene expression in the context of MI. Furthermore, they could be instrumental in guiding the development of targeted therapeutic interventions.

The functional enrichment analysis, utilizing both GO and KEGG pathways, shed light on the biological processes, cellular components, and molecular functions altered in MI (Figure 4). Particularly significant is the identification of pathways such as *MAPK*, *cAMP*, *PI3K-Akt*, and *RAS* signaling pathways in relation to MI-associated mRNAs. Notably, the *PI3K/Akt* pathway is known to regulate the growth and survival of cardiomyocytes and plays a critical role in the pathophysiology of MI [40]. Similarly, the *cAMP* signaling pathway and its compartmentalization are pivotal in cardiac physiology [41]. The *MAPK* is involved in the proliferation of cardiac fibroblast and interaction between fibroblasts and cardiomyocytes [42], while *RAS* signaling stimulates cardiomyocyte hypertrophy and fibroblast proliferation [43]. Thus, the functional enrichment analysis (Figure 4) corroborates the findings of numerous previous studies. These pathways are implicated in various aspects of cardiac function and pathology, including cell survival, proliferation, and apoptosis. This underscores the potential of identified miRNAs as therapeutic targets or biomarkers in the context of cardiac health and disease.

4.4. Functional Assay

The meticulous selection of miRNAs for in vitro functional studies, based on their differential expression and prior associations with MI, represents a systematic approach to uncovering novel factors in MI pathology (Figure 5). By deliberately excluding miRNAs that are already well-established roles in MI research, or those exhibiting low expression levels, this study concentrated on potentially novel miRNAs. This strategy aimed at revealing new insights into the mechanisms of MI. Consequently, a set of 20 miRNAs were identified as promising candidates for further investigation in the in vitro functional study, potentially acting as causative factors in MI.

Primary cardiac cells or cardiac cell lines exposed to hypoxic stress are often used as in vitro models of myocardial infarction [44–46], because AMI causes hypoxic stress in cardiac cells [47]. In this study, primary cardiomyocytes and fibroblasts as in vitro models of myocardial infarction were used. The mammalian adult heart is composed of various cell types, including cardiomyocyte, fibroblast, endothelial cells, and peri-vascular cells [48].

Studies by Bannerjee et al. reported that the rat heart comprises 30% cardiomyocyte, 64% fibroblast, and 6% endothelial cells. In contrast, the mouse heart consists of 54% cardiomyocyte, 26% fibroblast, and 6% endothelial cells [49]. Based on this cellular composition, this study primarily utilized cardiomyocyte and fibroblasts to investigate the functional role of miRNAs. The in vitro experiments, conducted under hypoxic conditions on primary cardiomyocytes and fibroblasts, simulated the MI environment, thereby providing insights into the protective roles of selected miRNAs (Figure 6).

Figure 6 illustrates that 19 and 12 miRNAs significantly inhibited hypoxic stress-induced cell death in primary cardiomyocytes and fibroblasts, respectively. Notably, 11 miRNAs demonstrated protective effects against hypoxic cell death in both cell types. Interestingly, most of the 20 miRNAs selected had no previously reported association with the heart. However, there are a few studies on some of these miRNAs in different contexts. For example, miR-30c-1-3p was significantly downregulated in retinas of mice with oxygen-induced retinopathy [50], and miR-149 was shown to enhance the myocardial differentiation of mouse bone marrow stem cells [51]. Additionally, miR-706 was reported to block oxidative stress-induced activation of liver in fibrogenesis [52]. The observation that most of the selected miRNAs significantly reduced hypoxic stress-induced cell death in both cardiomyocytes and fibroblasts (Figure 6) is a promising indication of their potential therapeutic utility in treating MI.

4.5. Limitations, Strength, and Perspectives of This Study

The limitations of this study include its reliance on in vitro and animal models, which may not fully replicate in vivo the human condition of AMI. Additionally, while miRNAs that can inhibit hypoxia-induced cell death were identified in this study, limitations to the sensitivity and specificity of a single miRNA still exist. Further research is required to validate these findings in human subjects and explore the therapeutic potential of these miRNAs in clinical settings.

On the other hand, a notable aspect of this study is its focus on miRNAs showing reduced expression in the MI group. This approach facilitated the exploration of potentially novel miRNAs in the context of MI, extending beyond those already well-characterized in this disease. The in vitro functional studies revealed that selected miRNAs significantly mitigated hypoxic stress-induced cell death in primary cardiomyocytes and fibroblasts, suggesting their protective roles in the context of MI and highlighting their potential as therapeutic targets or biomarkers. Furthermore, the strengths of this study lie in derivation of miRNAs from exosomes secreted from heart tissue directly affected by MI. As these miRNAs closely reflect the heart's condition during MI, the study's results realistically portray the characteristics of MI-secreted exosomes. There is a similar report about plasma exosomal miRNAs in human AMI samples, although the origin of species and tissues differ [53]. This report, which examined miRNA profiles from the plasma of 118 subjects and identified 18 miRNAs as biomarkers for early AMI diagnosis, highlights both the advantages and disadvantages of the current study.

This discovery not only broadens understanding of miRNA-mediated regulation in cardiac tissues but also emphasizes their potential as therapeutic targets for AMI. Future research should aim at the clinical translation of these findings, striving to improve the diagnosis, treatment, and prognosis of AMI.

5. Conclusions

This study offers a comprehensive analysis of exoRNAs within an MI model, underlining the dynamic alterations in miRNA expression and exploring their potential functional roles. By integrating RNA sequencing data with functional in vitro assays, a robust framework for elucidating the molecular mechanisms underlying MI has been established, pinpointing novel therapeutic targets. Looking ahead, it is imperative to extend this research by validating these findings in human samples. Doing so would not only reinforce the relevance of these results but also bridge the gap between experimental models and clinical applications. Furthermore, investigating the therapeutic potential of these miR-NAs in clinical settings stands as a crucial next step. This would involve evaluating their efficacy and safety in human subjects, potentially opening new avenues for MI treatment and management.

Author Contributions: Conceptualization, S.W.K. and J.-W.C.; data curation, S.E.J. and J.-W.C.; formal analysis, S.W.K. and J.-W.C.; investigation, S.E.J. and J.-W.C.; methodology, S.E.J. and J.-W.C.; resources, S.E.J., S.W.K. and J.-W.C.; writing—original draft, S.E.J. and J.-W.C.; writing—review and editing, S.W.K. All authors have read and agreed to the published version of the manuscript.

Funding: This work was supported by the Basic Science Research Program through the National Research Foundation of Korea NRF, funded by the Ministry of Education (NRF-2020R1I1A2073643; funder, Sang Woo Kim) and the NRF grant funded by the Korea government (MSIT) (NRF-2021R1A2C1005280; funder, Jung-Won Choi).

Institutional Review Board Statement: All surgical procedures on experimental animals were conducted with the approval and in accordance with the guidelines and regulations of the Committee for the Care and Use of Laboratory Animals of the Catholic Kwandong University College of Medicine (approval numbers: CKU-01-2020-017 (approval date, 1 November 2020) for the establishment of the MI model, and CKU-01-2022-006 (approval date, 13 December 2022) for the isolation of primary cardiomyocytes and fibroblasts).

Informed Consent Statement: Not applicable.

Data Availability Statement: The data that support the findings of this study are available on request from the corresponding author.

Conflicts of Interest: The authors declare no conflicts of interest.

References

1. Reed, G.W.; Rossi, J.E.; Cannon, C.P. Acute Myocardial Infarction. *Lancet* **2017**, *389*, 197–210. [CrossRef]
2. Sachdeva, P.; Kaur, K.; Fatima, S.; Mahak, F.; Noman, M.; Siddenthi, S.M.; Surksha, M.A.; Munir, M.; Fatima, F.; Sultana, S.S.; et al. Advancements in Myocardial Infarction Management: Exploring Novel Approaches and Strategies. *Cureus* **2023**, *15*, e45578. [CrossRef]
3. Sun, T.; Dong, Y.H.; Du, W.; Shi, C.Y.; Wang, K.; Tariq, M.A.; Wang, J.X.; Li, P.F. The Role of MicroRNAs in Myocardial Infarction: From Molecular Mechanism to Clinical Application. *Int. J. Mol. Sci.* **2017**, *18*, 745. [CrossRef]
4. Kadesjo, E.; Roos, A.; Siddiqui, A.; Desta, L.; Lundback, M.; Holzmann, M.J. Acute versus Chronic Myocardial Injury and Long-term Outcomes. *Heart* **2019**, *105*, 1905–1912. [CrossRef]
5. Chapman, A.R.; Adamson, P.D.; Mills, N.L. Assessment and Classification of Patients with Myocardial Injury and Infarction in Clinical Practice. *Heart* **2017**, *103*, 10–18. [CrossRef]
6. Yasuda, S.; Shimokawa, H. Acute Myocardial Infarction: The Enduring Challenge for Cardiac Protection and Survival. *Circ. J.* **2009**, *73*, 2000–2008. [CrossRef]
7. Ounpuu, S.; Negassa, A.; Yusuf, S. INTER-HEART: A Global Study of Risk Factors for Acute Myocardial Infarction. *Am. Heart J.* **2001**, *141*, 711–721. [CrossRef]
8. Soares, R.O.S.; Losada, D.M.; Jordani, M.C.; Evora, P.; Castro, E.S.O. Ischemia/Reperfusion Injury Revisited: An Overview of the Latest Pharmacological Strategies. *Int. J. Mol. Sci.* **2019**, *20*, 5034. [CrossRef]
9. Harishkumar, M.; Radha, M.; Yuichi, N.; Muthukaliannan, G.K.; Kaoru, O.; Shiomori, K.; Sakai, K.; Nozomi, W. Designer Exosomes: Smart Nano-communication Tools for Translational Medicine. *Bioengineering* **2021**, *8*, 158. [CrossRef]
10. Kalluri, R.; LeBleu, V.S. The Biology, Function, and Biomedical Applications of Exosomes. *Science* **2020**, *367*, eaau6977. [CrossRef] [PubMed]
11. Wang, J.; Yue, B.L.; Huang, Y.Z.; Lan, X.Y.; Liu, W.J.; Chen, H. Exosomal RNAs: Novel Potential Biomarkers for Diseases—A Review. *Int. J. Mol. Sci.* **2022**, *23*, 2461. [CrossRef]
12. Narang, P.; Shah, M.; Beljanski, V. Exosomal RNAs in Diagnosis and Therapies. *Non-Coding RNA Res.* **2022**, *7*, 7–15. [CrossRef] [PubMed]
13. Dykes, I.M. Exosomes in Cardiovascular Medicine. *Cardiol. Ther.* **2017**, *6*, 225–237. [CrossRef] [PubMed]
14. Emanueli, C.; Shearn, A.I.; Angelini, G.D.; Sahoo, S. Exosomes and Exosomal MiRNAs in Cardiovascular Protection and Repair. *Vascul. Pharmacol.* **2015**, *71*, 24–30. [CrossRef] [PubMed]
15. Chopp, M.; Zhang, Z.G. Emerging Potential of Exosomes and Noncoding MicroRNAs for the Treatment of Neurological Injury/diseases. *Expert Opin. Emerg. Drugs* **2015**, *20*, 523–526. [CrossRef]

16. O'Brien, K.; Lowry, M.C.; Corcoran, C.; Martinez, V.G.; Daly, M.; Rani, S.; Gallagher, W.M.; Radomski, M.W.; MacLeod, R.A.; O'Driscoll, L. MiR-134 in Extracellular Vesicles Reduces Triple-negative Breast Cancer Aggression and Increases Drug Sensitivity. *Oncotarget* **2015**, *6*, 32774–32789. [CrossRef]
17. Tian, J.; Popal, M.S.; Zhao, Y.; Liu, Y.; Chen, K.; Liu, Y. Interplay between Exosomes and Autophagy in Cardiovascular Diseases: Novel Promising Target for Diagnostic and Therapeutic Application. *Aging Dis.* **2019**, *10*, 1302–1310. [CrossRef]
18. Xue, R.; Tan, W.; Wu, Y.; Dong, B.; Xie, Z.; Huang, P.; He, J.; Dong, Y.; Liu, C. Role of Exosomal miRNAs in Heart Failure. *Front. Cardiovasc. Med.* **2020**, *7*, 592412. [CrossRef]
19. Bartel, D.P. MicroRNAs: Genomics, Biogenesis, Mechanism, and Function. *Cell* **2004**, *116*, 281–297. [CrossRef]
20. Boon, R.A.; Dimmeler, S. MicroRNAs in Myocardial Infarction. *Nat. Rev. Cardiol.* **2015**, *12*, 135–142. [CrossRef] [PubMed]
21. Jiang, C.; Chen, J.; Zhao, Y.; Gao, D.; Wang, H.; Pu, J. A Modified Simple Method for Induction of Myocardial Infarction in Mice. *J. Vis. Exp.* **2021**, *3*, 178.
22. Forte, E.; Skelly, D.A.; Chen, M.; Daigle, S.; Morelli, K.A.; Hon, O.; Philip, V.M.; Costa, M.W.; Rosenthal, N.A.; Furtado, M.B. Dynamic Interstitial Cell Response during Myocardial Infarction Predicts Resilience to Rupture in Genetically Diverse Mice. *Cell Rep.* **2020**, *3*, 3149–3163.e6. [CrossRef] [PubMed]
23. Shin, S.; Choi, J.W.; Moon, H.; Lee, C.Y.; Park, J.H.; Lee, J.; Seo, H.H.; Han, G.; Lim, S.; Kim, S.W.; et al. Stimultaneous Suppression of Multiple Programmed Cell Death Pathways by miRNA-105 in Cardiac Ischemic Injury. *Mol. Ther. Nucleic Acids* **2019**, *1*, 438–449. [CrossRef]
24. Chang, X.; Zhang, K.; Zhou, R.; Luo, F.; Zhu, L.; Gao, J.; He, H.; Wei, T.; Yan, T.; Ma, C. Cardioprotective Effects of Salidroside on Myocardial Ischemia-reperfusion Injury in Coronary Artery Occlusion-induced Rats and Langendorff-perfused Rat Hearts. *Int. J Cardiol.* **2016**, *15*, 532–544. [CrossRef] [PubMed]
25. Lee, J.; Kim, S.R.; Lee, C.; Jun, Y.I.; Bae, S.; Yoon, Y.J.; Kim, O.Y.; Gho, Y.S. Extracellular Vesicles from In Vivo Liver Tissue Accelerate Recovery of Liver Necrosis Induced by Carbon Tetrachloride. *J. Extracell. Vesicles* **2021**, *10*, e12133. [CrossRef] [PubMed]
26. Zhan, X.; Yuan, W.; Zhou, Y.; Ma, R.; Ge, Z. Small RNA Sequencing and Bioinformatics Analysis of RAW264.7-derived Exosomes after Mycobacterium Bovis Bacillus Calmette-Guerin Infection. *BMC Genomics* **2022**, *7*, 355. [CrossRef] [PubMed]
27. Cizmar, P.; Yuana, Y. Detection and Characterization of Extracellular Vesicles by Transmission and Cryo-Transmission Electron Microscopy. *Methods Mol. Biol.* **2017**, *1660*, 221–232. [PubMed]
28. Choi, J.W.; Lim, S.; Kang, J.H.; Hwang, S.H.; Hwang, K.C.; Kim, S.W.; Lee, S. Proteome Analysis of Human Natural Killer Cell Derived Extracellular Vesicles for Identification of Anticancer Effectors. *Molecules* **2020**, *9*, 5216. [CrossRef] [PubMed]
29. Mishra, M.; Tiwari, S.; Gomes, A.V. Protein Purification and Analysis: Next Generation Western Blotting Techniques. *Expert Rev. Proteomics* **2017**, *14*, 1037–1053. [CrossRef]
30. Jung, S.E.; Kim, S.W.; Jeong, S.; Moon, H.; Choi, W.S.; Lim, S.; Lee, S.; Hwang, K.C.; Choi, J.W. MicroRNA-26a/b-5p Promotes Myocardial Infarction-induced Cell Death by Downregulation Cytochrome C Oxidase 5a. *Exp. Mol. Med.* **2021**, *53*, 1332–1343. [CrossRef]
31. Pokrowiecki, R.; Zaręba, T.; Szaraniec, B.; Pałka, K.; Mielczarek, A.; Menaszek, E.; Tyski, S. In Vitro Studies of Nanosilver-doped Titanium Implants for Oral and Maxillofacial Surgery. *Int. J. Nanomed.* **2017**, *6*, 4285–4297. [CrossRef]
32. Oliveria, S.R.; Dionisio, P.A.; Brito, H.; Franco, L.; Rodrigues, C.A.B.; Guedes, R.C.; Afonso, C.A.M.; Amaral, J.D.; Rodrigues C.M.P. Phenotypic Screening Identifies a New Oxazolone Inhibitor of Necroptosis and Neuroinflammation. *Cell Death. Dicov.* **2018**, *4*, 10. [CrossRef] [PubMed]
33. Yamashita, S.; Katsumata, O. Heat-Induced Antigen Retrieval in Immunohistochemistry: Mechanisms and Applications. *Methods Mol. Bio.* **2017**, *1630*, 147–161.
34. Wu, Y.; Yin, X.; Wijaya, C.; Huang, M.H.; McConnell, B.K. Acute Myocardial Infarction in Rats. *J. Vis. Exp.* **2011**, *16*, 2464.
35. Hashmi, S.; Al-Salam, S. Acute Myocardial Infarction and Myocardial Ischemia-reperfusion Injury: A Comparison. *Int. J. Clin. Exp. Pathol.* **2015**, *8*, 8786–8796.
36. Lindsey, M.L.; Brunt, K.R.; Kirk, J.A.; Kleinbongard, P.; Calvert, J.W.; de Castro Bras, L.E.; DeLeon-Pennell, K.Y.; Del Re, D.P.; Frangogiannis, N.G.; Frantz, S.; et al. Guidelines for In Vivo Mouse Models of Myocardial Infarction. *Am. J. Physiol. Heart Circ. Physiol.* **2021**, *321*, H1056–H1073. [CrossRef]
37. Weil, B.R.; Neelamegham, S. Selectins and Immune Cells in Acute Myocardial Infarction and Post-infarction Ventricular Remodeling: Pathophysiology and Novel Treatments. *Front. Immunol.* **2019**, *10*, 300. [CrossRef] [PubMed]
38. Thery, C.; Zitvogel, L.; Amigorena, S. Exosomes: Composition, Biogenesis and Function. *Nat. Rev. Immunol.* **2002**, *2*, 569–579. [CrossRef] [PubMed]
39. Hurwitz, S.N.; Olcese, J.M.; Meckes, D.G., Jr. Extraction of Extracellular Vesicles from Whole Tissue. *J. Vis. Exp.* **2019**, *144*, e59143.
40. Walkowski, B.; Kleibert, M.; Majka, M.; Wojciechowska, M. Insight into the Role of the *PI3K/Akt* Pathway in Ischemic Injury and Post-Infarct Left Ventricular Remodeling in Normal and Diabetic Heart. *Cells* **2022**, *11*, 1553. [CrossRef]
41. Colombe, A.S.; Pidoux, G. Cardiac cAMP-PKA Signaling Compartmentalization in Myocardial Infarction. *Cells* **2021**, *10*, 922. [CrossRef]
42. Guo, H.; Zhao, X.; Li, H.; Liu, K.; Jiang, H.; Zeng, X.; Chang, J.; Ma, C.; Fu, Z.; Lv, X.; et al. GDF15 Promotes Cardiac Fibrosis and Proliferation of Cardiac Fibroblasts via the *MAPK/ERK1/2* Pathway after Irradiation in Rats. *Radiat. Res.* **2021**, *196*, 183–191. [CrossRef] [PubMed]

13. Lyu, L.; Wang, H.; Li, B.; Qin, Q.; Qi, L.; Nagarkatti, M.; Nagarkatti, P.; Janicki, J.S.; Wang, X.L.; Cui, T. A Critical Role of Cardiac Fibroblast-derived Exosomes in Activating Renin Angiotensin System in Cardiomyocytes. *J. Mol. Cell. Cardiol.* **2015**, *89*, 268–279. [CrossRef] [PubMed]
14. Jin, H.; Yu, J. Lidocaine Protects H9c2 Cells from Hypoxia-induced Injury through Regulation of the *MAPK/ERK/NFκB* Signaling Pathway. *Exp. Ther. Med.* **2019**, *18*, 4125–4131. [PubMed]
15. Cai, Y.; Li, Y. Upregulation of MiR-29b-3p Protects Cardiomyocytes from Hypoxia-induced Apoptosis by Targeting *TRAF5*. *Cell. Mol. Biol. Lett.* **2019**, *11*, 27. [CrossRef] [PubMed]
16. Pyo, J.O.; Nah, J.; Kim, H.J.; Chang, J.W.; Song, Y.W.; Yang, D.K.; Jo, D.G.; Kim, H.R.; Chae, H.J.; Chae, S.W.; et al. Protection of Cardiomyocytes from Ischemic/hypoxia Cell Death via *Drbp1* and *pMe2GlyDH* in Cardio-specific *ARC* transgenic mice. *J. Biol. Chem.* **2008**, *7*, 30707–30714. [CrossRef]
17. Datta Chaudhuri, R.; Banik, A.; Mandal, B.; Sarkar, S. Cardia-specific overexpression of *HIF-1α* during acute myocardial infarction ameliorates cardiomyocyte apoptosis via differential regulation of hypoxia-inducible pro-apoptotic and anti-oxidative genes. *Biochem. Biophys. Res. Commun.* **2021**, *22*, 100–108. [CrossRef] [PubMed]
18. Zhou, P.; Pu, W.T. Recounting Cardiac Cellular Composition. *Circ. Res.* **2016**, *118*, 368–370. [CrossRef]
19. Banerjee, I.; Fuseler, J.W.; Price, R.L.; Borg, T.K.; Baudino, T.A. Determination of Cell Types and Numbers during Cardiac Development in the Neonatal and Adult Rat and Mouse. *Am. J. Physiol. Heart Circ. Physiol.* **2007**, *293*, H1883–H1891. [CrossRef]
20. Zhang, L.S.; Zhou, Y.D.; Peng, Y.Q.; Zeng, H.L.; Yoshida, S.; Zhao, T.T. Identification of Altered MicroRNAs in Retinas of Mice with Oxygen-induced Retinopathy. *Int. J. Ophthalmol.* **2019**, *12*, 739–745.
21. Lu, M.; Xu, L.; Wang, M.; Guo, T.; Luo, F.; Su, N.; Yi, S.; Chen, T. MiR-149 Promotes the Myocardial Differentiation of Mouse Bone Marrow Stem Cells by Targeting *Dab2*. *Mol. Med. Rep.* **2018**, *17*, 8502–8509. [CrossRef]
22. Yin, R.; Guo, D.; Zhang, S.; Zhang, X. MiR-706 Inhibits the Oxidative Stress-induced Activation of *PKCalpha/TAOK1* in Liver Fibrogenesis. *Sci. Rep.* **2016**, *6*, 37509. [CrossRef]
23. Guo, M.; Li, R.; Yang, L.; Zhu, Q.; Han, M.; Chen, Z.; Ruan, F.; Yuan, Y.; Liu, Z.; Huang, B.; et al. Evaluation of Exosomal MiRNAs as Potential Diagnostic Biomarkers for Acute Myocardial Infarction Using Next-generation Sequencing. *Ann. Transl. Med.* **2021**, *9*, 219. [CrossRef]

Disclaimer/Publisher's Note: The statements, opinions and data contained in all publications are solely those of the individual author(s) and contributor(s) and not of MDPI and/or the editor(s). MDPI and/or the editor(s) disclaim responsibility for any injury to people or property resulting from any ideas, methods, instructions or products referred to in the content.

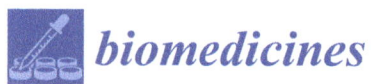

Article

Sex X Time Interactions in Lp(a) and LDL-C Response to Evolocumab

Federica Fogacci [1,†], Serra İlayda Yerlitaş [2,3,†], Marina Giovannini [1], Gökmen Zararsız [2,3], Paolo Lido [4], Claudio Borghi [1,5] and Arrigo F. G. Cicero [1,5,*]

1. Hypertension and Cardiovascular Risk Research Center, Medical and Surgical Sciences Department, Alma Mater Studiorum University of Bologna, 40100 Bologna, Italy; federica.fogacci@studio.unibo.it (F.F.); marina.giovannini3@unibo.it (M.G.); claudio.borghi@unibo.it (C.B.)
2. Department of Biostatistics, Erciyes University School of Medicine, 38039 Kayseri, Turkey; ilaydayerlitas340@gmail.com (S.İ.Y.); gokmen.zararsiz@gmail.com (G.Z.)
3. Drug Application and Research Center (ERFARMA), Erciyes University, 38280 Kayseri, Turkey
4. Italian Medicines Agency (AIFA), 00187 Rome, Italy; paulshore@virgilio.it
5. Unit of Cardiovascular Internal Medicine, Department of Cardiac, Thoracic, Vascular Pathology, IRCCS Azienda Ospedaliero-Universitaria di Bologna, 40100 Bologna, Italy
* Correspondence: arrigo.cicero@unibo.it; Tel.: +39-0516362224; Fax: +39-516826125
† These authors contributed equally to this work.

Abstract: The aim of this study was to evaluate whether there were significant sex x time interactions in lipoprotein(a) (Lp(a)) and low-density lipoprotein cholesterol (LDL-C) response to treatment with the Proprotein Convertase Subtilisin/Kexin type 9 inhibitor (PCSK9i) Evolocumab, in a real-life clinical setting. For this purpose, we pooled data from 176 outpatients (Men: 93; Women: 83) clinically evaluated at baseline and every six months after starting Evolocumab. Individuals who had been on PCSK9i for less than 30 months and nonadherent patients were excluded from the analysis. Over time, absolute values of Lp(a) plasma concentrations significantly decreased in the entire cohort (p-value < 0.001) and by sex (p-value < 0.001 in men and p-value = 0.002 in and women). However, there were no sex-related significant differences. Absolute plasma concentrations of LDL-C significantly decreased over time in the entire cohort and by sex (p-value < 0.001 always), with greater improvements in men compared to women. The sex x time interaction was statistically significant in LDL-C (all p-values < 0.05), while absolute changes in Lp(a) were not influenced by either sex or time (all p-value > 0.05). Our data partially reinforce the presence of differences in response to treatment to PCSK9i between men and women and are essential to gain a better understanding of the relationship between LDL-C and Lp(a) lowering in response to PCSK9i. Further research will clarify whether these sex-related significant differences translate into a meaningful difference in the long-term risk of ASCVD.

Keywords: lipoprotein(a); PCSK9; PCSK9 inhibitor; evolocumab; women's health

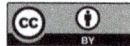

1. Introduction

The International guidelines for the prevention of atherosclerotic cardiovascular disease (ASCVD) recommend the use of proprotein convertase subtilisin/kexin type 9 (PCSK9) inhibitors (PCSK9i) in high-risk patients as second-line lipid-lowering agents in addition to the maximally tolerated statin dose [1]. A comprehensive meta-analysis of phase II and phase III clinical trials evaluating the effect of PCSK9i Evolocumab and Alirocumab on lipoprotein(a) (Lp(a)) concentration concluded significant improvements from baseline according to the comparator group (placebo: mean difference (MD): −27.9%, 95% confidence interval (CI): −31.1% to −24.6% versus ezetimibe: MD: −22.2%, 95% CI: −27.2% to −17.2, p-value: 0.04) and duration of treatment (≤12 weeks: MD: −30.9%, 95% CI: −34.7% to −27.1% versus >12 weeks: MD: −21.9%, 95% CI: −25.2% to −18.6%, p-value < 0.01) [2].

More recently, the small interfering ribonucleic acid (siRNA) Inclisiran has been shown to lower Lp(a) by an average of −20.9% (95% CI: −25.8% to −15.99%) [3], although the interindividual variation following treatment appears high [4].

In the last decade, substantial evidence from epidemiological and experimental studies clearly showed that high levels of Lp(a) are an independent and genetically determined risk factor for the development of atherosclerosis and ASCVD, such as coronary artery disease (CAD), stroke and aortic stenosis [5,6]. Thus, the absence of available therapeutic options for effectively managing patients with hyperlipoproteinemia(a) means that identifying the genetic determinants of individual response variability to PCSK9 pharmacological inhibition is a critical issue [7].

In real-world clinical settings, PCSK9i have been shown to be less effective in reducing LDL-C levels in women compared to men [8,9], with the underlying mechanisms to be clarified [9]. A tentative explanation for this observation could lie in the different PCSK9 concentrations between sexes [10], since large-scale clinical studies involving the collection of blood samples for the centralized measurement of PCSK9 showed that women have higher circulating PCSK9 than men [11]. Proposed alternative explanations for the unusual LDL-C response to PCSK9i include higher Lp(a) concentrations, which more commonly occur in postmenopausal women [9,12]. Treatment with PCSK9i has been shown to reduce LDL-C and Lp(a) in a 2:1 ratio (LDL-C approximately 50–60%: Lp(a) ≈25–30%), and often in a discordant manner (e.g., in >30% of individuals undergoing treatment, Lp(a) and LDL-C do not fall concordantly) [13,14]. In these cases, according to Warden et al., the reduced LDL-C response could be accounted for by the higher proportion of reported LDL-C consisting of Lp(a) particles, which are not cleared efficiently by the LDL receptor [12]. Unfortunately, unlike LDL-C, sex-dependent differences in the Lp(a)-lowering effect driven by PCSK9 inhibition have never been investigated before, neither in controlled clinical trials nor in real-world settings. Then, the aim of this study was to evaluate whether there were significant sex x time interactions in Lp(a) and LDL-C response to treatment with the PCSK9i Evolocumab.

2. Methods

2.1. Study Design and Participants

This is a subanalysis of an ongoing prospective observational study, whose protocol was approved by the Ethics Committee of the University of Bologna (Code: LLD-RP2018). The study followed the Declaration of Helsinki and its amendments, and all individuals signed an informed consent to participate.

Data were pooled from hypercholesterolemic patients recruited at the Lipid Clinic of the S. Orsola-Malpighi University Hospital, Bologna, Italy. Enrolled individuals were eligible for treatment with PCSK9i according to the recommendations of the European Society of Cardiology (ESC) and the European Atherosclerosis Society (EAS) [15], as well as the criteria released by the Italian Regulatory Agency (AIFA) [16,17]. Additional inclusion criteria were ≥18 years of age and being on maximum tolerated oral lipid-lowering therapy (statin and ezetimibe or ezetimibe monotherapy) for ≥6 months before starting Evolocumab, with no planned dose change.

Patients were clinically evaluated at baseline and every six months after starting Evolocumab (Figure 1). Individuals who had been on PCSK9i for less than 30 months and noncompliant patients were excluded from the analysis.

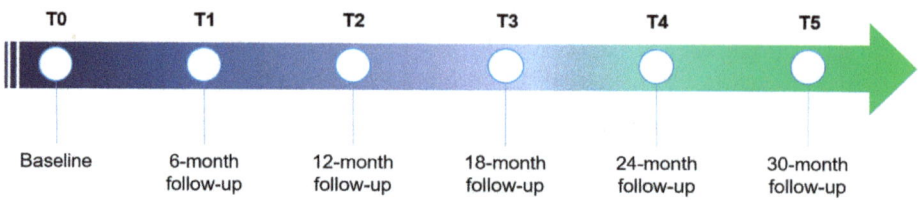

Figure 1. Study timeline.

2.2. Assessments

2.2.1. Clinical Data and Physical Assessments

Each patient's personal history was evaluated paying particular attention to ASCVD, smoking habit and ongoing pharmacological treatments. Genetic screening for the presence of an FH-causing variant was done in case of clinical suspicion. Height and weight were measured to the nearest 0.1 cm and 0.1 kg, respectively, with patients standing erect with eyes directed straight, wearing light clothes and with bare feet. Body mass index (BMI) was calculated as body weight in kilograms, divided by height squared in meters (kg/m^2) [18].

2.2.2. Laboratory Analysis

Laboratory analyses were performed to investigate complete blood count (CBC), total cholesterol (TC), high-density lipoprotein cholesterol (HDL-C), triglycerides (TG), Lp(a), apolipoprotein B (Apo-B), apolipoprotein A1 (Apo-A1), fasting plasma glucose (FPG), serum uric acid (SUA), creatinine (Cr), total bilirubin and fractions, alanine transaminase (ALT), aspartate transaminase (AST), gamma-glutamyl transferase (gamma-GT), creatinine phosphokinase (CPK) and thyroid-stimulating hormone (TSH). Venous blood samples were obtained from each patient after overnight fasting. Lp(a) concentrations were measured using an immunoturbidimetric assay. LDL-C was calculated by the Friedewald formula [19]. The glomerular filtration rate (eGFR) was estimated by the Chronic Kidney Disease Epidemiology Collaboration (CKD-epi) equation [20].

2.3. Statistical Analysis

Data distribution was assessed by histograms, q-q plots and Shapiro–Wilk's test. Continuous variables were summarized using arithmetic mean ± standard deviation, median and 1st/3rd quartiles and n (%). For two-group comparisons of descriptive clinical parameters, an independent two-sample t-test, Mann–Whitney U test and Pearson chi-squared test were used. To identify the main and interaction effects of sex and time points, nonparametric analysis of longitudinal data was applied for Lp(a) and LDL-C. Experimental results were summarized with Wald statistics, degrees of freedom and p-values. The Mann–Whitney U test was used for sex comparisons at each time point, separately. The Friedman test was used to compare the change over time in Lp(a) and LDL-C according to sex. Bonferroni and Nemenyi tests were applied for multiple comparisons. Area under the curve (AUC) values of Lp(a), LDL-C, percent change from baseline in Lp(a) and LDL-C were also calculated, and the median AUC values were compared by sex, using the Mann–Whitney U test. A p-value of <0.05 was considered statistically significant. All analyses were conducted using R 4.2.1 (www.r-project.org) software.

3. Results

According to the prespecified inclusion and exclusion criteria, we pooled data from 176 patients (Men: n = 93; Women: n = 83), who, in October 2022, had been treated with Evolocumab for at least 30 months. Baseline characteristics of the enrolled patients are reported in Table 1. The mean age and history of ASCVD were significantly higher in men than in women (p-value < 0.05). Following the classification of the American College of Cardiology (ACC) and the American Heart Association (AHA), the intensity of background statin therapy was reported as divided into 3 categories [21]. High-intensity statin use was defined as atorvastatin ≥ 40 mg or rosuvastatin ≥ 20 mg; moderate-intensity statin use was defined as atorvastatin ≤ 20 mg, rosuvastatin ≤ 10 mg, simvastatin ≥ 20 mg, pravastatin ≥ 40 mg, lovastatin ≥ 40 mg or fluvastatin 80 mg; low-intensity statin use was defined as simvastatin 10 mg, pravastatin ≤ 20 mg, lovastatin ≤ 20 mg or fluvastatin ≤ 40 mg. As reported in Table 1, the overall distribution of statin treatment was not different across men and women at the baseline (p-value > 0.05). The use of ezetimibe as background lipid-lowering therapy was higher in women than men (p-value < 0.05). The median values of TC, HDL-C, eGFR, ALT and gamma-GT were significantly higher in men than women (p-values < 0.05). In women, LDL-C, AST and CPK were higher (p-values < 0.05).

Table 1. Baseline characteristics of the patients enrolled in the study.

Characteristics	All Patients (n = 176)	Men (n = 93)	Women (n = 83)	p-Values
Age (years)	63.4 ± 10.1	63.4 ± 10.5	61.9 ± 10.3	0.012
History of ASCVD (n; %)	105 (59.7)	53 (57.0)	52 (62.7)	0.021
Type 2 Diabetes Mellitus (n; %)	21 (11.9)	12 (12.9)	9 (10.8)	0.409
Familial Hypercholesterolemia (n; %)	64 (36.6)	30 (32.3)	34 (41.5)	0.207
Hypertension (n; %)	117 (66.5)	58 (62.4)	59 (71.1)	0.308
Background lipid-lowering therapy				
Statin (n; %)	75 (42.6)	36 (38.7)	39 (47)	0.188
High-intensity dosage (n; %)	28 (38.4)	14 (33.3)	14 (45.2)	
Moderate-intensity dosage (n; %)	45 (61.6)	28 (66.7)	17 (54.8)	
Low-intensity dosage (n; %)	0 (0)	0 (0)	0 (0)	
Ezetimibe (n; %)	119 (67.6)	54 (58.1)	65 (78.3)	0.012
BMI (kg/m^2)	27 ± 4	26.8 ± 4.4	27.4 ± 4.3	0.122
TC (mg/dL)	214 (190–251)	216 (190–261.5)	205.5 (190–242.5)	0.003
LDL-C (mg/dL)	132.2 (111.2–166.8)	131.6 (111.3–173.8)	137 (111.2–161.8)	0.050
HDL-C (mg/dL)	53.8 ± 12.6	58.7 ± 11.9	48.9 ± 10	<0.001
TG (mg/dL)	132 (93.5–179)	139 (87.5–191.5)	119 (98.5–162.8)	0.842
Lp(a) (mg/dL)	39.2 (11.9–107)	39.2 (9.7–110.7)	36.3 (12–95.7)	0.722
eGFR (mL/min)	80 ± 18.7	82.6 ± 19.9	80.8 ± 20.6	0.030
AST (U/L)	25 (21–30)	25 (21.3–30)	26 (20–30.5)	0.001
ALT (U/L)	24 (17–32.5)	25 (18–31)	24 (16.3–33.8)	<0.001
Gamma-GT (U/L)	24.5 (17–35.3)	25 (17–39)	24 (16.5–33)	<0.001
CPK (U/L)	140.5 (85.8–236.8)	126 (84–206)	156 (91.5–262.5)	<0.001

ALT = Alanine transaminase; ASCVD = Atherosclerotic cardiovascular disease; AST = Aspartate transaminase; BMI = Body mass index; CPK = Creatinine phosphokinase; eGFR = Estimated glomerular filtration rate; Gamma-GT = Gamma-glutamyl transferase; HDL-C = High-density lipoprotein cholesterol; LDL-C = Low-density lipoprotein cholesterol; Lp(a) = Lipoprotein(a); n = Number of patients; TC = Total cholesterol; TG = Triglycerides. Values are expressed as mean ± standard deviation, median (1st/3rd quartiles) and n (%).

Absolute and percentage changes in LDL-C and Lp(a) for all patients and by sex are shown in Figure 2. A positive and moderate correlation was observed between the over-time change trends of Lp(a) and LDL-C measurements in women (ρ = 0.600). The relationship between these two measurement trends was observed to be quite weak in men (ρ = 0.086).

Nonparametric analysis of longitudinal data in factorial experiments for changes in plasma concentrations in Lp(a) and LDL-C is given in Table 2. The main effects and the interaction of the sex and time were found to be statistically significant in LDL-C (all p-values < 0.05). On the contrary, absolute changes in Lp(a) were influenced neither by sex nor by time (all p-value > 0.05) (Table 2).

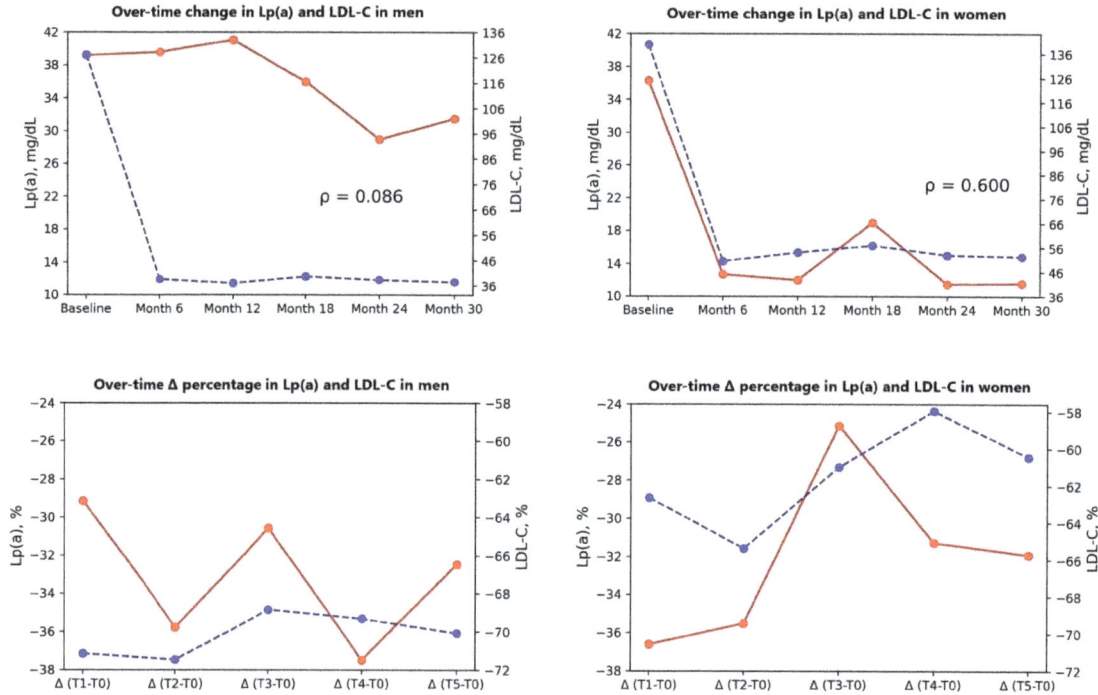

Figure 2. Longitudinal trends in LDL-C and Lp(a) plasma concentrations over time. LDL-C = Low-density lipoprotein cholesterol; Lp(a) = Lipoprotein(a). Dashed blue line: LDL-C; Solid red line: Lpa(a); ρ: Spearman correlation coefficient.

Table 2. Nonparametric analysis of longitudinal data in factorial experiments for changes in plasma concentrations in Lp(a) and LDL-C.

Source of Variation	df	Wald	p-Values
Lp(a)			
Sex	1	2.839	0.092
Time	5	10.965	0.052
Time × Sex	5	2.869	0.720
LDL-C			
Sex	1	16.843	<0.001
Time	5	855.501	<0.001
Time × Sex	5	14.005	0.016

df = Degrees of freedom; LDL-C = Low-density lipoprotein cholesterol; Lp(a) = Lipoprotein(a).

Absolute values of Lp(a) plasma concentrations significantly decreased in the entire cohort (p-value < 0.001), without any difference among sex over time (p-value < 0.001 in men and p-value = 0.002 in women) (Table 3). No sex-related significant differences were detected at any time point (p-value > 0.05). Moreover, no statistically significant difference was found in the percentage changes between sexes (p-value > 0.05) (Table 3).

Table 3. Between-sex changes in Lp(a) concentrations over time. Values are expressed as median (1st/3rd quartiles).

Time Points	All Patients (n = 176)	Men (n = 93)	Women (n = 83)	p-Values [†]
Lp(a)				
Baseline (T0)	39.2 (11.9/107) [a]	39.2 (9.7/110.7) [ab]	36.3 (12/95.7) [a]	0.722
6 Months (T1)	30.1 (6.4/79.7) [b]	39.6 (8.4/101.9) [ab]	12.7 (5.2/64.9) [ab]	0.063
12 Months (T2)	24.3 (8.1/72.9) [b]	41.1 (10.5/79.1) [a]	12 (6.6/68.6) [b]	0.054
18 Months (T3)	28.5 (8.6/74.3) [b]	36 (10.8/91.7) [b]	19 (5.9/65.4) [ab]	0.091
24 Months (T4)	22.9 (6.4/83.7) [b]	29 (6.9/97.5) [b]	11.5 (5.9/64.8) [b]	0.134
30 Months (T5)	27.6 (8.1/87.3) [b]	31.5 (9.2/103.2) [b]	11.6 (6.5/85.4) [b]	0.176
p-value [‡]	<0.001	<0.001	0.002	
AUC	1290.60 (316.50/3146.70)	2255.55 (489.15/3721.43)	1237.80 (1057.80/1932.60)	0.125
Delta %				
T1-T0	−33.62 (−43.56/−14.71)	−29.15 (−43.08/−16.34)	−36.60 (−45.34/−9.09)	0.865
T2-T0	−35.64 (−52.28/−13.71)	−35.78 (−52.36/−16.78)	−35.51 (−52.10/−8.68)	0.722
T3-T0	−29.22 (−45.04/−10.31)	−30.56 (−42.03/−15.17)	−25.13 (−46.53/0.89)	0.605
T4-T0	−36.36 (−61.08/−13.55)	−37.5 (−62.05/−14.41)	−31.27 (−52.69/−8.11)	0.681
T5-T0	−32.24 (−56.34/−17.89)	−32.47 (−54.73/−12.42)	−31.91 (−56.34/−18)	0.988

AUC = Area under the curve; Lp(a) = Lipoprotein(a); n: Number of patients. Delta % = 100 × ((Ti-T0)/T0). [†]: between-group comparison; [‡]: within-group comparisons. Different lowercase letters ([a,b]) in the same column indicate a statistically significant difference between the time points.

Absolute plasma concentrations of LDL-C significantly decreased over time, in the entire cohort (p-value < 0.001) and by sex (p-value < 0.001 in men and women) (Table 4). LDL-C concentrations remained significantly higher in women than men at each time point (p-values < 0.05 always); similarly, the AUC was higher in women than men (p-value = 0.017). LDL-C percentage significantly decreased more in men than in women at each time point (p-value < 0.01 always) (Table 4).

Table 4. Between-sex changes in LDL-C concentrations over time. Values are expressed as median (1st/3rd quartiles).

Time Points	All Patients (n = 176)	Men (n = 93)	Women (n = 83)	p-Values [†]
Baseline (T0)	132.2 (111.2/166.8) [a]	127.2 (107/156.2) [a]	139.8 (113.9/177.7) [a]	0.049
6 Months (T1)	45.4 (28.6/69.4) [b]	38.6 (22.6/56.1) [b]	50.6 (36.4/78.3) [b]	0.002
12 Months (T2)	44.8 (27.4/72) [b]	37 (24.6/56) [b]	54.1 (33.6/93.8) [b]	0.001
18 Months (T3)	42.7 (30.2/67.7) [b]	39.8 (25.8/55.2) [b]	57 (34.6/78.3) [b]	0.001
24 Months (T4)	47.6 (31.3/69.1) [b]	38.4 (24.7/60.9) [b]	53 (40/87) [b]	0.002
30 Months (T5)	44.3 (28.7/64.5) [b]	37.6 (23.6/54) [b]	52.4 (41.4/80) [b]	<0.001
p-value [‡]	<0.001	<0.001	<0.001	
AUC	1543.20 (1113.60/2245.65)	747.6 (228.9/1583.4)	1915.8 (1324.2/2623.2)	0.017
Delta %				
T1-T0	−67.8 (−76.43/−55.46)	−71.14 (−81.26/−60.54)	−62.65 (−71.44/−51.3)	0.004
T2-T0	−68.15 (−77.29/−50.75)	−71.46 (−79.41/−59.06)	−65.38 (−75.82/−37.93)	0.007
T3-T0	−66.6 (−75.25/−55.1)	−68.85 (−78.02/−61.84)	−60.99 (−73.35/−45.88)	0.006
T4-T0	−65.44 (−76.02/−49.91)	−69.32 (−79.37/−53.25)	−57.95 (−70.02/−49.1)	0.010
T5-T0	−65.77 (−75.5/−53.77)	−70.07 (−79.96/−58.23)	−60.46 (−72.18/−44.88)	0.006

AUC = Area under the curve; LDL-C = Low-density lipoprotein cholesterol; n: Number of patients. Delta % = 100 × ((T1-T0)/T0). [†]: between-group comparison; [‡]: within-group comparisons. Significant p-values are shown in bold. Different lowercase letters ([a,b]) in the same column indicate a statistically significant difference between time points.

Treatment with the PCSK9i was well tolerated. No serious adverse event was registered during the follow-up.

4. Discussion

Over the last 30 years, there was an overall declining trend in age-standardized disability-adjusted life years (DALY) rate as regards ASCVD, with larger declines among women compared to men [22]. Today, the identification of sex-related differences in determinants of individual CV risk continues to receive considerable attention from the scientific community, to plan and implement prevention policies and programs, also regarding the early diagnosis and management of dyslipidemia [23].

The controversy about whether women benefit to the same extent as men from lipid-lowering treatment is mainly attributable to a relative lack of information about the effects on women from individual clinical trials [24]. This bias is secondarily due to sampling errors that led to the enrollment disparity difference between the proportion of women with prevalent ASCVD and the proportion of women enrolled in the studies [25].

Early-phase drug investigations have historically excluded women of childbearing age due to physiological hormonal fluctuations and concerns of safety for the mother and fetus if the woman had become pregnant after enrollment [26]. Women are also well known to develop CHD on average 10 years later than men, being more likely to be excluded due to age requirements from clinical studies enrolling individuals with ASCVD [27].

In addition to improving enrollment, another critical issue is to develop strategies to foster the retention of women participants [28], since women are more likely to withdraw consent from the trials and discontinue study drugs compared to men [29].

Available data are conflicting about the existence of long-term differences between women and men in response to PCSK9i Evolocumab. It has been assumed that a role could be played by Lp(a), whose plasmatic concentrations are affected by estrogen fluctuations [30,31] This assumption has yet to be proven, and new data on the relationship between changes in Lp(a) and ASCVD risk reduction in women will come from the ongoing clinical trials testing the emergent Lp(a)-lowering drugs.

The siRNA agents (olpasiran, LY3819469 and SLN360) and the second-generation antisense oligopeptide pelacarsen are being developed to specifically interfere with Lp(a) synthesis in the liver by blocking the translation of apo(a) messenger RNA (mRNA) in apo(a) [32], and in the next years, the phase III pivotal CV outcome trials (CVOT)—Lp(a)HORIZON and OCEAN(a)—will definitively clarify whether lowering Lp(a) translates into improved ASCVD outcomes. However, according to the findings of a recently published dose–response meta-analysis providing a comprehensive overview of the association between circulating Lp(a) and all-cause and cause-specific mortality, the risk of death from ASCVD increases by 31% for each 50 mg/dL rise in Lp(a) plasma levels [33] Then, in the absence of treatment options currently available for the effective management of patients with high Lp(a) levels [34], the Lp(a)-lowering effect driven by PCSK9 inhibition is particularly interesting.

The FLOREY (Effects on Lipoprotein Metabolism From PCSK9 Inhibition Utilizing a Monoclonal Antibody) Study firstly suggested that Evolocumab reduces Lp(a) through the inhibition of the synthesis of apo(a) and the upregulation of the LDLR activity [35] A tentative explanation could be that Lp(a) can compete more favorably for the LDLR when LDL-C levels in plasma are very low [36]. However, if PCSK9 inhibition lowers Lp(a) exclusively through LDLR-mediated clearance, the Lp(a) response would likely be proportional to the LDL-C response, and this does not happen [14].

In our cohort of outpatients, there were no remarkable sex-related significant differences in Lp(a) response to Evolocumab. However, plasma concentrations of LDL-C significantly decreased over 2.5 years in the entire cohort and by sex, with greater improvements in men compared to women. The sex x time interaction was statistically significant in LDL-C, while absolute changes in Lp(a) were not influenced by either sex or time. Then, our analysis answers an important and clinically relevant question that was left open by the pivotal studies and subsequent research [14]. Overall, these observations are essential to gain a better understanding of the relationship between LDL-C and Lp(a) lowering in response to Evolocumab, since our findings are unlikely to be explained by non-sex differences in baseline characteristics between men and women. In addition, sex differences in response to treatment with Evolocumab are likely to be driven by a sex-hormone-independent mechanism, since our cohort consisted of postmenopausal women with none of them being on hormone replacement therapy or anti-estrogen therapy for breast cancer. According to this hypothesis, it is possible that PCSK9 inhibition modifies the composition of gut microbiota by interfering with the bile acids excretion differently in men and women, whereas gut dysbiosis could increase PCSK9 expression. All these mechanisms could be influenced by sex, with a consequent impact on LDL-C plasma levels unlike Lp(a), and a different response to PCSK9 inhibition [37]. Furthermore, PCSK9 inhibitors could exert different effects on inflammation in men and women and, consequently, on LDL-C. However, unlike other lipid-lowering drugs, PCSK9 inhibitors have no or marginal impact on the circulating levels of high-sensitivity C-reactive protein (hs-CRP) [38]. In the FOURIER (Further Cardiovascular Outcomes Research with PCSK9 Inhibition in Subjects with Elevated Risk) study, there was a stepwise risk increment according to the values of hs-CRP: +9% (<1 mg/L), +10.8% (1–3 mg/L) and +13.1% (>3 mg/L) even in patients with extremely low levels of LDL-C; however, no subanalysis by sex was carried out on the relationship between hs-CRP levels and changes in Lp(a) levels in men and women [39]. The reason why LDL-C decreased more in men than women in response to treatment with Evolocumab while Lp(a) similarly changed is yet to be elucidated.

Of course, our study has some limitations that need to be acknowledged. Firstly, background oral lipid-lowering therapy was heterogeneous in the cohort, and patients received the maximum tolerated dose of statin and/or ezetimibe or no treatment, based on the tolerability threshold. However, it is well known that statins and ezetimibe have no impact on Lp(a) levels. Additional limitations are that PCSK9 levels and apolipoprotein(a) (apo(a)) isoform size were not assessed. For this reason, the association between PCSK9 and LDL-C or Lp(a) cannot be investigated in this study. Moreover, we cannot establish whether the relative expression of apo(a) isoforms changes after the Lp(a) levels are lowered using Evolocumab. It is not even possible to ascertain that the size of the apo(a) is an independent determinant of the treatment response, even if one published study suggests that each additional kringle domain is with a 3% additional reduction in Lp(a) [40].

During follow-up, no major CV event or serious adverse event was registered, probably because all modifiable CV risk factors were strictly monitored throughout the observation period and optimized. However, it should be noted that the selection criteria of the analysis required an adherence rate to treatment of 100%. This may have led to an underestimation of adverse events as adverse events occurrence is one of the factors that most influence treatment nonadherence and discontinuation. Finally, this study was performed in a single center, and this may have had an impact on the sample size. However, all patients were treated according to the national PCSK9i reimbursement criteria, so our results are representative of individuals using PCSK9i in Italy.

5. Conclusions

In conclusion, our data partially reinforce the presence of differences in response to treatment to PCSK9i between men and women and are essential to gain a better understanding of the relationship between LDL-C and Lp(a) lowering in response to PCSK9i. Further research will clarify whether these sex-related significant differences translate into a meaningful difference in the long-term risk of ASCVD.

Author Contributions: Conceptualization, F.F. and A.F.G.C.; methodology, S.İ.Y., G.Z. and A.F.G.C.; software, S.İ.Y.; validation, G.Z.; formal analysis, S.İ.Y.; investigation, F.F., M.G. and A.F.G.C.; resources, A.F.G.C.; data curation, F.F, M.G. and S.İ.Y.; writing—original draft preparation, F.F., S.İ.Y., G.Z. and A.F.G.C.; writing—review and editing, M.G., P.L. and C.B.; visualization, F.F. and S.İ.Y.; supervision, A.F.G.C.; project administration, C.B. All authors have read and agreed to the published version of the manuscript.

Funding: This research received no external funding.

Institutional Review Board Statement: The study was conducted in accordance with the Declaration of Helsinki and approved by the Institutional Ethics Committee of the University of Bologna (Code: LLD-RP2018).

Informed Consent Statement: Written informed consent was obtained from all patients involved in the study.

Data Availability Statement: Data supporting the findings of this analysis are available from the University of Bologna. Data are available from the authors with the permission of the University of Bologna.

Acknowledgments: The views expressed in this work are personal and may not be understood or quoted as being made on behalf of or reflecting the position of the Italian Medicines Agency (AIFA) or one of their committees or working parties.

Conflicts of Interest: The authors declare no conflict of interest.

References

1. Raschi, E.; Casula, M.; Cicero, A.F.G.; Corsini, A.; Borghi, C.; Catapano, A. Beyond statins: New pharmacological targets to decrease LDL-cholesterol and cardiovascular events. *Pharmacol. Ther.* **2023**, *250*, 108507. [CrossRef] [PubMed]
2. Farmakis, I.; Doundoulakis, I.; Pagiantza, A.; Zafeiropoulos, S.; Antza, C.; Karvounis, H.; Giannakoulas, G. Lipoprotein(a) Reduction with Proprotein Convertase Subtilisin/Kexin Type 9 Inhibitors: A Systematic Review and Meta-analysis. *J. Cardiovasc. Pharmacol.* **2021**, *77*, 397–407. [CrossRef] [PubMed]
3. Cicero, A.F.G.; Fogacci, F.; Zambon, A.; Toth, P.P.; Borghi, C. Efficacy and safety of inclisiran a newly approved FDA drug: A systematic review and pooled analysis of available clinical studies. *Am. Heart J.* **2022**, *13*, 100127. [CrossRef]
4. Banerjee, Y.; Pantea Stoian, A.; Cicero, A.F.G.; Fogacci, F.; Nikolic, D.; Sachinidis, A.; Rizvi, A.A.; Janez, A.; Rizzo, M. Inclisiran: A small interfering RNA strategy targeting PCSK9 to treat hypercholesterolemia. *Expert Opin. Drug Saf.* **2022**, *21*, 9–20. [CrossRef] [PubMed]
5. Kronenberg, F. Lipoprotein(a) and cardiovascular disease: Make use of the knowledge we have. *Atherosclerosis* **2022**, *363*, 75–77. [CrossRef] [PubMed]
6. Fogacci, F.; Cicero, A.F.; D'Addato, S.; D'Agostini, L.; Rosticci, M.; Giovannini, M.; Bertagnin, E.; Borghi, C.; Brisighella Heart Study Group. Serum lipoprotein(a) level as long-term predictor of cardiovascular mortality in a large sample of subjects in primary cardiovascular prevention: Data from the Brisighella Heart Study. *Eur. J. Intern. Med.* **2017**, *37*, 49–55. [CrossRef] [PubMed]
7. Pasławska, A.; Tomasik, P.J. Lipoprotein(a)-60 Years Later-What Do We Know? *Cells* **2023**, *12*, 2472. [CrossRef]
8. Galema-Boers, A.M.H.; Mulder, J.W.C.M.; Steward, K.; Roeters van Lennep, J.E. Sex differences in efficacy and safety of PCSK9 mono-clonal antibodies: A real-world registry. *Atherosclerosis* **2023**, *384*, 117108. [CrossRef]
9. Paquette, M.; Faubert, S.; Saint-Pierre, N.; Baass, A.; Bernard, S. Sex differences in LDL-C response to PCSK9 inhibitors: A real world experience. *J. Clin. Lipidol.* **2023**, *17*, 142–149. [CrossRef]
10. Jia, F.; Fei, S.F.; Tong, D.B.; Xue, C.; Li, J.J. Sex difference in circulating PCSK9 and its clinical implications. *Front. Pharmacol.* **2022**, *13*, 953845. [CrossRef]
11. Lakoski, S.G.; Lagace, T.A.; Cohen, J.C.; Horton, J.D.; Hobbs, H.H. Genetic and metabolic determinants of plasma PCSK9 levels. *J. Clin. Endocrinol. Metab.* **2009**, *94*, 2537–2543. [CrossRef] [PubMed]
12. Warden, B.A.; Miles, J.R.; Oleaga, C.; Ganda, O.P.; Duell, P.B.; Purnell, J.Q.; Shapiro, M.D.; Fazio, S. Unusual responses to PCSK9 inhibitors in a clinical cohort utilizing a structured follow-up protocol. *Am. J. Prev. Cardiol.* **2020**, *1*, 100012. [CrossRef] [PubMed]
13. Edmiston, J.B.; Brooks, N.; Tavori, H.; Minnier, J.; Duell, B.; Purnell, J.Q.; Kaufman, T.; Wojcik, C.; Voros, S.; Fazio, S.; et al. Discordant response of low-density lipoprotein cholesterol and lipoprotein(a) levels to monoclonal antibodies targeting proprotein convertase subtilisin/kexin type 9. *J. Clin. Lipidol.* **2017**, *11*, 667–673. [CrossRef] [PubMed]
14. Shapiro, M.D.; Minnier, J.; Tavori, H.; Kassahun, H.; Flower, A.; Somaratne, R.; Fazio, S. Relationship Between Low-Density Lipoprotein Cholesterol and Lipoprotein(a) Lowering in Response to PCSK9 Inhibition with Evolocumab. *J. Am. Heart Assoc.* **2019**, *8*, e010932. [CrossRef]
15. Catapano, A.L.; Graham, I.; De Backer, G.; Wiklund, O.; Chapman, M.J.; Drexel, H.; Hoes, A.W.; Jennings, C.S.; Landmesser, U.; Pedersen, T.R.; et al. 2016 ESC/EAS Guidelines for the Management of Dyslipidaemias. *Rev. Esp. Cardiol. (Engl. Ed.)* **2017**, *70*, 115. [CrossRef]
16. AIFA (Italian Medicines Agency). Classificazione del Medicinale per uso Umano «Repatha», ai Sensi Dell'art. 8, Comma 10, Della Legge 24 Dicembre 1993, n. 537. (Determina n. 172/2017). Available online: https://www.gazzettaufficiale.it/eli/id/2017/02/07/17A01047/s#:~:text=%C2%ABRepatha%C2%BB%20e%E2%80%99%20indicato%20nei,C%20target%20con%20la%20dose (accessed on 2 December 2022).

7. Fogacci, F.; Giovannini, M.; Grandi, E.; Imbalzano, E.; Degli Esposti, D.; Borghi, C.; Cicero, A.F.G. Management of High-Risk Hypercholesterolemic Patients and PCSK9 Inhibitors Reimbursement Policies: Data from a Cohort of Italian Hypercholesterolemic Outpatients. *J. Clin. Med.* **2022**, *11*, 4701. [CrossRef]
8. Cicero, A.F.G.; Fogacci, F.; Veronesi, M.; Strocchi, E.; Grandi, E.; Rizzoli, E.; Poli, A.; Marangoni, F.; Borghi, C. A randomized Placebo-Controlled Clinical Trial to Evaluate the Medium-Term Effects of Oat Fibers on Human Health: The Beta-Glucan Effects on Lipid Profile, Glycemia and inTestinal Health (BELT) Study. *Nutrients* **2020**, *12*, 686. [CrossRef]
9. Friedewald, W.T.; Levy, R.I.; Fredrickson, D.S. Estimation of the concentration of low-density lipoprotein cholesterol in plasma, without use of the preparative ultracentrifuge. *Clin. Chem.* **1972**, *18*, 499–502. [CrossRef]
10. Levey, A.S.; Stevens, L.A.; Schmid, C.H.; Zhang, Y.L.; Castro, A.F., 3rd; Feldman, H.I.; Kusek, J.W.; Eggers, P.; Van Lente, F.; Greene, T.; et al. A new equation to estimate glomerular filtration rate. *Ann. Intern. Med.* **2009**, *150*, 604–612. [CrossRef]
11. Grundy, S.M.; Stone, N.J.; Bailey, A.L.; Beam, C.; Birtcher, K.K.; Blumenthal, R.S.; Braun, L.T.; de Ferranti, S.; Faiella-Tommasino, J.; Forman, D.E.; et al. 2018 AHA/ACC/AACVPR/AAPA/ABC/ACPM/ADA/AGS/APhA/ASPC/NLA/PCNA Guideline on the Management of Blood Cholesterol: Executive Summary: A Report of the American College of Cardiology/American Heart Association Task Force on Clinical Practice Guidelines. *Circulation* **2019**, *139*, e1046–e1081. [CrossRef]
12. Andrade, C.A.S.; Mahrouseh, N.; Gabrani, J.; Charalampous, P.; Cuschieri, S.; Grad, D.A.; Unim, B.; Mechili, E.A.; Chen-Xu, J.; Devleesschauwer, B.; et al. Inequalities in the burden of non-communicable diseases across European countries: A systematic analysis of the Global Burden of Disease 2019 study. *Int. J. Equity Health* **2023**, *22*, 140. [CrossRef] [PubMed]
13. Roeters van Lennep, J.E.; Tokgözoğlu, L.S.; Badimon, L.; Dumanski, S.M.; Gulati, M.; Hess, C.N.; Holven, K.B.; Kavousi, M.; Kayıkçıoğlu, M.; Lutgens, E.; et al. Women, lipids, and atherosclerotic car-diovascular disease: A call to action from the European Atherosclerosis Society. *Eur. Heart J.* **2023**, *44*, 4157–4173. [CrossRef] [PubMed]
14. Thakkar, A.; Agarwala, A.; Michos, E.D. Secondary Prevention of Cardiovascular Disease in Women: Closing the Gap. *Eur. Cardiol.* **2021**, *16*, e41. [CrossRef] [PubMed]
15. Ogungbe, O.; Grant, J.K.; Ayoola, A.S.; Bansah, E.; Miller, H.N.; Plante, T.B.; Sheikhattari, P.; Commodore-Mensah, Y.; Turkson-Ocran, R.N.; Juraschek, S.P.; et al. Strategies for Improving Enrollment of Diverse Populations with a Focus on Lipid-Lowering Clinical Trials. *Curr. Cardiol. Rep.* **2023**, *25*, 1189–1210. [CrossRef] [PubMed]
16. Fogacci, F.; Borghi, C.; Cicero, A.F.G. The short-circuit evidence on lipid-lowering drugs use in pregnancy. *Atherosclerosis* **2023**, *368*, 12–13. [CrossRef] [PubMed]
17. Khan, S.U.; Khan, M.Z.; Raghu Subramanian, C.; Riaz, H.; Khan, M.U.; Lone, A.N.; Khan, M.S.; Benson, E.M.; Alkhouli, M.; Blaha, M.J.; et al. Participation of Women and Older Participants in Randomized Clinical Trials of Lipid-Lowering Therapies: A Systematic Review. *JAMA Netw. Open* **2020**, *3*, e205202. [CrossRef]
18. Michos, E.D.; Reddy, T.K.; Gulati, M.; Brewer, L.C.; Bond, R.M.; Velarde, G.P.; Bailey, A.L.; Echols, M.R.; Nasser, S.A.; Bays, H.E.; et al. Improving the enrollment of women and racially/ethnically diverse populations in cardiovascular clinical trials: An ASPC practice statement. *Am. J. Prev. Cardiol.* **2021**, *8*, 100250. [CrossRef]
19. Lau, E.S.; Braunwald, E.; Morrow, D.A.; Giugliano, R.P.; Antman, E.M.; Gibson, C.M.; Scirica, B.M.; Bohula, E.A.; Wiviott, S.D.; Bhatt, D.L.; et al. Sex, Permanent Drug Discontinuation, and Study Retention in Clin-ical Trials: Insights from the TIMI trials. *Circulation* **2021**, *143*, 685–695. [CrossRef]
20. Masson, W.; Barbagelata, L.; Lobo, M.; Lavalle-Cobo, A.; Corral, P.; Nogueira, J.P. Plasma Lipoprotein(a) Levels in Polycystic Ovary Syndrome: A Systematic Review and Meta-analysis. *High Blood Press. Cardiovasc. Prev.* **2023**, *30*, 305–317. [CrossRef]
21. Anagnostis, P.; Galanis, P.; Chatzistergiou, V.; Stevenson, J.C.; Godsland, I.F.; Lambrinoudaki, I.; Theodorou, M.; Goulis, D.G. The effect of hormone replacement therapy and tibolone on lipoprotein (a) concentrations in postmenopausal women: A systematic review and meta-analysis. *Maturitas* **2017**, *99*, 27–36. [CrossRef]
22. Fogacci, F.; Di Micoli, V.; Avagimyan, A.; Giovannini, M.; Imbalzano, E.; Cicero, A.F.G. Assessment of Apolipoprotein(a) Isoform Size Using Phenotypic and Genotypic Methods. *Int. J. Mol. Sci.* **2023**, *24*, 13886. [CrossRef]
23. Amiri, M.; Raeisi-Dehkordi, H.; Verkaar, A.J.C.F.; Wu, Y.; van Westing, A.C.; Berk, K.A.; Bramer, W.M.; Aune, D.; Voortman, T. Circulating lipoprotein (a) and all-cause and cause-specific mortality: A systematic review and dose-response meta-analysis. *Eur. J. Epidemiol.* **2023**, *38*, 485–499. [CrossRef] [PubMed]
24. Bhatia, H.S.; Becker, R.C.; Leibundgut, G.; Patel, M.; Lacaze, P.; Tonkin, A.; Narula, J.; Tsimikas, S. Lipoprotein(a), platelet function and cardiovascular disease. *Nat. Rev. Cardiol.* **2023**; *Epub ahead of print*. [CrossRef]
25. Watts, G.F.; Chan, D.C.; Somaratne, R.; Wasserman, S.M.; Scott, R.; Marcovina, S.M.; Barrett, P.H.R. Controlled study of the effect of proprotein convertase subtilisin—kexin type 9 inhibition with evolocumab on lipoprotein(a) particle kinetics. *Eur. Heart J.* **2018**, *39*, 2577–2585. [CrossRef] [PubMed]
26. Raal, F.J.; Giugliano, R.P.; Sabatine, M.S.; Koren, M.J.; Blom, D.; Seidah, N.G.; Honarpour, N.; Lira, A.; Xue, A.; Chiruvolu, P.; et al. PCSK9 inhibition—mediated reduction in Lp(a) with evolocumab: An analysis of 10 clinical trials and the LDL receptor's role. *J. Lipid Res.* **2016**, *57*, 1086–1096. [CrossRef] [PubMed]
27. Morelli, M.B.; Wang, X.; Santulli, G. Functional role of gut microbiota and PCSK9 in the pathogenesis of diabetes mellitus and cardiovascular disease. *Atherosclerosis* **2019**, *289*, 176–178. [CrossRef]
28. Sahebkar, A.; Di Giosia, P.; Stamerra, C.A.; Grassi, D.; Pedone, C.; Ferretti, G.; Bacchetti, T.; Ferri, C.; Giorgini, P. Effect of monoclonal antibodies to PCSK9 on high-sensitivity C-reactive protein levels: A meta-analysis of 16 randomized controlled treatment arms. *Br. J. Clin. Pharmacol.* **2016**, *81*, 1175–1190. [CrossRef]

39. Ruscica, M.; Tokgözoğlu, L.; Corsini, A.; Sirtori, C.R. PCSK9 inhibition and inflammation: A narrative review. *Atherosclerosis* **2019**, *288*, 146–155. [CrossRef]
40. Blanchard, V.; Chemello, K.; Hollstein, T.; Hong-Fong, C.C.; Schumann, F.; Grenkowitz, T.; Nativel, B.; Coassin, S.; Croyal, M.; Kassner, U.; et al. The size of apolipoprotein (a) is an independent determinant of the reduction in lipoprotein (a) induced by PCSK9 inhibitors. *Cardiovasc. Res.* **2022**, *118*, 2103–2111. [CrossRef]

Disclaimer/Publisher's Note: The statements, opinions and data contained in all publications are solely those of the individual author(s) and contributor(s) and not of MDPI and/or the editor(s). MDPI and/or the editor(s) disclaim responsibility for any injury to people or property resulting from any ideas, methods, instructions or products referred to in the content.

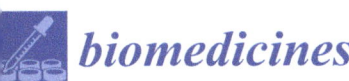

Article

Predictive Value of Fatty Liver Index for Long-Term Cardiovascular Events in Patients Receiving Liver Transplantation: The COLT Study

Alfredo Caturano [1,2,*,†], Gaetana Albanese [1,†], Anna Di Martino [1,3], Carmine Coppola [3], Vincenzo Russo [4,5], Raffaele Galiero [1], Luca Rinaldi [6], Marcellino Monda [2], Raffaele Marfella [1], Ferdinando Carlo Sasso [1,‡] and Teresa Salvatore [7,‡]

1. Department of Advanced Medical and Surgical Sciences, University of Campania Luigi Vanvitelli, 80138 Naples, Italy; raffaele.marfella@unicampania.it (R.M.)
2. Department of Experimental Medicine, University of Campania Luigi Vanvitelli, 80138 Naples, Italy
3. Area Stabiese Hospital, 80053 Naples, Italy
4. Sbarro Institute for Cancer Research and Molecular Medicine, Center for Biotechnology, College of Science and Technology, Temple University, Philadelphia, PA 19122, USA
5. Division of Cardiology, Department of Medical Translational Sciences, University of Campania Luigi Vanvitelli, 80131 Naples, Italy
6. Department of Medicine and Health Sciences "Vincenzo Tiberio", University of Molise, 86100 Campobasso, Italy
7. Department of Precision Medicine, University of Campania Luigi Vanvitelli, 80138 Naples, Italy
* Correspondence: alfredo.caturano@unicampania.it; Tel.: +39-3338616985
† These authors contributed equally to this work.
‡ These authors contributed equally to this work.

Abstract: Background and aims: Cardiovascular disease (CVD) is the leading cause of early mortality in orthotopic liver transplantation (OLT) patients. The fatty liver index (FLI) is strongly associated with carotid and coronary atherosclerosis, as well as cardiovascular mortality, surpassing traditional risk factors. Given the lack of data on FLI as a predictor of cardiovascular events in OLT recipients, we conducted a retrospective study to examine this topic. Methods and results: We performed a multicenter retrospective analysis of adult OLT recipients who had regular follow-up visits every three to six months (or more frequently if necessary) from January 1995 to December 2020. The minimum follow-up period was two years post-intervention. Anamnestic, clinical, anthropometric and laboratory data were collected, and FLI was calculated for all patients. Clinical trial.gov registration ID NCT05895669. A total of 110 eligible patients (median age 57 years [IQR: 50–62], 72.7% male) were followed for a median duration of 92.3 months (IQR: 45.7–172.4) post-liver transplantation. During this period, 16 patients (14.5%) experienced at least one adverse cardiovascular event (including fatal and non-fatal myocardial infarction and stroke). Receiver Operating Characteristic (ROC) analysis identified a cut-off value of 66.0725 for predicting cardiovascular events after OLT, with 86.7% sensitivity and 63.7% specificity (68% vs. 31%; $p = 0.001$). Kaplan–Meier analysis showed that patients with FLI > 66 had significantly reduced cardiovascular event-free survival than those with FLI ≤ 66 (log-rank: 0.0008). Furthermore, multivariable Cox regression analysis demonstrated that FLI > 66 and pre-OLT smoking were independently associated with increased cardiovascular risk. Conclusions: Our findings suggest that FLI > 66 and pre-OLT smoking predict cardiovascular risk in adult OLT recipients.

Keywords: fatty liver index; orthotopic liver transplantation; cardiovascular disease; myocardial infarction; stroke

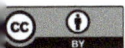

1. Introduction

Cardiovascular disease (CVD) represents a major concern for individuals who have undergone orthotopic liver transplantation (OLT), with statistics indicating that it is the leading cause of early mortality post-OLT, accounting for approximately 40% of such cases. Following CVD, infections and graft failure stand as the second and third most common causes of early mortality, constituting 28% and 12%, respectively [1]. Beyond the immediate post-transplant period, CVD, along with malignancies and end-stage kidney disease, continues to pose a significant threat, contributing significantly to long-term non-graft-related morbidity and mortality.

A decade ago, a comprehensive meta-analysis involving 12 studies shed light on the extent of this cardiovascular risk in OLT patients. The analysis revealed a substantial 10-year risk of 13.6% for cardiovascular events in these individuals [2]. Furthermore, a study conducted by Albeldawi et al. indicated cumulative risks of 4.5% and 10.1% for cardiovascular events within 1 and 3 years post-OLT, respectively [3]. Meanwhile, Fussner et al. found that over a longer time frame, 10.6%, 20.7%, and 30.3% of OLT recipients developed CVD within 1, 5, and 8 years after transplantation, respectively [4]. It is noteworthy that these frequencies are notably higher than what is observed in the general population, underscoring the unique cardiovascular challenges faced by OLT recipients.

Several factors are anticipated to further exacerbate the severity of cardiovascular risk in this population. One significant factor is the increasing age of OLT recipients, with a growing number of individuals aged over 65 undergoing transplantations. Moreover, improved OLT-related care has led to increased survival rates, resulting in a larger pool of long-term recipients at risk. The chronic use of immunosuppressive medications also contributes to heightened cardiovascular risk. Additionally, the rising prevalence of liver transplantation for nonalcoholic steatohepatitis (NASH) adds another layer of complexity to this issue [5–8].

Despite the growing awareness of the cardiovascular burden faced by post-OLT individuals, a consensus has yet to be reached regarding the optimal assessment of cardiovascular risk before intervention [9–11]. In particular, the distinct lack of a straightforward, accurate, and objective system for identifying patients at a higher risk of experiencing long-term cardiovascular events remains a notable research gap in the management of liver transplant recipients. The motivation lies in a number of factors, including the absence of consensus on outcome definition, incomplete knowledge, suboptimal data quality, and the uneven predictive accuracy of different non-invasive tests, as highlighted by a systematic review of the literature [12]. Preliminary findings from a recent study offer a glimmer of hope, suggesting that aortic pulse wave velocity, a surrogate marker of arterial stiffness, could serve as a valuable biomarker for assessing cardiovascular risk in OLT candidates [13]. In 2018, a predictive model known as the CAR-OLT score was developed to estimate the one-year global risk of death or hospitalization due to a significant cardiac or vascular event following OLT [14]. The CAR-OLT score is derived from easily accessible pre-transplant patients' characteristics and personal history. It serves as a valuable tool for healthcare professionals to facilitate on-the-spot conversations regarding the one-year risk of significant cardiac or vascular events. However, it is important to note that CAR-OLT still requires external validation and does not address the long-term cardiac risk associated with OLT. Therefore, CAR-OLT should not be utilized for making decisions related to transplant management. Instead, it should be used to provide valuable information during risk-related discussions.

Nonalcoholic fatty liver disease (NAFLD), currently the most prevalent chronic liver disorder, has emerged as a risk factor in the general population for both severe hepatic consequences, such as cirrhosis and hepatocellular carcinoma, and cardiovascular morbidity and mortality. This risk extends to transplant recipients, particularly those with NASH [15–19].

While liver biopsy remains the gold standard for diagnosing NAFLD, efforts have been made to explore non-invasive and non-imaging approaches, which can be more practical in clinical settings. Among these methodologies, the fatty liver index (FLI) has gained substantial recognition as a simple yet accurate tool for identifying the presence of steatosis in both the general population and patients with NAFLD [20–24]. Importantly,

FLI-assessed fatty liver has demonstrated a strong association with carotid and coronary atherosclerosis, as well as cardiovascular mortality, often surpassing the predictive power of traditional risk factors [25,26]. A recent study conducted in Korea, utilizing a large dataset, further confirmed the prognostic value of FLI in identifying in the general population those individuals at higher risk for cardiovascular events, including cardiovascular deaths [27].

Given the paucity of data regarding the significance of FLI, a well-validated surrogate marker of liver steatosis, as a predictor of cardiovascular events in OLT recipients, we have undertaken a comprehensive study to investigate this relevant topic. This research aims to shed light on the potential utility of FLI in assessing cardiovascular risk in the specific context of liver transplant recipients, with the ultimate goal of improving the management and outcomes of these individuals.

2. Patients and Methods

The "Cardiovascular outcomes in Orthotopic Liver Transplant patients study" (COLT study) is a multicenter retrospective cohort study. We considered 132 consecutive eligible adult patients who underwent liver transplantation, attending every three/six months (or more often when needed) from January 1995 to December 2020 and for at least two years after intervention, the "Chronic non-viral hepatitis clinic", pertaining to the U.O.C. of Internal Medicine, II Polyclinic of Naples, University of Campania "Luigi Vanvitelli", and the "Liver Transplant Clinic", pertaining to the Hepatology and Interventional Ultrasound Unit, Gragnano Hospital, ASL Naples 3 South.

The transplantation procedures were conducted at various hospitals spanning across different regions within Italy and, in some cases, even in other European hospital centers, where patients were generally followed for the first year after OLT. The aetiology of cirrhosis was inferred from the liver biopsy performed before OLT and/or the explant liver biopsy report. The causes of liver disease requiring OLT were distributed as follows: 34 (30.9%) viral cirrhosis, 32 (29.1%) non-viral causes (dysmetabolic, alcoholic and/or cryptogenic cirrhosis; hepatocellular carcinoma with and without cirrhosis), and 44 (40%) both viral and non-viral aetiology. All included patients were in the outpatient setting without evidence of acute graft rejection or dysfunction, technical complications, or active infections. Re-transplanted (n = 2) or multi-organ transplanted patients (n = 4), autoimmune hepatitis (n = 1) and hemochromatosis (n = 0) causes of OLT, and subjects with missing data (n = 8) were excluded from the study. In addition, the pre-OLT presenting symptoms suggestive of CVD, the pre-OLT history of documented cardiovascular events or coronary stent implantation (n = 2), as well as the presence of moderate–severe hydrosaline-retention (n = 5) compromising BMI and waist circumference (WC) evaluation were criteria for exclusion from the study. A total of 110 OLT recipient patients were finally included (Figure 1).

All information was obtained from electronic medical records and transferred to a Microsoft Excel table. In addition to age, sex, and cause of transplantation, the following clinical data were collected for each patient: self-reported personal history of pre-OLT angina pectoris, nonfatal MI, nonfatal stroke or symptoms suggestive of CVD; family history of CVD and type 2 diabetes (T2D); current pre/post-OLT smoking and alcohol abuse; pre/post-OLT co-morbidities such as arterial hypertension, T2D and dyslipidaemia with respective medications; anti-rejection therapy; pre/post-OLT measurement of body mass index (BMI), WC and blood values of glucose, triglycerides, cholesterol (total, LDL and HDL), creatinine, and γ-glutamyl transferase (GGT). Pre-OLT and post-OLT data were recorded within one month before surgery and during the last follow-up visit at our two clinics, respectively. For glucose and lipids, blood samples were obtained after an overnight fast. CKD-EPI creatinine formula (2021 update) was used to estimate the glomerular filtration rate (eGFR). Diabetes, arterial hypertension, and dyslipidaemia were diagnosed according to the 2016 European guidelines [28]. The criteria established by the National Cholesterol Education Program were used to diagnose metabolic syndrome (MetS): WC > 102 cm in men and >88 cm in women, Triglycerides levels > 150 mg/dL,

HDL < 40 mg/dL in men and <50 mg/dL in woman, blood pressure ≥ 130/≥ 80 or in treatment, fasting glucose ≥ 110 mg/dL [29]. For all patients, the pre- and post-OLT FLI was calculated according to the formula reported by Bedogni et al. (17): FLI = (exp[0.953 × loge (triglycerides) + 0.139 × BMI + 0.718 × loge (GGT + 0.053 × WC − 15.745])/(1 + exp[0.953 × loge (triglycerides) + 0.139 × BMI + 0.718 × loge (GGT) + 0.053 × WC − 15.745]) × 100, where levels of triglycerides are expressed as mmol/L and those of GGT as U/L, BMI calculated with the usual formula (weight in kilograms divided by height in meters squared) and WC measured to the nearest 0.1 cm at the end of a normal expiration in a standing position. The value of pre-OLT FLI was the mean of at least two measurements at the screening examination carried out during the three months preceding the transplantation The score of FLI ranges from 0 to 100 [20].

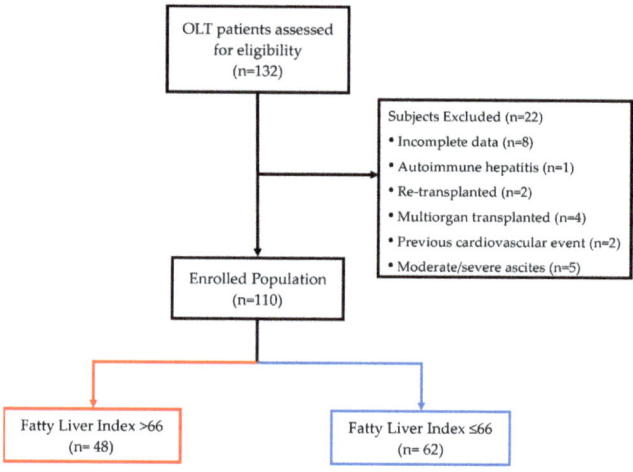

Figure 1. Study flow-chart.

The primary outcome of the study was the occurrence in the post-transplantation follow-up of myocardial infarction (MI) (documented instrumentally and/or enzymatically), ischemic stroke, and cardiovascular death. Deaths from non-cardiovascular causes were also registered. Subjects completed the study at the end of the follow-up period or on the date of eventual cardiovascular or non-cardiovascular death. All patients provided written informed consent for data storage and analysis. The study was conducted in accordance with the 1976 Declaration of Helsinki and was approved by the local ethics committees (University of Campania "Luigi Vanvitelli", Azienda Ospedaliera Universitaria, "Luigi Vanvitelli", Azienda Ospedaliera di Rilievo Nazionale "Ospedale dei Colli"; approval ID 12771/I; approval date 2 May 2023). Clinical trial.gov registration ID NCT05895669.

Statistical Analysis

The entire dataset was initially analyzed using descriptive statistical indices. For a comprehensive understanding, qualitative data were represented in terms of absolute and relative percentage frequencies. Conversely, for quantitative continuous data, we employed two different descriptive methods based on data distribution characteristics. Specifically, normally distributed data were described using the mean and standard deviation (SD), whereas non-normally distributed data were summarized using the median and interquartile range (IQR). To determine the normality of the data distribution, the Shapiro–Wilk test was conducted prior to further analysis.

To assess the predictive value of the pre-OLT FLI for the occurrence of post-OLT cardiovascular events, we conducted a Receiver Operating Characteristic (ROC) curve analysis. This analysis aimed to identify a potential cutoff value for the FLI that could effectively discriminate between patients at risk and those not at risk of cardiovascular events following transplantation. Based on the outcome of this analysis, participants were categorized into two distinct groups: those with FLI values above the determined cutoff and those with FLI values equal to or below the cutoff. Subsequently, we explored the differences between these two subgroups through appropriate statistical tests. For the analysis of qualitative variables, we employed either the Chi-squared test or, when applicable, the Fisher–Freeman–Haltob exact test. Continuous data, on the other hand, were compared using either the Student's t-test or the Mann–Whitney U test, depending on the underlying data distribution. To gauge the accuracy of our predictive model, we employed Harrel's C index, which is equivalent to the ROC curve and ranges from 0 to 1. Higher values of this index signify greater accuracy in predicting outcomes.

Our primary endpoint, defined as the first-event free survival following liver transplantation, was assessed using a Kaplan–Meier survival analysis. We employed the log-rank test to compare survival curves and determine if there were statistically significant differences among different groups.

Furthermore, Kaplan–Meier curves were generated to visually depict the survival estimates over time. To identify potential prognostic factors, whether negative or positive, that could influence survival outcomes, we utilized univariable and multivariable Cox proportional hazards regression models. These models provided us with hazard ratios (HR) and their corresponding 95% confidence intervals (CI), enabling us to assess the strength and significance of these factors in relation to the primary endpoint.

Statistical analyses were conducted using SPSS statistical software (version 24.0, SPSS, Chicago, IL, USA) and STATA 14.0 software (StataCorp, College Station, TX, USA).

3. Results

We identified 110 eligible Caucasian patients (median age 57 years [IQR: 50–62], 72.7% male) who were followed for a median of 92.3 months (IQR: 45.7–172.4) after liver transplantation.

The patient characteristics at pre-OLT and at the last post-OLT ambulatory visit are detailed in Table 1. The comparison between the two times showed a significantly higher prevalence of metabolic syndrome (MetS), type 2 diabetes (T2D), arterial hypertension, dyslipidaemia, as well as significantly higher blood levels of triglycerides, total cholesterol, LDL cholesterol, and HDL cholesterol. However, lower levels of GGT and estimated glomerular filtration rate (eGFR) were observed at the last follow-up visit. No significant differences were found for body mass index (BMI), waist circumference (WC), impaired fasting glucose, or FLI value. The prevalence of tobacco habit and alcohol abuse was higher at the pre-OLT stage. Harrel's C index for assessing the association between the FLI and cardiovascular outcomes was found to be 0.700 (CI 95% 0.599 to 0.801).

The receiver operating characteristic (ROC) analysis estimated a cutoff value of 66.0725 for predicting post-OLT cardiovascular events, with an 86.7% sensitivity and a 63.7% specificity (Figure 2). The area under the curve (AUC) for FLI in predicting post-OLT cardiovascular events was 0.7. Based on this cutoff, participants were classified into two groups: FLI $\leq$ 66 or FLI > 66.

At the pre-OLT stage, 48 out of 110 patients had FLI > 66 (Table 2), with higher BMI, WC, prevalence of obesity and overweight, and higher GGT levels when compared to the 62 patients with FLI $\leq$ 66. No differences were observed for the other parameters. As depicted in Table 3, there was no difference in median follow-up duration between patients with FLI $\leq$ 66 and those with FLI > 66. At the last clinic visit, patients with FLI > 66 exhibited higher BMI, WC, prevalence of obesity and overweight, as well as a significantly higher prevalence of MetS and a higher median FLI value compared to patients with FLI $\leq$ 66.

Table 1. Pre- and post-OLT characteristics of the study sample.

Parameter	Baseline (n = 110)	Follow-Up (n = 110)	p
Age, years, median [IQR]	57.0 [50.0–62.0]	67.0 [61.0–72.0]	**<0.001**
Sex, n (%)			
M	80 (72.7)		
F	30 (27.3)		
FLI, median [IQR]	59.5 [38.3–82.3]	55.3 [33.4–79.1]	0.324
BMI, kg/m^2, median [IQR]	26.6 [23.5–28.4]	26.5 [23.9–30.0]	0.505
Obese, n (%)	17 (16.0)	18 (16.4)	*0.098*
Overweight, n (%)	50 (45.5)	55 (55.0)	0.137
Waist circumference, cm, median [IQR]	103.0 [90.0–113.6]	100.0 [92.0–115.0]	0.893
Impaired fast glucose, n (%)	7 (6.6)	5 (4.5)	0.553
Diabetes, n (%)	15 (14.2)	43 (39.1)	**0.001**
Hypertension, n (%)	16 (14.5)	79 (71.8)	**<0.001**
Total cholesterol, mg/dL, median [IQR]	123.5 [105.0–165.5]	192.5 [160.0–225.0]	**<0.001**
LDL, mg/dL, median [IQR]	86.5 [66.0–105.0]	128.0 [100.0–155.0]	**<0.001**
HDL, mg/dL, median [IQR]	33.5 [28.0–44.0]	48.0 [39.0–59.5]	**<0.001**
Triglycerides, mg/dL, median [IQR]	89.0 [71.0–118.0]	123.0 [86.0–167.0]	**<0.001**
Dyslipidemia, n (%)	10 (9.1)	68 (63)	**<0.001**
Metabolic Syndrome, n (%)	15 (13.6)	44 (40)	**<0.001**
GGT, U/L, median [IQR]	57.5 [42.0–84.0]	28.5 [17.5–53.0]	**<0.001**
Smoking, n (%)	34 (32.1)	13 (11.8)	**0.0002**
Alcohol abuse, n (%)	24 (21.8)	2 (1.8)	**<0.001**
eGFR, mL/min/m^2, median [IQR]	91.9 [76.0–103.8]	69.2 [55.3–90.4]	**<0.001**

OLT: orthotopic liver transplantation; IQR: interquartile range; FLI: fatty liver index; BMI: body mass index; GGT: γ-glutamyltransferase; eGFR: estimated glomerular filtration rate.

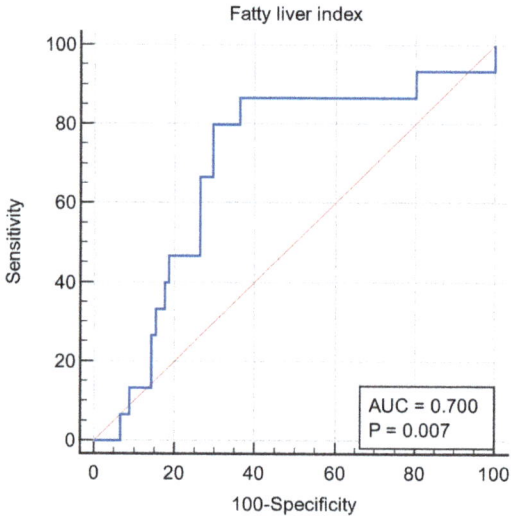

Figure 2. ROC curve for the definition of the fatty liver index cut-off value (sensitivity: 86.7%, specificity 63.7%).

Table 2. Pre-OLT characteristics of the study sample categorized using the fatty liver index.

Parameter	Overall (n = 110)	FLI ≤ 66 (n = 62)	FLI > 66 (n = 48)	p
Age, years, median [IQR]	57.0 [50.0–62.0]	56.5 [48.0–63.0]	57.0 [52.0–60.0]	0.845
Sex, n (%)				
M	80 (72.7)	41 (66.1)	39 (81.3)	0.079
F	30 (27.3)	21 (33.9)	9 (18.8)	
Family history of CVD, n (%)	10 (9.3)	3 (4.8)	7 (14.6)	0.095
Family history of diabetes, n (%)	12 (11.2)	3 (4.8)	9 (18.8)	0.144
Personal history of MI, n (%)	2 (1.8)	0	2 (4.2)	0.106
Personal history of Stroke, n (%)	3 (2.7)	2 (3.2)	1 (2.1)	0.716
FLI, median [IQR]	59.5 [38.3–82.3]	41 [26.3–56.6]	89.0 [74.6–95.3]	**<0.001**
BMI, kg/m^2, median [IQR]	26.6 [23.5–28.4]	24.5 [22.7–26.0]	27.8 [27.0–31.8]	**<0.001**
Obese, n (%)	17 (16.0)	0	17 (35.4)	**<0.001**
Overweight, n (%)	50 (45.5)	21 (33.9)	29 (60.4)	**0.008**
Waist circumference, cm, median [IQR]	103.0 [90.0–113.6]	92.0 [87.0–100.0]	116 [107.8–128.0]	**<0.001**
Impaired fast glucose, n (%)	7 (6.6)	4 (6.5)	3 (6.3)	0.935
Diabetes, n (%)	15 (14.2)	9 (14.5)	6 (12.5)	0.716
Hypertension, n (%)	16 (14.5)	10 (16.1)	6 (12.5)	0.594
Total cholesterol, mg/dL, median [IQR]	123.5 [105.0–165.5]	119.0 [103.0–152.0]	142.0 [116.8–185.8]	**0.032**
LDL, mg/dL, median [IQR]	86.5 [66.0–105.0]	76.0 [58.5–100.3]	99.0 [72.3–119.8]	*0.086*
HDL, mg/dL, median [IQR]	33.5 [28.0–44.0]	33.0 [28.0–36.8]	36.0 [25.8–47.0]	0.482
Triglycerides, mg/dL, median [IQR]	89.0 [71.0–118.0]	88.5 [69.0–102.0]	88.5 [70.0–142.0]	0.146
Dyslipidemia, n (%)	10 (9.1)	5 (8.1)	5 (10.4)	0.672
Metabolic Syndrome, n (%)	15 (14.0)	5 (8.1)	10 (20.8)	*0.068*
GGT, U/L, median [IQR]	57.5 [42.0–84.0]	51.0 [32.0–70.0]	63.5 [55.0–89.0]	**0.004**
Smoking, n (%)	34 (32.1)	21 (33.9)	13 (27.1)	0.387
Alcohol abuse, n (%)	24 (21.8)	16 (25.8)	8 (16.7)	0.252
eGFR, mL/min/m^2, median [IQR]	91.9 [76.0–103.8]	91.0 [81.0–104.0]	93.7 [73.3–102.5]	0.668

OLT: orthotopic liver transplantation; IQR: interquartile range; CVD: cardiovascular disease; MI: myocardial infraction; FLI: fatty liver index; BMI: body mass index; GGT: γ-glutamyltransferase; eGFR: estimated glomerular filtration rate.

During the follow-up period, 16 patients (14.5%) developed at least one adverse cardiovascular event. Among them, three experienced both non-fatal myocardial infarction (MI) and ischemic stroke. Despite the small number of events, the incidence of fatal and non-fatal stroke, particularly fatal and non-fatal MI, was significantly higher in the FLI > 66 group (27.1% vs. 4.8%; $p = 0.001$) (Table 4). Five patients died, with two deaths attributed to cardiovascular disease and three to non-cardiovascular causes (massive pulmonary bleeding due to Rendu-Osler Syndrome, complications during intensive care unit stay for COVID-19 infection, hepatocellular carcinoma relapse).

The Kaplan–Meier analysis revealed a worse cardiovascular event-free survival in patients with FLI > 66 compared to those with FLI ≤ 66 (log-rank: 0.0008) (Figure 3).

The univariate Cox regression analysis performed for all pre-OLT parameters showed that age, FLI > 66, BMI, WC, obesity, smoking, and history of CVD before transplantation were significantly associated with the incidence of new-onset cardiovascular events (Table 5).

Table 3. Post-OLT characteristics of the study sample categorized using the fatty liver index.

Parameter	Overall (n = 110)	FLI ≤ 66 (n = 62)	FLI > 66 (n = 48)	p
Age, years, median [IQR]	67.0 [61.0–72.0]	67.0 [60.8–71.3]	67.5 [62.5–73.5]	0.490
Follow-up months, median [IQR]	92.3 [45.6–172.4]	89.4 [45.7–172.4]	112.5 [54.7–214.8]	0.357
FLI, median [IQR]	55.3 [33.4–79.1]	41.8 [26.5–63.1]	75.0 [48.7–87.6]	<0.001
BMI, kg/m^2, median [IQR]	26.5 [23.9–30.0]	24.9 [23.4–27.4]	28.5 [26.0–32.9]	<0.001
Obese, n (%)	18 (16.4)	0	18 (37.5)	<0.001
Overweight, n (%)	55 (55.0)	25 (40.3)	30 (62.5)	0.022
Waist circumference, cm, median [IQR]	100.0 [92.0–115.0]	95.0 [88.0–100.0]	113.0 [103.5–125.5]	<0.001
Impaired fast glucose, n (%)	5 (4.5)	3 (4.8)	2 (4.2)	0.867
Diabetes, n (%)	43 (39.1)	22 (35.5)	21 (43.8)	0.380
Hypertension, n (%)	79 (71.8)	46 (74.2)	33 (68.8)	0.531
Total cholesterol, mg/dL, median [IQR]	192.5 [160.0–225.0]	190.0 [160.0–225.0]	194.0 [153.0–225.0]	0.939
LDL, mg/dL, median [IQR]	128.0 [100.0–155.0]	128.0 [97.0–151.0]	128.0 [106.0–156.0]	0.662
HDL, mg/dL, median [IQR]	48.0 [39.0–59.5]	49.0 [41.0–62.5]	46.0 [34.5–58.5]	0.144
Triglycerides, mg/dL, median [IQR]	123.0 [86.0–167.0]	112.0 [81.0–158.0]	129.5 [96.0–182.0]	0.128
Dyslipidemia, n (%)	68 (63)	36 (58.1)	32 (66.7)	0.336
Metabolic Syndrome, n (%)	44 (41.1)	19 (30.6)	25 (52.1)	0.039
GGT, U/L, median [IQR]	28.5 [17.5–53.0]	29.0 [16.0–53.0]	28.0 [18.0–46.0]	0.763
Smoking, n (%)	13 (11.8)	8 (12.9)	5 (10.4)	0.690
Alcohol abuse, n (%)	2 (1.8)	0	2 (4.2)	0.106
eGFR, mL/min/m^2, median [IQR]	69.2 [55.3–90.4]	73.1 [60.2–91.9]	65.5 [51.5–80.4]	0.078

OLT: orthotopic liver transplantation; IQR: interquartile range; FLI: fatty liver index; BMI: body mass index; GGT γ-glutamyltransferase; eGFR: estimated glomerular filtration rate.

Table 4. Post-OLT cardiovascular events and overall mortality in the study sample categorized using FLI.

Parameter	Overall (n = 110)	FLI ≤ 66 (n = 62)	FLI > 66 (n = 48)	p
Incident fatal and non-fatal MI, n (%)	16 (14.5)	3 (4.8)	13 (27.1)	0.001
Incident fatal and non-fatal Stroke, n (%)	3 (2.8)	0	3 (6.3)	0.047
Cardiovascular death, n (%)	2 (2.2)	1 (1.6)	1 (2.1)	0.739
Overall incident CV events, n (%)	16 (14.5)	3 (4.8)	13 (27.1)	0.001
Overall mortality, n (%)	5 (5.4)	2 (3.2)	3 (6.3)	0.663

MI: myocardial infarction; CV: cardiovascular.

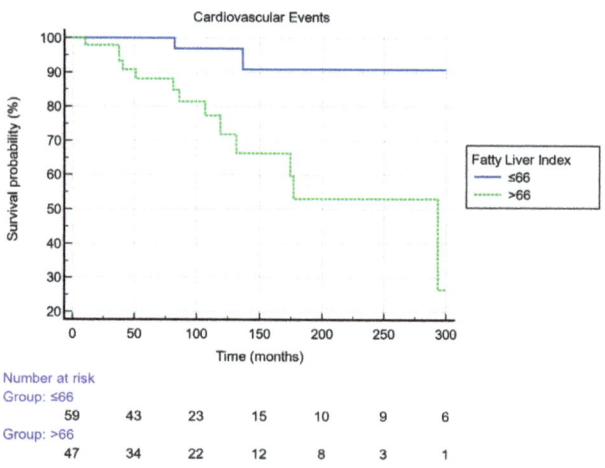

Figure 3. Kaplan–Meier survival analysis estimating the risk of cardiovascular events among OLT patients according to FLI.

Table 5. Univariable Cox regression model.

Parameter	Univariable Analysis			
	HR	95% CI		p
Age	1.07	1.00	1.15	**0.049**
Sex				
M (ref)				
F		0.09	1.25	0.104
Family history of MI	1.59	0.70	3.61	0.267
Family history of diabetes	1.52	0.34	6.78	0.580
Personal history of MI	12.29	1.36	110.80	**0.025**
Personal history of Stroke	0.00	0.00	inf	0.960
Fatty liver index				
≤66	1			
>66	6.34	1.78	22.56	**0.004**
BMI	1.13	1.03	1.24	**0.011**
Waist circumference	1.05	1.02	1.08	**0.002**
Obese	5.02	1.38	18.32	**0.015**
Overweight	1.25	0.47	3.39	0.648
Impaired fast glucose	1.19	0.15	9.20	0.866
Diabetes	1.83	0.40	8.40	0.439
Hypertension	0.70	0.09	5.35	0.728
Total cholesterol	0.99	0.98	1.02	0.996
LDL	0.99	0.96	1.03	0.811
HDL	1.05	0.95	1.16	0.313
Triglycerides	0.99	0.99	1.01	0.976
Dyslipidemia	2.84	0.81	9.97	0.104
Metabolic Syndrome	0.48	0.06	3.65	0.480
GGT	0.99	0.98	1.01	0.729
Smoking	3.00	1.06	8.49	**0.038**
Alcohol Abuse	1.72	0.55	5.35	0.350
eGFR	1.01	0.98	1.04	0.482

MI: myocardial infraction; BMI: body mass index; GGT: γ-glutamyltransferase; eGFR: estimated glomerular filtration rate.

Considering the limited number of recorded cardiovascular events, only variables that showed significance in the univariate analysis were included in the multivariate analysis. Additionally, BMI and WC were not considered to be these parameters already included in the calculation of FLI and obesity was already represented by these measures. Ultimately, the two variables independently associated with cardiovascular risk were FLI > 66 and smoking habits at the pre-OLT stage, while the role of age and pre-OLT CVD was not significant (Table 6).

Table 6. Multivariable Cox regression model.

Parameter	Multivariable Analysis			
	HR	95% CI		p
Age	1.06	0.97	1.15	0.185

Table 6. Cont.

Parameter	Multivariable Analysis			
	HR	95% CI		p
Fatty liver index				
≤66	1			
>66	5.50	0.51	59.85	**0.010**
Smoking	3.20	1.01	10.12	**0.048**
Personal history of MI	3.04	0.31	30.17	0.343

MI: myocardial infraction.

4. Discussion

The present cohort study investigated, for the first time, the relationship between the FLI, a well-validated surrogate marker of nonalcoholic fatty liver disease (NAFLD), and the risk of cardiovascular events in a population of individuals who underwent liver transplantation. The main finding of this investigation was the significant independent predictive value of FLI for the long-term post-OLT occurrence of the composite outcome of MI, ischemic stroke, and cardiovascular mortality, irrespective of age and personal history of previous cardiovascular events. Specifically, the study identified an FLI cutoff value > 66 as an accurate indicator of higher cardiovascular risk in the late post-transplantation period, with an incidence of cardiovascular events 5.5 times higher than in patients with FLI ≤ 66. This FLI cutoff value may serve as an appropriate threshold for non-invasive stress testing before liver transplantation in patients without cardiovascular symptoms and for enhanced surveillance of cardio-metabolic risk following OLTm facilitating early intervention for preventive purposes.

Our FLI cutoff value closely corresponds to the previously established threshold of ≥60, documented in this study as a reliable predictor of arterial hypertension in individuals who have not yet been exposed to antihypertensive medications [30]. The same FLI threshold has also been associated with significant clinical conditions, such as the onset of left ventricular remodelling and diastolic dysfunction [31,32]. Of noteworthy significance is a recent extensive population-based cohort investigation that may underscore the clinical relevance of our findings [33]. In this study, persistent NAFLD, as defined by a FLI score of ≥60, emerged as a potent predictor of adverse outcomes such as all-cause mortality, MI, and stroke when compared to those with either no NAFLD or sporadic, intermittent NAFLD [33].

Patients who are diagnosed with end-stage liver disease are often thought to possess a relatively improved cardiovascular risk profile. This presumption stems from several key peculiarities of this type of subject. First, liver insufficiency reduces the production of cholesterol, which notoriously plays a crucial role in the development of atherosclerosis. Second, these patients frequently exhibit peripheral vasodilation coupled with normal to lower arterial blood pressure, contributing to a decreased risk of cardiovascular events. Additionally, increased estrogen levels, commonly observed in this population, are believed to exert protective effects against atherosclerotic plaque formation, further suggesting a reduced susceptibility to cardiovascular complications [34–36]. However, it is worth noting that despite these apparent protective mechanisms, the prevalence of coronary heart disease in patients awaiting liver transplantation is unexpectedly higher than anticipated, as evidenced by various studies [37,38]. Furthermore, once liver transplantation has taken place, coronary heart disease emerges as a substantial contributor to post-transplant morbidity and mortality [39]. These findings align well with the observations made in our study, underscoring the importance of the cardiovascular risk in patients with end-stage liver disease that makes the cardiovascular assessment an essential component of pre-OLT evaluation despite controversies about the methodological approach to be used.

Given the substantial impact of OLT on cardiovascular mortality, especially over the long term [5], the availability of a novel risk stratification tool, derived from a mere quartet of straightforward clinical variables readily obtainable in any healthcare or nursing setting, holds significant promise in mitigating the medical and economic burden associated with the screening and diagnosis of CVD within this patient population. The intriguing revelation from our study is the predictive efficacy of the FLI value assessed prior to transplantation, independently of advancing age and escalating burden of cardiovascular risk factors developed in the post-OLT. This highlights the potential utility of the FLI as a valuable tool for early risk assessment in liver transplant candidates, offering a means to proactively identify individuals at heightened risk of cardiovascular complications in advance of the transplantation procedure and potentially enabling more targeted and cost-effective interventions to safeguard the cardiovascular health of these patients.

It is well known that FLI encompasses some traditional cardiovascular risk factors such as BMI, triglyceride levels, and WC. Thus, the resulting index value may reflect the worsening of these variables, specifically BMI. Nevertheless, the intricate interplay between the pathophysiological mechanisms underpinning hepatic steatosis and atherosclerosis must not be neglected. NAFLD demonstrates a close association with the hallmarks of metabolic syndrome, encompassing insulin resistance, lipotoxicity, oxidative stress, and altered adipocytokine secretion. These factors collectively contribute to a condition of chronic low-grade inflammation, which in turn leads to the simultaneous accumulation of fat in the liver and the formation of atheroma in the intimal layer of the arterial wall. Intriguingly, NAFLD has been demonstrated to elevate the risk of vascular endothelial dysfunction and the progression of atherosclerosis, even independently of metabolic syndrome and its individual components [40,41]. In this context, numerous pieces of evidence emphasize the main role of endothelial dysfunction as a common pathogenic factor in NAFLD and NAFLD-associated atherosclerosis [42].

In addition to pre-OLT FLI, the pre-OLT smoking habit also has been shown to independently predict the long-term cardiovascular risk in adult OLT recipients we studied, being associated with a threefold increase in the risk of cardiovascular events, despite the fact that the majority of patients stopped tobacco use after surgery. Notably, the prevalence of tobacco use among liver transplant recipients is noteworthy, with reported rates spanning from 14.7% to as high as 75% [43]. However, it must be admitted that our comprehension of the potential implications of cigarette smoking on morbidity and mortality following liver transplantation remains relatively underexplored within the realm of research. As such, a significant knowledge gap persists regarding the intricate relationship between cigarette smoking and health outcomes post-liver transplantation, warranting comprehensive investigation and scrutiny. This finding, though intriguing, poses a challenge in terms of interpretation, particularly in light of the limited literature available for comparison. The existing body of research presents varying perspectives on the association between smoking and post-OLT outcomes. For instance, one study found no independent link between active smoking one year after liver transplantation and vascular events [44]. By contrast, in a separate study, individuals who were active smokers at the time of listing for OLT procedures were found to have an independent association with the development of cardiovascular disease in the post-OLT period, with a hazard ratio of 10.91 (95% confidence interval 1.22–97.92) [45]. Conversely, another study has presented evidence indicating that active smokers presented a 79% higher risk of mortality than those who had never smoked or quit smoking before OLT [46].

Cardiovascular disease is reported as a complication of chronic immunosuppression, which can negatively affect long-term survival and quality of life in liver transplantation [8]. Due to the very different extension of follow-up in our patients, multiple combination regimens and newly introduced drugs may have occurred over the years, making it difficult to adequately evaluate the eventual impact of various immunosuppressive agents on CVD [47,48].

In conclusion, this study emphasizes the critical importance of assessing cardiovascular risk in liver transplant candidates, given the absence of a standardized method. The FLI emerges as a valuable screening tool, predicting potentially fatal cardiovascular events. Its consistency suggests potential clinical utility, although integration into routine assessments must be approached cautiously. Further validation through extensive, multicenter studies is crucial to establish its reliability across diverse populations.

Future research should explore FLI-guided interventions for hepatic steatosis and investigate smoking's specific impact on cardiovascular health in liver transplant recipients. While FLI shows promise, its clinical application requires a careful, evidence-driven approach.

The quest for improved cardiovascular care and outcomes in liver transplant candidates continues to be a complex and evolving challenge, demanding further investigation and innovation in the field.

Limitations

The study suffers from various limitations that need to be acknowledged. Firstly, its retrospective design inherently carries important biases. Secondly, the sample size was relatively modest, which may have influenced the statistical power to detect certain associations, as well as the number of recorded cardiovascular events during the follow-up period was relatively low. The Caucasian race of our whole population limits the generalizability of the findings to other ethnic groups. Furthermore, our reliance on self-reported information regarding the history or status of pre-transplant cardiovascular disease introduces potential recall bias and may not capture all relevant clinical details accurately. Additionally, exhaustive information on smoking habits was not available, which could affect the precision of our analysis, as smoking is a well-known complex and multifactorial risk factor for cardiovascular events. Finally, we could not manage to assess the impact of immunosuppressive treatment on cardiovascular outcomes due to the variations in the duration of follow-up periods and the utilization of diverse combination regimens and modifications.

Author Contributions: Conceptualization, A.C., C.C., G.A., T.S. and F.C.S.; investigation, A.C., G.A. A.D.M. and C.C.; formal analysis, A.C.; writing, original draft preparation, A.C., G.A. and T.S. writing, review and editing, A.C., G.A., R.G., T.S., L.R., V.R. and F.C.S.; supervision, R.M., T.S., M.M and F.C.S. All authors have read and agreed to the published version of the manuscript.

Funding: This research received no external funding.

Institutional Review Board Statement: The study was conducted in accordance with the Declaration of Helsinki, and approved by the Institutional Review Board (or Ethics Committee) of University of Campania "Luigi Vanvitelli", Azienda Ospedaliera Universitaria, "Luigi Vanvitelli", Azienda Ospedaliera di Rilievo Nazionale "Ospedale dei Colli" (protocol code 12771/I and date of approval 2 May 2023). Clinical trial.gov registration ID NCT05895669.

Informed Consent Statement: All patients signed a written informed consent to participate in the study

Data Availability Statement: The data that support the findings of this study are available upon reasonable request from the corresponding author.

Conflicts of Interest: The authors declare no conflict of interest.

Abbreviations

CVD = cardiovascular disease; FLI = fatty liver index; BMI = body mass index; WC = waist circumference; MI = myocardial infarction; eGFR = estimated glomerular filtration rate; GGT = γ-glutamyltransferase; MetS = metabolic syndrome; NASH = nonalcoholic steatohepatitis; NAFLD = Nonalcoholic fatty liver disease; OLT = orthotopic liver transplantation; T2D = type 2 diabetes.

References

1. Van Wagner, L.B.; Lapin, B.; Levitsky, J.; Wilkins, J.T.; Abecassis, M.M.; Skaro, A.I.; Lloyd-Jones, D.M. High early cardiovascular mortality after liver transplantation. *Liver Transplant.* **2014**, *20*, 1306–1316. [CrossRef] [PubMed]
2. Madhwal, S.; Atreja, A.; Albeldawi, M.; Lopez, R.; Post, A.; Costa, M.A. Is liver transplantation a risk factor for cardiovascular disease? A meta-analysis of observational studies. *Liver Transplant.* **2012**, *18*, 1140–1146. [CrossRef] [PubMed]

1. Albeldawi, M.; Aggarwal, A.; Madhwal, S.; Cywinski, J.; Lopez, R.; Eghtesad, B.; Zein, N.N. Cumulative risk of cardiovascular events after orthotopic liver transplantation. *Liver Transplant.* **2012**, *18*, 370–375. [CrossRef] [PubMed]
2. Fussner, L.A.; Heimbach, J.K.; Fan, C.; Dierkhising, R.; Coss, E.; Leise, M.D.; Watt, K.D. Cardiovascular disease after liver transplantation: When, What, and Who Is at Risk. *Liver Transplant.* **2015**, *21*, 889–896. [CrossRef]
3. Koshy, A.N.; Gow, P.J.; Han, H.C.; Teh, A.W.; Jones, R.; Testro, A.; Lim, H.S.; McCaughan, G.; Jeffrey, G.P.; Crawford, M.; et al. Cardiovascular mortality following liver transplantation: Predictors and temporal trends over 30 years. *Eur. Heart J. Qual. Care Clin. Outcomes* **2020**, *6*, 243–253. [CrossRef]
4. Kwong, A.J.; Devuni, D.; Wang, C.; Boike, J.; Jo, J.; VanWagner, L.; Serper, M.; Jones, L.; Sharma, R.; Verna, E.C.; et al. Outcomes of liver transplantation among older recipients with nonalcoholic steatohepatitis in a large multicenter us cohort: The re-evaluating age limits in transplantation consortium. *Liver Transplant.* **2020**, *26*, 1492–1503. [CrossRef]
5. Wong, R.J.; Singal, A.K. Trends in liver disease etiology among adults awaiting liver transplantation in the United States, 2014–2019. *JAMA Netw. Open* **2020**, *3*, e1920294. [CrossRef]
6. Pérez-Escobar, J.; Jimenez, J.V.; Rodríguez-Aguilar, E.F.; Servín-Rojas, M.; Ruiz-Manriquez, J.; Safar-Boueri, L.; Carrillo-Maravilla, E.; Navasa, M.; García-Juárez, I. Immunotolerance in liver transplantation: A primer for the clinician. *Ann. Hepatol.* **2023**, *28*, 100760. [CrossRef]
7. Martin, P.; DiMartini, A.; Feng, S.; Brown, R., Jr.; Fallon, M. Evaluation for liver transplantation in adults: 2013 practice guideline by the American Association for the Study of Liver Diseases and the American Society of Transplantation. *Hepatology* **2014**, *59*, 1144–1165. [CrossRef]
10. Lentine, K.L.; Costa, S.P.; Weir, M.R.; Robb, J.F.; Fleisher, L.A.; Kasiske, B.L.; Carithers, R.L.; Ragosta, M.; Bolton, K.; Auerbach, A.D.; et al. Cardiac disease evaluation and management among kidney and liver transplantation candidates: A scientific statement from the American Heart Association and the American College of Cardiology Foundation. *J. Am. Coll. Cardiol.* **2012**, *60*, 434–480. [CrossRef]
11. Alexander, S.; Teshome, M.; Patel, H.; Chan, E.Y.; Doukky, R. The diagnostic and prognostic utility of risk factors defined by the AHA/ACCF on the evaluation of cardiac disease in liver transplantation candidates. *BMC Cardiovasc. Disord.* **2019**, *19*, 102. [CrossRef] [PubMed]
12. Konerman, M.A.; Fritze, D.; Weinberg, R.L.; Sonnenday, C.J.; Sharma, P. Incidence of and risk assessment for adverse cardiovascular outcomes after liver transplantation: A systematic review. *Transplantation* **2017**, *101*, 1645–1657. [CrossRef] [PubMed]
13. Sastre, L.; García, R.; Gándara, J.G.; Fernández-Llama, P.; Amor, A.J.; Sierra, C.; Escudé, L.; Ruiz, P.; Colmenero, J.; Ortega, E.; et al. The role of arterial stiffness in the estimation of cardiovascular risk in liver transplant recipients. *Transplant. Direct* **2021**, *8*, e1272. [CrossRef] [PubMed]
14. VanWagner, L.B.; Ning, H.; Whitsett, M.; Levitsky, J.; Uttal, S.; Wilkins, J.T.; Abecassis, M.M.; Ladner, D.P.; Skaro, A.I.; Lloyd-Jones, D.M. A point-based prediction model for cardiovascular risk in orthotopic liver transplantation: The CAR-OLT score. *Hepatology* **2017**, *66*, 1968–1979. [CrossRef]
15. Targher, G.; Byrne, C.D.; Lonardo, A.; Zoppini, G.; Barbui, C. Non-alcoholic fatty liver disease and risk of incident cardiovascular disease: A meta-analysis. *J. Hepatol.* **2016**, *65*, 589–600. [CrossRef]
16. Salvatore, T.; Galiero, R.; Caturano, A.; Vetrano, E.; Rinaldi, L.; Coviello, F.; Di Martino, A.; Albanese, G.; Colantuoni, S.; Medicamento, G.; et al. Dysregulated epicardial adipose tissue as a risk factor and potential therapeutic target of heart failure with preserved ejection fraction in diabetes. *Biomolecules* **2022**, *12*, 176. [CrossRef]
17. Sinn, D.H.; Kang, D.; Chang, Y.; Ryu, S.; Cho, S.J.; Paik, S.W.; Song, Y.B.; Pastor-Barriuso, R.; Guallar, E.; Cho, J.; et al. Non-alcoholic fatty liver disease and the incidence of myocardial infarction: A cohort study. *J. Gastroenterol. Hepatol.* **2020**, *35*, 833–839. [CrossRef]
18. Acierno, C.; Caturano, A.; Pafundi, P.C.; Nevola, R.; Adinolfi, L.E.; Sasso, F.C. Nonalcoholic fatty liver disease and type 2 diabetes: Pathophysiological mechanisms shared between the two faces of the same coin. *Explor. Med.* **2020**, *1*, 287–306. [CrossRef]
19. Piazza, N.A.; Singal, A.K. Frequency of cardiovascular events and effect on survival in liver transplant recipients for cirrhosis due to alcoholic or nonalcoholic steatohepatitis. *Exp. Clin. Transplant.* **2016**, *14*, 79–85.
20. Bedogni, G.; Bellentani, S.; Miglioli, L.; Masutti, F.; Passalacqua, M.; Castiglione, A.; Tiribelli, C. The Fatty Liver Index: A simple and accurate predictor of hepatic steatosis in the general population. *BMC Gastroenterol.* **2006**, *6*, 33. [CrossRef]
21. Galiero, R.; Caturano, A.; Vetrano, E.; Cesaro, A.; Rinaldi, L.; Salvatore, T.; Marfella, R.; Sardu, C.; Moscarella, E.; Gragnano, F.; et al. Pathophysiological mechanisms and clinical evidence of relationship between Nonalcoholic fatty liver disease (NAFLD) and cardiovascular disease. *Rev. Cardiovasc. Med.* **2021**, *22*, 755–768. [CrossRef] [PubMed]
22. Caturano, A.; Acierno, C.; Nevola, R.; Pafundi, P.C.; Galiero, R.; Rinaldi, L.; Salvatore, T.; Adinolfi, L.E.; Sasso, F.C. Non-alcoholic fatty liver disease: From pathogenesis to clinical impact. *Processes* **2021**, *9*, 135. [CrossRef]
23. Salvatore, T.; Pafundi, P.C.; Morgillo, F.; Di Liello, R.; Galiero, R.; Nevola, R.; Marfella, R.; Monaco, L.; Rinaldi, L.; Adinolfi, L.E.; et al. Metformin: An old drug against old age and associated morbidities. *Diabetes Res. Clin. Pract.* **2020**, *160*, 108025. [CrossRef] [PubMed]
24. Fedchuk, L.; Nascimbeni, F.; Pais, R.; Charlotte, F.; Housset, C.; Ratziu, V.; LIDO Study Group. Performance and limitations of steatosis biomarkers in patients with nonalcoholic fatty liver disease. *Aliment. Pharmacol. Ther.* **2014**, *40*, 1209–1222. [CrossRef]
25. Pais, R.; Giral, P.; Khan, J.F.; Rosenbaum, D.; Housset, C.; Poynard, T.; Ratziu, V.; LIDO Study Group. Fatty liver is an independent predictor of early carotid atherosclerosis. *J. Hepatol.* **2016**, *65*, 95–102. [CrossRef]

26. Pais, R.; Redheuil, A.; Cluzel, P.; Ratziu, V.; Giral, P. Relationship among fatty liver, specific and multiple-site atherosclerosis, and 10-year Framingham score. *Hepatology.* **2019**, *69*, 1453–1463. [CrossRef] [PubMed]
27. Kim, J.H.; Moon, J.S.; Byun, S.J.; Lee, J.H.; Kang, D.R.; Sung, K.C.; Kim, J.Y.; Huh, J.H. Fatty liver index and development of cardiovascular disease in Koreans without pre-existing myocardial infarction and ischemic stroke: A large population-based study. *Cardiovasc. Diabetol.* **2020**, *19*, 51. [CrossRef]
28. Piepoli, M.F.; Hoes, A.W.; Agewall, S.; Albus, C.; Brotons, C.; Catapano, A.L.; Cooney, M.T.; Corrà, U.; Cosyns, B.; Deaton, C.; et al. 2016 European Guidelines on cardiovascular disease prevention in clinical practice: The Sixth Joint Task Force of the European Society of Cardiology and Other Societies on Cardiovascular Disease Prevention in Clinical Practice (constituted by representatives of 10 societies and by invited experts) Developed with the special contribution of the European Association for Cardiovascular Prevention & Rehabilitation (EACPR). *Eur. Heart J.* **2016**, *37*, 2315–2381.
29. Expert panel on detection, evaluation, and treatment of high blood cholesterol in adults. executive summary of the third report of the national cholesterol education program (ncep) expert panel on detection, evaluation, and treatment of high blood cholesterol in adults (adult treatment panel III). *JAMA.* **2001**, *285*, 2486–2497. [CrossRef]
30. Siafi, E.; Andrikou, I.; Thomopoulos, C.; Konstantinidis, D.; Kakouri, N.; Tatakis, F.; Kariori, M.; Filippou, C.; Zamanis, I.; Manta, E.; et al. Fatty liver index and cardiovascular outcomes in never-treated hypertensive patients: A prospective cohort. *Hypertens. Res.* **2023**, *46*, 119–127. [CrossRef]
31. Li, X.; Heiskanen, J.S.; Ma, H.; Heianza, Y.; Guo, Y.; Kelly, T.N.; He, H.; Fonseca, V.A.; Chen, W.; Harville, E.W.; et al. Fatty liver index and left ventricular mass: Prospective associations from two independent cohorts. *J. Hypertens.* **2021**, *39*, 961–969. [CrossRef] [PubMed]
32. Furuhashi, M.; Muranaka, A.; Yuda, S.; Tanaka, M.; Koyama, M.; Kawamukai-Nishida, M.; Takahashi, S.; Higashiura, Y.; Miyamori, D.; Nishikawa, R.; et al. Independent association of fatty liver index with left ventricular diastolic dysfunction in subjects without medication. *Am. J. Cardiol.* **2021**, *158*, 139–146. [CrossRef] [PubMed]
33. Lee, C.H.; Han, K.D.; Kim, D.H.; Kwak, M.S. The repeatedly elevated fatty liver index is associated with increased mortality: A population-based cohort study. *Front. Endocrinol.* **2021**, *12*, 638615. [CrossRef] [PubMed]
34. Cicognani, C.; Malavolti, M.; Morselli-Labate, A.M.; Zamboni, L.; Sama, C.; Barbara, L. Serum lipid and lipoprotein patterns in patients with liver cirrhosis and chronic active hepatitis. *Arch. Intern. Med.* **1997**, *157*, 792–796. [CrossRef]
35. Blei, A.T.; Mazhar, S.; Davidson, C.J.; Flamm, S.L.; Abecassis, M.; Gheorghiade, M. Hemodynamic evaluation before liver transplantation: Insights into the portal hypertensive syndrome. *J. Clin. Gastroenterol.* **2007**, *41* (Suppl. S3), S323–S329. [CrossRef]
36. Kavanagh, K.; Davis, M.A.; Zhang, L.; Wilson, M.D.; Register, T.C.; Adams, M.R.; Rudel, L.L.; Wagner, J.D. Estrogen decreases atherosclerosis in part by reducing hepatic acyl-CoA:cholesterol acyltransferase 2 (ACAT2) in monkeys. *Arterioscler. Thromb. Vasc. Biol.* **2009**, *29*, 1471–1477. [CrossRef]
37. Parikh, K.; Appis, A.; Doukky, R. Cardiac imaging for the assessment of patients being evaluated for kidney or liver transplantation. *J. Nucl. Cardiol.* **2015**, *22*, 282–296. [CrossRef]
38. Carey, W.D.; Dumot, J.A.; Pimentel, R.R.; Barnes, D.S.; Hobbs, R.E.; Henderson, J.M.; Vogt, D.P.; Mayes, J.T.; Westveer, M.K.; Easley, K.A. The prevalence of coronary artery disease in liver transplant candidates over age 50. *Transplantation* **1995**, *59*, 859–864. [CrossRef]
39. Skaro, A.I.; Gallon, L.G.; Lyuksemburg, V.; Jay, C.L.; Zhao, L.; Ladner, D.P.; VanWagner, L.B.; De Wolf, A.M.; Flaherty, J.D.; Levitsky, J.; et al. The impact of coronary artery disease on outcomes after liver transplantation. *J. Cardiovasc. Med.* **2016**, *17*, 875–885. [CrossRef]
40. Ozturk, K.; Uygun, A.; Guler, A.K.; Demirci, H.; Ozdemir, C.; Cakir, M.; Sakin, Y.S.; Turker, T.; Sari, S.; Demirbas, S.; et al. Nonalcoholic fatty liver disease is an independent risk factor for atherosclerosis in young adult men. *Atherosclerosis* **2015**, *240*, 380–386. [CrossRef]
41. Caturano, A.; D'Angelo, M.; Mormone, A.; Russo, V.; Mollica, M.P.; Salvatore, T.; Galiero, R.; Rinaldi, L.; Vetrano, E.; Marfella, R.; et al. Oxidative Stress in Type 2 Diabetes: Impacts from Pathogenesis to Lifestyle Modifications. *Curr. Issues Mol. Biol.* **2023**, *45*, 6651–6666. [CrossRef]
42. Nasiri-Ansari, N.; Androutsakos, T.; Flessa, C.M.; Kyrou, I.; Siasos, G.; Randeva, H.S.; Kassi, E.; Papavassiliou, A.G. Endothelial cell dysfunction and nonalcoholic fatty liver disease (NAFLD): A concise review. *Cells* **2022**, *11*, 2511. [CrossRef] [PubMed]
43. Li, Q.; Wang, Y.; Ma, T.; Liu, X.; Wang, B.; Wu, Z.; Lv, Y.; Wu, R. Impact of cigarette smoking on early complications after liver transplantation: A single-center experience and a meta-analysis. *PLoS ONE* **2017**, *12*, e0178570. [CrossRef]
44. Borg, M.A.; van der Wouden, E.J.; Sluiter, W.J.; Slooff, M.J.; Haagsma, E.B.; van den Berg, A.P. Vascular events after liver transplantation: A long-term follow-up study. *Transpl. Int.* **2008**, *21*, 74–80. [CrossRef] [PubMed]
45. Leithead, J.A.; Ferguson, J.W.; Hayes, P.C. Smoking-related morbidity and mortality following liver transplantation. *Liver Transplant.* **2008**, *14*, 1159–1164. [CrossRef]
46. López-Lazcano, A.I.; Gual, A.; Colmenero, J.; Caballería, E.; Lligoña, A.; Navasa, M.; Crespo, G.; López, E.; López-Pelayo, H. Active smoking before liver transplantation in patients with alcohol use disorder: Risk factors and outcomes. *J. Clin. Med.* **2020**, *9*, 2710. [CrossRef]

7. Valente, G.; Rinaldi, L.; Sgambato, M.; Piai, G. Conversion from twice-daily to once-daily tacrolimus in stable liver transplant patients: Effectiveness in a real-world setting. *Transplant. Proc.* **2013**, *45*, 1273–1275. [CrossRef] [PubMed]
8. Di Francia, R.; Rinaldi, L.; Cillo, M.; Varriale, E.; Facchini, G.; D'Aniello, C.; Marotta, G.; Berretta, M. Antioxidant diet and genotyping as tools for the prevention of liver disease. *Eur. Rev. Med. Pharmacol. Sci.* **2016**, *20*, 5155–5163. [PubMed]

Disclaimer/Publisher's Note: The statements, opinions and data contained in all publications are solely those of the individual author(s) and contributor(s) and not of MDPI and/or the editor(s). MDPI and/or the editor(s) disclaim responsibility for any injury to people or property resulting from any ideas, methods, instructions or products referred to in the content.

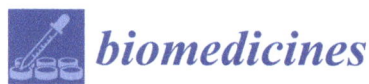

Article

A Comparison of Two Multi-Tasking Approaches to Cognitive Training in Cardiac Surgery Patients

Irina Tarasova *, Olga Trubnikova, Irina Kukhareva, Irina Syrova, Anastasia Sosnina, Darya Kupriyanova and Olga Barbarash

Department of Clinical Cardiology, Research Institute for Complex Issues of Cardiovascular Diseases, Sosnovy Blvd., 6, 650002 Kemerovo, Russia; truboa@kemcardio.ru (O.T.); syrova@kemcardio.ru (I.S.)
* Correspondence: iriz78@mail.ru

Abstract: Background: The multi-tasking approach may be promising for cognitive rehabilitation in cardiac surgery patients due to a significant effect on attentional and executive functions. This study aimed to compare the neuropsychological changes in patients who have undergone two variants of multi-tasking training and a control group in the early postoperative period of coronary artery bypass grafting (CABG). Methods: One hundred and ten CABG patients were divided into three groups: cognitive training (CT) I (a postural balance task with mental arithmetic, verbal fluency, and divergent tasks) (n = 30), CT II (a simple visual–motor reaction with mental arithmetic, verbal fluency, and divergent tasks) (n = 40), and control (n = 40). Results: Two or more cognitive indicators improved in 93.3% of CT I patients, in 72.5% of CT II patients, and in 62.5% of control patients, CT I patients differed from CT II and control (p = 0.04 and p = 0.008, respectively). The improving short-term memory and attention was found more frequently in the CT I group as compared to control (56.7% vs. 15%; p = 0.0005). The cognitive improvement of all domains (psychomotor and executive functions, attention, and short-term memory) was also revealed in CT I patients more frequently than CT II (46.7% vs. 20%; p = 0.02) and control (46.7% vs. 5%; p = 0.0005). Conclusions: The CT I multi-tasking training was more effective at improving the cognitive performance in cardiac surgery patients as compared to CT II training and standard post-surgery management. The findings of this study will be helpful for future studies involving multi-tasking training.

Keywords: cognitive training; multi-tasking; postoperative cognitive dysfunction; cardiac surgery

Citation: Tarasova, I.; Trubnikova, O.; Kukhareva, I.; Syrova, I.; Sosnina, A.; Kupriyanova, D.; Barbarash, O. A Comparison of Two Multi-Tasking Approaches to Cognitive Training in Cardiac Surgery Patients. *Biomedicines* **2023**, *11*, 2823. https://doi.org/10.3390/biomedicines11102823

Academic Editor: Alfredo Caturano

Received: 21 August 2023
Revised: 13 October 2023
Accepted: 13 October 2023
Published: 18 October 2023

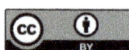

Copyright: © 2023 by the authors. Licensee MDPI, Basel, Switzerland. This article is an open access article distributed under the terms and conditions of the Creative Commons Attribution (CC BY) license (https://creativecommons.org/licenses/by/4.0/).

1. Introduction

It is known that cardiovascular disease is a significant pathophysiological background for the development of ischemic brain damage [1–3]. Vascular changes have been shown to cause brain tissue pathology well in advance of clinical manifestations of neurological or cognitive deficits [4–6]. Currently, cognitive deficit is considered as a marker not only of low quality of life in patients, but also of a decrease in life expectancy. The deterioration of cognitive health contributes to a decrease in the patient's adherence to treatment, which, in turn, can lead to the progression and worsening of the prognosis of cardiovascular disease [7]. Patients with cardiovascular disease and cognitive deficit who undergo cardiac surgery represent a distinct cohort that is difficult to manage [8,9]. Cardiopulmonary bypass surgery also contributes to an acute ischemic brain injury [10,11]. The most significant complications of cardiac surgery are stroke and postoperative cognitive deficit or dysfunction [POCD]. The prevalence of POCD is high and can reach 70% [12,13]. POCD development in cardiac surgery patients is associated with prolonged intensive care and hospital stay, as well as deterioration of rehabilitation procedures, ultimately reducing the effectiveness of surgery.

Currently, there are no clear approaches to POCD prevention and cognitive rehabilitation of cardiac surgery patients. High medical and social significance of POCD determines the need to develop new strategies for cognitive rehabilitation in cardiovascular disease patients that may preserve the quality of life and social status. Among nonpharmacological treatments for cognitive deficits, combined programs of physical and cognitive training are now becoming more widespread [14–16]. Recent studies show that physical and cognitive development are interdependent and closely related [16,17]. It has been established that neurogenesis continues even in adulthood [18], and physical activity is a key factor in neurogenesis, depending on the intensity and systemic effect [19]. At the same time, it should be noted that better cognitive functioning after training was based on a combination of physical and cognitive exercise compared with either alone [20].

People are often confronted with situations in daily life that require the concurrent performance of a motor and cognitive task or the concurrent processing of motor and cognitive information such as taking an incoming call when walking or dribbling a ball in basketball. In multi-tasking situations, individuals may have to switch between different task demands or perform two tasks simultaneously. It has also been shown that the performance of competing tasks promotes the activation of widespread areas of the brain, most often the frontal and parietal cortex, as key elements of the distribution of attention during information processing [21,22]. These areas of the brain are known to be the watersheds of the blood supply, at the borders between the vascular pools [23,24]. Chronic ischemia and/or episodes of acute cerebral ischemia during cardiac surgery have been established to have a greater impact on them than any other brain regions. The vulnerability of these regions, not only in the elderly but also in cardiovascular patients, requires professionals to find new approaches to protect and restore brain functions that are associated with them.

The use of a multi-tasking approach, which involves the simultaneous performance of motor and cognitive tasks, may be promising for cognitive rehabilitation in cardiac surgery patients due to the requirement of significant control of attentional and executive functions [25,26]. Previous studies have been reported that simultaneous cognitive–motor training can result in higher benefits in cognitive and motor performance than both training regimes (cognitive or motor training) alone [20]. Although the benefits of a multi-tasking approach have already been demonstrated in patients with Parkinson's and Alzheimer's disease, as well as in preventing the risk of falls in the elderly [27–29], studies involving cardiac surgery patients are extremely rare. The possibility of using a multi-tasking approach in patients after cardiac surgery is being actively discussed and requires special studies since there is no unequivocal opinion regarding their rehabilitation effect.

It should be taken into account that cardiac surgery patients commonly have a lower functional reserve and a risk of complications in the early postoperative period. It is, therefore, difficult to choose an approach for cognitive recovery due to the physical state of cardiac surgery patients. A multi-tasking approach should include tasks appropriate to their physical condition during the early postoperative period. However, it is also very important to gradually increase the level of difficulty of a cognitive task throughout the learning process. Preliminary evidence suggests that combined motor–cognitive training can provide effective cognitive recovery in patients with cardiovascular disease, optimize cognitive and physical functions, and improve quality of life [30].

Despite the evidence, the multi-tasking approach had not yet been sufficiently implemented into clinical practice. It is necessary to determine the cognitive and motor tasks that require the most activation of the functional reserves of the patients. The optimal training regime and duration of exercises is not certain. We hypothesized that incorporating multi-tasking-based cognitive trainings into the management of patients in the early postoperative period of coronary artery bypass grafting (CABG) will have a positive impact on their cognitive functioning. In addition, we would like to test the benefits of combinations of various cognitive and motor tasks. Thus, the aim of this study was to compare the neuropsychological changes in patients who have undergone two variants of multi-tasking training and a control group in the early postoperative period of coronary artery bypass grafting (CABG).

2. Materials and Methods

2.1. Data Collection and Sampling

One hundred and ten patients with stable coronary artery disease (CAD) were selected from the cohort of patients of the Cardiology Department Clinic of the Research Institute for Complex Issues of Cardiovascular Diseases. The study was carried out in accordance with the Helsinki Declaration (revised in 2013). The Ethics Committee of the Research Institute for Complex Issues of Cardiovascular Diseases has approved the study (protocol No. 10 dated 10 December 2020). In March 2020, the collection of patient data was initiated. The inclusion criteria were as follows: stable coronary artery disease (CAD), elective CABG, aged 45–75 years, and provided informed consent. The exclusion criteria were as follows: history of stroke, epilepsy, traumatic brain injury, depression, dementia; Montreal Cognitive Assessment Scale (MoCA) score ≤ 18 (30); Beck's Depression Inventory (BDI-II) score ≥ 8 (31); and non-cardiovascular decompensated comorbidities [30]. All of the patients met the study criteria and signed an informed consent form. Upon admission to hospital, all patients underwent neurological examination, as well as cognitive and depression screening. Reviewers were blinded regarding the participation of patients in the study.

A pseudo-randomization method was used to form three groups, comparable in terms of clinical characteristics. The study sample was divided into the groups: cognitive training (CT) I (n = 40), CT II (n = 40), and control (n = 40). The baseline clinical characteristics are given in Table 1. After initial examination, 10 patients were excluded from the CT I group for various reasons (see Figure 1). The overview of the study design can be seen in Figure 1.

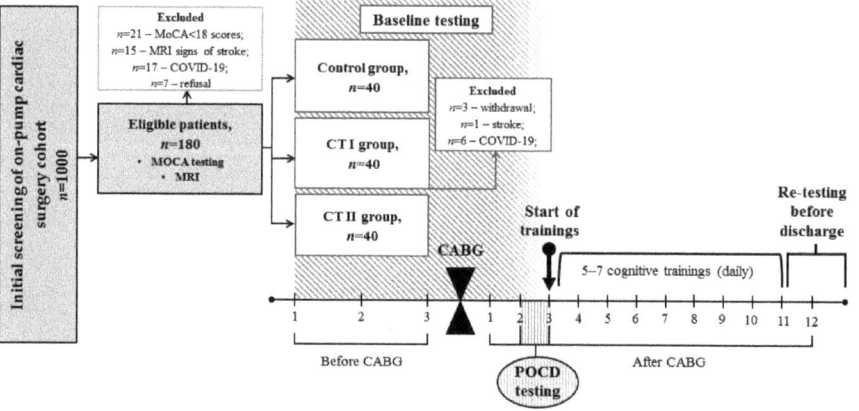

Figure 1. Overview of the study. MOCA, The Montreal Cognitive Assessment; MRI, Magnetic Resonance Imaging; CABG, Coronary Artery Bypass Grafting; POCD, Postoperative Cognitive Dysfunction.

Elective CABG was carried out in all groups using normothermic non-pulsatile cardiopulmonary bypass (CPB). Standard procedures for endotracheal anesthesia and infusion were used. An on-line monitoring of cerebral cortex oxygenation (rSO2) (INVOS-3100, Somanetics, Troy, MI, USA) was carried out. During the surgery time, oxygen saturation indicators were within the normal range. The mean CPB time and surgery time can be found in Table 1. After CABG, all patients were transferred to the intensive care unit for one to two days. The patients were transferred to the cardiology department for postoperative management after intensive care and discharged in 11–12 days.

Table 1. The clinical and anamnestic characteristics of all patients before cardiac surgery (n = 110).

Variable	Cognitive Training I (n = 30)	Cognitive Training II (n = 40)	Control (n = 40)	p-Value
Age, years, Me [Q25; Q75]	65 [60; 68]	65.5 [61; 70.5]	65 [61; 69]	0.37 *
MoCA, scores, Me [Q25; Q75]	25 [22; 26]	25 [24; 27]	26 [23; 27]	0.65 *
BDI-II, scores, Me [Q25; Q75]	5 [2; 6]	3 [2; 4]	4 [1; 5]	0.08 *
Educational attainment, years, Me [Q25; Q75]	12 [11; 16]	11 [10; 15]	12 [10; 15]	0.11 *
Functional class of angina, n (%) I–II / III	26 (86.7) / 4 (13.3)	29 (72.5) / 11 (27.5)	31 (77.5) / 9 (22.5)	0.41 #
Functional class NYHA, n (%) I–II / III	27 (90) / 3 (10)	39 (97.5) / 1 (2.5)	37 (92.5) / 3 (7.5)	0.46 #
History of myocardial infarction, n (%)	16 (53.3)	18 (45)	27 (67.5)	0.13 #
Fraction of left ventricle ejection, %, Me [Q25; Q75]	62 [52; 68]	64 [52.5; 66]	64 [58; 67]	0.81 #
Type 2 of diabetes mellitus, n (%)	9 (30)	10 (25)	16 (40)	0.65 #
CA stenosis < 50%, n (%)	17 (56.7)	22 (55)	12 (30)	0.14 #
Cardiopulmonary bypass time, min, Me [Q25; Q75]	85 [68; 102]	81 [68; 99]	72 [56; 103]	0.45 *
Surgery time, min, Me [Q25; Q75]	225 [175; 241]	220 [180; 245]	200 [180; 228]	0.49 *
Medication, n (%)				
ACEi	16 (53.3)	28 (70)	27 (67.5)	0.28 #
Statins	30 (100)	40 (100)	40 (100)	-
Beta-blockers	30 (100)	38 (95)	38 (95)	0.49 #
Antiplatelet drugs	30 (100)	40 (100)	40 (100)	-
CCB	7 (23.3)	10 (25)	11 (27.5)	0.53 #
ARB	7 (23.3)	9 (22.5)	8 (20)	0.91 #
Diuretics	24 (80)	32 (80)	30 (75)	0.80 #

ACEi, angiotensin-converting enzyme inhibitor; ARBs, angiotensin II receptor blockers; CA, carotid artery; CCB, calcium channel blocker; NYHA, heart failure according to the New York Heart Association. *—between-group differences by Kruskal–Wallis one-way analysis of variance; #—between-group differences by χ^2.

2.2. Neuropsychological Examination

Before study inclusion, the groups of patients (CTI, CT II, and control) were assessed by the screening scale MoCA in the validated Russian-modified version. Extensive neuropsychological testing was used to examine all participants of the study (see Table 2). The baseline testing was carried out 2–3 days before CABG. The first POCD testing was conducted at 2–3 days after surgery. Alternate versions of the neuropsychological tests were used in repeated measurements to minimize practice effects. POCD was determined for each patient individually, using the percentage of relative changes in postoperative indicators compared with a baseline using the following formula: (baseline value–postoperative value)/baseline value) × 100%. Negative values indicated an increase in the cognitive indicator compared to the baseline, positive values indicated a decrease, and the threshold value for cognitive decline was equal to 20% [30]. The examiners were standardized and unaware of the patients' participation in the study. Upon completion of the cognitive training course or approximately 11–12 days after the CABG, all patients were retested.

Table 2. Cognitive test battery for assessing cognitive function in cardiac surgery patients.

Cognitive Tests and Indicators	Description of the Procedure
Cognitive screening	
Montreal Cognitive Assessment Scale (MoCA), scores	30-point questionnaire for cognitive impairment and dementia screening (Russian-modified version).
Psychomotor and executive functions	
Complex visual–motor reaction Reaction time, ms Errors, n	Reaction latencies of the right and left hands to stimuli (different colors of rectangles) when the subject can choose one of the three presented signals (the number of signals in the test is 30).
Level of functional mobility of nervous processes: responses to feedback Reaction time, ms Errors, n Missed signals, n	Feedback mode is used for the performance of the previous test. The exposure time of the test signals (rectangles) is changed: the exposure of the next signal is shortened by 20 ms with each correct answer and extended by 20 ms with an incorrect answer. The test contains 120 signals. A missed signal is indicated by the absence of response to the test signal.
Attention	
The Bourdon's test Processed letters per min, n Processed letters per 4 min, n Attention ratio, scores	The subject is provided with the alphabetic version of Bourdon's test to highlight certain letters for a time of 4 min.
Attention span, scores	The subject is presented with a square grid of 16 equal cells. Crosses appear in different parts of the grid for a short time, and the subject must memorize their location and mark the corresponding cells with the left mouse button immediately after the stimulus disappears.
Short-term memory	
10 words memorizing test, n	To remember as many of 10 words presented one after another as possible.
10 numbers memorizing test, n	To remember as many of 10 numbers presented one after another as possible.
Figurative memory, n	The subject is presented with 10 figures, which must be remembered (30 s memory time). Next appears a set of 30 figures, among which it is necessary to find and mark with the left mouse button all previously remembered figures.

2.3. Multi-Tasking Training

All cognitive training courses were started 3–4 days after CABG, once daily for a period of 5–7 days. Before the start of the training, the presence of POCD was confirmed according to the above criteria in all patients included in the study. POCD was in 100% of patients in both groups.

2.4. CT I (A Postural Task with Mental Arithmetic and Divergent Tasks)

The original multi-tasking training protocol was developed using a postural balance task as a motor subtask, and cognitive subtasks included mental arithmetic, verbal fluency, and divergent tasks. For the postural balance task, trained patients stood on a balance platform to maintain the position of the center of pressure (CoP) at the same point using visual feedback. On the screen of the monitor, the CoP of the subject was presented as a marker, which had to be aligned with the target located in the center of the monitor. Simultaneously to the postural balance, one of the three cognitive tasks was conducted in sequence. The mental arithmetic task involved sequentially subtracting 7 from 100. In the verbal fluency task, the main goal was to produce as many words as possible that start in a given time (60 s). For the divergent task, the participants were asked to generate unusual uses for common objects (e.g., bricks, knives, and newspapers). Each of the cognitive tasks was performed sequentially with resting periods and exit from the balance platform.

2.5. CT II (A Simple Visual–Motor Reaction with Mental Arithmetic and Divergent Tasks)

For this training protocol, a simple visual–motor reaction was used as a motor subtask, while the cognitive subtasks were the same as in the CT I protocol. A motor subtask involved pushing the space button as soon as possible upon the appearance of different colors of rectangles on the laptop screen (the number of signals in the test was 30).

The daily training session lasted 20 min, was performed in the morning, and included a preparatory (2 min) and training (10–15 min) period for both CT I and CT II groups. The patient can request to reduce the duration of the training phase. The preparatory period was a discussion with a trainee specialist.

2.6. Statistical Analysis

All statistical analyses were conducted using the Statistica 10.0 software (StatSoft, Tulsa, OK, USA, SN: BXXR210F562022FA-A). The distribution of variables was assessed by the Shapiro–Wilk test. Most of the clinical and cognitive variables were not normally distributed. Thus, the parameters are presented as the median with IQR [25th; 75th percentile] and the number of observations (n, %). Continuous variables were evaluated using Kruskal–Wallis one-way analysis of variance and Wilcoxon tests. Continuity-corrected χ^2 tests were used to determine categorical variables and the percentage relative change in postoperative indicators. The statistical significance of the differences was determined at $p\ 0.05$.

3. Results

3.1. Cognitive Performance in CT I

Most patients with CT I training reported an acceptable level of subjective difficulty in performing multi-tasking. Thirty participants completed a course of training. The mean number of training sessions was 5.4. No participants requested a shorter session. The mean time of the training session was 16.0 min at the end of the training course. Cognitive performance changes are presented in Table 3.

Table 3. Cognitive performance changes in CT I patients.

Cognitive Indicator	Baseline Testing (n = 30)	Retesting (after Training) (n = 30)	p
	Complex visual–motor reaction		
Reaction time, ms	622.5 [584; 703]	555 [512; 601]	0.000005
Errors, n	1 [1; 2]	1 [1; 2]	0.84
	Level of functional mobility of nervous processes: responses to feedback		
Reaction time, ms	478.5 [447; 511]	475 [456; 516]	0.5
Errors, n	28 [23; 31]	26 [24; 30]	0.51
Missed signals, n	15 [10; 21]	13 [8; 20]	0.84
	Attention		
Bourdon's test			
Processed letters per min, n	71 [48; 89]	64 [51; 86]	0.4
Processed letters per 4 min, n	102 [78; 117.5]	102 [75; 117]	0.1
Attention ratio, scores	36 [28; 48]	38 [30; 53]	0.08
Attention span test, scores	5 [4; 8]	6 [5; 7]	0.27
	Short-term memory		
Figurative memory test, n	8 [6; 9]	9 [8; 10]	0.0004
10 words memorizing test, n	4 [4; 5]	4 [4; 5]	0.82
10 numbers memorizing test, n	4 [3; 5]	4 [3; 6]	0.1

Data are presented as the median with IQR [25th; 75th percentile].

As seen in Table 3, there was a statistically significant accelerating speed of psychomotor reactions and an increase in figurative memory after multi-tasking training. In addition, a tendency for an increase in the attention ratio in Bourdon's test and the attention span test was shown. An individual analysis of cognitive indicators carried out with the cutoff limit of 20% detected multidirectional changes after training. Of the 12 test battery indicators, 2 or more cognitive indicators increased by 20% in 28 patients (93.3%). A combination of improved attention and executive functions was found in 5 patients (16.7%), whereas a combination of improved short-term memory and attention was found in 17 patients (56.7%). An increase in parameters in all domains (psychomotor and executive functions, attention, and short-term memory) was observed in 14 cases (46.7%). Nevertheless, 60% of patients ($n = 18$) met the POCD criteria (a 20% decline in retesting parameters compared to baseline in three cognitive indicators of the test battery).

3.2. Cognitive Performance in CT II

The mean number of training sessions was 5.2. No participants requested a shorter session. The mean time of the training session was 15.4 min at the end of the training course. The cognitive performance data of the CT II group are presented in Table 4. Psychomotor speed after multi-tasking training compared to preoperative values was faster, and a tendency for an increase in errors in the executive function test was revealed. There was also an increase in figurative memory compared with preoperative values. An individual analysis of cognitive indicators showed that two or more cognitive indicators increased by 20% in 29 patients (72.5%). A combination of improved attention and executive functions was found in seven patients (17.5%). A combination of improved short-term memory and attention was found only in six patients (15%). An increase in parameters in all domains (psychomotor and executive functions, attention, and short-term memory) was observed in eight cases (20%). Twenty-six patients (65%) met the POCD criteria.

Table 4. Cognitive performance changes in CT II patients.

Cognitive Indicator	Baseline Testing ($n = 40$)	Retesting (after Training) ($n = 40$)	p
	Complex visual–motor reaction		
Reaction time, ms	677.5 [621; 756.5]	618 [547.5; 684]	0.0001
Errors, n	1 [0; 1,5]	1 [0.5; 3]	0.11
	Level of functional mobility of nervous processes responses to feedback		
Reaction time, ms	493.5 [473; 528]	486 [457; 536]	0.44
Errors, n	26 [21; 29]	25.5 [23; 29.5]	0.46
Missed signals, n	17.5 [10; 20.5]	14 [11; 19]	0.77
	Attention		
Bourdon's test			
Processed letters per min, n	65 [48; 79]	57.5 [47; 80]	0.25
Processed letters per 4 min, n	78 [57; 127]	80 [58; 111]	0.65
Attention ratio, scores	34 [29; 47]	29 [26; 39]	0.04
Attention span test, scores	5 [4; 6]	4.5 [4; 5.5]	0.32
	Short-term memory		
Figurative memory test, n	7 [6; 8]	8 [7; 9]	0.007
10 words memorizing test, n	4 [3; 5,5]	4 [3; 5]	0.86
10 numbers memorizing test, n	4 [3; 5,5]	4 [4; 5]	0.93

Data are presented as the median with IQR [25th; 75th percentile].

3.3. Control Group

At the first POCD testing (2–3 days after surgery), the presence of POCD was confirmed according to the above criteria in all control patients ($n = 40$) included in the study. Before discharge (11–12 days after the CABG), thirty-two patients (80%) met the POCD criteria. An individual analysis of cognitive results revealed that in 25 patients (62.5%), two or more cognitive indicators increased by 20%. Executive functions decreased in 21 patients (52.5%).

A combination of short-term memory and attention enhancement was more frequent and was observed in 20 patients (50%). An increase in parameters in all domains (psychomotor and executive functions, attention, and short-term memory) was observed in two cases (5%). The group data of control subjects are presented also in Table 5.

Table 5. Cognitive performance changes in the control group of patients.

Cognitive Indicator	Baseline Testing ($n = 40$)	Retesting (11–12 Days after the CABG) ($n = 40$)	p
Complex visual–motor reaction			
Reaction time, ms	631 [556; 684]	579 [536; 635]	0.0007
Errors, n	1 [0; 2]	1 [1; 3]	0.12
Level of functional mobility of nervous processes: responses to feedback			
Reaction time, ms	488 [455.5; 521.5]	488 [453.5; 542.5]	0.23
Errors, n	25 [22.5; 29]	28.5 [24; 29.5]	0.05
Missed signals, n	16 [10; 23]	14 [9; 18]	0.1
Attention			
Bourdon's test			
Processed letters per min, n	66 [42; 99]	68 [49.5; 89.5]	0.43
Processed letters per 4 min, n	82 [69; 112.5]	90 [67; 109.5]	0.69
Attention ratio, scores	34 [27; 47]	37 [27; 50]	0.15
Attention span test, scores	5 [4; 7]	5 [4; 6]	0.96
Short-term memory			
Figurative memory test, n	8 [6; 9]	8 [6.5; 9]	0.14
10 words memorizing test, n	4.5 [3; 5]	4 [4; 5]	0.35
10 numbers memorizing test, n	4 [3; 6]	4 [3; 5]	0.86

Data are presented as the median with IQR [25th; 75th percentile].

3.4. Between-Group Differences

Before surgery, between-group differences in cognitive performance were not observed.

The re-testing revealed that there was only a tendency for differences in POCD incidence between CT I (60%) and the control group (80%) at 11–12 days after the CABG: OR = 2.7; 95% CI: 0.92–7.73; z statistic = 1.805; $p = 0.07$. Additionally, CT II (65%) differed from the control patients (80%) not significantly: OR = 2.2; 95% CI: 0.78–5.92; z statistic = 1.487; $p = 0.14$.

Between-group differences in cognitive performance after multi-tasking training and re-testing are illustrated in Figure 2. This analysis (see Figure 2a) revealed the differences in psychomotor speed with lower values in the CT II group compared to CT I. The control group did not differ with regard to psychomotor speed from CT I and CT II groups.

In addition, differences between CT I and CT II groups were in figurative memory (Figure 2c) and attention indicators (Figure 2b,d). These differences were due to better cognitive performance in CT I patients compared to CT II after multi-tasking training. The results of control patients were the same with CT II and lower compared with CT I, but there were no significant differences.

As a result of an individual analysis of cognitive performance, it was established that CT I patients demonstrated an improvement of two or more cognitive indicators in a larger number of cases (93.3% vs. 72.5%), OR = 5.31, 95% CI = 1.1–26.1, Z = 2.05, $p = 0.04$, as compared to the CT II group. There were significant differences in the improvement of two or more cognitive indicators (93.3% vs. 62.5%), OR = 8.40, 95% CI = 1.75–40.41, Z = 2.66, $p = 0.008$, between CT I and the control group.

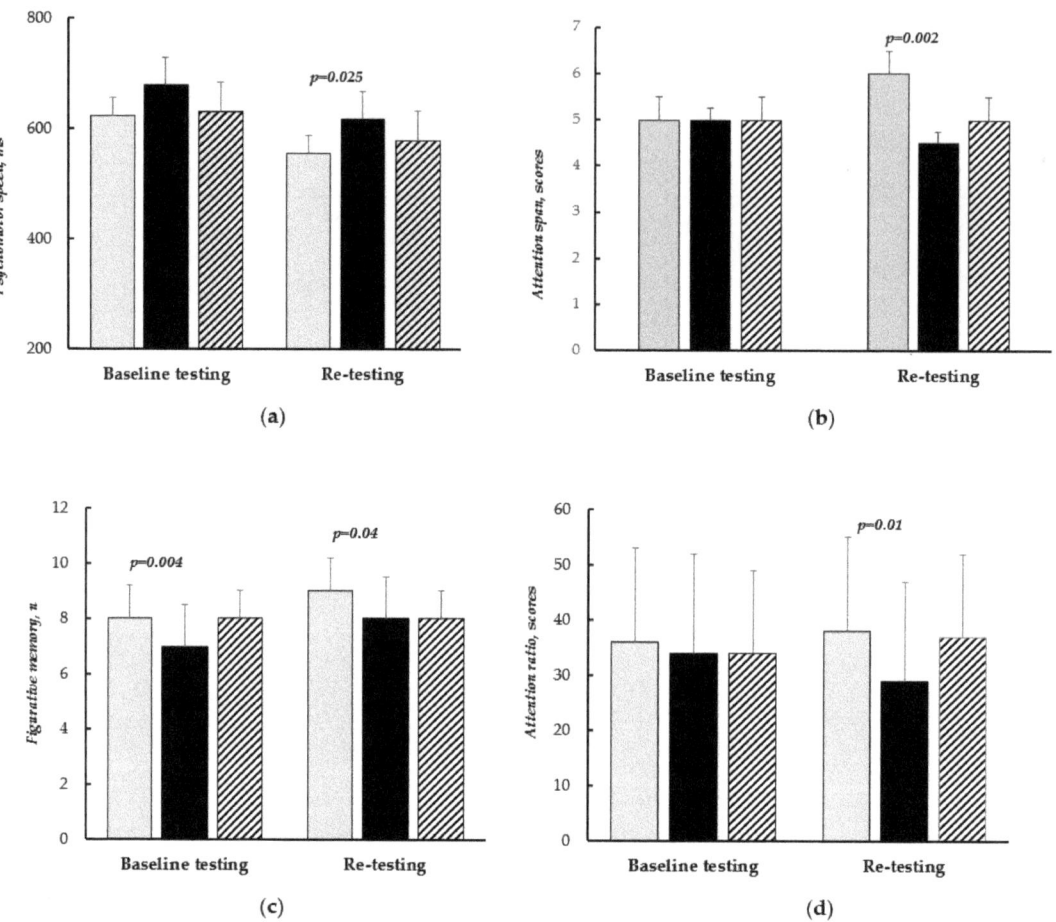

Figure 2. Between-group differences in cognitive performance after multi-tasking training (re-testing) (**a**)—psychomotor speed; (**b**)—attention span; (**c**)—figurative memory; (**d**)—attention ratio. Light bars—CT I patients; dark bars—CT II, shaded bars—control group. Data are presented as the median with IQR [25th; 75th percentile].

In addition, the combination of improved short-term memory and attention was found more frequently in the CT I group compared to CT II (56.7% vs. 15%), OR = 7.41, 95% CI = 2.4–22.9, Z = 3.48, p = 0.0005. There was no difference between the CT I and control patients in the combination of improved short-term memory and attention (56.7% vs. 50%), OR = 1.31, 95% CI = 0.5–3.4, Z = 0.55, p = 0.58. CT II patients demonstrated the combination of improved short-term memory and attention in a fewer number of cases (15% vs. 50%) in comparison to control patients, OR = 0.18, 95% CI = 0.6–0.51, Z = 3.19, p = 0.001. The cognitive improvement of all domains (psychomotor and executive functions, attention, and short-term memory) was also revealed in CT I patients more frequently compared with CT II and control groups (46.7% vs. 20%, OR = 3.5, 95% CI = 3.38–81.74, Z = 2.33, p = 0.02 and 46.7% vs. 5%, OR = 16.63, 95% CI = 1.22–10.1, Z = 3.46, p = 0.0005), respectively.

4. Discussion

The study results showed positive effects of the multi-tasking training on cognitive functions in cardiac surgery patients. In 93.3% of cases in CT I patients, there was an improvement in two or more cognitive indicators, which is significantly higher than in the

CT II group (72.5%). In addition, the CT I group demonstrated the improvement of two or more cognitive indicators in a larger number of cases in comparison with control patients (93.3% vs. 62.5%). A combination of improved short-term memory and attention was also found more frequently in the CT I group compared to the CT II patients (56.7% vs. 15%). However, the cognitive improvement of all domains was in a larger number of cases in the CT I and CT II patients in comparison to the control group (46.7% and 20% vs. 5%). This was shown by an individual analysis of cognitive indicators.

The advantages of the CT I multi-tasking approach were also demonstrated in comparison to CT II in the results of between-group comparisons. CT I patients had better figurative memory, psychomotor speed, and attention indicators than CT II after multi-tasking training. Thus, the combination of a postural task with mental arithmetic and divergent tasks has a more beneficial effect on cognitive performance in cardiac surgery patients.

As shown previously, a successful option for multi-tasking may be a combination of motor training and attention or executive function tasks [16,31,32]. Some authors have pointed to the positive effect of their inclusion in the rehabilitation course [28–30]. It was also reported that these elements have a positive effect on cognitive abilities and recommend a cautious increase in task complexity, depending on the individual abilities of the subject [31]. However, this applies to cognitively and clinically intact individuals. The early postoperative period with pain syndrome, asthenia, and other surgical complications can restrict the physical status of cardiac surgery patients. Therefore, the motor component selection for the dual task is limited. We opted for postural training and a simple visual–motor task to ensure maximum tolerance in the difficult cohort of patients. Dual tasks including postural training were previously used to restore cognitive function in traumatic brain damage [33]. In fact, in our study, the training with a postural motor task (CT I) demonstrated better results than CT II with a simple visual–motor reaction task.

It should be noted, however, that the multi-tasking training conducted in the early postoperative period of CABG had a limited impact on the cognitive performance in the patients of both groups in terms of POCD incidence. The frequency of POCD was quite high (60% in CT I and 65% in CT II). According to the literature, POCD frequency can reach 70–80% [12–14]. Our previous study found that patients who underwent standard recovery therapy had a POCD frequency of 79.5% in the early postoperative period of cardiac surgery [14].

It was shown that the performance of each of the components of the dual task can be impaired by interference processes [28,33,34]. In our study, the insignificant clinical effect of the multi-tasking paradigms chosen can be explained by the interference interactions between cognitive and motor components. It has been demonstrated that for older people, performing competitive tasks causes cognitive component deterioration in a combination of complex cognitive tasks and any motor task, and motor tasks are performed less by them combined with complex cognitive tasks [35]. Since the divergent task used in this study as a cognitive component can be classified as a complex cognitive task, the limited cognitive resources of patients in the early postoperative period of CABG did not allow them to cope effectively with the proposed version of the training.

Multi-tasking difficulties have been established in the aging population [21,36,37]. A number of studies have also shown interference effects during the concurrent performance of motor tasks involving postural control and cognitive tasks, with pronounced effects in the elderly [32,38,39]. The study of Brahms et al. [40] investigated the effects of cognitive-motor multi-tasking interventions on postural stability and cognitive performance in healthy older adults. These findings showed that the simultaneous performance of cognitive and postural tasks was moderated by modality compatibility mapping, workload memory, and increased postural demands. However, postural and cognitive performance did not change as a result of training. Bohle and his colleagues showed an age-related decline in cognitive performance at high cognitive–postural task demands [41].

Nevertheless, the CT I version of multi-tasking cognitive training can be effective in improving the cognitive state of cardiac surgery patients, as it provides a greater transfer effect (improvement in short-term memory and attention in the post-training period compared to the baseline). Previously, it was found that the effect of the transfer varies depending on the complexity and modality of the task performed [42]. It is suggested that the effectiveness of the multi-tasking approach in the recovery of cognitive functions is ensured by more effective coordination of cognitive processes.

It should also be noted that, in this study, multi-tasking training was used as a short course (5–7 training sessions). The obtained data indicate the formation of beneficial effects on cognitive functions in a short time period after CABG, which is especially important in patients to establish medical adherence and optimization of rehabilitation procedures in general. In most previous studies, short-term effects of multi-tasking training were not studied, especially in the cardiac cohort of patients [40,41,43]. It can be assumed that if the duration of the course is extended, it would have a greater positive impact on cognitive performance in cardiac surgery patients. Therefore, future studies should separately consider the impact of the length of the course of multi-tasking training on the involvement of different cognitive domains. The sustainability of the positive effects of short-term cognitive training on the preservation of the patient's overall intellectual functions also requires careful study. It is necessary to further improve approaches to multi-tasking postoperative training with an intensification load and individual support for cardiac surgery patients in the long-term postoperative period.

New technologies may offer new opportunities for medical research and practice, including virtual reality (VR) [15,44,45]. The manipulation of experimental parameters in VR software has great potential for new forms of intervention and treatment of cognitive and motor disorders in patients with different pathology, including ischemic brain damage. Further studies in the field of adapting successful multi-tasking trainings to the VR interface to the effective training of memory, executive functioning, and attention are needed.

5. Limitations

When interpreting the findings, it is important to take into account the limitations of our study. The study's observational nature was a limitation, and the effectiveness of CT for patients was assessed through an individual analysis of cognitive performance. Additionally, only a short early postoperative period of CABG was used for training. The other limitation was the small sample of patients, as we only recruited consecutive ones. Thus, we performed this pilot study to plan a larger and more comprehensive prospective study.

6. Conclusions

The CT I multi-tasking training was more effective in improving the cognitive performance in the early postoperative period of CABG in comparison to CT II training and standard post-surgery management of patients. The combination of a postural task with mental arithmetic and divergent tasks provided a greater transfer effect (better results in short-term memory and attention). The findings of this study raise important questions regarding the effectiveness of multi-tasking interventions and will be helpful for designing and implementing future studies involving multi-tasking training. Consequently, future studies should investigate interventions with different lengths of the multi-tasking training course in larger samples.

Author Contributions: Conceptualization, I.T., O.T. and O.B.; methodology, I.T. and O.T.; validation, I.T. and O.T.; formal analysis, I.T. and A.S.; investigation, D.K., I.K., I.S. and A.S.; data curation, D.K., I.K., I.S. and A.S.; writing—original draft preparation, I.T.; writing—review and editing, O.T. and O.B.; project administration, O.T.; funding acquisition, O.T. All authors have read and agreed to the published version of the manuscript.

Funding: This research was funded by the Russian Science Foundation No. 23-15-00379, https://rscf.ru/en/project/23-15-00379/, accessed on 15 May 2023.

Institutional Review Board Statement: The study was conducted in accordance with the Declaration of Helsinki and approved by the Institutional Ethics Committee of the Research Institute for Complex Issues of Cardiovascular Diseases (01/2011-2520). The study was registered on ClinicalTrials.gov (NCT05172362).

Informed Consent Statement: Informed consent was obtained from all subjects involved in the study.

Data Availability Statement: Not applicable.

Conflicts of Interest: The authors declare no conflict of interest. The funder had no role in the design of the study; in the collection, analyses, or interpretation of data; in the writing of the manuscript; or in the decision to publish the results.

References

1. Gorelick, P.B.; Scuteri, A.; Black, S.E.; Decarli, C.; Greenberg, S.M.; Iadecola, C.; Launer, L.J.; Laurent, S.; Lopez, O.L.; Nyenhuis, D.; et al. Vascular contributions to cognitive impairment and dementia: A statement for healthcare professionals from the American heart association/American stroke association. *Stroke* **2011**, *42*, 2672–2713. [CrossRef]
2. Stefanidis, K.B.; Askew, C.D.; Greaves, K.; Summers, M.J. The Effect of non-stroke cardiovascular disease states on risk for cognitive decline and dementia: A systematic and meta-analytic review. *Neuropsychol. Rev.* **2018**, *28*, 1–15. [CrossRef]
3. Giang, K.W.; Jeppsson, A.; Karlsson, M.; Hansson, E.C.; Pivodic, A.; Skoog, I.; Lindgren, M.; Nielsen, S.J. The risk of dementia after coronary artery bypass grafting in relation to age and sex. *Alzheimers Dement.* **2021**, *17*, 1042–1050. [CrossRef] [PubMed]
4. Barbay, M.; Taillia, H.; Nedelec-Ciceri, C.; Arnoux, A.; Puy, L.; Wiener, E.; Canaple, S.; Lamy, C.; Godefroy, O.; Roussel, M.; et al. Vascular cognitive impairment: Advances and trends. *Rev. Neurol.* **2017**, *173*, 473–480. [CrossRef] [PubMed]
5. de la Torre, J. The vascular hypothesis of Alzheimer's disease: A key to preclinical prediction of dementia using neuroimaging. *J. Alzheimers Dis.* **2018**, *63*, 35–52. [CrossRef] [PubMed]
6. Fisher, R.A.; Miners, J.S.; Love, S. Pathological changes within the cerebral vasculature in Alzheimer's disease: New perspectives. *Brain Pathol.* **2022**, *32*, e13061. [CrossRef]
7. Zuo, W.; Wu, J. The interaction and pathogenesis between cognitive impairment and common cardiovascular diseases in the elderly. *Ther. Adv. Chronic Dis.* **2022**, *13*, 20406223211063020. [CrossRef]
8. Indja, B.; Seco, M.; Seamark, R.; Kaplan, J.; Bannon, P.G.; Grieve, S.M.; Vallely, M.P. Neurocognitive and psychiatric issues post cardiac surgery. *Heart Lung Circ.* **2017**, *26*, 779–785. [CrossRef]
9. Tarasova, I.V.; Trubnikova, O.A.; Syrova, I.D.; Barbarash, O.L. Long-term neurophysiological outcomes in patients undergoing coronary artery bypass grafting. *Braz. J. Cardiovasc. Surg.* **2021**, *36*, 629–638. [CrossRef]
10. Hu, W.S.; Lin, C.L. Postoperative ischemic stroke and death prediction with CHA2DS2-VASc score in patients having coronary artery bypass grafting surgery: A nationwide cohort study. *Int. J. Cardiol.* **2017**, *241*, 120–123. [CrossRef]
11. Bukauskienė, R.; Širvinskas, E.; Lenkutis, T.; Benetis, R.; Steponavičiūtė, R. The influence of blood flow velocity changes to postoperative cognitive dysfunction development in patients undergoing heart surgery with cardiopulmonary bypass. *Perfusion* **2020**, *35*, 672–679. [CrossRef] [PubMed]
12. Fink, H.A.; Hemmy, L.S.; MacDonald, R.; Carlyle, M.H.; Olson, C.M.; Dysken, M.W.; McCarten, J.R.; Kane, R.L.; Garcia, S.A.; Rutks, I.R.; et al. Intermediate-and long-term cognitive outcomes after cardiovascular procedures in older adults: A systematic review. *Ann. Intern. Med.* **2015**, *163*, 107–117. [CrossRef] [PubMed]
13. Patel, N.; Minhas, J.S.; Chung, E.M.L. Risk factors associated with cognitive decline after cardiac surgery: A systematic review. *Cardiovasc. Psychiatry Neurol.* **2015**, *2015*, 370612. [CrossRef] [PubMed]
14. Trubnikova, O.A.; Tarasova, I.V.; Moskin, E.G.; Kupriyanova, D.S.; Argunova, Y.A.; Pomeshkina, S.A.; Gruzdeva, O.V.; Barbarash, O.L. Beneficial effects of a short course of physical prehabilitation on neurophysiological functioning and neurovascular biomarkers in patients undergoing coronary artery bypass grafting. *Front. Aging Neurosci.* **2021**, *13*, 699259. [CrossRef]
15. Nobari, H.; Rezaei, S.; Sheikh, M.; Fuentes-García, J.P.; Pérez-Gómez, J. Effect of virtual reality exercises on the cognitive status and dual motor task performance of the aging population. *Int. J. Environ. Res. Public Health* **2021**, *18*, 8005. [CrossRef]
16. Hassandra, M.; Galanis, E.; Hatzigeorgiadis, A.; Goudas, M.; Mouzakidis, C.; Karathanasi, E.M.; Petridou, N.; Tsolaki, M.; Zikas, P.; Evangelou, G.; et al. A virtual reality app for physical and cognitive training of older people with mild cognitive impairment: Mixed methods feasibility study. *JMIR Serious Games* **2021**, *9*, e24170. [CrossRef]
17. Stillman, C.M.; Esteban-Cornejo, I.; Brown, B.; Bender, C.M.; Erickson, K.I. Effects of exercise on brain and cognition across age groups and health states. *Trends Neurosci.* **2020**, *43*, 533–543. [CrossRef]
18. Landry, T.; Huang, H. Mini Review: The relationship between energy status and adult hippocampal neurogenesis. *Neurosci. Lett.* **2021**, *765*, 136261. [CrossRef]
19. Yu, H.; Zhang, C.; Xia, J.; Xu, B. Treadmill exercise ameliorates adult hippocampal neurogenesis possibly by adjusting the APP proteolytic pathway in APP/PS1 transgenic mice. *Int. J. Mol. Sci.* **2021**, *22*, 9570. [CrossRef]
20. Petrigna, L.; Thomas, E.; Gentile, A.; Paoli, A.; Pajaujiene, S.; Palma, A.; Bianco, A. The evaluation of dual-task conditions on static postural control in the older adults: A systematic review and meta-analysis protocol. *Syst. Rev.* **2019**, *8*, 188. [CrossRef]

21. Stelzel, C.; Bohle, H.; Schauenburg, G.; Walter, H.; Granacher, U.; Rapp, M.A.; Heinzel, S. Contribution of the lateral prefrontal cortex to cognitive-postural multi-tasking. *Front. Psychol.* **2018**, *9*, 1075. [CrossRef] [PubMed]
22. Lim, S.B.; Peters, S.; Yang, C.L.; Boyd, L.A.; Liu-Ambrose, T.; Eng, J.J. Frontal, sensorimotor, and posterior parietal regions are involved in dual-task walking after stroke. *Front. Neurol.* **2022**, *13*, 904145. [CrossRef] [PubMed]
23. Erdoes, G.; Rummel, C.; Basciani, R.M.; Verma, R.; Carrel, T.; Banz, Y.; Eberle, B.; Schroth, G. Limitations of current near-infrared spectroscopy configuration in detecting focal cerebral ischemia during cardiac surgery: An observational case-series study. *Artif. Organs.* **2018**, *42*, 1001–1009. [CrossRef]
24. Safan, A.S.; Imam, Y.; Akhtar, N.; Al-Taweel, H.; Zakaria, A.; Quateen, A.; Own, A.; Kamran, S. Acute ischemic stroke and convexity subarachnoid hemorrhage in large vessel atherosclerotic stenosis: Case series and review of the literature. *Clin. Case Rep.* **2022**, *10*, e5968. [CrossRef] [PubMed]
25. Heath, M.; Weiler, J.; Gregory, M.A.; Gill, D.P.; Petrella, R.J. A six-month cognitive-motor and aerobic exercise program improves executive function in persons with an objective cognitive impairment: A pilot investigation using the anti-saccade task. *J. Alzheimers Dis.* **2016**, *54*, 923–931. [CrossRef] [PubMed]
26. Hsu, C.L.; Best, J.R.; Davis, J.C.; Nagamatsu, L.S.; Wang, S.; Boyd, L.A.; Hsiung, G.R.; Voss, M.W.; Eng, J.J.; Liu-Ambrose, T. Aerobic exercise promotes executive functions and impacts functional neural activity among older adults with vascular cognitive impairment. *Br. J. Sports Med.* **2018**, *52*, 184–191. [CrossRef]
27. Ansai, J.H.; Andrade, L.P.; Rossi, P.G.; Almeida, M.L.; Carvalho Vale, F.A.; Rebelatto, J.R. Association between gait and dual task with cognitive domains in older people with cognitive impairment. *J. Mot. Behav.* **2018**, *50*, 409–415. [CrossRef]
28. Kleiner, A.F.R.; Souza Pagnussat, A.; Pinto, C.; Redivo Marchese, R.; Salazar, A.P.; Galli, M. Automated mechanical peripheral stimulation effects on gait variability in individuals with Parkinson disease and freezing of gait: A double-blind, randomized controlled trial. *Arch. Phys. Med. Rehabil.* **2018**, *99*, 2420–2429. [CrossRef]
29. Commandeur, D.; Klimstra, M.D.; MacDonald, S.; Inouye, K.; Cox, M.; Chan, D.; Hundza, S.R. Difference scores between single task and dual-task gait measures are better than clinical measures for detection of fall-risk in community-dwelling older adults. *Gait Posture* **2018**, *66*, 155–159. [CrossRef]
30. Syrova, I.D.; Tarasova, I.V.; Trubnikova, O.A.; Kupriyanova, D.S.; Sosnina, A.S.; Temnikova, T.B.; Barbarash, O.L. A multitask approach to prevention of the cognitive decline after coronary artery bypass grafting: A prospective randomized controlled study. *J. Xiangya Med.* **2023**, *8*, 2. [CrossRef]
31. Law, L.L.; Barnett, F.; Yau, M.K.; Gray, M.A. Effects of combined cognitive and exercise interventions on cognition in older adults with and without cognitive impairment: A systematic review. *Ageing Res. Rev.* **2014**, *15*, 61–75. [CrossRef] [PubMed]
32. Wiśniowska, J.; Łojek, E.; Olejnik, A.; Chabuda, A. The characteristics of the reduction of interference effect during dual-task cognitive-motor training compared to a single task cognitive and motor training in elderly: A randomized controlled trial. *Int. J. Environ. Res. Public Health* **2023**, *20*, 1477. [CrossRef]
33. Zhavoronkova, L.A.; Maksakova, O.A.; Shevtsova, T.P.; Moraresku, S.I.; Kuptsova, S.V.; Kushnir, E.M.; Iksanova, E.M. Dvoĭnye zadachi–indikator osobennosteĭ kognitivnogo defitsita u patsientov posle cherepno-mozgovoĭ travmy [Dual-tasks is an indicator of cognitive deficit specificity in patients after traumatic brain injury]. *Zh. Nevrol. Psikhiatr. Im. S. S. Korsakova.* **2019**, *119*, 46–52. [CrossRef] [PubMed]
34. Wajda, D.A.; Mirelman, A.; Hausdorff, J.M.; Sosnoff, J.J. Intervention modalities for targeting cognitive-motor interference in individuals with neurodegenerative disease: A systematic review. *Expert. Rev. Neurother.* **2017**, *17*, 251–261. [CrossRef] [PubMed]
35. Ozdemir, R.A.; Contreras-Vidal, J.L.; Lee, B.C.; Paloski, W.H. Cortical activity modulations underlying age-related performance differences during posture-cognition dual tasking. *Exp. Brain Res.* **2016**, *234*, 3321–3334. [CrossRef]
36. Anguera, J.A.; Boccanfuso, J.; Rintoul, J.L.; Al-Hashimi, O.; Faraji, F.; Janowich, J.; Kong, E.; Larraburo, Y.; Rolle, C.; Johnston, E.; et al. Video game training enhances cognitive control in older adults. *Nature* **2013**, *501*, 97–101. [CrossRef]
37. Nguyen, L.; Murphy, K.; Andrews, G. Cognitive and neural plasticity in old age: A systematic review of evidence from executive functions cognitive training. *Ageing Res. Rev.* **2019**, *53*, 100912. [CrossRef]
38. Wollesen, B.; Voelcker-Rehage, C. Differences in cognitive-motor interference in older adults while walking and performing a visual-verbal stroop task. *Front. Aging Neurosci.* **2019**, *10*, 426. [CrossRef]
39. Mack, M.; Stojan, R.; Bock, O.; Voelcker-Rehage, C. Cognitive-motor multi-tasking in older adults: A randomized controlled study on the effects of individual differences on training success. *BMC Geriatr.* **2022**, *22*, 581. [CrossRef]
40. Brahms, M.; Heinzel, S.; Rapp, M.; Reisner, V.; Wahmkow, G.; Rimpel, J.; Schauenburg, G.; Stelzel, C.; Granacher, U. Cognitive-Postural Multi-tasking Training in Older Adults—Effects of Input-Output Modality Mappings on Cognitive Performance and Postural Control. *J. Cogn.* **2021**, *4*, 20. [CrossRef]
41. Bohle, H.; Rimpel, J.; Schauenburg, G.; Gebel, A.; Stelzel, C.; Heinzel, S.; Rapp, M.; Granacher, U. Behavioral and neural correlates of cognitive-motor interference during multi-tasking in young and old adults. *Neural. Plast.* **2019**, *2019*, 9478656. [CrossRef] [PubMed]
42. Heinzel, S.; Rimpel, J.; Stelzel, C.; Rapp, M.A. Transfer effects to a multimodal dual-task after working memory training and associated neural correlates in older adults—A pilot study. *Front. Hum. Neurosci.* **2017**, *11*, 85. [CrossRef] [PubMed]
43. Li, K.Z.H.; Bherer, L.; Mirelman, A.; Maidan, I.; Hausdorff, J.M. Cognitive Involvement in balance, gait and dual-tasking in aging: A focused review from a neuroscience of aging perspective. *Front. Neurol.* **2018**, *9*, 913. [CrossRef] [PubMed]

4. Maggio, M.G.; De Luca, R.; Molonia, F.; Porcari, B.; Destro, M.; Casella, C.; Salvati, R.; Bramanti, P.; Calabro, R.S. Cognitive rehabilitation in patients with traumatic brain injury: A narrative review on the emerging use of virtual reality. *J. Clin. Neurosci.* **2019**, *61*, 1–4. [CrossRef] [PubMed]
5. Liao, Y.Y.; Chen, I.H.; Lin, Y.J.; Chen, Y.; Hsu, W.C. Effects of virtual reality-based physical and cognitive training on executive function and dual-task gait performance in older adults with mild cognitive impairment: A randomized control trial. *Front. Aging Neurosci.* **2019**, *11*, 162. [CrossRef] [PubMed]

Disclaimer/Publisher's Note: The statements, opinions and data contained in all publications are solely those of the individual author(s) and contributor(s) and not of MDPI and/or the editor(s). MDPI and/or the editor(s) disclaim responsibility for any injury to people or property resulting from any ideas, methods, instructions or products referred to in the content.

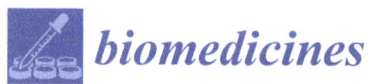

Article

Antidiabetic Molecule Efficacy in Patients with Type 2 Diabetes Mellitus—A Real-Life Clinical Practice Study

Teodor Salmen [1,*], Ali Abbas Rizvi [2,*], Manfredi Rizzo [3], Valeria-Anca Pietrosel [4], Ioana-Cristina Bica [1], Cosmina Theodora Diaconu [1], Claudia Gabriela Potcovaru [1], Bianca-Margareta Salmen [1], Oana Andreia Coman [5], Anca Bobircă [6], Roxana-Adriana Stoica [7] and Anca Pantea Stoian [4,7]

1 Doctoral School of Carol Davila, University of Medicine and Pharmacy, 020021 Bucharest, Romania
2 Department of Medicine, University of Central Florida College of Medicine, Orlando, FL 32827, USA
3 School of Medicine, Department of Health Promotion Sciences Maternal and Infantile Care, Internal Medicine and Medical Specialties (Promise), University of Palermo, 90133 Palermo, Italy
4 Department of Diabetes, Nutrition and Metabolic Diseases, "Prof. Dr N.C. Paulescu" National Institute of Diabetes, Nutrition and Metabolic Diseases, 030167 Bucharest, Romania
5 Department of Pharmacology and Pharmacotherapy, Faculty of Medicine, Carol Davila University of Medicine and Pharmacy, 020021 Bucharest, Romania
6 Internal Medicine and Rheumatology Department, Carol Davila University of Medicine and Pharmacy, 050474 Bucharest, Romania
7 Department of Diabetes, Nutrition and Metabolic Diseases, Carol Davila University of Medicine and Pharmacy, 050474 Bucharest, Romania
* Correspondence: teodor.salmen@drd.umfcd.ro (T.S.); ali.rizvi@ucf.edu (A.A.R.)

Citation: Salmen, T.; Rizvi, A.A.; Rizzo, M.; Pietrosel, V.-A.; Bica, I.-C.; Diaconu, C.T.; Potcovaru, C.G.; Salmen, B.-M.; Coman, O.A.; Bobircă, A.; et al. Antidiabetic Molecule Efficacy in Patients with Type 2 Diabetes Mellitus—A Real-Life Clinical Practice Study. *Biomedicines* **2023**, *11*, 2455. https://doi.org/10.3390/biomedicines11092455

Academic Editors: Alfredo Caturano and Antonio Andrés

Received: 3 August 2023
Revised: 25 August 2023
Accepted: 31 August 2023
Published: 4 September 2023

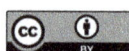

Copyright: © 2023 by the authors. Licensee MDPI, Basel, Switzerland. This article is an open access article distributed under the terms and conditions of the Creative Commons Attribution (CC BY) license (https:// creativecommons.org/licenses/by/ 4.0/).

Abstract: In this paper, we aim to evaluate the efficacy of antidiabetic cardioprotective molecules such as Sodium-Glucose Cotransporter-2 Inhibitors (SGLT-2i) and Glucagon-like Peptide 1 Receptor Agonists (GLP-1 RAs) when used with other glucose-lowering drugs, lipid-lowering, and blood pressure (BP)-lowering drugs in a real-life setting. A retrospective, observational study on 477 patients admitted consecutively in 2019 to the outpatient clinic of a tertiary care unit for Diabetes Mellitus was conducted. Body mass index (BMI), blood pressure (BP) (both systolic and diastolic), and metabolic parameters, as well as A1c hemoglobin, fasting glycaemia and lipid profile, including total cholesterol (C), HDL-C, LDL-C, and triglycerides), were evaluated at baseline and two follow-up visits were scheduled (6 months and 12 months) in order to assess the antidiabetic medication efficacy. Both SGLT-2i and GLP-1 RAs were efficient in terms of weight control reflected by BMI; metabolic control suggested by fasting glycaemia and A1c; and the diastolic component of BP control when comparing the data from the 6 and 12-month visits to the baseline, and when comparing the 12-month visit to the 6-month visit. Moreover, when comparing SGLT-2i and GLP-1 RAs with metformin, there are efficacy data for SGLT-2i at baseline in terms of BMI, fasting glycaemia, and HbA1c. In this retrospective study, both classes of cardioprotective molecules, when used in conjunction with other glucose-lowering, antihypertensive, and lipid-lowering medications, appeared to be efficient in a real-life setting for the management of T2DM.

Keywords: treatment; real-life; diabetes mellitus; sodium-glucose cotransporter-2 inhibitors; glucagon-like peptide-1 receptor agonist

1. Introduction

Modern society is facing an accelerating rate of obesity and type 2 diabetes mellitus (DM) due to changes in diet and lifestyle [1,2]. Longer lifespans and sedentary living are leading to an increase in chronic illnesses that require multiple medications [2]. In this context, polypharmacy is generally referred to as the use of more than five medications per day per patient [3,4]. The high numbers of administered drugs oblige healthcare providers to carefully choose them and, more importantly, to recommend efficient and personalized treatments [5].

Type 2 DM (T2DM) is a complex disease characterized by a hyperglycaemic state with an increased risk of microvascular complications, such as retinopathy, nephropathy, or neuropathy; macrovascular complications such as atherosclerotic disease (peripheral artery disease, ischemic stroke, or coronary artery disease); and cognitive impairment or adverse reactions (AR) from the antidiabetic drugs [6], which all lead to an overwhelming burden. Given the high risk for complications, need for hospitalization, and the all-cause mortality, the current recommendations are to personalize the treatment in order to achieve individualized metabolic targets while addressing the patients' concomitant comorbidities [6,7].

DM and especially T2DM are characterized by heterogeneity both in pathophysiological and in clinical features, a fact that is emphasized by the recent tendency to cluster patients into subgroups based on disease progression and onset of DM-related complications, including retinopathy, neuropathy, chronic kidney disease, cardiovascular (CV) disease, and NAFLD. Therefore, personalized management of cases, including prevention and treatment methods, should be pursued, but more studies in this direction are required [8].

SGLT-2i and GLP-1 RAs are antidiabetic drugs that are proven to be efficient in achieving glycaemic, metabolic, and weight control, and in reducing the risk of a composite of CV death, nonfatal myocardial infarction (MI), and nonfatal stroke—together referred to as major adverse cardiovascular events (MACE) [9,10].

Randomized control trials (RCTs) represent the gold standard in providing directions for adjusting a patient's management. Despite their significant usefulness, they require plentiful resources and they offer information on only a select cohort of patients in a more or less controlled setting; therefore, real-life studies are needed in order to provide complementary data to RCTs [11,12].

The aim of this study was to evaluate the efficacy of two classes of glucose-lowering medications, namely SGLT-2i and GLP-1 RAs, for the treatment of T2DM when used in a real-life clinical practice with other glucose, blood pressure (BP), and lipid-lowering medication.

2. Materials and Methods

This retrospective, observational study was conducted in accordance with the Declaration of Helsinki and approved by the Institutional Ethics Committee of N Paulescu National Institute for Diabetes Mellitus, Nutrition and Metabolic Disorders, Bucharest, Romania (protocol number 5591, from 17 November 2022). From the 477 patients that were consecutively admitted in 2019 to the "N. Paulescu" National Institute for Diabetes Mellitus, Nutrition and Metabolic Disorders' Outpatient Department, 16 patients discontinued their treatment early due to AR, 56 patients refused or were unable to attend baseline visits, and at least one of the control visits and 405 patients met the inclusion criteria. Figure 1 synthetizes the analysis of those patients who was intended to receive treatment, the pre-study drop-outs, those lost for follow-up, and those who discontinued treatment due to AR.

The inclusion criteria are extensively presented in Table 1 and comprise adult patients with at least a 6-month duration of T2DM prior to admission, treated in a standard-of-care regimen for 6 months prior to the baseline visit, and who received at least one of the BP-lowering or lipid-lowering drugs of interest. The included patients had to attend at minimum two of the three visits of interest which were, respectively, a baseline visit (mandatory) (V0M), a plus 6-month visit (V6M) or a plus 12-month visit (V12M), or both a plus V6M and V12M. Furthermore, patients were assigned to one of three groups depending on their non-insulinic treatment for DM which were, respectively, metformin, metformin plus SGLT-2i, and metformin plus GLP-1 Ra. The exclusion criteria are also presented in Table 1 and include non-adult patients with other types of DM.

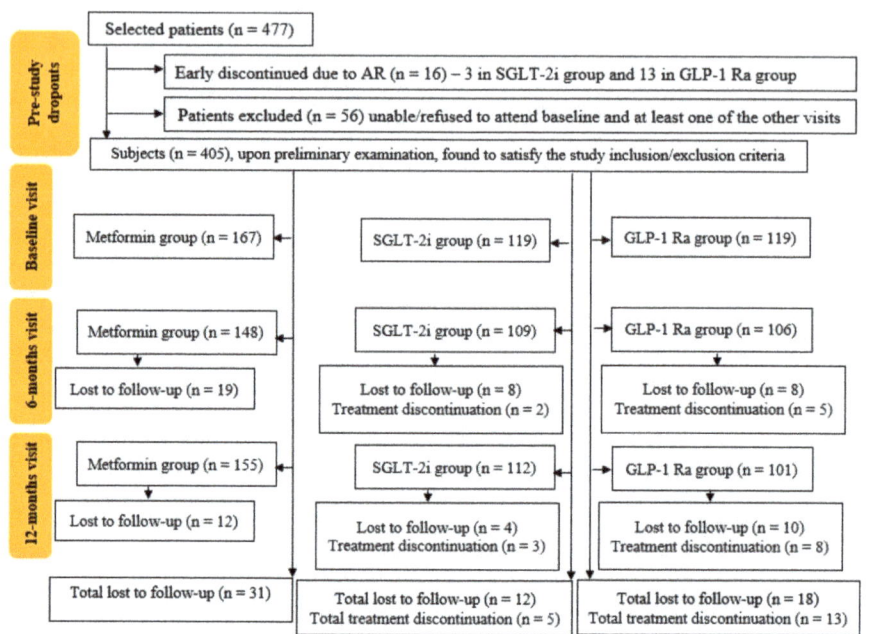

Figure 1. Patient selection and inclusion process. AR—adverse reaction; SGLT-2i—sodium glucose loop transporter 2 inhibitor; GLP-1 RA—glucagon-like peptide 1 receptor agonist.

Table 1. Inclusion and exclusion criteria.

Inclusion Criteria	Exclusion Criteria
Adults > 18 years old	Younger than 18 years old
Duration of T2DM > 6 months	Type 1 DM or secondary DM
Standard-of-care treatment for T2DM with maximum tolerated doses > 6 months prior to inclusion	Severe/acute heart failure, renal insufficiency or hepatic insufficiency
At least two visits from V0M, V6M and V12M	
Treatment with BB and/or CCB and/or ARB/ACEI and/or statin	

DM—diabetes mellitus; T2DM—type 2 diabetes mellitus; V0M—baseline visit; V6M—6 months visit; V12M—12 months visit; BB—beta-blockers; CCB—calcium-channel blockers; ARB—angiotensin receptor blockers; ACEI—angiotensin converting enzyme inhibitors.

The drugs of interest from the SGLT-2i and GLP-1 RA classes are the ones that were available and approved by the National Drug Association at the time of the study, beginning with empagliflozin and dapagliflozin for SGLT-2i, and dulaglutide, lixisenatide, and exenatide for GLP-1 RAs.

Patients' real-life data regarding their demographic parameters (e.g., age, gender, and settlement), clinical examination (BMI, heart rate-HR, systolic, and diastolic BP), comorbidities (e.g., high BP and dyslipidemia, etc.), paraclinical profile (fasting glycaemia, A1c, total-C, HDL-C, LDL-C, and TG), and data about the treatment (antidiabetic, BP-lowering, and lipid-lowering drugs) at V0M, V6M, and V12M were collected from the electronic database of the N. Paulescu National Institute for Diabetes Mellitus, Nutrition and Metabolic Disorders, Bucharest, Romania. Using Excel software 2019th version and SPSS software, 20th version, the data were statistically analyzed using the Kolmogorov–Smirnov test for normality, ANOVA test for baseline characteristics comparison, and student t-test for comparison between visits if the variables had normal distribution, as well as a Wilcoxon test and Kruskal–Wallis tests for non-normal distributions.

3. Results

Detailed data regarding the included patients' participation, demographics, comorbidities, and treatment for the molecules of interest are shown in Table 2. The Romanian standard–of–care treatment regarding the maximum tolerated dose for T2DM for the metformin group is represented by metformin, or metformin plus insulin; in the SGLT-2i group by metformin plus SGLT-2i or metformin plus SGLT-2i plus insulin; in the GLP-1 RA group by metformin plus GLP-1 RAs plus insulin, as shown in Table 2; and, alongside with CV treatment of interest, respectively, beta-blockers (BB), calcium-channel blockers (CCB), angiotensin-converting enzyme inhibitors/angiotensin receptor blockers (ACEI/ARB) or statins and, when needed, diuretics.

Table 2. Data about the patient's participation at visits, demographic and standard-of-care treatment for T2DM and cardiovascular (CV) treatment of interest.

	Metformin	SGLT-2i	GLP-1Ras	
No of patients (% of total)	167 (41.2%)	119 (29.4%)	119 (29.4%)	
No of patients at V6M (% of group)	148 (88.62%)	109 (91.59%)	106 (89.07%)	
No of patients at V12M (% of group)	155 (92.81%)	112 (94.11%)	101 (84.87%)	
Insulin treatment (%)	16 (9.58%)	15 (12.6%)	61 (51.26%)	$p < 0.001$, $\eta^2 = 0.24$
Female (%)	65 (38.9%)	34 (71.4%)	57 (47.9%)	$p = 0.009$, $\eta^2 = 0.023$
Mean age (years) [mean ± SD]	57 ± 10	56 ± 10	59 ± 9	$p = 0.185$, $\eta^2 = 0.008$
Urban settlement (%)	113 (67.66%)	98 (82.35%)	88 (73.95%)	$p < 0.001$, $\eta^2 < 0.001$
Active smoker (%)	29 (17.36%)	15 (12.6%)	27 (22.68%)	$p = 0.281$, $\eta^2 = 0.006$
Chronic kidney disease (%)	14 (8.38%)	15 (12.6%)	20 (16.80%)	$p = 0.097$, $\eta^2 = 0.012$
Heart failure (%)	10 (5.98%)	14 (11.76%)	8 (6.72%)	$p = 0.174$, $\eta^2 = 0.009$
BB (%)	94 (56.28%)	78 (65.54%)	74 (62.18%)	$p = 0.268$, $\eta^2 = 0.007$
CCB (%)	43 (25.74%)	28 (23.52%)	28 (23.52%)	$p = 0.818$, $\eta^2 = 0.01$
ACEI/ARB (%)	104 (62.27%)	84 (70.58%)	94 (78.98%)	$p = 0.01$, $\eta^2 = 0.023$
Statin (%)	135 (80.83%)	104 (87.39%)	106 (89%)	$p = 0.112$, $\eta^2 = 0.011$
Diuretics (%)	73 (43.71%)	36 (30.25%)	43 (36.13%)	$p = 0.181$, $\eta^2 = 0.008$

SGLT-2i—sodium glucose loop transporter 2 inhibitor; GLP-1 Ras—glucagon-like peptide 1 receptor agonist; V6M—6-month visit; V12M—12-month visits; BB—beta-blockers; CCB—calcium channel blockers; ACEI—angiotensin converting enzyme inhibitors; ARB—angiotensin receptor blockers; SD—standard deviation.

The baseline visit (V0M) parameters of interest are the clinical parameters—Body mass index (BMI), heart rate (HR), systolic and diastolic BP, and the metabolic parameters—fasting glycaemia, total-cholesterol (total-C), HDL-cholesterol (HDL-C), LDL-cholesterol (LDL-C) and triglycerides (TG); these are shown in Table 3.

Table 3. The V0M parameters of interest for clinical (BMI, HR, systolic and diastolic BP) and metabolic parameters (fasting glycaemia, total-C, HDL-C, LDL-C and TG).

	Metformin (n = 167)		SGLT-2i (n = 119)		GLP-1Ras (n = 119)		
BMI (kg/m^2) [mean ± SD]	31.8 ± 5.8	$p = 0.672$	35.5 ± 6.5	$p = 0.209$	32.1 ± 6.1	$p = 0.022$	$p < 0.001$, $\eta^2 = 0.067$
Systolic BP (mmHg) [mean ± SD]	133.4 ± 12.8	$p = 0.004$	131.7 ± 13.4	$p = 0.009$	131.4 ± 1	$p = 0.022$	$p = 0.377$, $\eta^2 = 0.05$
Diastolic BP (mmHg) [mean ± SD]	80.4 ± 8.7	$p < 0.001$	79.7 ± 12.7	$p < 0.001$	79.3 ± 8.8	$p < 0.001$	$p = 0.63$, $\eta^2 = 0.002$
HR (beat per minute) [mean ± SD]	78 ± 11	$p < 0.001$	77 ± 12	$p = 0.009$	73 ± 8	$p = 0.23$	$p < 0.001$, $\eta^2 = 0.041$
Fasting glycaemia (mg/dL) [mean ± SD]	155.4 ± 48.4	$p = 0.026$	170.6 ± 66.1	$p = 0.006$	155.7 ± 49.5	$p = 0.003$	$p = 0.041$, $\eta^2 = 0.016$
HbA1c (%) [mean ± SD]	7.4 ± 1.2	$p = 0.006$	8.1 ± 1.5	$p = 0.068$	7.4 ± 1.4	$p = 0.044$	$p < 0.001$, $\eta^2 = 0.05$

Table 3. Cont.

	Metformin (n = 167)		SGLT-2i (n = 119)		GLP-1Ras (n = 119)		
Total-C (mg/dL) *	172 (52)	$p = 0.236$	161 (61)	$p = 0.595$	168 (60)	$p = 0.654$	$p = 0.215, \eta^2 = 0.008$
HDL-C (mg/dL) [mean ± SD]	46 ± 12	$p = 0.008$	43 ± 16	$p < 0.001$	44 ± 13	$p = 0.11$	$p = 0.182, \eta^2 = 0.008$
LDL-C (mg/dL) *	92 (41)	$p = 0.232$	98 (47)	$p = 0.168$	91 (53)	$p = 0.403$	$p = 0.816, \eta^2 = 0.001$
TG (mg/dL) *	170 (103)	$p = 0.004$	172 (115)	$p = 0.002$	170 (82)	$p < 0.001$	$p = 0.419, \eta^2 = 0.004$

SGLT-2i—sodium glucose loop transporter 2 inhibitor; GLP-1 RA—glucagon like peptide 1 receptor agonist; total-cholesterol—total-C; HDL-cholesterol—HDL-C; LDL-cholesterol—LDL-C; TG—triglycerides; SD—standard deviation. *—where the baseline distribution was not normal, we reported the data as median and interquartile range.

The 6-month visit (V6M) parameters of interest are the clinical parameters—BMI, HR, systolic and diastolic BP, and the metabolic parameters—fasting glycaemia, total-C, HDL-C, LDL-C and TG; these are shown in Table 4.

Table 4. The V6M parameters of interest for clinical (BMI, HR, systolic and diastolic BP) and metabolic parameters (fasting glycaemia, total-C, HDL-C, LDL-C, TG).

	Metformin (n = 148)		SGLT-2i (n = 109)		GLP-1Ras (n = 106)	
BMI (kg/m^2) [mean ± SD]	31.3 ± 5.9	$p = 0.756$	31.6 ± 5.5	$p = 0.96$	31.5 ± 5.8	$p = 0.022$
Systolic BP (mmHg) [mean ± SD]	133.1 ± 12.8	$p = 0.004$	133.1 ± 12.8	$p = 0.017$	130.7 ± 16.1	$p = 0.08$
Diastolic BP (mmHg) [mean ± SD]	80.8 ± 9.9	$p < 0.001$	81.6 ± 10.1	$p < 0.001$	76.9 ± 9.7	$p < 0.001$
HR (beat per minute) [mean ± SD]	77 ± 9	$p = 0.009$	76 ± 9	$p = 0.015$	73 ± 8	$p = 0.782$
Fasting glycaemia (mg/dL) [mean ± SD]	136.8 ± 36.1	$p = 0.357$	133.9 ± 35.3	$p = 0.282$	135.4 ± 35.3	$p = 0.099$
HbA1c (%) [mean ± SD]	7.1 ± 1.2	$p = 0.002$	7 ± 1.2	$p = 0.027$	7.1 ± 1.3	$p = 0.02$
Total-C (mg/dL) *	170 (60)	$p = 0.32$	167 (61)	$p = 0.23$	164 (55)	$p = 0.345$
HDL-C (mg/dL) [mean ± SD]	46 ± 11	$p = 0.029$	47 ± 12	$p = 0.117$	45 ± 11	$p = 0.855$
LDL-C (mg/dL) *	92 (52)	$p = 0.425$	88 (50)	$p = 0.266$	90 (50)	$p = 0.081$
TG (mg/dL) *	156 (120)	$p = 0.132$	142 (123)	$p = 0.171$	154 (91)	$p = 0.026$

SGLT-2i—sodium glucose loop transporter 2 inhibitor; GLP-1 RA—glucagon like peptide 1 receptor agonist; total-cholesterol—total-C; HDL-cholesterol—HDL-C; LDL-cholesterol—LDL-C; TG—triglycerides; SD—standard deviation. *—where the baseline distribution was not normal, we reported the data as median and interquartile range.

The 12-month visit (V12M) parameters of interest are the clinical parameters—BMI, HR, systolic and diastolic BP, and the metabolic parameters—fasting glycaemia, total-C, HDL-C, LDL-C, and TG; these are shown in Table 5.

Table 5. The V12M parameters of interest for clinical (BMI, HR, systolic and diastolic BP) and metabolic parameters (fasting glycaemia, total-C, HDL-C, LDL-C, TG).

	Metformin (n = 155)		SGLT-2i (n = 112)		GLP-1RAs (n = 101)	
BMI (kg/m^2) [mean ± SD]	31.0 ± 5.8	$p = 0.582$	31.2 ± 5.4	$p = 0.78$	31.3 ± 5.7	$p = 0.05$
Systolic BP (mmHg) [mean ± SD]	133.2 ± 13.0	$p = 0.005$	132 ± 12.7	$p = 0.011$	130 ± 13.6	$p = 0.029$
Diastolic BP (mmHg) [mean ± SD]	79.9 ± 10.7	$p < 0.001$	80.3 ± 11.4	$p < 0.001$	76.5 ± 10.3	$p < 0.001$
HR (beat per minute) [mean ± SD]	77 ± 9	$p = 0.063$	77 ± 9	$p = 0.03$	73 ± 9	$p = 0.327$
Fasting glycaemia (mg/dL) [mean ± SD]	142.9 ± 39.5	$p = 0.157$	139.2 ± 36.8	$p = 0.262$	146 ± 50.7	$p = 0.007$
HbA1c (%) [mean ± SD]	7.1 ± 1.1	$p = 0.01$	7 ± 1	$p = 0.073$	7.1 ± 1	$p = 0.023$
Total-C (mg/dL) *	173 (57)	$p = 0.035$	165 (58)	$p = 0.053$	166 (62)	$p = 0.508$
HDL-C (mg/dL) [mean ± SD]	47 ± 12	$p = 0.019$	48 ± 12	$p = 0.096$	45 ± 13	$p = 0.212$
LDL-C (mg/dL) *	92 (43)	$p = 0.064$	87 (39)	$p = 0.091$	91 (50)	$p = 0.504$
TG (mg/dL) *	162 (103)	$p = 0.017$	140 (100)	$p = 0.095$	152 (85)	$p = 0.017$

SGLT-2i—sodium glucose loop transporter 2 inhibitor; GLP-1 RA—glucagon like peptide 1 receptor agonist; total-cholesterol—total-C; HDL-cholesterol—HDL-C; LDL-cholesterol—LDL-C; TG—triglycerides; SD—standard deviation. *—where the baseline distribution was not normal, we reported the data as median and interquartile range.

The patients were evaluated both clinically (BMI, systolic and diastolic BP, and HR) and paraclinically (fasting glycaemia, HbA1c, total-C, HDL-C, LDL-C, and TG) at V6M and at V12M as compared to V0M, and at V12M as compared to V6M; the results are synthetized in Table 6. They had at least one statistically significant value with $p < 0.05$, while for systolic BP, HR, total-C, and HDL-C there were no significant differences.

Table 6. Clinical (BMI, diastolic BP) and paraclinical (fasting glycaemia, HbA1c, HDL-cholesterol and tryglicerides) at V6M and at V12M as compared to V0M, and at V12M as compared to V6M.

	Metformin		SGLT-2i		GLP-1 RAs	
	Mean Difference		Mean Difference		Mean Difference	
	V6M compared to V0M					
BMI (kg/m^2)	0.5 ± 0.09	$p < 0.001$	3.9 ± 0.78	$p < 0.001$	0.6 ± 0.1	$p < 0.001$
Diastolic BP (mmHg)	0.4 ± 0.8	$p = 0.380$	1.9 ± 1.3	$p = 0.151$	2.4 ± 0.8	$p = 0.013$
Fasting glycaemia (mg/dL)	18.6 ± 3.8	$p < 0.001$	36.7 ± 7.4	$p < 0.001$	20.3 ± 4.6	$p < 0.001$
HbA1c (%)	0.3 ± 0.1	$p = 0.018$	1.1 ± 0.2	$p < 0.001$	0.3 ± 0.1	$p = 0.01$
HDL-cholesterol (mg/dL)	0 ± 0.6	$p = 0.765$	4 ± 2	$p < 0.001$	0 ± 0.8	$p = 0.895$
Triglycerides (mg/dL)	4 ± 8.3	$p = 0.38$	30 ± 12.5	$p = 0.023$	2 ± 12.2	$p = 0.258$
	V12M compared to V0M					
BMI (kg/m^2)	0.3 ± 0.1	$p < 0.001$	4.3 ± 0.75	$p < 0.001$	0.8 ± 0.1	$p < 0.001$
Diastolic BP (mmHg)	0.9 ± 0.9	$p = 0.728$	0.6 ± 1.3	$p = 0.314$	2.8 ± 1.1	$p = 0.008$
Fasting glycaemia (mg/dL)	6.1 ± 4	$p = 0.018$	31.4 ± 7.2	$p = 0.001$	9.7 ± 5.2	$p = 0.05$
HbA1c (%)	0 ± 0.08	$p = 0.195$	1.1 ± 0.1	$p < 0.001$	0.3 ± 0.1	$p = 0.075$
HDL-cholesterol (mg/dL)	1 ± 0.7	$p = 0.056$	5 ± 2	$p < 0.001$	1 ± 0.6	$p = 0.283$
Triglycerides (mg/dL)	8 ± 8.1	$p = 0.906$	32 ± 7.2	$p = 0.019$	28 ± 12.9	$p = 0.099$
	V12M compared to V6M					
BMI (kg/m^2)	0.8 ± 0.08	$p = 0.04$	4.3 ± 0.09	$p = 0.086$	0.2 ± 0.09	$p = 0.083$
Diastolic BP (mmHg)	0.5 ± 1	$p = 0.67$	1.3 ± 1.3	$p = 0.759$	0.4 ± 1.1	$p = 0.322$
Fasting glycaemia (mg/dL)	12.5 ± 3	$p = 0.024$	31.4 ± 3.3	$p = 0.045$	10.6 ± 3.5	$p = 0.025$
HbA1c (%)	0.3 ± 0.07	$p = 0.426$	0 ± 0.9	$p = 0.952$	0 ± 0	$p = 0.24$
HDL-cholesterol (mg/dL)	1 ± 0.6	$p = 0.342$	1 ± 0.6	$p = 0.536$	1 ± 0.8	$p = 0.442$
Triglycerides (mg/dL)	6 ± 0.1	$p = 0.51$	2 ± 12.5	$p = 0.974$	16 ± 8.1	$p = 0.798$

SGLT-2i—sodium glucose loop transporter 2 inhibitor; GLP-1 RAs—glucagon like peptide 1 receptor agonist; V0M—baseline visit; V6M—6-month visit; V12M—12-month visit; BMI—body mass index; BP- blood pressure; HR—heart rate; Chol -cholesterol; TG—triglycerides.

Moreover, a comparison of the SGLT-2i and GLP-1 RA groups with the metformin group for efficacy, looking at BMI, HR, systolic and diastolic BP, HbA1c, fasting glycaemia, total-C, HDL-C, LDL-C, and TG at V0M, at V6M and at V12M are statistically significant only for BMI (3.69 ± 0.73 kg/m^2, $p < 0.001$), fasting glycaemia (15.27 ± 6.79 mg/dL, $p = 0.025$), and HbA1c (0.72 ± 0.16%, $p < 0.001$) at V0M when comparing SGLT-2i to metformin. Meanwhile, no parameter was efficient when comparing GLP-1 RAs to metformin.

To summarize our results, both SGLT-2i and GLP-1 RA are efficient in terms of weight control, reflected by patients significantly lowering their BMIs after 6 months, with a benefit that was maintained until 12 months. Additionally, metabolic control evaluated by fasting glycaemia and HbA1c improved when comparing the data from V6M and V12M to V0M, and when comparing V12M to V6M; however, only fasting glycemia had a significant decrease after 6 months. Moreover, when comparing SGLT-2i and GLP-1 RAs with metformin, efficacy data were only found for SGLT-2i at V0M for BMI, fasting glycaemia, and HbA1c as compared to metformin.

4. Discussion

Our real-world study confirms that, compared to metformin, the antidiabetic non-insulin drugs SGLT-2i and GLP-1 RAs confer extra benefits when administered in standard-of-care treatment and in association with CV drugs used for the treatment of High BP (HBP), such as BB, CCB, ACEI, or ARB, or for the treatment of dyslipidaemia, such as statins. It is important to emphasize that the two classes are reported to have cardioprotective benefits, but the complex mechanisms that lie beyond this property are still being studied.

CVOTs reported that the standard-of-care treatment that included SGLT-2i could provide benefits such as metabolic control by reducing HbA1c [13–15], ameliorating hyperglycaemia [14,16], lowering body weight [13,15,16], reducing systolic and diastolic BP [13,14,16], and ameliorating the lipid profile by reducing TG levels [13].

CVOTs that evaluated GLP-1 RAs with the standard-of-care treatment demonstrated that this class has beneficial effects on the reduction of HbA1c [17–19], fasting glycaemia [17–20], body weight [17–19], systolic and diastolic BP [17,19], and amelioration of the lipid profile [17,19] by reducing LDL-C, total-C, and TG levels.

Metformin has been used in T2DM as a first-line standard-of-care treatment for several decades [21]. Its benefits were not evaluated by CVOTs [22] because it was widely available with no severe AR, and due to its easy affordability and tolerability [23]. It has beneficial CV effects, as shown in the United Kingdom Prospective Diabetes Study (UKPDS) [23]. It is efficacious in reducing fasting glycaemia [24,25], HbA1c [25], and body weight [25,26], and has modest effects on the lipid profile, especially LDL-C and TG [26]. The following is a narrative comparison of the actions of metformin versus the GLP-1RAs and SGLT-2i agents as reported in the literature and a parallel to our study.

4.1. BMI

Metformin, one of the first-line treatment options in T2DM treatment, is reported to reduce weight by inducing satiety and improving insulin sensitivity [25–27]. For example, Zyrek et al. [28] reported a reduction in the BMI of patients with T2DM from baseline (27.29 ± 2.1 kg/m^2) to the 3-month visit (28.27 ± 2.71 kg/m^2), $p < 0.0001$, which is similar to the findings in our study when comparing BMI at V6M to V0M; V12M to V0M; and V12M to V6M (Tables 3–5).

The GLP-1 RAs are a class of antidiabetic drugs used in the treatment of T2DM and have multiple benefits such as increased satiety, reduced appetite and food intake with weight loss, and concomitant gastrointestinal effects such as slowing the gastric emptying rate and small intestinal peristalsis [17,19,20,29]. For this class, Tofé et al. [30] reported a decrease in BMI for patients with T2DM treated with GLP-1 RAs at 6 months (37.05 ± 6.1 kg/m^2) and at 12 months (37.21 ± 6.8 kg/m^2) as compared to their initial visit (38.56 ± 6.6 kg/m^2), $p < 0.001$, results that are similar to the ones from our study when comparing V6M to V0M and V12M to V0M (Tables 3–5).

Another aspect is the lack of a significant decrease in BMI between V6M and V12M. This confirms the results of previous studies [31], where the maximum decrease in BMI under GLP-1 RAs is observed after 30 weeks and then is maintained over time.

Another class of antidiabetic drugs with cardioprotective benefits that is used in the treatment of T2DM along with GLP-1 RAs are the SGLT-2i that block SGLT-2-mediated glucose reabsorption in the kidneys, resulting in glycosuria and weight loss [13,15,16,32]. In a study by Sawada et al. [33], there was a decrease in the BMI of patients with T2DM treated with SGLT-2i (without specifying the duration of treatment administration) from 30.3 ± 6.1 kg/m^2 to 29.2 ± 5.7 kg/m^2, $p < 0.001$. In our study, SGLT-2i was efficient in terms of reducing BMI at V6M as compared to V0M and at V12M as compared to V0M (Tables 3–5).

4.2. Blood Pressure

GLP-1 RAs in T2DM are reported to lower BP secondary to weight loss, increase in natriuresis, and provide better regulation of the renin–angiotensin–aldosterone system [17,19,29,34,35]. In a study by Hu et al. [35] a reduction in diastolic BP of -0.898 mmHg, $p < 0.001$, was reported in patients with T2DM treated with GLP-1 RAs, consistent with our study results, where we found a reduction at V6M as compared to V0M and V12M as compared to V0M (Tables 3–5).

BP reduction in the SGLT-2i class of patients with T2DM can be explained by decreased sodium reabsorption in the proximal renal tubule, increase in diuresis with a reduction in the plasma volume, improved arterial stiffness, and by the indirect effect of weight reduction [36,37]. The data reported by Sawada et al. [33] showed a decrease in diastolic BP in patients with T2DM treated with SGLT-2i from 74 ± 12 mmHg before initiation to 71 ± 12 mmHg afterwards, $p = 0.332$, but they did not state the duration of the follow-up.

4.3. Fasting Glycaemia

Metformin ameliorates fasting glycaemia in patients with T2DM by decreasing the hepatic glucose production and the production of reactive oxygen species, resulting in an improvement in cerebral memory and cognitive performance, along with glycaemic control [24,25,38]. In a study by Rosenstock et al. [39], there was a reported reduction in plasma glycaemic levels in patients with T2DM treated with metformin (191 ± 49 mg/dL) as compared to levels during the 26-week visit (mean reduction -35 ± 3 mg/dL). Interestingly, this is similar to our results from V6M as compared to V0M; V12M as compared to V0M; and at V12M as compared to V6M (Tables 3–5).

SGLT-2i reduces proximal glucose reabsorption in the kidney, leading to a decrease in blood glucose levels when used in patients with T2DM [40]. Singh et al. [41] reported that SGLT-2i used in the treatment of T2DM has durable efficiency in reducing glycaemic levels, which is consistent with our findings at V6M as compared to V0M; at V12M as compared to V0M; and at V12M as compared to V6M (Tables 3–5).

GLP-1 RAs ameliorate the glycaemic profile in patients with T2DM by increasing the secretion of insulin and synthesis of pancreatic islet cells, in parallel with a decrease in glucagon secretion and β-cell apoptosis [17–20,34]. In a study conducted by Tofé et al. [30] in patients with T2DM, treatment with GLP-1 RAs was efficient in reducing fasting glycaemia at 6 months (145 ± 51 mg/dL) and at 12 months (153 ± 53 mg/dL) as compared to the initial visit (177 ± 59 mg/dL), $p < 0.0001$. In our study, the differences in terms of glycaemic control were encountered at V6M as compared to V0M; at V12M as compared to V0M; and at V12M as compared to V6M (Tables 3–5).

4.4. HbA1c

Metformin reduces HbA1c in patients with T2DM [25]. Rosenstock et al. [39] reported that in patients with T2DM with initial HbA1C $\geq 8\%$, metformin therapy led to a reduction in HbA1c from $8.70 \pm 0.033\%$ to $7.57 \pm 0.08\%$ at 3 months, $p < 0.0001$, which is consistent with our results showing HbA1c at V6M as compared to V0M (Tables 3–5).

GLP-1 RAs are credited with glucose-lowering effects and with an approximately 1% reduction in HbA1c when used in patients with T2DM [17–19,34]. Tofé et al. [30] reported that GLP-1 RA therapy reduced HbA1c at 6 months ($7.24 \pm 1.45\%$) and at 12 months ($7.29 \pm 1.51\%$) as compared to the initial visit ($8.18 \pm 1.53\%$), $p < 0.0001$, in subjects with T2DM—results that are similar to our study when comparing V6M to V0M (Tables 3–5).

SGLT-2is are reported to reduce HbA1c in patients with T2DM with values that range from 0.5% to 1% [42], but the reduction can be larger as, for example, in a meta-analysis by Masson W et al., where they reported a reduction in HbA1c of -0.94% 95% CI (-1.69, -0.18), $p = 0.002$ [43], results that are similar to our study when comparing V6M with V0M and V12M with V6M.

It is important to emphasize that a possible explanation for the lower improvement in HbA1c between V12M and V6M as compared to V6M as compared to baseline could be secondary to the lower HbA1c from the baseline.

4.5. SGLT-2i, GLP-1 RAs and Metformin Comparison

Optimal management of T2DM frequently requires combination therapy with several glucose-lowering drugs. Since metformin has a long track record, it has been generally accepted as a safe and effective first-line therapy by international consensus guidelines and recommendations. Our study showed the efficacy of both SGLT-2i and GLP-1 RAs only for fasting glycaemia when compared to metformin in the treatment of T2DM as standard-of-care in patients with T2DM. The data from the literature indicate that they are also efficient for metabolic control (HbA1c, fasting glycaemia), body weight, BP lowering, and improving the lipid profile. A systematic review and meta-analysis by Milder et al. [44] compared the combination of SGLT-2i and metformin with metformin alone in the treatment of T2DM. Differences in efficacy were observed for HbA1c, with a 95% confidence interval (95% CI) of −0.55% (−0.67, −0.43), body weight with a 95% CI of −2 kg (−2.34, −1.66), and systolic and diastolic BP reduction. In a meta-analysis that also compared the differences in efficacy between SGLT-2i plus metformin with metformin alone in the treatment of T2DM, Jinfang et al. [45] reported a reduction in HbA1c with 95% CI of −0.50% (−0.62, −0.38), weight gain with a 95% CI of −1.72kg (−2.05, −1.39), systolic BP with a 95% CI of −4.44 mm Hg (−5.45, −3.43), and diastolic BP with a 95% CI of −1.74 mm Hg (−2.40, −1.07), as well as fasting plasma glucose levels of −20.16 mg/dL with a 95% CI of (−24.84, −15.66). The DISCOVER study by Khunti et al. [46] evaluated the association of metformin with sulphonylurea (SU), dipeptidyl peptidase-4 (DPP-4) inhibitors, SGLT-2i, or GLP-1 RAs and reported a significantly reduction in HbA1c and body weight for the last three groups as compared to the first one.

In a study by Hutmacher et al. [47], GLP-1 RAs plus basal insulin reduced HbA1c by −0.7% (95% CI −1.2, −0.2) when compared with basal insulin and placebo; the effects of long-acting GLP-1 RAs (−1.0%, 95% CI −1.2, −0.8) and of short-acting GLP-1 RAs (−0.5%, 95% CI −1.2, −0.8) were similar. However, it is generally believed that long-acting GLP-1 RAs are more efficient in terms of reduction in HbA1c, fasting plasma glycaemia, and body weight when compared to short-acting GLP-1 RAs.

A systematic review and meta-analysis by Patoulias et al. [48] reported that GLP-1 RAs offered better HbA1c reduction with −0.38% (95% CI −0.55, −0.22) as compared to SGLT-2i, but with similar improvements in body weight −0.29 kg (95% CI −1.24, 0.66) and fasting plasma glycaemia in T2DM. GLP-1 RAs are not superior to SGLT-2i for systolic BP 0.98 (95% CI −1, 2.97) and for diastolic BP 1.01 (95% CI −0.25, 2.27).

4.6. Future Perspectives in Efficacy of Cardioprotective Molecules

Taking into consideration the evolution of modern medicine towards precision treatment, including in the case of DM and especially in T2DM, we should not forget that the efficacy of any treatment should be reported to the type of the patient [8]. Future studies should analyze if the drugs provide different grades of efficacy due to their variable curves of efficacy or due to different cut-offs until which the patients respond, or due to the different pathophysiology of DM, different DM evolution patterns, complication onsets, or comorbidities of the patients [49,50].

Moreover, in addition to the present real-life clinical practice results in efficacy for cardioprotective antidiabetic drugs, we reported in a previous paper [51] data about their safety as part of the same research project. Clinical inertia may be the main cause for low rates of success in achieving metabolic control. However, in this project, we did not select the included patients, but enrolled them consecutively, and clinicians tend to indirectly select the patients that receive these drugs based on their medical judgement, despite the guideline recommendations and the need to move the paradigm from HbA1c control to a comprehensive metabolic control that targets weight control, lipid profile, or BP control [52], which allow for a reduction in CV risk.

Thus, there is hope for patients with T2DM because recently, in randomized multicenter, clinical studies, it was reported that the reduction in MACEs and mortality is incrementally related to the number of risk factors that reached the recommended targets [53,54].

The strengths of our study rely on gaining real-life clinical practice data for molecules that once more proves their benefits in body weight and BP control, and in helping to achieve a lipid profile and metabolic profile closer to the recommended ones as compared to the CVOT data, where the patients are more carefully selected, monitored, and treated. On the other hand, the limitations of our study include that, despite a robust association, its observational design precludes establishing a definite causal relationship, along with a relatively small number of subjects. The short period of follow-up of a maximum of three visits in a one-year duration can also explain why the only discontinuation cause was AR, while the real-life conditions brought up dietary and physical activity variation between patients, as well as different grades of adherence, which are difficult to quantify, but may influence the results; the baseline differences between treatment groups and patient selection by the diabetologists may include preferential selection of patients who are more adherent to the medical recommendations, due to the high financial burden that the treatment represents for the national health system. However, our results are promising and provide the basis for larger, randomized studies in this therapeutic area and in real-life settings, which can be performed on a longer duration to evaluate the maintenance of the effect in time or to figure out several explanations for poor efficacy, including the segregation by clusters of T2DM patients.

5. Conclusions

The present real-life study presents two classes of noninsulin antidiabetic agents, namely GLP-1 RAs and the SGLT-2i, which appear to be efficacious in the reduction in body weight reflected by BMI at 6 and 12 months as compared to baseline, along with metabolic control reflected by reducing fasting glycaemia at 6 and 12 months as compared to baseline and at 12 months as compared to the 6-month visit, and by reducing HbA1c at 6 months as compared to baseline visit when used in a real-life clinical practice setting for patients with T2DM, even in combination with therapeutic agents for treating HBP (BB, CCB, ACEI, or ARB) or for the treatment of dyslipidaemia with statins. Therefore, this study adds to the body of literature, and is close to real-world, clinical, and translational care, showing that the resultant multifactorial reduction in CV risk may prove to be highly beneficial in reducing morbidity and mortality in patients with T2DM.

Author Contributions: Conceptualization, T.S. and V.-A.P.; methodology, A.P.S. and O.A.C.; software, I.-C.B.; validation, A.A.R., M.R. and C.T.D.; formal analysis, T.S. and R.-A.S.; investigation, C.G.P. and A.B.; resources, B.-M.S.; data curation, A.P.S.; writing—original draft preparation, T.S., V.-A.P. and I.-C.B.; writing—review and editing, A.A.R., C.G.P. and C.T.D.; visualization, M.R., R.-A.S. and B.-M.S.; supervision, A.P.S.; project administration, T.S. All authors have read and agreed to the published version of the manuscript.

Funding: This research received no external funding.

Institutional Review Board Statement: The study was conducted in accordance with the Declaration of Helsinki, and approved by the Ethics Committee of the N Paulescu National Institute for Diabetes Mellitus, Nutrition and Metabolic Disorders, Bucharest, Romania (protocol number 5591, from 17 November 2022).

Informed Consent Statement: Not applicable.

Data Availability Statement: Data available on request from the corresponding authors.

Conflicts of Interest: Anca Pantea Stoian is currently the President of the Romanian National Diabetes Committee, and she has given lectures, received honoraria and research support, and participated in conferences, advisory boards, and clinical trials sponsored by many companies, including Amgen, AstraZeneca, Boehringer Ingelheim, Medtronic, MSD, Medochemie, Eli Lilly, Merck, Novo Nordisk, Novartis, Roche Diagnostics, Servier and Sanofi. Roxana Adriana Stoica has given lectures, received honoraria, and participated in conferences, sponsored by AstraZeneca, Boehringer Ingelheim, Eli Lilly, Novo Nordisk, Novartis, and Sanofi.

References

1. Matheson, G.O.; Klügl, M.; Engebretsen, L.; Bendiksen, F.; Blair, S.N.; Börjesson, M.; Budget, R.; Derman, W.; Erdener, U.; Ioannidis, J.; et al. Prevention and management of non-communicable disease: The IOC consensus statement, Lausanne 2013. *Sports Med.* **2013**, *43*, 1075–1088. [CrossRef]
2. Jakovljevic, M.; Cerda, A.A.; Liu, Y.; García, L.; Timofeyev, Y.; Krstic, K.; Fontanesi, J. Sustainability Challenge of Eastern Europe—Historical Legacy, Belt and Road Initiative, Population Aging and Migration. *Sustainability* **2021**, *13*, 11038. [CrossRef]

3. Villén, N.; Guisado-Clavero, M.; Fernández-Bertolín, S.; Troncoso-Mariño, A.; Foguet-Boreu, Q.; Amado, E.; Pons-Vigués, M.; Roso-Llorach, A.; Violán, C. Multimorbidity patterns, polypharmacy and their association with liver and kidney abnormalities in people over 65 years of age: A longitudinal study. *BMC Geriatr.* **2020**, *20*, 206. [CrossRef]
4. Papotti, B.; Marchi, C.; Adorni, M.P.; Potì, F. Drug-drug interactions in polypharmacy patients: The impact of renal impairment. *Curr. Res. Pharmacol. Drug Discov.* **2021**, *2*, 100020. [CrossRef]
5. Diaconu, C.C.; Cozma, M.A.; Dobrică, E.C.; Gheorghe, G.; Jichitu, A.; Ionescu, V.A.; Nicolae, A.C.; Drăgoi, C.M.; Găman, M.A. Polypharmacy in the Management of Arterial Hypertension-Friend or Foe? *Medicina* **2021**, *57*, 1288. [CrossRef]
6. Peron, E.P.; Ogbonna, K.C.; Donohoe, K.L. Antidiabetic medications and polypharmacy. *Clin. Geriatr. Med.* **2015**, *31*, 17–27. [CrossRef]
7. Al-Musawe, L.; Martins, A.P.; Raposo, J.F.; Torre, C. The association between polypharmacy and adverse health consequences in elderly type 2 diabetes mellitus patients; a systematic review and meta-analysis. *Diabetes Res. Clin. Pract.* **2019**, *155*, 107804. [CrossRef] [PubMed]
8. Herder, C.; Roden, M. A novel diabetes typology: Towards precision diabetology from pathogenesis to treatment. *Diabetologia* **2022**, *65*, 1770–1781. [CrossRef]
9. Marx, N.; McGuire, D.K.; Perkovic, V.; Woerle, H.J.; Broedl, U.C.; von Eynatten, M.; George, J.T.; Rosenstock, J. Composite Primary End Points in Cardiovascular Outcomes Trials Involving Type 2 Diabetes Patients: Should Unstable Angina Be Included in the Primary End Point? *Diabetes Care* **2017**, *40*, 1144–1151. [CrossRef]
10. Hupfeld, C.; Mudaliar, S. Navigating the "MACE" in Cardiovascular Outcomes Trials and decoding the relevance of Atherosclerotic Cardiovascular Disease benefits versus Heart Failure benefits. *Diabetes Obes. Metab.* **2019**, *21*, 1780–1789. [CrossRef]
11. Blonde, L.; Khunti, K.; Harris, S.B.; Meizinger, C.; Skolnik, N.S. Interpretation and Impact of Real-World Clinical Data for the Practicing Clinician. *Adv. Ther.* **2018**, *35*, 1763–1774. [CrossRef] [PubMed]
12. Katkade, V.B.; Sanders, K.N.; Zou, K.H. Real world data: An opportunity to supplement existing evidence for the use of long-established medicines in health care decision making. *J. Multidiscip. Healthc.* **2018**, *11*, 295–304. [CrossRef] [PubMed]
13. Brown, E.; Wilding, J.P.H.; Alam, U.; Barber, T.M.; Karalliedde, J.; Cuthbertson, D.J. The expanding role of SGLT2 inhibitors beyond glucose-lowering to cardiorenal protection. *Ann. Med.* **2021**, *53*, 2072–2089. [CrossRef]
14. Muscoli, S.; Barillà, F.; Tajmir, R.; Meloni, M.; Della Morte, D.; Bellia, A.; Di Daniele, N.; Lauro, D.; Andreadi, A. The New Role of SGLT2 Inhibitors in the Management of Heart Failure: Current Evidence and Future Perspective. *Pharmaceutics* **2022**, *14*, 1730. [CrossRef]
15. Jiang, Y.; Yang, P.; Fu, L.; Sun, L.; Shen, W.; Wu, Q. Comparative Cardiovascular Outcomes of SGLT2 Inhibitors in Type 2 Diabetes Mellitus: A Network Meta-Analysis of Randomized Controlled Trials. *Front. Endocrinol.* **2022**, *13*, 802992. [CrossRef]
16. Ni, L.; Yuan, C.; Chen, G.; Zhang, C.; Wu, X. SGLT2i: Beyond the glucose-lowering effect. *Cardiovasc. Diabetol.* **2020**, *19*, 98. [CrossRef] [PubMed]
17. Caruso, I.; Cignarelli, A.; Sorice, G.P.; Natalicchio, A.; Perrini, S.; Laviola, L.; Giorgino, F. Cardiovascular and Renal Effectiveness of GLP-1 Receptor Agonists vs. Other Glucose-Lowering Drugs in Type 2 Diabetes: A Systematic Review and Meta-Analysis of Real-World Studies. *Metabolites* **2022**, *12*, 183. [CrossRef]
18. Sheahan, K.H.; Wahlberg, E.A.; Gilbert, M.P. An overview of GLP-1 agonists and recent cardiovascular outcomes trials. *Postgrad. Med. J.* **2020**, *96*, 156–161. [CrossRef]
19. Andreasen, C.R.; Andersen, A.; Knop, F.K.; Vilsbøll, T. Understanding the place for GLP-1RA therapy: Translating guidelines for treatment of type 2 diabetes into everyday clinical practice and patient selection. *Diabetes Obes. Metab.* **2021**, *23*, 40–52. [CrossRef]
20. Melo, M.; Gavina, C.; Silva-Nunes, J.; Andrade, L.; Carvalho, D. Heterogeneity amongst GLP-1 RA cardiovascular outcome trials results: Can definition of established cardiovascular disease be the missing link? *Diabetol. Metab. Syndr.* **2021**, *13*, 81. [CrossRef]
21. Top, W.M.C.; Kooy, A.; Stehouwer, C.D.A. Metformin: A Narrative Review of Its Potential Benefits for Cardiovascular Disease, Cancer and Dementia. *Pharmaceuticals* **2022**, *15*, 312. [CrossRef] [PubMed]
22. Jorsal, A.; Persson, F.; Bruun, J.M. Comments on the 2019 ESC Guidelines on diabetes, pre-diabetes, and cardiovascular diseases. *Eur. Heart J.* **2020**, *41*, 328. [CrossRef] [PubMed]
23. Harrington, J.L.; de Albuquerque Rocha, N.; Patel, K.V.; Verma, S.; McGuire, D.K. Should Metformin Remain First-Line Medical Therapy for Patients with Type 2 Diabetes Mellitus and Atherosclerotic Cardiovascular Disease? An Alternative Approach. *Curr. Diabetes Rep.* **2018**, *18*, 64. [CrossRef] [PubMed]
24. Kheniser, K.G.; Kashyap, S.R.; Kasumov, T. A systematic review: The appraisal of the effects of metformin on lipoprotein modification and function. *Obes. Sci. Pract.* **2019**, *5*, 36–45. [CrossRef]
25. Jenkins, A.J.; Welsh, P.; Petrie, J.R. Metformin, lipids and atherosclerosis prevention. *Curr. Opin. Lipidol.* **2018**, *29*, 346–353. [CrossRef]
26. Petrie, J.R.; Rossing, P.R.; Campbell, I.W. Metformin and cardiorenal outcomes in diabetes: A reappraisal. *Diabetes Obes. Metab.* **2020**, *22*, 904–915. [CrossRef]
27. Muscogiuri, G.; Barrea, L.; Faggiano, F.; Maiorino, M.I.; Parrillo, M.; Pugliese, G.; Ruggeri, R.M.; Scarano, E.; Savastano, S.; Colao, A.; et al. Obesity in Prader-Willi syndrome: Physiopathological mechanisms, nutritional and pharmacological approaches. *J. Endocrinol. Investig.* **2021**, *44*, 2057–2070. [CrossRef]
28. Ziyrek, M.; Kahraman, S.; Ozdemir, E.; Dogan, A. Metformin monotherapy significantly decreases epicardial adipose tissue thickness in newly diagnosed type 2 diabetes patients. *Rev. Port. De Cardiol.* **2019**, *38*, 419–423. [CrossRef]

29. Greco, E.V.; Russo, G.; Giandalia, A.; Viazzi, F.; Pontremoli, R.; De Cosmo, S. GLP-1 Receptor Agonists and Kidney Protection. *Medicina* **2019**, *55*, 233. [CrossRef]
30. Tofé, S.; Argüelles, I.; Mena, E.; Serra, G.; Codina, M.; Urgeles, J.R.; García, H.; Pereg, V. Real-world GLP-1 RA therapy in type 2 diabetes: A long-term effectiveness observational study. *Endocrinol. Diabetes Metab.* **2018**, *2*, e00051. [CrossRef]
31. Marso, S.P.; Bain, S.C.; Consoli, A.; Eliaschewitz, F.G.; Jódar, E.; Leiter, L.A.; Lingvay, I.; Rosenstock, J.; Seufert, J.; Warren, M.L.; et al. Semaglutide and Cardiovascular Outcomes in Patients with Type 2 Diabetes. *N. Engl. J. Med.* **2016**, *375*, 1834–1844. [CrossRef]
32. Khan, A.; Ross, H.M.; Parra, N.S.; Chen, S.L.; Chauhan, K.; Wang, M.; Yan, B.; Magagna, J.; Beiriger, J.; Shah, Y.; et al. Risk Prevention and Health Promotion for Non-Alcoholic Fatty Liver Diseases (NAFLD). *Livers* **2022**, *2*, 264–282. [CrossRef]
33. Sawada, K.; Karashima, S.; Kometani, M.; Oka, R.; Takeda, Y.; Sawamura, T.; Fujimoto, A.; Demura, M.; Wakayama, A.; Usukura, M.; et al. Effect of sodium glucose cotransporter 2 inhibitors on obstructive sleep apnea in patients with type 2 diabetes. *Endocr. J.* **2018**, *65*, 461–467. [CrossRef]
34. Rojano Toimil, A.; Ciudin, A. GLP-1 Receptor Agonists in Diabetic Kidney Disease: From Physiology to Clinical Outcomes. *J. Clin. Med.* **2021**, *10*, 3955. [CrossRef]
35. Hu, M.; Cai, X.; Yang, W.; Zhang, S.; Nie, L.; Ji, L. Effect of Hemoglobin A1c Reduction or Weight Reduction on Blood Pressure in Glucagon-Like Peptide-1 Receptor Agonist and Sodium-Glucose Cotransporter-2 Inhibitor Treatment in Type 2 Diabetes Mellitus: A Meta-Analysis. *J. Am. Heart Assoc.* **2020**, *9*, e015323. [CrossRef]
36. Benham, J.L.; Booth, J.E.; Sigal, R.J.; Daskalopoulou, S.S.; Leung, A.A.; Rabi, D.M. Systematic review and meta-analysis: SGLT2 inhibitors, blood pressure and cardiovascular outcomes. *Int. J. Cardiol. Heart Vasc.* **2021**, *33*, 100725. [CrossRef]
37. Palmiero, G.; Cesaro, A.; Vetrano, E.; Pafundi, P.C.; Galiero, R.; Caturano, A.; Moscarella, E.; Gragnano, F.; Salvatore, T.; Rinaldi, L.; et al. Impact of SGLT2 Inhibitors on Heart Failure: From Pathophysiology to Clinical Effects. *Int. J. Mol. Sci.* **2021**, *22*, 5863. [CrossRef]
38. Malin, S.K.; Stewart, N.R. Metformin May Contribute to Inter-individual Variability for Glycemic Responses to Exercise. *Front. Endocrinol.* **2020**, *11*, 519. [CrossRef]
39. Rosenstock, J.; Chuck, L.; González-Ortiz, M.; Merton, K.; Craig, J.; Capuano, G.; Qiu, R. Initial Combination Therapy With Canagliflozin Plus Metformin Versus Each Component as Monotherapy for Drug-Naïve Type 2 Diabetes. *Diabetes Care* **2016**, *39*, 353–362. [CrossRef]
40. Brown, E.; Rajeev, S.P.; Cuthbertson, D.J.; Wilding, J.P.H. A review of the mechanism of action, metabolic profile and haemodynamic effects of sodium-glucose co-transporter-2 inhibitors. *Diabetes Obes. Metab.* **2019**, *21*, 9–18. [CrossRef]
41. Singh, A.K.; Unnikrishnan, A.G.; Zargar, A.H.; Kumar, A.; Das, A.K.; Saboo, B.; Sinha, B.; Gangopadhyay, K.K.; Talwalkar, P.G.; Ghosal, S.; et al. Evidence-Based Consensus on Positioning of SGLT2i in Type 2 Diabetes Mellitus in Indians. *Diabetes Ther.* **2019**, *10*, 393–428. [CrossRef]
42. Tentolouris, A.; Vlachakis, P.; Tzeravini, E.; Eleftheriadou, I.; Tentolouris, N. SGLT2 Inhibitors: A Review of Their Antidiabetic and Cardioprotective Effects. *Int. J. Environ. Res. Public Health* **2019**, *16*, 2965. [CrossRef]
43. Masson, W.; Lavalle-Cobo, A.; Nogueira, J.P. Effect of SGLT2-Inhibitors on Epicardial Adipose Tissue: A Meta-Analysis. *Cells* **2021**, *10*, 2150. [CrossRef]
44. Milder, T.Y.; Stocker, S.L.; Abdel Shaheed, C.; McGrath-Cadell, L.; Samocha-Bonet, D.; Greenfield, J.R.; Day, R.O. Combination Therapy with an SGLT2 Inhibitor as Initial Treatment for Type 2 Diabetes: A Systematic Review and Meta-Analysis. *J. Clin. Med.* **2019**, *8*, 45. [CrossRef]
45. Jingfan, Z.; Ling, L.; Cong, L.; Ping, L.; Yu, C. Efficacy and safety of sodium-glucose cotransporter-2 inhibitors in type 2 diabetes mellitus with inadequate glycemic control on metformin: A meta-analysis. *Arch. Endocrinol. Metab.* **2019**, *63*, 478–486. [CrossRef]
46. Khunti, K.; Charbonnel, B.; Cooper, A.; Gomes, M.B.; Ji, L.; Leigh, P.; Nicolucci, A.; Rathmann, W.; Shestakova, M.V.; Siddiqui, A.; et al. Associations between second-line glucose-lowering combination therapies with metformin and HbA1c, body weight, quality of life, hypoglycaemic events and glucose-lowering treatment intensification: The DISCOVER study. *Diabetes Obes. Metab.* **2021**, *23*, 1823–1833. [CrossRef]
47. Huthmacher, J.A.; Meier, J.J.; Nauck, M.A. Efficacy and Safety of Short- and Long-Acting Glucagon-Like Peptide 1 Receptor Agonists on a Background of Basal Insulin in Type 2 Diabetes: A Meta-analysis. *Diabetes Care* **2020**, *43*, 2303–2312. [CrossRef]
48. Patoulias, D.; Katsimardou, A.; Kalogirou, M.S.; Zografou, I.; Toumpourleka, M.; Imprialos, K.; Stavropoulos, K.; Stergiou, I.; Papadopoulos, C.; Doumas, M. Glucagon-like peptide-1 receptor agonists or sodium-glucose cotransporter-2 inhibitors as add-on therapy for patients with type 2 diabetes? A systematic review and meta-analysis of surrogate metabolic endpoints. *Diabetes Metab.* **2020**, *46*, 272–279. [CrossRef]
49. Sachinidis, A.; Nikolic, D.; Stoian, A.P.; Papanas, N.; Tarar, O.; Rizvi, A.A.; Rizzo, M. Cardiovascular outcomes trials with incretin-based medications: A critical review of data available on GLP-1 receptor agonists and DPP-4 inhibitors. *Metabolism* **2020**, *111*, 154343. [CrossRef]
50. Dardano, A.; Miccoli, R.; Bianchi, C.; Daniele, G.; Del Prato, S. Invited review. Series: Implications of the recent CVOTs in type 2 diabetes: Which patients for GLP-1RA or SGLT-2 inhibitor? *Diabetes Res. Clin. Pract.* **2020**, *162*, 108112. [CrossRef]
51. Salmen, T.; Bobirca, F.-T.; Bica, I.-C.; Mihai, D.-A.; Pop, C.; Stoian, A.P. The Safety Profile of Sodium-Glucose Cotransporter-2 Inhibitors and Glucagon-like Peptide-1 Receptor Agonists in the Standard of Care Treatment of Type 2 Diabetes Mellitus. *Life* **2023**, *13*, 839. [CrossRef] [PubMed]

52. Schernthaner, G.; Shehadeh, N.; Ametov, A.S.; Bazarova, A.V.; Ebrahimi, F.; Fasching, P.; Janež, A.; Kempler, P.; Konrāde, I.; Lalić, N.M.; et al. Worldwide inertia to the use of cardiorenal protective glucose-lowering drugs (SGLT2i and GLP-1 RA) in high-risk patients with type 2 diabetes. *Cardiovasc. Diabetol.* **2020**, *19*, 185. [CrossRef] [PubMed]
53. Sasso, F.C.; Pafundi, P.C.; Simeon, V.; De Nicola, L.; Chiodini, P.; Galiero, R.; Rinaldi, L.; Nevola, R.; Salvatore, T.; Sardu, C.; et al. Efficacy and durability of multifactorial intervention on mortality and MACEs: A randomized clinical trial in type-2 diabetic kidney disease. *Cardiovasc. Diabetol.* **2021**, *20*, 145. [CrossRef] [PubMed]
54. Sasso, F.C.; Simeon, V.; Galiero, R.; Caturano, A.; De Nicola, L.; Chiodini, P.; Rinaldi, L.; Salvatore, T.; Lettieri, M.; Nevola, R.; et al. The number of risk factors not at target is associated with cardiovascular risk in a type 2 diabetic population with albuminuria in primary cardiovascular prevention. Post-hoc analysis of the NID-2 trial. *Cardiovasc. Diabetol.* **2022**, *21*, 235. [CrossRef]

Disclaimer/Publisher's Note: The statements, opinions and data contained in all publications are solely those of the individual author(s) and contributor(s) and not of MDPI and/or the editor(s). MDPI and/or the editor(s) disclaim responsibility for any injury to people or property resulting from any ideas, methods, instructions or products referred to in the content.

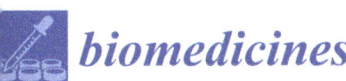

Article

Handgrip Strength Is Associated with Specific Aspects of Vascular Function in Individuals with Metabolic Syndrome

Juan Carlos Sánchez-Delgado [1,2,*], Daniel D. Cohen [1,3], Paul A. Camacho-López [4], Javier Carreño-Robayo [1], Alvaro Castañeda-Hernández [1], Daniel García-González [2], Daniel Martínez-Bello [1], Gustavo Aroca-Martinez [5], Gianfranco Parati [6] and Patricio Lopez-Jaramillo [1,*]

1. Universidad de Santander, Facultad de Ciencias Médicas y de la Salud, Bucaramanga 680003, Colombia; danielcohen1971@gmail.com (D.D.C.); javi.carreno.19@gmail.com (J.C.-R.); al.castaneda@mail.udes.edu.co (A.C.-H.); dan.martinez@mail.udes.edu.co (D.M.-B.)
2. Grupo de Investigación Ser Cultura y Movimiento, Universidad Santo Tomás-Bucaramanga, Santander 680001, Colombia; daniel.garcia@ustabuca.edu.co
3. Department of Physical Education and Sport Sciences, Faculty of Education and Health Sciences, University of Limerick, V94T9PX Limerick, Ireland
4. Fundación Oftalmológica de Santander, Floridablanca 811004, Colombia; paul.camacho@foscal.com.co
5. Facultad de Ciencias de la Salud, Universidad Simón Bolívar, Barranquilla 080002, Colombia; garoca1@hotmail.com
6. Istituto Auxologico Italiano & University of Milano-Bicocca, Department of Medicine and Surgery, Piazza Brescia, 20149 Milan, Italy; gianfranco.parati@unimib.it
* Correspondence: juancarlossanchezd@gmail.com (J.C.S.-D.); jplopezj@gmail.com (P.L.-J.)

Abstract: Background: Metabolic syndrome (MetS) is a disorder associated with an increased risk for the development of diabetes mellitus and its complications. Lower isometric handgrip strength (HGS) is associated with an increased risk of cardiometabolic diseases. However, the association between HGS and arterial stiffness parameters, which are considered the predictors of morbidity and mortality in individuals with MetS, is not well defined. Objective: To determine the association between HGS and HGS asymmetry on components of vascular function in adults with MetS. Methods: We measured handgrip strength normalized to bodyweight (HGS/kg), HGS asymmetry, body composition, blood glucose, lipid profile, blood pressure, pulse wave velocity (PWV), reflection coefficient (RC), augmentation index @75 bpm (AIx@75) and peripheral vascular resistance (PVR) in 55 adults with a diagnosis of MetS between 25 and 54 years old. Results: Mean age was 43.1 ± 7.0 years, 56.3% were females. HGS/kg was negatively correlated with AIx@75 (r = −0.440), $p < 0.05$, but these associations were not significant after adjusting for age and sex. However, when interaction effects between sex, HGS/kg and age were examined, we observed an inverse relationship between HGS/kg and AIx@75 in the older adults in the sample, whereas in the younger adults, a weak direct association was found. We also found a significant association between HGS asymmetry and PVR (beta = 30, 95% CI = 7.02; 54.2; $p < 0.012$). Conclusions: Our findings suggest that in people with MetS, maintaining muscle strength may have an increasingly important role in older age in the attenuation of age-related increases in AIx@75—a marker of vascular stiffness—and that a higher HGS asymmetry could be associated with a greater vascular resistance.

Keywords: handgrip; metabolic syndrome; blood pressure; isometric strength; vascular stiffness; muscle strength dynamometer

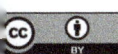

1. Introduction

Metabolic syndrome (MetS) is associated with an increased risk of type 2 diabetes and cardiovascular diseases (CVDs). MetS is defined by the presence of at least three of the following risk factors: high waist circumference, hypertriglyceridemia, low HDL cholesterol, hypertension and dysglycemia [1]. Between 20% and 30% of the adult population can be characterized as having metabolic syndrome, which is considered a clinical picture associated with an increased incidence of arterial hypertension, atherosclerosis, left ventricular hypertrophy, diastolic dysfunction as well as an increase in premature mortality from coronary and cerebrovascular diseases [2].

While it is well established that a higher adiposity increases the risk of MetS, recent evidence also supports an association between lower muscle strength and mass, and the development of MetS and CVDs in adults [1–4] as well as a poorer metabolic risk profile in children [5]. Skeletal muscle loss and fat accumulation share a combination of factors, including increased oxidative stress, elevated inflammatory cytokines, mitochondrial dysfunction and insulin resistance (IR) [6]. It is believed that a persistent condition of these factors, particularly IR, justifies the close association between MetS and sarcopenia [7]. This can be substantiated by considering that one of the main causes of this syndrome is the increase in IR, which can be significantly exacerbated by the reduction in skeletal muscle mass—a tissue responsible for approximately 80% of glucose clearance [8]. Another reason that underscores this association is that IR is accompanied by an increase in the release of free fatty acids and the inhibition of the growth hormone (GH)–insulin-like growth factor 1 (IGF1) axis. This inhibition further hampers skeletal muscle protein synthesis Additionally, it is believed that hyperinsulinemia caused by IR also augments the amount of myostatin, which acts to diminish skeletal muscle [8,9].

MetS is associated with an increased arterial stiffness across all age groups. This is thought to be mainly due to hormonal and metabolic abnormalities present from the onset of a state of insulin resistance—a preponderant factor that commonly accelerates vascular aging. Arterial stiffness is characterized by the loss of the elastic properties of the arteries, and while a consequence of physiological vascular aging, it can also be accelerated in a variety of pathological conditions [10,11]. Specifically, the mechanisms that promote arterial stiffness are an increase in the collagen/elastin ratio, oxidative stress, endothelial dysfunction, vascular smooth muscle proliferation, calcification, metabolic alterations, genetic mutations, epigenetic abnormalities, sympathetic activation and renin-angiotensin–aldosterone system. The increase in cardiovascular risk in patients with MetS has been associated with changes in arterial parameters, including those that determine the degree of arterial stiffness. Specifically, some studies estimate that individuals with higher arterial stiffness are estimated to have a 48% higher risk of developing cardiovascular disease [10–13].

Decreased arterial compliance and elasticity leads to an increase in arterial stiffness, a common risk factor for the development of atherosclerotic cardiovascular diseases [12,13] The augmentation increase index (AIx) and PWV are considered the main markers of systemic arterial stiffness in the general population, and provide an estimation of vascular aging in patients with Mest. These can be measured non-invasively by tonometry, oscillometry, ultrasound, magnetic resonance imaging, with elevated values indicative of an increased arterial stiffness. The PWV is considered the "gold standard" non-invasive parameter for measuring arterial stiffness. AIx has also shown independent associations with cardiovascular events and all-cause mortality [14,15].

Some studies report an inverse relationship between muscle strength and arterial stiffness in healthy populations and in older adults, and it is suggested that endothelial dysfunction and arterial stiffness could mediate the association between muscle strength and cardiovascular events [14–20]. However, the association between strength and variables that relate to arterial stiffness in subjects with MetS has not been described. Furthermore, studies examining associations between strength and components of vascular function have a typically measured dynamic strength using equipment that, due either to cost and/or to time requirement for implementing the assessment, are not practical to implement in clinical settings [21]. In contrast, isometric handgrip dynamometry assessment is a relatively low cost, portable and rapid means to obtain a measure of maximal strength [22]. Handgrip strength (HGS) is the measure most commonly used in studies showing associations between low strength and the current metabolic risk profile and the risk of future CVD disease and mortality, including associations with hypertension [23–27]. Although HGS measures in these studies focus on the maximum HGS, interest in HGS asymmetry has increased due to evidence showing that its inclusion in analyses increases the predictive power of HGS on health outcomes such as falls, limitations functions, cognitive alterations, future chronic disease risk events and mortality [28–32].

Studies examining the association between HGS and arterial stiffness have found inconsistent results [20,33,34]. Furthermore, to the best of our knowledge, neither this association nor HGS asymmetry have been investigated in a MetS population. The present study aims to determine the association between maximal HGS, HGS asymmetry and aspects of vascular function in individuals with MetS.

2. Methodology

The present study was a cross-sectional analysis of fifty-five men and women between 25 and 54 years of age diagnosed with MetS according to the criteria of the International Diabetes Federation (three or more of the following factors: abdominal obesity (>80 cm in women/>90 cm in men), blood pressure ($\geq$130/85 mmHg) or taking antihypertensive drugs, a fasting blood glucose between 100 and 125 mg/dL, elevated triglycerides (>150 mg/dL) and a decreased HDL (<40 mg/dL in men/<50 mg/dL in women) or taking lipid-lowering medications) [1,35]. The sample was selected through a non-probabilistic convenience sampling of the employees of two health institutions in Bucaramanga, Colombia. The participants were a subsample of subjects recruited for a randomized clinical trial of isometric strength training (EEFIT). A physiotherapist and/or nurse approached each of the potential participants in the workplace to implement the first stage of screening, which consisted of measuring the abdominal circumference with a measuring tape and blood pressure with a validated digital blood pressure monitor (Omron HEM 705 CP, **Omron** Healthcare Inc., Lake Forest, IL, US) to confirm two of the inclusion criteria before performing analyses of blood biochemistry. Those that fulfilled at least one of the additional criteria (fasting blood glucose, triglycerides or HDL) were then invited to participate, and the same professionals performed other hemodynamic and anthropometric measures and assessment of HGS. Evaluations were carried out between the months of October 2019 and January 2020.

2.1. Procedures

After a 15 min rest period, sitting, without crossing the legs, arterial stiffness parameters were assessed using the Mobil-O-Graph® 24Hpwa device (IEM, Stolberg, Germany). The device cuff was placed on the non-dominant arm and with the arm supported at the level of the heart. The equipment initially measures blood pressure. The cuff is then inflated for approximately 10 s to the level of diastolic pressure to allow the measurement of pulse waves of the brachial artery from which several arterial stiffness parameters are indirectly estimated using the ARCSolver® algorithm (Austrian Institute of Technology, Vienna, Austria). The following parameters were estimated and used in further analysis: pulse wave velocity (PWV); defined as the time difference between the start of the forward pulse wave and the beginning of the reflected wave, augmentation index at 75 bpm (AIx@75); the difference between the second and first systolic peaks, also representing the intensity of the reflection of the pulse waves, reflection coefficient (RC); the relationship between the amplitude of the reflected pulse wave and the incident pulse wave, and peripheral vascular resistance (PVR); the resistance in the circulatory system that contributes to blood pressure [36]. Height was measured using a standard height rod graduated in centimeters (cm) and millimeters (mm), to the nearest 0.1 cm. Body weight was measured using a digital scale with a precision of 100 g, and body mass index (BMI = kg/m^2) was calculated. Fat mass (kg) and % fat was estimated using bioimpedance (BC—554 Ironman®, Tanita, Tokyo, Japan). Isometric HGS was evaluated using a hydraulic hand dynamometer (JAMAR®—5030J1, Chicago, IL, USA) with the participant seated, shoulders adducted and without rotation, with the elbow flexed at 90°, forearm and wrist in neutral position with an extension between 0 and 30° and with an ulnar deviation of 0°–15°. Three maximal voluntary contractions were performed in each hand and the highest of the three attempts was used in further analysis after normalizing for bodyweight (HGS/kg). HGS was measured alternately in the right and left hand, with a rest period of approximately one minute between measurements of the same hand [37].

We calculated an asymmetry ratio by dividing the higher HGS by the lower HGS, irrespective of hand "dominance", to generate an absolute % magnitude value (independent of direction).

2.2. Statistical Analysis

Data were analyzed using Stata 12.0 (Stata Corp LCC, College Station, TX, USA). Measures of central tendency and dispersion were calculated for the quantitative variables, and absolute and relative frequencies for categorical variables. Gender differences in variables were assessed using the student's *t*-test. We determined correlations between HGS/Kg, HGS asymmetry and arterial stiffness parameters. A multiple linear regression model was performed using three levels of interaction where HGS/Kg, age and sex were used as predictors and Aix @75, RVP, PWV, RC as response variables. An additional multiple linear analysis was performed between the arterial stiffness variables and HGS asymmetry, adjusting for gender, age, BMI, fat mass, triglycerides, glucose and HDL. An alpha level of 5% was set as significant for all analyses.

3. Results

The general characteristics and the metabolic profile of the study population are described in Table 1. The mean age was 43 years and 56% were women, who presented significantly lower values of grip strength (difference = -18.09 ± 4.1 Kg, $p < 0.001$), relative handgrip strength (difference = -0.06 ± 0.09 Kg/kg, $p < 0.05$), diastolic blood pressure (difference = -7 ± 10 mmHg, $p = 0.001$), systolic blood pressure (difference = -6 ± 4 mmHg, $p < 0.001$) and waist circumference (difference = -9 ± 5.4 cm, $p = 0.001$); men showed lower fat percentage (difference = -10 ± 4, $p < 0.05$), HDL (difference = -9 ± 6.1 mg/dL, $p < 0.001$) and AIx@75 (difference = -13 ± 7, $p < 0.001$).

Table 1. Characteristics of the study population.

Variable	Female (n = 31) Mean (SD)	Male (n = 24) Mean (SD)	Total (n = 55) Mean (SD)
Age (years) %	44.48 (6.92)	41.42 (7.02)	43.15 (7.07)
BMI (kg/m^2)	29.25 (4.93)	29.10 (2.80)	29.18 (4.10)
Waist circumference (cm)	89.27 (9.02)	98.52 (6.69) *	93.31 (9.26)
Fat mass (%)	37.13 (6.44)	27.36 (3.98) *	32.86 (7.33)
Handgrip strength (kg)	25.74 (6.17)	43.83 (6.68) *	33.64 (11.05)
Relative handgrip strength (kg/weight in kg)	0.36 (0.10)	0.52 (0.09) *	0.43 (0.12)
Handgrip strength asymmetry (%)	15.8 (17.1)	11.8 (11.4)	14.0 (14.9)
Glucose (mg/dL)	99.25 (10.37)	101.70 (10.45)	100.32 (10.38)
TC (mg/dL)	196.31 (37.69)	190.97 (36.62)	193.98 (36.98)
LDL (mg/dL)	131.13 (33.42)	123.88 (28.35)	127.97 (31.24)
HDL (mg/dL)	44.69 (10.37)	36.48 (7.29) *	41.11 (9.97)
Triglycerides (mg/dL)	183.56 (73.39)	244.07 (174.98)	209.97 (130.20)
Systolic blood pressure (mm/Hg)	113.61 (7.89)	121.58 (10.12) *	117.09 (9.70)
Diastolic blood pressure (mm/Hg)	72.74 (6.93)	78.96 (6.52) *	75.45 (7.38)
RHR (bpm)	74.23 (7.93)	72.25 (7.16)	73.36 (7.60)

Table 1. Cont.

Variable	Female (n = 31) Mean (SD)	Male (n = 24) Mean (SD)	Total (n = 55) Mean (SD)
PVR (s.mmHg/mL)	1.28 (0.20)	1.22 (0.17)	1.25 (0.19)
Reflection coefficient (%)	61.23 (6.94)	57.62 (13.57)	59.65 (10.42)
Aix@75 (%)	25.65 (11.17)	12.96 (9.22) *	20.11 (12.08)
Pulse wave velocity (m/s)	6.50 (0.87)	6.41 (0.62)	6.46 (0.77)

SD: Standard deviation; PVR: peripheral vascular resistance; Aix@75: augmentation index at 75 bpm; BMI: body mass index; LDL: low-density lipoprotein; HDL: high-density lipoprotein; RHR: resting heart rate; TC: total cholesterol; * $p < 0.05$, t-test.

Figure 1 shows negative correlations (Pearson) between HGS/kg and Aix@75 (r = −0.440, p = 0.0008) and PVR (r = −0.260, p = 0.050), and a positive correlation between HGS asymmetry and PVR (r = 0.322, p = 0.016). The linear regression analysis, adjusted for sex and age, and the model of covariance with three levels of interaction were not significant. The two-level interaction effect regression model showed an inverse association between HGS/kg and Aix@75 as age increased in the population ($p < 0.05$) (Table 2).

Table 2. Univariate and multivariate linear regression coefficients of HGS/kg, age and sex with indicators of arterial stiffness.

Response	Characteristic	Univariate SS (CI 95%), p value	Multivariate SS (CI 95%), p Value
Aix@75	Male	−12.69 (−18.34 to −7.03), p < 0.001 *	−73.71 (−127.11 to −20.31), p = 0.008 *
	Age	0.16 (−0.31 to 0.63), p = 0.488	2.42 (0.61 to 4.23), p = 0.010 *
	HGS	−43.96 (−68.66 to −19.25), p = 0.001 *	314.56 (76.48 to 552.63), p = 0.011 *
	I-HGS_Age	−0.73 (−1.24 to −0.22), p = 0.006 *	−7.40 (−12.51 to −2.28), p = 0.005 *
	I-HGS_Sex	−23.66 (−34.43 to −12.88), p < 0.001 *	3.24 (−59.33 to 65.80), p = 0.918
	I-Sex_Age	−0.29 (−0.43 to −0.16), p < 0.001 *	1.42 (0.21 to 2.62), p = 0.022 *
PVR	Male	−0.07 (−0.17 to 0.03), p = 0.187	−0.93 (−1.92 to 0.05), p = 0.064
	Age	0.00 (−0.00 to 0.01), p = 0.516	0.03 (−0.01 to 0.06), p = 0.125
	HGS	−0.40 (−0.81 to 0.01), p = 0.055	2.90 (−1.50 to 7.30), p = 0.192
	I-HGS _Age	−0.01 (−0.01 to 0.00), p = 0.135	−0.08 (−0.17 to 0.02), p = 0.108
	I-HGS_Sex	−0.12 (−0.31 to 0.07), p = 0.206	0.44 (−0.72 to 1.60), p = 0.449
	I-Sex_Age	−0.00 (−0.00 to 0.00), p = 0.243	0.02 (−0.01 to 0.04), p = 0.138

β = Coefficient for linear regression; HGS: body weight-normalized handgrip strength; Aix@75 = augmentation index at 75 bpm; PVR: peripheral vascular resistance. I-HGS_Age: Interaction between HGS and age adjusted for sex; I-HGS_Sex: interaction between HGS and sex; I-Sex_Age: interaction between sex and age. * $p < 0.05$.

Multiple linear regression analysis adjusted for gender, age, BMI, fat mass, triglycerides, glucose and HDL showed a significant association between HGS asymmetry and PVR values (beta = 30; 95% CI = 7.02;54.2; p = 0.012) (Table 3).

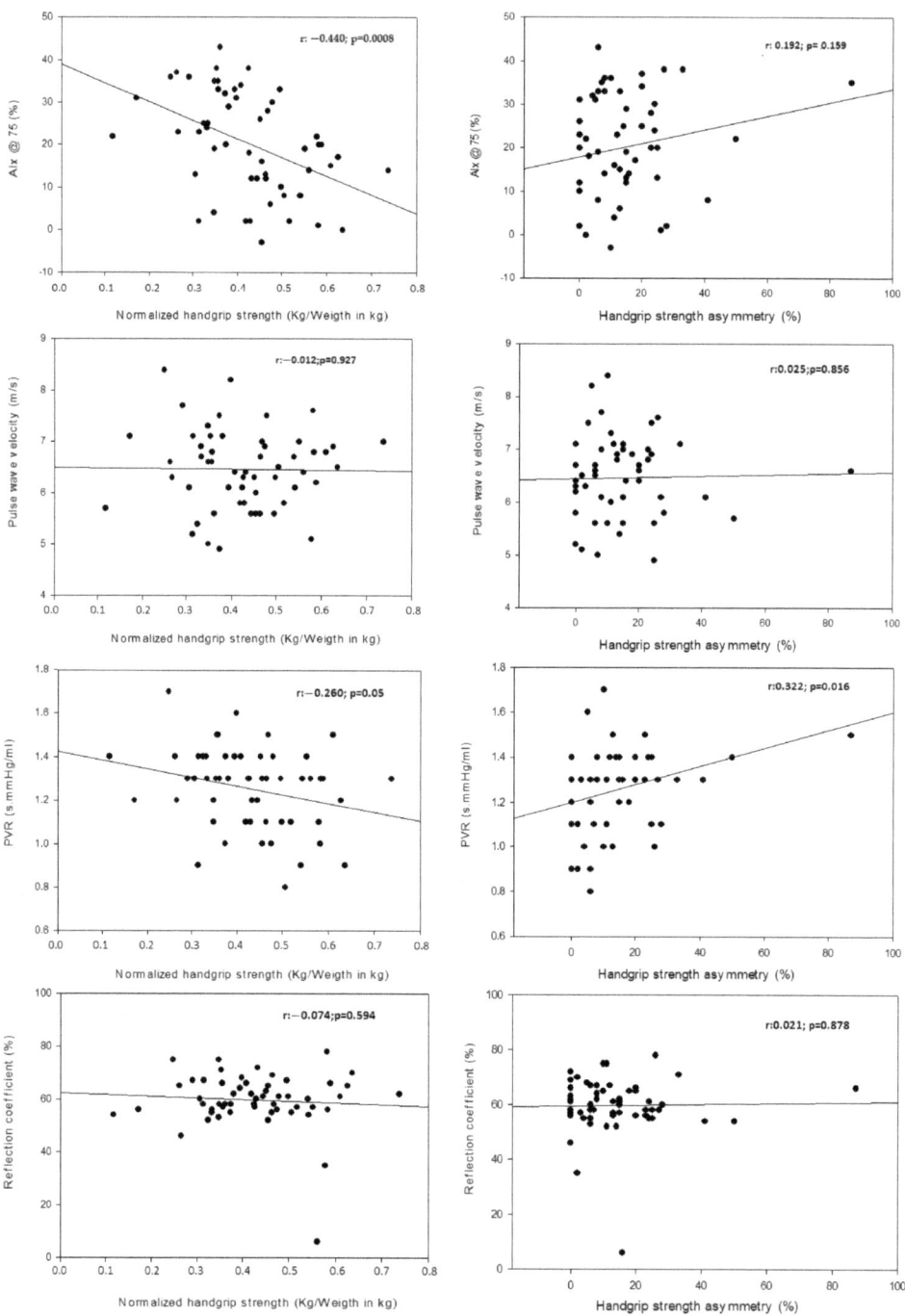

Figure 1. Analysis of the correlation between HGS/Kg, HGS asymmetry and indicators of arterial stiffness in individuals with MetS. Aix@75 = augmentation index at 75 bpm; PVR = peripheral vascular resistance.

Table 3. Univariate and multivariate linear regression coefficients of handgrip asymmetry with indicators of arterial stiffness.

Variable	Crude Model	Fully Adjusted Models [†]
	SS (CI 95%), *p*-Value	OR (95%CI), *p*-Value
Aix@75 (%)	0.23 (−0.09; 0.57), 0.159	0.25 (−0.16; 0.68), 0.227
PWV (m/s)	0.48 (−4.87; 5.84), 0.856	10 (−0.94; 21.5), 0.072
RC (%)	0.03 (−0.36; 0.42), 0.878	0.04 (0.39; 0.48), 0.824
PVR (s.mmHg/mL)	26 (4.94; 46.7), 0.016 *	30 (7.02; 54.2), 0.012 *

CI: Confidence interval; Aix@75 = augmentation index at 75 bpm; PVR: peripheral vascular resistance; † fully adjusted models controlled for age, sex, BMI, fat mass, triglycerides, glucose; HDL: high-density lipoprotein. * $p < 0.05$.

4. Discussion

In the present analysis of associations between HGS and markers of vascular function in middle-aged adults with MetS, there were three principal findings. First, after adjusting for age and sex, relative strength (HGS/Kg) was not associated with any marker of vascular function. Second, we found a significant interaction effect between HGS/Kg and AIx@75 as a function of age, such that, in the older study participants (aged between 40 and 55 years old), a greater HGS/kg was inversely associated with this marker—an indicator of the state of the muscular or peripheral arteries. Third, those subjects with high HGS asymmetry were shown to be more likely to present high PVR values. This suggests that inadequate muscle strength with increasing age, as well as elevated strength asymmetry, could be predictors of arterial stiffness, at least in people with metabolic syndrome.

Women presented lower values of handgrip strength, blood pressure, lower adiposity and arterial stiffness than men. The differences evidenced in body composition, muscle strength and blood pressure between the men and women analyzed are commonly described in the literature [38]. However, the higher AIx@75 values found in the women in the present study conflict with the findings of Ogola et al. [39], who observed lower levels than in men of the same age. This may be related to the majority of women in their study being of reproductive age. Although the protective mechanisms on arterial stiffness in women of reproductive age are not fully elucidated, it is believed that hormonal factors, specifically those in relation to estrogen levels, as well as the density of their receptors, have a significant influence on vascular health. Despite this, it is important to note that the decrease in the levels of this hormone does not occur exactly at 50 years of age, which is the average age considered for the onset of menopause; therefore, the deleterious effects of estrogen decline on the cardiovascular system may begin before the natural cessation of menstruation, and could partly explain our results [40].

To our knowledge, only two studies have evaluated the association between HGS/Kg and AIx@75%, in hypertensive and diabetic subjects with a mean age of 58 and 61 years, respectively. These studies showed both lower values of grip strength and higher values of AIx@75% than those obtained in the present study, consistent with their older age and their a diagnosis with two of the chronic pathologies that are commonly associated with an increased arterial stiffness. They observed a negative correlation between HGS/Kg and AIx@75% [20,33]. Another study found a negative correlation between maximum dynamic strength and AIx@75% in individuals with mobility limitations and a mean age of 68 years [41]. This may be explained by the association between muscle function and capillary density, an important determinant of microvascular function [21,42,43].

It is also known that there is an inverse relationship between the augmentation index and the bioavailability of nitric oxide (NO), a potent vasodilator and anti-atherogenic substance produced in the vascular endothelium [44]. Aging is accompanied by a reduction in the bioavailability of NO and by an increase in the formation of peroxynitrite in smooth and skeletal muscle. The former limits blood perfusion to muscle fibers [45,46] while the latter decreases contractile force and increases susceptibility to muscular fatigue, [43] providing potential explanations for the observed associations between muscle function and AIx@75% as age increases in people with Mets. Alternatively, microvascular blood flow is a determinant of anabolic processes, and as such, a diminished vascular function might accelerate the ageing-related losses of muscle mass, and as a consequence, a reduction in muscle strength and function. In addition, microvascular dysfunction can alter metabolism, mainly developing insulin resistance, a factor that affects arterial stiffness and accelerates arterial aging [18,47–49].

Another of the possible mechanisms that explain the relationship between HGS and markers of stiffness observed relates to the understanding of muscle as an endocrine organ, having a better state and which can promote the production of myokines (such as interleukin-15, myostatin and irisin), which improve the processes of the regulation of fats and carbohydrates, thus favoring endothelial function and neovascularization, which in turn is accompanied by lower values of arterial stiffness [50]. In addition, arterial stiffness, as well as the attenuation of NO bioavailability that commonly accompanies it, could reduce blood flow to resting muscle tissue and hyperemia due to physical exercise by approximately 45%, which leads to a reduced supply of oxygen and nutrients to the muscle, thus limiting its contractile ability [41,51] These conditions have also been shown to affect satellite cell activation and therefore the hypertrophy of skeletal muscle fibers [52]. Additionally, the literature reports that a decrease in NO synthesis may negatively affect muscle excitation–contraction coupling, by reducing the activity of dihydropyridine receptors located in the T-tubules of the cytoplasmic membrane, as well as the activity of the enzyme calcium—ATPase—and the release of calcium from the sarcoplasmic reticulum through an alteration in ryanodine receptors [53–55].

The average asymmetry of HGS in the studied population was 14%, showing above the 10% threshold considered to be significant asymmetry by a number of studies [28–32]. Based on this cut-point, 51% of those evaluated presented an elevated asymmetry, similar to that reported previously in samples over 50 years of age [28,56]. However, it is important to highlight that there is no unified diagnostic criterion for asymmetry, considering the limited epidemiological information on this topic. The association between HGS asymmetry and PVR may be related to the finding that increased asymmetry has been shown to be a marker of decreased muscle function [28,57], a condition that may be accompanied by endothelial and smooth muscle vascular deterioration, mainly at the arteriolar level where peripheral vascular resistance is regulated [42,43,58]. In addition, individuals with a reduced muscle function are likely to also present with a lower capillary density [59], a factor that could also promote an increase in PVR [60]. While potential mechanisms linking strength asymmetry and cardiovascular disease risk are not clear, several studies have shown that a higher HGS asymmetry is associated with poorer cardiovascular health outcomes [61]. Our findings align with this and supports the need for the inclusion of asymmetry measures in the further investigation of potential associations between strength and cardiovascular health in those with, and without MetS.

The methodology and results of the present study do not permit us to determine the physiological and/or molecular mechanisms that describe the influence of HGS on arterial stiffness. However, there are common factors that may contribute to low muscle strength, as well as an increased arterial stiffness, including oxidative stress, insulin resistance, increased body fat percentage, endothelial dysfunction and the presence of higher levels of circulating inflammatory markers (elevated levels of C-reactive protein, interleukin-6, D-dimer, factor VIII) [33,62–64].

Amongst the other results that emerged in the interaction analysis, there was a direct relationship between HGS/kg and AIx@75% in people aged 25 to 40 years, an association that was stronger in women. This finding is contrary to the prior literature, showing that regardless of age, higher strength is related to a better vascular status [21,65–67]. Associations between grip strength and PWV are reported primarily in subjects older than 50 years, a potential explanation for the lack of association in the present study [14,18,48,65–70]. In addition, as this marker is more representative of lower-body arterial stiffness, it may be more associated with measures of lower body strength than with HGS, which correlates more strongly with upper extremity strength [71,72].

Studies that reported associations similar to that of the present investigation used diverse evaluation modalities. Most evaluated vascular health status using tonometry and plethysmography [21,41,65–67], while one used oscillometry [20], which is the modality employed in the present study and which is shown to have good psychometric properties compared to invasive and non-invasive evaluation methods [73,74]. Despite the predictive value shown by arterial stiffness and grip strength on cardiovascular health status, as well as the adequate psychometric properties of the different tools used to assess these markers, their use is mainly described in the research context, with little applicability in clinical practice. There is therefore a need to determine if the data obtained with these tools can facilitate clinical decisions, considering that they are economical and versatile. In addition, they have shown to be useful for the early identification of biological aging before cardiovascular disease is evident, making their use as a screening/preventive tool attractive—HGS in particular, as it is highly reproducible and is faster and less prone to errors. Therefore, further research examining the association between the two variables of interest analyzed in this study might further develop our understanding of the relationship between HGS and CVD in subjects with MetS. Furthermore, it is conceivable that targeted interventions and/or advice to improve muscle strength in those diagnosed with low HGS may contribute to an improved arterial health [18,41,75–77]. Particularly promising are the results of low-intensity isometric exercise in reducing systolic blood pressure [78,79], with some evidence that improvements in specific aspects of vascular function contribute to this effect [80].

5. Study Limitations

The study's limitations include the small sample size, which may have limited our ability to confirm other associations, the lack of control over the use of antihypertensive drugs or hormone replacement therapies—a potential confounding influence on the associations observed—and finally, the cross-sectional design, which prevents us from establishing causality. However, recognizing that HGS, HGS asymmetry and arterial stiffness are markers of biological age, it is possible that there is not a unilateral or bilateral causal relationship between these variables, and the possible association observed is due to them measuring the same characteristic.

6. Conclusions

Our findings suggest that in people with MetS with increasing age, a lower relative handgrip strength is increasingly associated with higher AIx@75; moreover, HGS asymmetry could also be a marker of arterial stiffness. The causality and direction of causality remain to be determined. In this population, at an elevated risk of diabetes and CVDs, further studies are needed to examine whether isometric exercise interventions that promote the development of strength or reduce strength asymmetry can improve AIx and/or other markers of vascular function/stiffness and whether these changes may have an impact on the outcome. In addition, the positive interaction between HGS/kg and Aix observed in the younger participants warrants further investigation. Finally, further work is needed to understand causality and the pathophysiological mechanisms involved.

Author Contributions: Conceptualization, J.C.S.-D., D.D.C., D.M.-B., P.A.C.-L., J.C.-R., A.C.-H., D.G.-G., G.A.-M., G.P. and P.L.-J.; methodology, J.C.S.-D., D.D.C. and D.G.-G.; formal analysis, J.C.S.-D., D.D.C., D.M.-B. and P.L.-J.; investigation, P.A.C.-L. and J.C.-R.; data curation, D.M.-B.; writing—original draft preparation, J.C.S.-D., D.D.C., D.M.-B., P.A.C.-L., J.C.-R., A.C.-H., D.G.-G., G.A.-M., G.P. and P.L.-J.; writing—review and editing, J.C.S.-D., D.D.C. and G.P.; supervision, D.D.C., P.A.C.-L. and G.A.-M.; project administration, J.C.-R., A.C.-H., G.A.-M. and P.L.-J. All authors have read and agreed to the published version of the manuscript.

Funding: This research was funded by [Minciencias] grant number [129980764353].

Institutional Review Board Statement: The protocol was approved by the Bioethics committee of the University of Santander (Approval code 010-CBU; Approval date: 15 May 2018). Informed consent was obtained from the patients following the ethical standards of the committee and the World Medical Association and the Declaration of Helsinki.

Informed Consent Statement: Informed consent was obtained from all subjects involved in the study

Data Availability Statement: Data are available upon request due to privacy/ethical restrictions.

Acknowledgments: Thanks to Minciencias who financed this project.

Conflicts of Interest: The authors have no conflicts of interest to disclose.

References

1. Wilson, P.W.; D'Agostino, R.B.; Parise, H.; Sullivan, L.; Meigs, J.B. Metabolic syndrome as a precursor of cardiovascular disease and type 2 diabetes mellitus. *Circulation* **2005**, *112*, 3066–3072. [CrossRef]
2. Lawman, H.G.; Troiano, R.P.; Perna, F.M.; Wang, C.Y.; Fryar, C.D.; Ogden, C.L. Associations of Relative Handgrip Strength and Cardiovascular Disease Biomarkers in U.S. Adults, 2011–2012. *Am. J. Prev. Med.* **2016**, *50*, 677–683. [CrossRef]
3. Ramírez-Vélez, R.; Correa-Bautista, J.E.; Lobelo, F.; Izquierdo, M.; Alonso-Martínez, A.; Rodríguez-Rodríguez, F.; Cristi-Montero, C. High muscular fitness has a powerful protective cardiometabolic effect in adults: Influence of weight status. *BMC Public Health* **2016**, *16*, 1012.
4. Leong, D.P.; Teo, K.K.; Rangarajan, S.; Lopez-Jaramillo, P.; Avezum, A.; Orlandini, A.; Seron, P.; Ahmed, S.H.; Rosengren, A.; Kelishadi, R.; et al. Prognostic value of grip strength: Findings from the Prospective Urban Rural Epidemiology (PURE) study. *Lancet* **2015**, *386*, 266–273.
5. Cohen, D.D.; Gómez-Arbeláez, D.; Camacho, P.A.; Pinzon, S.; Hormiga, C.; Trejos-Suarez, J.; Duperly, J.; Lopez-Jaramillo, P. Low muscle strength is associated with metabolic risk factors in Colombian children: The ACFIES study. *PLoS ONE* **2014**, *9*, e93150.
6. Rubio-Ruiz, M.E.; Guarner-Lans, V.; Pérez-Torres, I.; Soto, M.E. Mechanisms Underlying Metabolic Syndrome-Related Sarcopenia and Possible Therapeutic Measures. *Int. J. Mol. Sci.* **2019**, *20*, 647. [CrossRef]
7. Gluvic, Z.; Zaric, B.; Resanovic, I.; Obradovic, M.; Mitrovic, A.; Radak, D.; RIsenovic, E. Link between Metabolic Syndrome and Insulin Resistance. *Curr. Vasc. Pharmacol.* **2017**, *15*, 30–39. [CrossRef]
8. Nishikawa, H.; Asai, A.; Fukunishi, S.; Nishiguchi, S.; Higuchi, K. Metabolic Syndrome and Sarcopenia. *Nutrients* **2021**, *13*, 3519 [CrossRef]
9. Baczek, J.; Silkiewicz, M.; Wojszel, Z.B. Myostatin as a Biomarker of Muscle Wasting and other Pathologies-State of the Art and Knowledge Gaps. *Nutrients* **2020**, *12*, 2401. [CrossRef]
10. McEniery, C.M.; Yasmin, N.; Maki-Petaja, K.M.; McDonnell, B.J.; Munnery, M.; Hickson, S.S.; Franklin, S.S.; Cockcroft, J.R.; Wilkinson, I.B. The impact of cardiovascular risk factors on aortic stiffness and wave reflections depends on age: The Anglo-Cardiff Collaborative Trial (ACCT III). *Hypertension* **2010**, *56*, 591–597. [CrossRef]
11. Zieman, S.J.; Melenovsky, V.; Kass, D.A. Mechanisms, pathophysiology, and therapy of arterial stiffness. *Arterioscler. Thromb. Vasc. Biol.* **2005**, *25*, 932–943.
12. Miyoshi, T.; Ito, H. Arterial stiffness in health and disease: The role of cardio-ankle vascular index. *J. Cardiol.* **2021**, *78*, 493–501 [PubMed]
13. Cecelja, M.; Chowienczyk, P. Role of arterial stiffness in cardiovascular disease. *JRSM Cardiovasc. Dis.* **2012**, *1*, 1–10.
14. Fahs, C.A.; Thiebaud, R.S.; Rossow, L.M.; Loenneke, J.P.; Bemben, D.A.; Bemben, M.G. Relationships between central arterial stiffness, lean body mass, and absolute and relative strength in young and older men and women. *Clin. Physiol. Funct. Imaging* **2018**, *38*, 676–680.
15. Yang, M.; Zhang, X.; Ding, Z.; Wang, F.; Wang, Y.; Jiao, C.; Chen, J.H. Low skeletal muscle mass is associated with arterial stiffness in community-dwelling Chinese aged 45 years and older. *BMC Public Health* **2020**, *20*, 226.
16. Ben-Shlomo, Y.; Spears, M.; Boustred, C.; May, M.; Anderson, S.G.; Benjamin, E.J.; Boutouyrie, P.; Cameron, J.; Chen, C.H.; Cruickshank, J.K.; et al. Aortic pulse wave velocity improves cardiovascular event prediction: An individual participant meta-analysis of prospective observational data from 17,635 subjects. *J. Am. Coll. Cardiol.* **2014**, *63*, 636–646.
17. Heusinkveld, M.H.; Delhaas, T.; Lumens, J.; Huberts, W.; Spronck, B.; Hughes, A.D.; Reesink, K.D. Augmentation index is not a proxy for wave reflection magnitude: Mechanistic analysis using a computational model. *J. Appl. Physiol.* **2019**, *127*, 491–500.
18. König, M.; Buchmann, N.; Seeland, U.; Spira, D.; Steinhagen, E.; Demuth, I. Low muscle strength and increased arterial stiffness go hand in hand. *Sci. Rep.* **2021**, *11*, 2906.
19. Fahs, C.A.; Heffernan, K.S.; Ranadive, S.; Jae, S.Y.; Fernhall, B. Muscular strength is inversely associated with aortic stiffness in young men. *Med. Sci. Sports Exerc.* **2010**, *42*, 1619–1624.
20. Lima-Junior, D.D.; Farah, B.Q.; Germano-Soares, A.H.; Andrade-Lima, A.; Silva, G.O.; Rodrigues, S.L.C.; Ritti-Dias, R. Association between handgrip strength and vascular function in patients with hypertension. *Clin. Exp. Hypertens.* **2019**, *41*, 692–695.
21. Dvoretskiy, S.; Lieblein-Boff, J.C.; Jonnalagadda, S.; Atherton, P.J.; Phillips, B.E.; Pereira, S.L. Exploring the Association between Vascular Dysfunction and Skeletal Muscle Mass, Strength and Function in Healthy Adults: A Systematic Review. *Nutrients* **2020**, *12*, 715. [PubMed]

2. Bohannon, R.W. Considerations and Practical Options for Measuring Muscle Strength: A Narrative Review. *Biomed. Res. Int.* **2019**, *2019*, 8194537.
3. Shen, C.; Lu, J.; Xu, Z.; Xu, Y.; Yang, Y. Association between handgrip strength and the risk of new-onset metabolic syndrome: A population-based cohort study. *BMJ Open* **2020**, *10*, e041384. [PubMed]
4. Lopez-Lopez, J.P.; Cohen, D.D.; Ney-Salazar, D.; Martinez, D.; Otero, J.; Gomez-Arbelaez, D.; Camacho, P.A.; Sanchez-Vallejo, G.; Arcos, E.; Narvaez, C.; et al. The prediction of Metabolic Syndrome alterations is improved by combining waist circumference and handgrip strength measurements compared to either alone. *Cardiovasc. Diabetol.* **2021**, *20*, 68.
5. Araújo, C.; Amaral, T.L.M.; Monteiro, G.T.R.; de Vasconcellos, M.T.L.; Portela, M.C. Factors associated with low handgrip strength in older people: Data of the Study of Chronic Diseases (Edoc-I). *BMC Public Health* **2020**, *20*, 395.
6. Ji, C.; Zheng, L.; Zhang, R.; Wu, Q.; Zhao, Y. Handgrip strength is positively related to blood pressure and hypertension risk: Results from the National Health and nutrition examination survey. *Lipids Health Dis.* **2018**, *17*, 86.
7. Hao, G.; Chen, H.; Ying, Y.; Wu, M.; Yang, G.; Jing, C. The Relative Handgrip Strength and Risk of Cardiometabolic Disorders: A Prospective Study. *Front. Physiol.* **2020**, *11*, 719.
8. Klawitter, L.; Vincent, B.M.; Choi, B.J.; Smith, J.; Hammer, K.D.; Jurivich, D.A.; Dahl, L.J.; McGrath, R. Handgrip Strength Asymmetry and Weakness Are Associated with Future Morbidity Accumulation in Americans. *J. Strength Cond. Res.* **2022**, *36*, 106–112.
9. McGrath, R.; Clark, B.C.; Cesari, M.; Johnson, C.; Jurivich, D.A. Handgrip strength asymmetry is associated with future falls in older Americans. *Aging Clin. Exp. Res.* **2021**, *33*, 2461–2469.
10. McGrath, R.; Cawthon, P.M.; Cesari, M.; Al Snih, S.; Clark, B.C. Handgrip Strength Asymmetry and Weakness Are Associated with Lower Cognitive Function: A Panel Study. *J. Am. Geriatr. Soc.* **2020**, *68*, 2051–2058.
11. Collins, K.; Johnson, N.; Klawitter, L.; Waldera, R.; Stastny, S.; Kraemer, W.J.; Christensen, B.; McGrath, R. Handgrip Strength Asymmetry and Weakness are Differentially Associated with Functional Limitations in Older Americans. *Int. J. Environ. Res. Public Health* **2020**, *17*, 3231. [CrossRef] [PubMed]
12. McGrath, R.; Tomkinson, G.R.; LaRoche, D.P.; Vincent, B.M.; Bond, C.W.; Hackney, K.J. Handgrip Strength Asymmetry and Weakness May Accelerate Time to Mortality in Aging Americans. *J. Am. Med. Dir. Assoc.* **2020**, *21*, 2003–2007.e1. [CrossRef] [PubMed]
13. Hamasaki, H.; Yanai, H. Handgrip strength is inversely associated with augmentation index in patients with type 2 diabetes. *Sci. Rep.* **2023**, *13*, 1125. [CrossRef]
14. Van Dijk, S.C.; Swart, K.M.A.; Ham, A.C.; Enneman, A.W.; Van Wijngaarden, J.P.; Feskens, E.J.; Geleijnse, J.M.; De Jongh, R.T.; Blom, H.J.; Dhonukshe-Rutten, R.A.M. Physical fitness, activity and hand-grip strength are not associated with arterial stiffness in older individuals. *J. Nutr. Health Aging* **2015**, *19*, 779–784. [CrossRef] [PubMed]
15. Alberti, K.G.; Eckel, R.H.; Grundy, S.M.; Zimmet, P.Z.; Cleeman, J.I.; Donato, K.A.; Fruchart, J.C.; James, W.P.T.; Loria, C.M.; Smith, S.C., Jr. Harmonizing the Metabolic Syndrome: A joint Interim Statement of the International Diabetes Federation Task Force on Epidemiology and Prevention; National Heart, Lung, and Blood Institute; American Heart Association; World Heart Federation; International Atherosclerosis Society; and International Association for the Study of Obesity. *Circulation* **2009**, *120*, 1640–1645.
16. Berukstis, A.; Jarasunas, J.; Daskeviciute, A.; Ryliskyte, L.; Baranauskas, A.; Steponeniene, R.; Laucevicius, A. How to interpret 24-h arterial stiffness markers: Comparison of 24-h ambulatory Mobil-O-Graph with SphygmoCor office values. *Blood Press. Monit.* **2019**, *24*, 93–98. [CrossRef] [PubMed]
17. Bahannon, R.W.; Peolsson, A.; Massy-Westropp, N.; Desrosiers, J.; Bear-Lehman, J. Reference values for adult grip strength measured with a Jamar dynamometer: A descriptive meta-analysis. *Physiotherapy* **2006**, *92*, 11–15. [CrossRef]
18. Colineaux, H.; Neufcourt, L.; Delpierre, C.; Kelly-Irving, M.; Lepage, B. Explaining biological differences between men and women by gendered mechanisms. *Emerg. Themes Epidemiol.* **2023**, *20*, 2. [CrossRef]
19. Ogola, B.O.; Zimmerman, M.A.; Clark, G.L.; Abshire, C.M.; Gentry, K.M.; Miller, K.S.; Lindsey, S.H. New insights into arterial stiffening: Does sex matter? *Am. J. Physiol. Heart Circ. Physiol.* **2018**, *315*, H1073–H1087. [CrossRef]
20. El Khoudary, S.R.; Aggarwal, B.; Beckie, T.M.; Hodis, H.N.; Johnson, A.E.; Langer, R.D.; Limacher, M.C.; Manson, J.E.; Stefanick, M.L.; Allison, M.A.; et al. Menopause Transition and Cardiovascular Disease Risk: Implications for Timing of Early Prevention: A Scientific Statement from the American Heart Association. *Circulation* **2020**, *142*, e506–e532. [CrossRef]
21. Heffernan, K.S.; Chalé, A.; Hau, C.; Cloutier, G.J.; Phillips, E.M.; Warner, P.; Nickerson, H.; Reid, K.F.; Kuvin, J.T.; Fielding, R.A. Systemic vascular function is associated with muscular power in older adults. *J. Aging Res.* **2012**, *2012*, 386387. [CrossRef] [PubMed]
22. Mendes-Pinto, D.; Rodrigues-Machado, M. Aplicabilidade dos marcadores de rigidez arterial na doença arterial periférica. *J. Vasc. Bras.* **2019**, *18*, e20180093. [CrossRef] [PubMed]
23. Rodriguez, A.J.; Karim, M.N.; Srikanth, V.; Ebeling, P.R.; Scott, D. Lower muscle tissue is associated with higher pulse wave velocity: A systematic review and meta-analysis of observational study data. *Clin. Exp. Pharmacol. Physiol.* **2017**, *44*, 980–992. [CrossRef]
24. Lopez-Jaramillo, P.; Gonzalez, M.C.; Palmer, R.M.; Moncada, S. The crucial role of physiological Ca^{2+} concentrations in the production of endothelial nitric oxide and the control of vascular tone. *Br. J. Pharmacol.* **1990**, *101*, 489–493. [CrossRef] [PubMed]
25. Maréchal, G.; Gailly, P. Effects of nitric oxide on the contraction of skeletal muscle. *Cell Mol. Life Sci.* **1999**, *55*, 1088–1102. [CrossRef]

46. Ibrahim, M.Y.; Ashour, O.M. Changes in nitric oxide and free radical levels in rat gastrocnemius muscle during contraction and fatigue. *Clin. Exp. Pharmacol. Physiol.* **2011**, *38*, 791–795. [CrossRef]
47. Townsend, R.R.; Wilkinson, I.B.; Schiffrin, E.L.; Avolio, A.P.; Chirinos, J.A.; Cockcroft, J.R.; Heffernan, K.S.; Lakatta, E.G.; McEniery, C.M.; Mitchell, G.F.; et al. Recommendations for improving and standardizing vascular research on arterial stiffness: A scientific statement from the American Heart Association. *Hypertension* **2015**, *66*, 698–722. [CrossRef]
48. Seals, D.R.; Jablonski, K.L.; Donato, A.J. Aging and vascular endothelial function in humans. *Clin. Sci.* **2011**, *120*, 357–375. [CrossRef]
49. Hasegawa, N.; Fujie, S.; Horii, N.; Miyamoto-Mikami, E.R.I.; Tsuji, K.; Uchida, M.; Hamaoka, T.; Tabata, I.; Iemitsu, M. Effects of Different Exercise Modes on Arterial Stiffness and Nitric Oxide Synthesis. *Med. Sci. Sports Exerc.* **2018**, *50*, 1177–1185. [CrossRef]
50. Severinsen, M.C.K.; Pedersen, B.K. Muscle-Organ Crosstalk: The Emerging Roles of Myokines. *Endocr. Rev.* **2021**, *42*, 97–99. [CrossRef]
51. Yu, Z.; Li, P.; Zhang, M.; Hannink, M.; Stamler, J.S.; Yan, Z. Fiber type-specific nitric oxide protects oxidative myofibers against cachectic stimuli. *PLoS ONE.* **2008**, *3*, e2086. [CrossRef]
52. Mendonca, G.V.; Pezarat-Correia, P.; Vaz, J.R.; Silva, L.; Heffernan, K.S. Impact of Aging on Endurance and Neuromuscular Physical Performance: The Role of Vascular Senescence. *Sports Med.* **2017**, *47*, 583–598. [CrossRef]
53. Van Der Loo, B.; Labugger, R.; Skepper, J.N.; Bachschmid, M.; Kilo, J.; Powell, J.M.; Palacios-Callender, M.; Erusalimsky, J.D.; Quaschning, T.; Malinski, T.; et al. Enhanced peroxynitrite formation is associated with vascular aging. *J. Exp. Med.* **2000**, *192*, 1731–1744. [CrossRef]
54. Lamb, G.D.; Westerblad, H. Acute effects of reactive oxygen and nitrogen species on the contractile function of skeletal muscle. *J. Physiol.* **2011**, *589 Pt 9*, 2119–2127. [CrossRef]
55. Hare, J.M. Nitric oxide and excitation-contraction coupling. *J. Mol. Cell Cardiol.* **2003**, *35*, 719–729. [CrossRef]
56. Liu, M.; Liu, S.; Sun, S.; Tian, H.; Li, S.; Wu, Y. Sex Differences in the Associations of Handgrip Strength and Asymmetry with Multimorbidity: Evidence from the English Longitudinal Study of Ageing. *J. Am. Med. Dir Assoc.* **2022**, *23*, 493–498.e1. [CrossRef]
57. McGrath, R.; Lang, J.J.; Ortega, F.B.; Chaput, J.P.; Zhang, K.; Smith, J.; Vincent, B.; Piñero, J.C.; Garcia, M.C.; Tomkinson, G.R. Handgrip strength asymmetry is associated with slow gait speed and poorer standing balance in older Americans. *Arch. Gerontol. Geriatr.* **2022**, *102*, 104716. [CrossRef]
58. Delong, C.; Sharma, S. Physiology, Peripheral Vascular Resistance. In *StatPearls*; StatPearls Publishing: Treasure Island, FL, USA, 2023.
59. Hendrickse, P.; Degens, H. The role of the microcirculation in muscle function and plasticity. *J. Muscle Res. Cell Motil.* **2019**, *40*, 127–140. [CrossRef]
60. Cheng, C.; Daskalakis, C.; Falkner, B. Association of capillary density and function measures with blood pressure, fasting plasma glucose, and insulin sensitivity. *J. Clin. Hypertens.* **2010**, *12*, 125–135. [CrossRef]
61. Lin, S.; Wang, F.; Huang, Y.; Yuan, Y.; Huang, F.; Zhu, P. Handgrip strength weakness and asymmetry together are associated with cardiovascular outcomes in older outpatients: A prospective cohort study. *Geriatr. Gerontol. Int.* **2022**, *22*, 759–765. [CrossRef]
62. Starzak, M.; Stanek, A.; Jakubiak, G.K.; Cholewka, A.; Cieślar, G. Arterial Stiffness Assessment by Pulse Wave Velocity in Patients with Metabolic Syndrome and Its Components: Is It a Useful Tol in Clinical Practice? *Int. J. Environ. Res. Public Health* **2022**, *19*, 10368. [CrossRef] [PubMed]
63. Amarasekera, A.T.; Chang, D.; Schwarz, P.; Tan, T.C. Does vascular endothelial dysfunction play a role in physical frailty and sarcopenia? A systematic review. *Age Ageing* **2021**, *50*, 725–732. [CrossRef] [PubMed]
64. Tuttle, C.S.L.; Thang, L.A.N.; Maier, A.B. Markers of inflammation and their association with muscle strength and mass: A systematic review and meta-analysis. *Ageing Res. Rev.* **2020**, *64*, 101185. [CrossRef]
65. Loenneke, J.P.; Fahs, C.A.; Heffernan, K.S.; Rossow, L.M.; Thiebaud, R.S.; Bemben, M.G. Relationship between thigh muscle mass and augmented pressure from wave reflections in healthy adults. *Eur. J. Appl. Physiol.* **2013**, *113*, 395–401. [CrossRef] [PubMed]
66. Lee, D.; Byun, K.; Hwang, M.-H.; Lee, S. Augmentation Index Is Inversely Associated with Skeletal Muscle Mass, Muscle Strength, and Anaerobic Power in Young Male Adults: A Preliminary Study. *Appl. Sci.* **2021**, *11*, 3146. [CrossRef]
67. Aminuddin, A.; Noor Hashim, M.F.; Mohd Zaberi, N.A.S.; Zheng Wei, L.; Ching Chu, B.; Jamaludin, N.A.; Salamt, N.; Che Roos, N.A.; Ugusman, A. The Association Between Arterial Stiffness and Muscle Indices Among Healthy Subjects and Subjects with Cardiovascular Risk Factors: An Evidence-Based Review. *Front. Physiol.* **2021**, *12*, 742338. [CrossRef]
68. Zhang, L.; Guo, Q.; Feng, B.L.; Wang, C.Y.; Han, P.P.; Hu, J.; Sun, X.D.; Zeng, W.F.; Zheng, Z.X.; Li, H.S.; et al. Cross-Sectional Study of the Association between Arterial Stiffness and Sarcopenia in Chinese Community-Dwelling Elderly Using the Asian Working Group for Sarcopenia Criteria. *J. Nutr. Health Aging* **2019**, *23*, 195–201. [CrossRef]
69. Chung, J.; Kim, M.; Jin, Y.; Kim, Y.; Hong, J. Fitness as a determinant of arterial stiffness in healthy adult men: A cross-sectional study. *J. Sports Med. Phys. Fit.* **2018**, *58*, 150–156. [CrossRef]
70. Wong, A.; Figueroa, A.; Son, W.M.; Chernykh, O.; Park, S.Y. The effects of stair climbing on arterial stiffness, blood pressure, and leg strength in postmenopausal women with stage 2 hypertension. *Menopause* **2018**, *25*, 731–737. [CrossRef]
71. Watanabe, Y.; Masaki, H.; Yunoki, Y.; Tabuchi, A.; Morita, I.; Mohri, S.; Tanemoto, K. Ankle-brachial index, toe-brachial index, and pulse volume recording in healthy young adults. *Ann. Vasc. Dis.* **2015**, *8*, 227–235. [CrossRef]

2. Kuh, D.; Bassey, E.J.; Butterworth, S.; Hardy, R.; Wadsworth, M.E. Musculoskeletal Study Team: Grip strength, postural control, and functional leg power in a representative cohort of British men and women: Associations with physical activity, health status, and socioeconomic conditions. *J. Gerontol. A Biol. Sci. Med. Sci.* **2005**, *60*, 224–231. [CrossRef] [PubMed]
3. Weiss, W.; Gohlisch, C.; Harsch-Gladisch, C.; Tölle, M.; Zidek, W.; Van Der Giet, M. Oscillometric estimation of central blood pressure: Validation of the Mobil-O-Graph in comparison with the SphygmoCor device. *Blood Press Monit.* **2012**, *17*, 128–131. [CrossRef]
4. Papaioannou, T.G.; Argyris, A.; Protogerou, A.D.; Vrachatis, D.; Nasothimiou, E.G.; Sfikakis, P.P.; Stergiou, G.S.; Stefanadis, C.I. Non-invasive 24 hour ambulatory monitoring of aortic wave reflection and arterial stiffness by a novel oscillometric device: The first feasibility and reproducibility study. *Int. J. Cardiol.* **2013**, *169*, 57–61. [CrossRef]
5. Hamasaki, H. What can hand grip strength tell us about type 2 diabetes?: Mortality, morbidities and risk of diabetes. *Expert Rev. Endocrinol. Metab.* **2021**, *16*, 237–250. [CrossRef] [PubMed]
6. Cruz-Jentoft, A.J.; Sayer, A.A. Sarcopenia. *Lancet* **2019**, *393*, 2636–2646. [CrossRef] [PubMed]
7. González, D.E.G.; Robayo, J.H.C.; Pérez, P.A.M.; López, P.A.C.; Cohen, D.D.; Ardila, E.S.M.; Delgado, J.C.S. Efectos del entrenamiento de fuerza prensil y su asociación sobre la función vascular en sujetos con criterios diagnósticos de síndrome metabólico: Una revisión de tema. *Rev. Cuba. Investig. Biomed.* **2022**, *41*, e1411.
8. Taylor, K.A.; Wiles, J.D.; Coleman, D.A.; Leeson, P.; Sharma, R.; O'Driscoll, J.M. Neurohumoral and ambulatory haemodynamic adaptations following isometric exercise training in unmedicated hypertensive patients. *J. Hypertens.* **2019**, *37*, 827–836. [CrossRef]
9. Cohen, D.D.; Aroca-Martinez, G.; Carreño-Robayo, J.; Castañeda-Hernández, A.; Herazo-Beltran, Y.; Camacho, P.A.; Otero, J.; Martinez-Bello, D.; Lopez-Lopez, J.P.; Lopez-Jaramillo, P. Reductions in systolic blood pressure achieved by hypertensives with three isometric training sessions per week are maintained with a single session per week. *J. Clin. Hypertens.* **2023**, *25*, 380–387. [CrossRef]
10. Edwards, J.J.; Wiles, J.; O'Driscoll, J. Mechanisms for blood pressure reduction following isometric exercise training: A systematic review and meta-analysis. *J. Hypertens.* **2022**, *40*, 2299–2306. [CrossRef]

Disclaimer/Publisher's Note: The statements, opinions and data contained in all publications are solely those of the individual author(s) and contributor(s) and not of MDPI and/or the editor(s). MDPI and/or the editor(s) disclaim responsibility for any injury to people or property resulting from any ideas, methods, instructions or products referred to in the content.

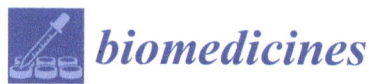

Communication

Macrophages of the Cardiorenal Axis and Myocardial Infarction

Maria Kercheva [1,2,*], Vyacheslav Ryabov [1,2,3], Aleksandra Gombozhapova [1,2], Ivan Stepanov [2] and Julia Kzhyshkowska [3,4]

[1] Cardiology Division, Siberian State Medical University, 2 Moscovsky Trakt, 634055 Tomsk, Russia
[2] Cardiology Research Institute, Tomsk National Research Medical Center of the RAS, 111a Kievskaya Street, 634012 Tomsk, Russia
[3] Laboratory of Translational and Cellular Biomedicine, National Research Tomsk State University, 36 Lenin Avenue, 634050 Tomsk, Russia
[4] Institute of Transfusion Medicine and Immunology, University of Heidelberg, 1-3 Theodor-Kutzer Ufer, 68167 Mannheim, Germany
* Correspondence: mariiakercheva@mail.ru; Tel.: +7-3822-561232

Abstract: The aim of our study was to compare the features of macrophage (mf) composition of the kidneys in patients with fatal myocardial infarction (MI) and in patients without cardiovascular diseases (CVD). We used kidney fragments taken during autopsy. Macrophage infiltration was assessed by immunohistochemistry: antibodies CD68 were used as a common mf marker, CD80—M1 type mf marker, CD163, CD206, and stabilin-1—M2 type. Macrophage composition of the kidneys in patients with fatal MI was characterized by the predominance of CD163+ cells among studied cells and the control group was characterized by the predominance of CD163+, CD206+, and CD68+. In patients with MI, biphasic response from kidney cells was characterized for CD80+ and CD206+: their number decreased by the long-term period of MI; other cells did not show any dynamics. The exact number of CD80+ cells in kidneys of individuals without CVD was slightly higher than in patients with MI, and the number of CD206+—strikingly predominant. Subsequent analysis of CD80+ and CD206+ cells in a larger sample, as well as comparison of data with results obtained from survivors of MI, may bring us closer to understanding whether the influence on these cells can serve as a new target in personalized therapy in postinfarction complications.

Keywords: myocardial infarction; cardiac remodeling; cardiac macrophages; kidney macrophages; inflammation

Citation: Kercheva, M.; Ryabov, V.; Gombozhapova, A.; Stepanov, I.; Kzhyshkowska, J. Macrophages of the Cardiorenal Axis and Myocardial Infarction. *Biomedicines* **2023**, *11*, 1843. https://doi.org/10.3390/biomedicines11071843

Academic Editor: Alfredo Caturano

Received: 31 May 2023
Revised: 21 June 2023
Accepted: 22 June 2023
Published: 27 June 2023

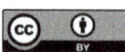

Copyright: © 2023 by the authors. Licensee MDPI, Basel, Switzerland. This article is an open access article distributed under the terms and conditions of the Creative Commons Attribution (CC BY) license (https://creativecommons.org/licenses/by/4.0/).

1. Introduction

Impaired hemodynamics and inadequate renal perfusion cause the formation of cardiorenal syndrome (CRS) in myocardial infarction (MI) [1]. Acute impairment of kidney function in patients with MI develops in 7.1–29.3% of cases, worsens both short-term and long-term prognosis in this cohort of patients, and increases hospitalization time [2]. The existing understanding of CRS within its classification according to clinical and anamnestic data can detect cardiorenal dysfunction but does not change disease management and prognosis [3,4]. The cardiorenal relationships at the cellular level are poorly studied [5] and the existing experimental data are not sufficient to affect the course of the disease. Recently, it has become evident that cells of innate immunity are important to maintain a balanced relationship between the heart and the kidneys [5,6]. Changed polarization of macrophages (mf) in the kidneys induced by ischemia enhances the release of granulocyte–macrophage colony-stimulating factor into the bloodstream, which in turn causes subsequent polarization of myocardial mf into the regenerative M2 type and is associated with the development of fibrosis and adaptive myocardial hypertrophy [5]. However, clinical data on this interaction of innate immune cells along the heart–kidney axis are limited [7,8]. In our previous study, we investigated the composition of mf in the kidneys and its relationship with changes in mf infiltration into the heart, and with an adverse course of the disease in patients with fatal MI. A pronounced heterogeneity of the mf composition in the kidneys with the predominance of CD163+ cells was revealed in this cohort of patients. Among all studied cells we revealed two types—CD206+ and CD80+, which showed significant quantitative dynamics in the late period after MI and a number of relationships with both adverse prognosis and cardiac macrophages [9]. Yet, it remains unclear whether our data indicate changes in the mf composition of the kidneys in response to myocardial ischemia, and whether these changes can affect the course and prognosis of the disease. In this regard, the aim of the study was to compare data on the features of the mf composition in the kidneys in patients with fatal MI and in patients from the control group without a history of cardiovascular diseases (CVD).

2. Materials and Methods

2.1. Clinical and Anamnestic Characteristics

The study involved patients with fatal type 1 MI. The exclusion criteria were type II–V MI, oncological disorders, infectious complications (sepsis, pneumonia), and valvular defects requiring surgical intervention. The study protocol was approved by the Biomedical Ethics Committee of Cardiology Research Institute (Tomsk, Russia), protocol No. 128, of 23 December 2014. The study was conducted in accordance with the principles of the Declaration of Helsinki. Pathological autopsy was carried out in accordance with the order of the Ministry of Health of the Russian Federation of 6 June 2013, No. 354n, on the procedure of postmortem examinations. In this study, informed consent could not be obtained, yet this did not contradict the principles for conducting the study in accordance with the Declaration of Helsinki (informed consent, paragraph 32).

The study object was kidney fragments taken from MI patients (n = 30) and from patients in the control group (n = 8) during autopsy. The control group consisted of people who died from fatal injuries and did not have CVD (aged from 18 to 55). An autopsy was performed within 24 h after death. The material was fixed in 10% buffered formalin for 1 day. The material for histological examination was prepared by standard method using a Thermo Scientific Excelsior AS (Thermo Fisher Scientific, Waltham, MA, USA). After that, the material was embedded in paraffin using a Tissue-Tek® TEC™ 6 embedding console system (Sakura, Tokyo, Japan). The results were obtained using the equipment of the Center for Collective Use "Medical Genomics", Tomsk National Medical Research Center.

To study the spatiotemporal pattern of accumulation of mf in the kidneys and their phenotypes, the patients with MI were divided into groups depending on infarction duration: group 1 involved those who died during the first three days after MI, within 72 h; group 2 included patients who died on day 4–28.

We have already reported clinical and anamnestic data on these groups of patients [9]. It should be noted that the average age of the examined patients was 74.8 ± 9.8. The time from the onset of the disease to admission to the hospital was 180 min (120–720 min.). Circular MI was recorded in 40% of cases, and recurrent MI was observed in half of the patients. Heart failure (HF) in anamnesis occurred in 50% of patients. Cardiogenic shock was the main death factor; other reasons were cardiac rupture and arrhythmogenic shock.

2.2. Immunohistochemical Analysis

To perform an immunohistochemical analysis with a rotary microtome (HM 355S, Thermo Fisher Scientific, Waltham, MA, USA), kidney sections were prepared: 10 sections from each block. The material was then applied to L-polylysine-coated slides, two sections per slide. The study was performed using an automated immunostainer (Leica Bond-Max, Wetzlar, Germany) in accordance with a standard protocol [10]. The study used antibodies against mf markers. CD68 was used as a common mf marker. CD80 was used as M1 type mf marker. CD163 and CD206 were used as classical M2 type mf markers, and stabilin-1 was used as an additional M2 type mf marker. We used mouse monoclonal antibodies against CD68 (Cell Marque, 1:500 dilution), antibodies against CD163 (Cell Marque, Rocklin, CA, USA, 1:50 dilution), antibodies against CD80 (Invitrogen, Waltham, MA, USA, 1:600

dilution), mouse monoclonal antibodies against CD206 (Santa Cruz, 1:100 dilution), and antibodies against stabilin-1 RS1 (1:1000 dilution) synthesized in the Laboratory of Innate Immunity and Immunological Tolerance (University of Heidelberg).

The studied markers were visualized using the BOND Polymer Refine Detection system (Leica, Wetzlar, Germany). BOND Polymer Refine Detection contains a peroxide block, post-primary, polymer reagent, DAB chromogen, and hematoxylin counterstain. Two independent experts counted positively stained mfs in the kidney and analyzed 10 randomly chosen fields of view (40× objective) using a Zeiss Axio Imager M2 microscope, bright field.

2.3. Statistical Analysis

The obtained data were analyzed using the STATISTICA 12.0 software package. The quantitative data were tested for normality using the Shapiro–Wilk test. All quantitative indicators that showed abnormal distribution were described by the median (Me) and interquartile interval (Q1; Q3). The Mann–Whitney test was used to compare quantitative indicators in independent groups, Kendall rank correlation coefficient and Wilcoxon signed-rank test were used to dependent groups. Statistical hypotheses were tested with the significance value $p = 0.05$.

3. Results

The features of mf composition in the kidneys and its dynamics in MI patients were revealed through the analysis of the data obtained from both the control group and MI patients at different time periods—early and late periods after MI (Table 1).

Table 1. Features of macrophage composition in the kidneys in patients with fatal MI and in patients from the control group (number of positive stained macrophages counted per histology section area of interest and analyzed in 10 randomly chosen fields of view).

Cells	All Patients (n = 30)	Control (n = 8)	p1	Group 1 (n = 17)	Group 2 (n = 13)	p2	p3	p4
CD163+	55 (32; 97)	47 (34; 68)	0.5	55 (34; 72)	58 (32; 97)	0.5	0.9	0.4
CD68+	30 (23; 51) *	41 (33;48)	0.45	30 (24; 49) *	35(23; 51) *	0.7	0.4	0.7
CD206+	4 (2; 6) *, **	30 (27; 35)	0.0005	6 (5; 8) *,**	2 (1; 2) *, **	0.01	0.005	0.0001
Stabilin-1+	2 (1; 3) *, **, ***	2 (1; 3) *, **, ***	0.8	1 (1; 4) *, **, ***	2 (1; 2) *, **	0.3	0.9	0.7
CD80+	3 (2; 5) *, **, ***	6 (6; 7) *, **, ***, ****	0.0003	5 (3; 5) *, **, ***	2 (1;2) *, **	0.01	0.0005	0.0007

Note: MI—myocardial infarction. p1—Significant difference between the group with fatal MI and the control group; p2—significant difference between patients with fatal MI from group 1 and group 2; p3—significant difference between patients with control group from group 1; p4—significant difference between patients with control group from group 2. *—Significant difference in the group between the number of CD163+ cells and other cells; **—significant difference in the group between the number of CD68+ cells and other cells; ***—significant difference in the group between the number of CD206+ cells and other cells; ****—significant difference in the group between the number of stabilin-1+ cells and other cells.

CD163+ cells were predominant in the kidneys of MI patients; however, in the control group these cells were predominant with CD68+ and CD206+ cells (Figures 1 and 2).

Interestingly, among the studied kidney cells, CD206+ and CD80+ were the types of cells that had dynamics that changed depending on the MI period (Table 1). The number of these cells in the kidneys decreased in the late period after MI. The number of these cells in the kidneys of patients from the control group exceeded that in MI patients (Table 1, Figure 2). Other kidney cells neither changed over time nor differed from those in patients from the control group.

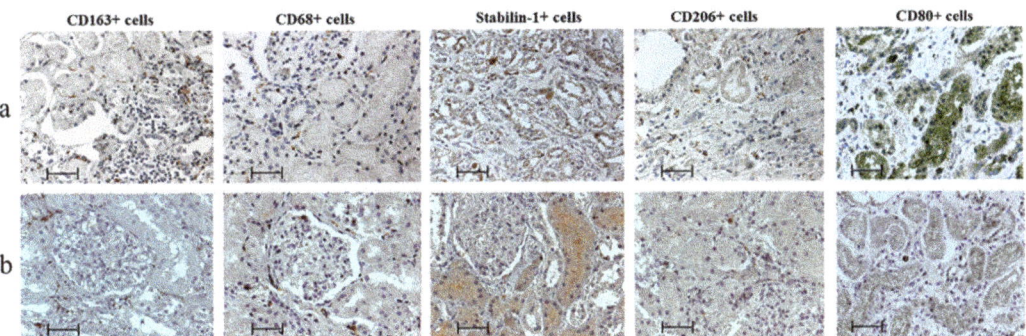

Figure 1. Features of macrophage infiltration of kidneys (**a**) in patients with myocardial infarction and (**b**) of control group, immunohistochemistry; scale bar: 50 μm.

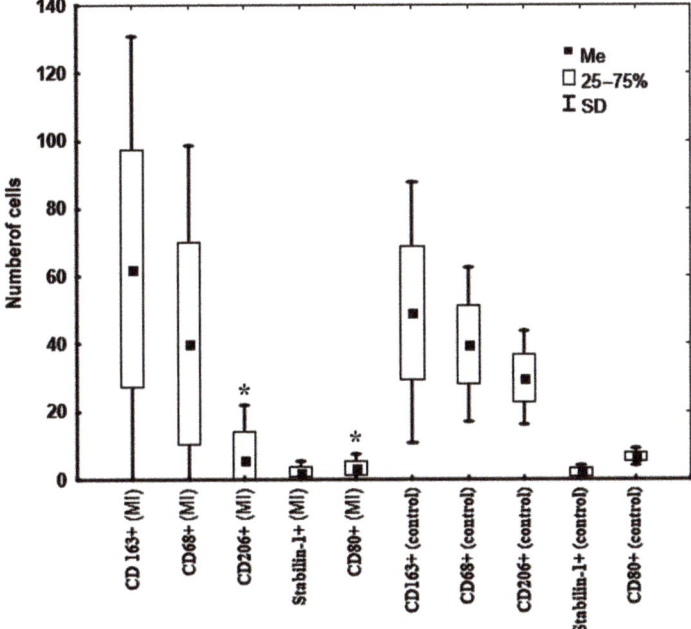

Figure 2. Features of the macrophage composition in the kidneys in patients with fatal MI (n = 30) and in patients from the control group (n = 8). Note: *—significant difference between patients with fatal MI from group 1 and group 2. Abbreviation: MI—myocardial infarction.

4. Discussion

Our data are unique and novel since we are the first to reveal the features of changes in the kidney mf composition in MI patients, and show the relationship between these changes and unfavorable outcome through comparison of these changes with the results obtained for patients without CVD. However, the results mainly indicate pathophysiological processes that occur under experimental ischemic conditions in animals.

Among all the studied cells, CD163+ predominate in terms of their number in the kidneys of patients with MI and they serve as one of the leading cell types in the control group. The CD163 cellular receptor is actively expressed on both monocytes and mf, and serves as a marker for alternatively activated M2 mf [11]. Monocytes are known to express a small amount of CD163. However, mf, particularly in the inflammation resolution phase, exhibit a high expression of CD163 [12]. As previously reported, a high concentration of these cell types in kidney biopsy specimens from patients with lupus nephritis [13] was due to the unfavorable course and prognosis of the disease. Similar data were reported for patients with IgA nephropathy [14] and for patients after kidney transplantation [15]. A high concentration of these cells in the myocardium in the late postinfarction period was also due to unfavorable outcome [16]. However, we assume that these cells are most likely involved in tissue homeostasis, immunological regulation, and tissue regeneration in case of any injury, and initiation, which explains their high and comparable concentration in kidney tissues in both groups [7].

The number of CD68+ cells is the next largest in the group of MI and they also serve as one of the leading cell types in the control group. CD68 is an immunohistochemical marker of the common population of mf, of which the main function is the absorption of apoptotic and damaged cells [17]. This can be the cause of a high concentration of these cells in MI patients. A high concentration of this cell type in kidneys in the late observation period probably shows their involvement in a prolonged inflammatory reaction and is associated with unfavorable prognosis, which indicates involvement of the innate immune system in postinfarction kidney regeneration. In a number of studies, concentration of CD68+ cells correlated with albuminuria and unfavorable outcome [18]. The number of these cells in MI patients from the studied group was comparable to the number of CD68+ cells in the kidneys of patients with a reduced glomerular filtration rate and the presence of lupus nephritis [19]. Yet, the number of cells was similar to that in healthy individuals, which may indirectly indicate the lack of the impact of this cell type on cardiorenal relationships in MI patients.

One of the most widely studied markers of M1 mf is CD80 [20]. M1 mf secrete pro-inflammatory cytokines, cathepsins, and matrix metalloproteinases, which induce the elimination of cellular debris and apoptotic cells and the beginning of the repair process [21]. The decrease in the level of these cells in patients with MI by the late period of MI determines the physiological course of the inflammatory response [21]. However, the fact that the level of CD80 cells is lower in individuals with MI than in the control group, along with a decrease in the level of M2 mf– CD206+ cells by the late period of MI and becoming comparable with CD80+ and stabilin-1 cells, may cause an adverse course of the disease. An inadequate weak inflammatory response, along with an inadequate low-intensity regeneration phase, can cause an unfavorable outcome of MI.

The study of the concentration of stabilin-1+ cells in the kidneys of patients with MI and without CVD showed single stabilin+ cells. Studies on the role of stabilin-1+ cells in cardiovascular pathology are insufficient [16,22]. Some data were obtained for patients with cancer [23]. The study of these cells in the kidneys of MI patients has not been performed. A low content of cells in the renal tissue of the examined MI patients probably indicates a negligible impact, or lack thereof, of these cells on the cardiorenal relationships. The data obtained in this study show inadequacy of the dichotomous model for assessing mf and their functions with regard to their conditional division into two phenotypes—pro- and anti-inflammatory. The behavior of all the studied M2 type mf is completely different. They are different in their concentration in tissues and in their response to myocardial ischemia.

In our opinion, among all the studied kidney mf, CD206+ cells belonging to M2 type mf are most interesting and promising for further research [24]. This is the type of mf that showed significant dynamics in renal tissue in the late period after MI, as well as a significantly lower concentration in patients with fatal MI. A number of researchers reported data that are partly comparable to our data. In particular, comparison of the number of these cells in the kidneys of patients with acute interstitial nephritis and in a cohort of patients with acute tubular necrosis showed a lower number of CD206+ cells in patients with acute tubular necrosis [25]. This type of cells was referred to as a resident type of mf [25] involved in renal tissue homeostasis; therefore, their number can reduce under ischemic conditions and trigger an unfavorable course of the disease. In addition, according to the experimental data on rodents [5], the polarization of kidney mf under ischemic conditions, including CD206+ cells, stimulates the polarization of myocardial mf into M2 type, followed by the development of adaptive left ventricular hypertrophy and myocardial fibrosis. The effect of these processes on the disease outcome remained unclear. However, it should be noted that IL-4, IL-13, and IL-10 play a central role in the polarization of mfs in the direction of the M2 type [7]. We cannot currently confirm or deny these data, because the lack of a comprehensive, systematic analysis, including an analysis of the microenvironment, as well as the level of circulating markers, is a limitation of our study, the elimination of which is planned by us in the subsequent data collection. In addition to the influence of the microenvironment on the cell phenotype, a metabolic factor such as hypoxia may explain the low functional activity of CD206+ cells in kidneys tissue in patients with MI, which was different from that in patients without CVD [26]. It is interesting that the number of CD206+ cells in persons with MI was several times lower than in persons from the control group. An adequate/greater number of M2 mf in the kidneys may be required to change the polarization of cardiac mf in the early period after MI, which may affect the inflammatory response in the early postinfarction period and lead to unfavorable outcome. The number of these cells in MI patients was twice as low as that in patients with tubulointerstitial necrosis [25], which may indicate active involvement of this cell type in cardiorenal relationships under ischemic conditions. According to our previous data, the number of CD206+ cells in MI patients with CKD+ and CKD- was different, and the results of the multivariate analysis confirm our assumption about the relevance of studying this cell type as one of the key components of cardiorenal relationships under ischemic conditions [9]. The subsequent detailed analysis of the most pronounced pathological mf, and comparison of the data obtained on the autopsy material with those obtained for patients who have successfully come through MI, will help identify a specific target. This will contribute to targeted therapy and improve the prognosis for patients with MI affecting the development, course, and progression of postinfarction heart and renal failure.

Limitation

This study was conducted as a single-center trial and the size of a sample was small. In addition, the ratio of kidney/myocardial mf at a given time period was not a static indicator. Nowadays, this work is of a fundamental and descriptive nature. Therefore, one promising direction for future research is the changes in the amount of cells with these phenotypes in vivo in patients with MI and favorable outcome. Future investigation needs to have a complex systematic approach, accessing the cells and microenvironments changes in the heart and comparing them with the changes in target organs, with a connection with circulated biomarkers and unfavorable outcomes of MI. For these reasons, further studies are required.

5. Conclusions

Macrophage composition of the kidneys in patients with fatal MI among all the cells studied by us was characterized by the predominance of CD163+ cells, the control group characterized by the predominance of CD163+, CD206+, and CD68+. In patients with fatal MI, biphasic response from kidney macrophages was characterized for CD80+ and CD206+ cells: their number decreased by the long-term period of MI; other cells did not show any dynamics. Moreover, the exact number of CD80+ cells in kidneys of individuals without cardiovascular disease was slightly higher than in fatal MI, and the number of CD206+ cells was strikingly predominant. Subsequent analysis of CD80+ and CD206+ cells in a larger sample, as well as comparison of data with results obtained from survivors of MI, may bring us closer to understanding whether the influence on these cells can serve as a new target in personalized therapy in postinfarction complications.

Author Contributions: Conceptualization, V.R. and J.K.; methodology, V.R. and J.K.; formal analysis, M.K., A.G. and I.S.; data curation, A.G. and M.K.; investigation, V.R., A.G., M.K. and I.S.; writing, original draft preparation, M.K.; project administration, M.K.; supervision, V.R. and J.K. All authors have read and agreed to the published version of the manuscript.

Funding: The study was conducted in the framework of the fundamental research No. 122020300043-1, Tomsk NRMC.

Institutional Review Board Statement: The study was approved by the Biomedical Ethics Committee of the Research Institute of Cardiology, Tomsk National Research Medical Center (Protocol No. 128) and was conducted in accordance with the principles of the Declaration of Helsinki. Autopsy was performed in accordance with the order of the Ministry of Health of the Russian Federation No. 354n, dated 6 June 2013.

Informed Consent Statement: A signed informed consent of the patients was not taken, which did not contradict the principles for conducting the study according to the Declaration of Helsinki ("informed consent", para. 32).

Data Availability Statement: The data presented in this study are available upon request from the corresponding author.

Conflicts of Interest: The authors declare no conflict of interest.

References

1. Wang, C.; Pei, Y.-Y.; Ma, Y.-H.; Ma, X.-L.; Liu, Z.-W.; Zhu, J.-H.; Li, C.-S. Risk factors for acute kidney injury in patients with acute myocardial infarction. *Chin. Med. J.* **2019**, *132*, 1660–1665. [CrossRef] [PubMed]
2. Shacham, Y.; Steinvil, A.; Arbel, Y. Acute kidney injury among ST elevation myocardial infarction patients treated by primary percutaneous coronary intervention: A multifactorial entity. *J. Nephrol.* **2016**, *29*, 169–174. [CrossRef] [PubMed]
3. Farhan, S.; Vogel, B.; Tentzeris, I.; Jarai, R.; Freynhofer, M.K.; Smetana, P.; Egger, F.; Kautzky-Willer, A.; Huber, K. Contrast induced acute kidney injury in acute coronary syndrome patients: A single centre experience. *Eur. Heart J. Acute Cardiovasc. Care* **2016**, *5*, 55–61. [CrossRef]
4. Ronco, C.; Haapio, M.; House, A.A.; Anavekar, N.; Bellomo, R. Cardiorenal syndrome. *J. Am. Coll. Cardiol.* **2008**, *52*, 1527–1539. [CrossRef] [PubMed]
5. Fujiu, K.; Shibata, M.; Nakayama, Y.; Ogata, F.; Matsumoto, S.; Noshita, K.; Iwami, S.; Nakae, S.; Komuro, I.; Nagai, R.; et al. A heart-brain-kidney network controls adaptation to cardiac stress through tissue macrophage activation. *Nat. Med.* **2017**, *23*, 611–622. [CrossRef]
6. Silljé, H.H.W.; de Boer, R.A. Heart failure: Macrophages take centre stage in the heart-brain-kidney axis. *Nat. Rev. Nephrol.* **2017**, *13*, 388–390. [CrossRef]
7. Guiteras, R.; Flaquer, M.; Cruzado, J.M. Macrophage in chronic kidney disease. *Clin. Kidney J.* **2016**, *9*, 765–771. [CrossRef]
8. Kercheva, M.; Ryabov, V. Role of macrophages in cardiorenal syndrome development in patients with myocardial infarction. *Russ. J. Cardiol.* **2021**, *26*, 4309. (In Russian) [CrossRef]
9. Kercheva, M.; Ryabov, V.; Gombozhapova, A.; Rebenkova, M.; Kzhyshkowska, J. Macrophages of the "Heart-Kidney" Axis: Their Dynamics and Correlations with Clinical Data and Outcomes in Patients with Myocardial Infarction. *J. Pers. Med.* **2022**, *12*, 127. [CrossRef]
10. Ryabov, V.; Gombozhapova, A.; Rogovskaya, Y.; Kzhyshkowska, J.; Rebenkova, M.; Karpov, R. Cardiac CD68+ and stabilin-1+ macrophages in wound healing following myocardial infarction: From experiment to clinic. *Immunobiology* **2018**, *223*, 413–421. [CrossRef]
11. Fischer-Riepe, L.; Daber, N.; Schulte-Schrepping, J.; De Carvalho, B.C.V.; Russo, A.; Pohlen, M.; Fischer, J.; Chasan, A.I.; Wolf, M.; Barczyk-Kahlert, K.; et al. CD163 expression defines specific, IRF8-dependent, immune-modulatory macrophages in the bone marrow. *J. Allergy Clin. Immunol.* **2020**, *146*, 1137–1151. [CrossRef] [PubMed]
12. Evans, B.J.; Haskard, D.O.; Sempowksi, G.; Landis, R.C. Evolution of the Macrophage CD163 Phenotype and Cytokine Profiles in a Human Model of Resolving Inflammation. *Int. J. Inflamm.* **2013**, *2013*, 780502. [CrossRef] [PubMed]
13. Olmes, G.; Büttner-Herold, M.; Ferrazzi, F.; Distel, L.; Amann, K.; Daniel, C. CD163+ M2c-like macrophages predominate in renal biopsies from patients with lupus nephritis. *Arthritis Res. Ther.* **2016**, *18*, 90. [CrossRef]
14. Guillén-Gómez, E.; Guirado, L.; Belmonte, X.; Maderuelo, A.; Santín, S.; Juarez, C.; Ars, E.; Facundo, C.; Ballarín, J.A.; Díaz-Encarnación, M.M.; et al. Renal macrophage infiltration is associated with a poor outcome in IgA nephropathy. *Clinics* **2012**, *67*, 697–703.
15. Guillén-Gómez, E.; Guirado, L.; Belmonte, X.; Maderuelo, A.; Santín, S.; Juarez, C.; Ars, E.; Facundo, C.; Ballarín, J.A.; Vidal, S.; et al. Monocyte implication in renal allograft dysfunction. *Clin. Exp. Immunol.* **2014**, *175*, 323–331. [CrossRef]
16. Gombozhapova, A.; Rogovskaya, Y.; Rebenkova, M.; Ryabov, V. Phenotypic heterogeneity of cardiac macrophages during wound healing following myocardial infarction: Perspectives in clinical research. *Sib. J. Clin. Exp. Med.* **2018**, *33*, 70–76. [CrossRef]
17. Chistiakov, D.A.; Killingsworth, M.C.; Myasoedova, V.A.; Orekhov, A.N.; Bobryshev, Y.V. CD68/macrosialin: Not just a histochemical marker. *Lab. Investig.* **2017**, *97*, 4–13. [CrossRef]
18. Marks, S.D.; Williams, S.J.; Tullus, K.; Sebire, N.J. Glomerular expression of monocyte chemoattractant protein-1 is predictive of poor renal prognosis in pediatric lupus nephritis. *Nephrol. Dial. Transplant.* **2008**, *23*, 3521–3526. [CrossRef]

29. Dias, C.B.; Malafronte, P.; Lee, J.; Resende, A.; Jorge, L.; Pinheiro, C.C.; Malheiros, D.; Woronik, V. Role of renal expression of CD68 in the long-term prognosis of proliferative lupus nephritis. *J. Nephrol.* **2017**, *30*, 87–94. [CrossRef]
30. Ryabov, V.V.; Gombozhapova, A.E.; Rogovskaya, Y.V.; Rebenkova, M.S.; Alekseeva, Y.V.; Kzhyshkowska, Y.G. Inflammation as a universal pathogenetic link between injury, repair and regeneration, in acute coronary syndrome. From experiment to clinic. *Kardiologiia* **2019**, *59*, 15–23. [CrossRef]
31. Frangogiannis, N.G. The inflammatory response in myocardial injury, repair, and remodelling. *Nat. Rev. Cardiol.* **2014**, *11*, 255–265. [CrossRef] [PubMed]
32. Mosig, S.; Rennert, K.; Krause, S.; Kzhyshkowska, J.; Neunübel, K.; Heller, R.; Funke, H. Different functions of monocyte subsets in familial hypercholesterolemia: Potential function of CD14+ CD16+ monocytes in detoxification of oxidized LDL. *FASEB J.* **2009**, *23*, 866–874. [CrossRef] [PubMed]
33. Kzhyshkowska, J. Multifunctional receptor stabilin-1 in homeostasis and disease. *Sci. World J.* **2010**, *10*, 2039–2053. [CrossRef] [PubMed]
34. Wen, Y.; Yan, H.R.; Wang, B.; Liu, B.C. Macrophage Heterogeneity in Kidney Injury and Fibrosis. *Front. Immunol.* **2021**, *12*, 681748. [CrossRef]
35. Li, J.; Liu, C.H.; Xu, D.L.; Gao, B. Clinicopathological significance of CD206-positive macrophages in patients with acute tubulointerstitial disease. *Int. J. Clin. Exp. Pathol.* **2015**, *8*, 11386–11392.
36. Staples, K.J.; Sotoodehnejadnematalahi, F.; Pearson, H.; Frankenberger, M.; Francescut, L.; Ziegler-Heitbrock, L.; Burke, B. Monocytederived macrophages matured under prolonged hypoxia transcriptionally up-regulate HIF-1α mRNA. *Immunobiology* **2011**, *216*, 832–839. [CrossRef]

Disclaimer/Publisher's Note: The statements, opinions and data contained in all publications are solely those of the individual author(s) and contributor(s) and not of MDPI and/or the editor(s). MDPI and/or the editor(s) disclaim responsibility for any injury to people or property resulting from any ideas, methods, instructions or products referred to in the content.

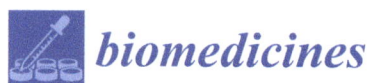

Article

Fibroblast Growth Factor 23: Potential Marker of Invisible Heart Damage in Diabetic Population

Anna Kurpas [1], Karolina Supel [1,*], Paulina Wieczorkiewicz [1], Joanna Bodalska Duleba [2] and Marzenna Zielinska [1]

[1] Department of Interventional Cardiology, Medical University of Lodz, 251 Pomorska Street, 92-213 Lodz, Poland; a.lipinska.a@gmail.com (A.K.); paulina.wieczorkiewicz@umed.lodz.pl (P.W.); marzenna.zielinska@umed.lodz.pl (M.Z.)
[2] Diabetes Outpatient Clinic 'Poradnia Nowa', 90-631 Lodz, Poland; j.bodalska.duleba@gmail.com
* Correspondence: karolina.supel@umed.lodz.pl; Tel.: +48-42-201-42-60

Abstract: Two-dimensional speckle-tracking echocardiography (2DSTE) detects myocardial dysfunction despite a preserved left ventricular ejection fraction. Fibroblast growth factor 23 (FGF23) has become a promising biomarker of cardiovascular risk. This study aimed to determine whether FGF23 may be used as a marker of myocardial damage among patients with diabetes mellitus type 2 (T2DM) and no previous history of myocardial infarction. The study enrolled 71 patients with a median age of 70 years. Laboratory data were analyzed retrospectively. Serum FGF23 levels were determined using a sandwich enzyme-linked immunosorbent assay. All patients underwent conventional echocardiography and 2DSTE. Baseline characteristics indicated that the median time elapsed since diagnosis with T2DM was 19 years. All subjects were divided into two groups according to left ventricular diastolic function. Individuals with confirmed left ventricular diastolic dysfunction had significantly lower levels of estimated glomerular filtration rate and higher values of hemoglobin A1c. Global circumferential strain (GCS) was reduced in the majority of patients. Only an epicardial GCS correlated significantly with the FGF23 concentration in all patients. The study indicates that a cardiac strain is a reliable tool for a subtle myocardial damage assessment. It is possible that FGF23 may become an early diagnostic marker of myocardial damage in patients with T2DM.

Keywords: fibroblast growth factor 23; two-dimensional speckle-tracking echocardiography; left ventricular diastolic dysfunction; diabetes mellitus

Citation: Kurpas, A.; Supel, K.; Wieczorkiewicz, P.; Bodalska Duleba, J.; Zielinska, M. Fibroblast Growth Factor 23: Potential Marker of Invisible Heart Damage in Diabetic Population. *Biomedicines* 2023, 11, 1523. https://doi.org/10.3390/biomedicines11061523

Academic Editor: Alfredo Caturano

Received: 12 April 2023
Revised: 22 May 2023
Accepted: 23 May 2023
Published: 25 May 2023

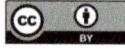

Copyright: © 2023 by the authors. Licensee MDPI, Basel, Switzerland. This article is an open access article distributed under the terms and conditions of the Creative Commons Attribution (CC BY) license (https://creativecommons.org/licenses/by/4.0/).

1. Introduction

Diabetes mellitus (DM) poses a serious challenge to the world's health. Despite global efforts to tackle the diabetes pandemic, the number of adults living with DM is on the rise. The International Diabetes Federation reported that the number of adults with DM has already surpassed 537 million and is predicted to rise to 643 million by 2030 [1]. Even more frightening, is the fact that there are another 541 million people with impaired glucose tolerance, who are at high risk of type 2 diabetes mellitus (T2DM). T2DM accounts for approximately 90% of all cases of DM [2].

Cardiovascular disease (CVD) is the most prevalent cause of morbidity and mortality in a diabetic population [3]. DM is associated with a 2- to 3-fold increased risk of myocardial infarction (MI) and stroke [4]. The dreadful combination of DM and ischemic heart disease (IHD) has always put a severe strain on diabetologists and cardiologists. An increased prevalence of IHD in patients with DM contributes to the greater incidence of heart failure (HF). The risk of HF in diabetic patients is more than twice that of the nondiabetic population [5,6].

Nearly 50 years ago, Rubler et al. introduced the concept of diabetic cardiomyopathy (DCM), which is considered a primary myocardial disease in diabetic patients [7,8]. DCM was defined as abnormal cardiac structure and performance in the absence of IHD, arterial hypertension (HA), or significant valvular disease. Despite the importance of this entity, the mechanisms underlying DCM pathogenesis have remained poorly elucidated. Dysregulated glucose and lipid metabolism causes increased oxidative and inflammation stress, which both mediate pathological cardiac remodeling, characterized by left ventricular (LV) concentric hypertrophy and increased myocardial fibrosis [9]. Subsequently, the gradual decline in LV function (diastolic often precedes systolic) may be observed [10]. Therefore, a diabetic population is particularly susceptible to a long-standing subclinical myocardial dysfunction before development of overt HF.

DM claims lives and triggers disability. Patients with DM have unfavorable prognoses due to multiple diabetic complications and frequent comorbidities, worse cardiovascular (CV) outcomes, and higher rates of hospitalization compared to their healthy counterparts [5,6,11]. Numerous studies indicate that poor glycemic control is associated with an increased risk of exacerbation of IHD and HF [12,13]. DM combined with cardiac diseases is frequently related to a poorer quality of life and the burden of high medical costs.

Transthoracic echocardiography (TTE) is the most fundamental method for a cardiac function evaluation of patients with DM. Although reduced left ventricular ejection fraction (LVEF) indicates HF among symptomatic patients, a considerable proportion of patients with HF still have preserved LVEF [14]. The latter cannot be efficiently detected by traditional echocardiographic parameters. Hence, development of other techniques, particularly noninvasive, objectively identifying myocardial dysfunction is highly desirable.

In 1973, Mirsky and Parmley described the concept of evaluating myocardial stiffness by using a measure of deformation (i.e., strain) [15]. Myocardial strain was defined as the percent change in the length of a myocardial segment relative to its resting length and considered an indicator of LV function [16]. Two-dimensional speckle-tracking echocardiography (2DSTE) is a new technique, which enables reliable evaluation of regional deformation in three directions: longitudinal, circumferential, and radial [17]. Due to 2DSTE, it is feasible to identify patients with a preserved LVEF, no previous history of CVD, and asymptomatic LV systolic or diastolic dysfunction.

In recent years, fibroblast growth factor 23 (FGF23) has gained wide attention in many fields of medicine and has become a promising biomarker linking chronic kidney disease (CKD) with CV morbidity and mortality [18,19]. FGF23, as an endocrine-acting phosphaturic hormone, plays a pivotal role in calcium-phosphate metabolism and interorgan signaling. Apart from its physiologic actions, an elevated FGF23 level is also associated with pathologic effects, such as left ventricular hypertrophy, and mediates cardiac remodeling [20]. Some data indicate that FGF23 triggers production of inflammatory markers (e.g., transforming growth factor β), which promotes development of myocardial fibrosis [21,22]. Multiple publications have indicated that FGF23 is a novel biomarker of CV risk; however, most of them have promoted a clear relationship between FGF23 level and CV mortality and morbidity in patients with HF rather than IHD [23,24]. In our previous study, we reported consistent results with recent findings. We did not provide the evidence for any correlation between FGF level and either overt IHD (33% of study population) or LVEF (56%, interquartile range (IQR) 52–60) [25]. Therefore, in furtherance of our earlier research, we aimed to determine whether FGF23 may be used as a marker of early myocardial damage among patients with long-standing T2DM and no previous history of MI. The utility of FGF23 was assessed with reference to the global longitudinal (GLS) and global circumferential strain (GCS). An early detection of DCM is pivotal to the enhancement of outcomes in a diabetic population.

2. Materials and Methods

2.1. Study Design and Population

For the present analysis, we included 71 consecutive patients. Data of all individuals were obtained from a Diabetes Outpatient Clinic (Lodz, Poland) database between 2019 and 2021. Patients had the following inclusion criteria: (1) T2DM duration of >10 years; (2) regular follow-up care by a mutual diabetologist; and (3) hemoglobin A1c (HbA1c) ≤ 8% were enrolled in the study, whereas subjects with any of the following conditions were excluded: (1) age < 18 years; (2) previous history of MI; (3) active infection; (4) malignant tumor; (5) no electronic TTE data available for retrospective analysis; or (6) missing key clinical data. Afterwards, participants were divided into two groups according to a diagnosis of left ventricular diastolic dysfunction (LVDD): Group 1 (non-LVDD, n = 46) or Group 2 (LVDD, n = 25). A flowchart of the study is shown in Figure 1.

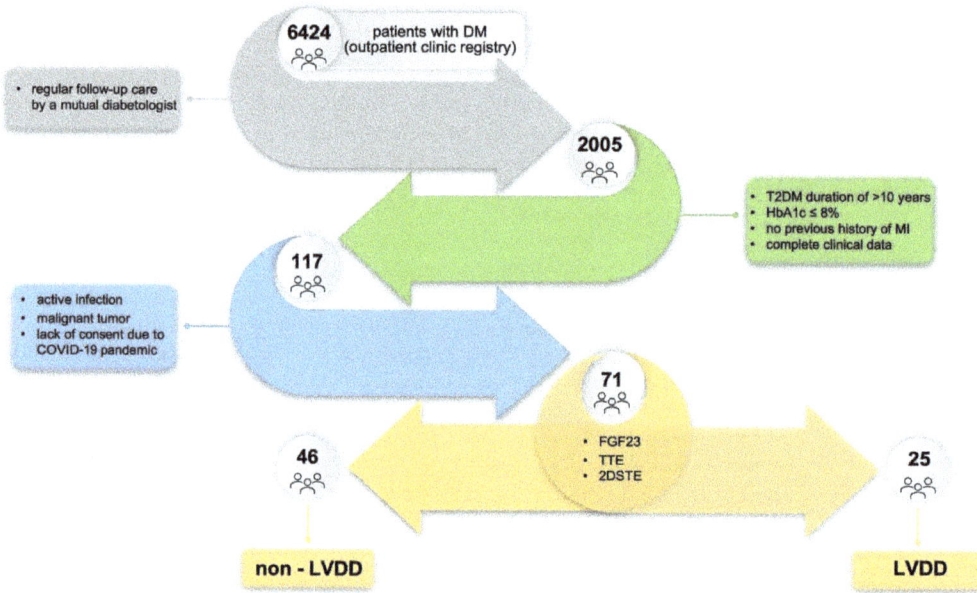

Figure 1. Study flow chart. Abbreviations: DM, diabetes mellitus; T2DM, type 2 diabetes mellitus; HbA1c, hemoglobin A1c; COVID-19, coronavirus disease 2019; FGF23, fibroblast growth factor 23; TTE, transthoracic echocardiography; 2DSTE, two-dimensional speckle-tracking echocardiography; LVDD, left ventricular diastolic dysfunction.

Demographic and clinical characteristics were collected during a structured interview, and included, among others: sex, age, height, body weight, body mass index (BMI), T2DM duration, and smoking history. Data related to comorbidities (e.g., HA, arrythmias), cardiovascular hospitalization, and family history of heart disease or DM were obtained from all participants as well. Diaries of self-control were used to verify home blood pressure monitoring. Laboratory examination data, such as HbA1c (%), creatinine (Cr; mg/dL), estimated glomerular filtration rate (eGFR) (mL/min/1.73m^2), total cholesterol (TC) (mg/dL), high-density lipoprotein cholesterol (HDL-C) (mg/dL), low-density lipoprotein cholesterol (LDL-C) (mg/dL), non-high-density lipoprotein cholesterol (non-HDL-C) (mg/dL), and triglycerides (TG) (mg/dL), were analyzed retrospectively.

The study protocol was in accordance with the Declaration of Helsinki and approved by the Ethics Committee of the District Medical Chamber in Lodz (No. K.B.-10/18, 11 April 2018). Written informed consent was obtained for inclusion of the patients.

2.2. FGF23 Measurement

Serum levels of intact FGF23 (iFGF23) were measured using a sandwich enzyme-linked immunosorbent assay (ELISA) with a FGF23 ELISA kit (SunRed Biological Technology, Shanghai, China). All blood samples were collected in the morning after an overnight fast (minimum 10 h), during previously scheduled appointments at the Diabetes Outpatient

Clinic, and stored at −80 °C before analysis. The reference range for serum iFGF23 level in healthy adults is 8.2–54.3 pg/mL [26].

2.3. Conventional Echocardiography

All patients underwent two-dimensional (2D) TTE using a commercially available ultrasound system (Vivid E9, General-Electric Healthcare, Horten, Norway) equipped with a 3.5-Mhz transducer. Participants were evaluated with 2D, M-mode, color Doppler, pulse Doppler, and continue Doppler echocardiographic examinations in the left lateral decubitus position. To achieve optimal image quality, we adjusted gain, compression, depth, and sector width. The images were acquired in the apical (four- and two-chamber and apical long-axis views) and parasternal views (long- and short-axis views) at the basal, papillary, and apical LV levels at high frame rates of 70–90 frames/s.

LV volumes were measured from the apical four- and two-chamber views. LVEF was calculated in the apical four-chamber view using the modified Simpson's rule. LVDD was defined in accordance with the most recent guidelines [27]. To determine whether a diastolic function is normal or abnormal, analysis of four variables with the following cutoff values was performed: (1) annular e' velocity (septal e' < 7cm/s, lateral e' < 10cm/s); (2) average E/e' ratio > 14; (3) peak tricuspid regurgitation velocity > 2.8 m/s; and (4) left atrial volume index > 34 mL/m^2. If more than two parameters met the above-mentioned cutoff values, LVDD was diagnosed, as shown in Figure 2.

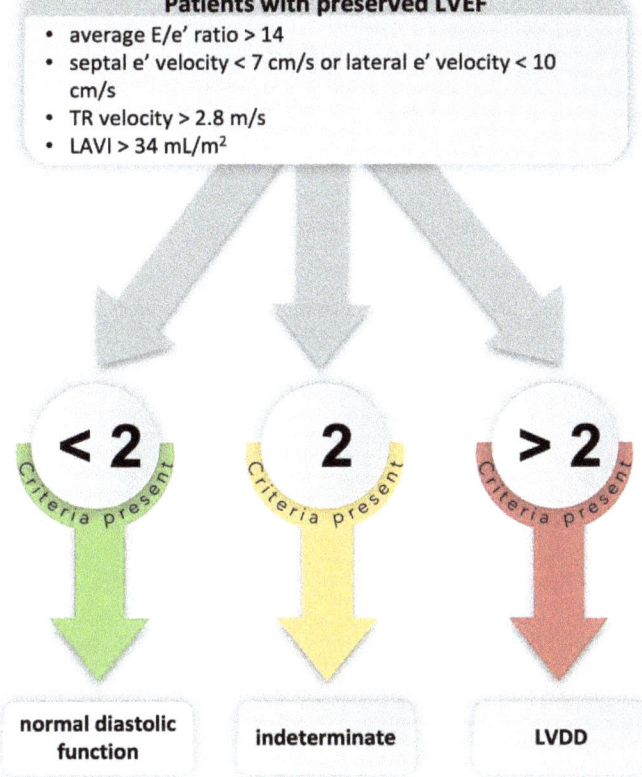

Figure 2. Algorithm for diagnosis of LVDD in patients with preserved LVEF. Abbreviations: LVEF, left ventricular ejection fraction; TR, tricuspid regurgitation; LAVI, left atrial volume index; LVDD, left ventricular diastolic dysfunction.

2.4. Two-Dimensional Speckle-Tracking Echocardiography

LV function was further evaluated with 2DSTE using a software package (EchoPAC Horten, Norway, version 201 software, General-Electric Medical Systems) by two experienced and independent observers. In each plane, three consecutive cardiac cycles were captured during a breath hold at the end-expiration and stored in a cine-loop format for offline analysis. 2DSTE is a relatively new technique of cardiac imaging based on frame by-frame tracking of ultrasonic speckles in gray scale. It allows accurate assessment of myocardial deformation in two dimensions. Two different patterns [i.e., circumferential strain (CS) and longitudinal strain (LS)] may be evaluated using the apical and parasternal short-axis views. LS shows systolic shortening in the long-axis plane, while CS represents systolic shortening but in a short-axis plane. During systole, LS and CS are anticipated to be negative values. Moreover, we analyzed CS in three myocardial layers: epicardium, mid-wall, and endocardium, under the assumption that the alterations among diabetic population may appear layer-specific. The software automatically divided the region of interest (ROI) into six equal segments and provided the time–strain curves for each myocardial segment. If necessary, ROI was manually adjusted using a point-and-click approach to enhance tracking quality. Curves of regional and global peak systolic strain, previously calculated by segmental averaging, were obtained. The reference range for GLS and GCS strain values are based on Nagata et al. [28].

2.5. Statistical Analysis

All statistical analyses were performed using STATISTICA v. 14 software (StatSoft Polska, Kraków, Poland). A p-value of 0.05 was used as the threshold of statistical significance. The normality assumption was verified using the Shapiro–Wilk test. Categorical variables are expressed as the number of observations (N) with the corresponding percentages (%), whereas quantitative variables as median and IQR. Pearson's χ^2 test was used to determine differences between categorical variables. If the number of cases were less than 5, Yates's correction for continuity was used. Continuous variables were analyzed with a nonparametric test. The Mann–Whitney U test was used to compare two independent trials Spearman's rank correlation coefficient was used for assessment of correlation strength.

3. Results

A total of 71 individuals with T2DM and no prior history of MI were enrolled in the study. There were 36 women (51%) and 35 men (49%) with a median age of 70 years (IQR 66–74). Baseline characteristics indicated that the median time elapsed since diagnosis with T2DM was 19 years (IQR 13–24). According to the results, the median BMI of the study population was 29.7 kg/m^2. Patients were diagnosed with various diseases, among others. arterial hypertension (83%), atrial fibrillation (AF) (5%), and stroke (7%). Furthermore, we assessed the frequency of chronic complications of DM, such as retinopathy (17%), neuropathy (10%), and diabetic foot syndrome (4%). Nearly two-thirds (66%) of the patients were either current or former smokers. As many as 15% of the patients were hospitalized due to CVD at least once in their lifetime. Family history of heart disease and DM were, respectively, reported in 49% and 66% patients. Table 1 presents demographic and clinical data according to the presence or absence of LVDD. As shown, there are no statistically significant differences between the two groups of patients.

Table 1. Baseline characteristics.

Variable	Total N = 71	Without LVDD N = 46	With LVDD N = 25	p Value
Age, years	70 (66–74)	67.5 (65–74)	70 (69–74)	0.061
Female sex	36 (51)	22 (49)	14 (56)	0.511
T2DM duration, years	19 (13–24)	18 (13–22)	19 (14–27)	0.446

Table 1. Cont.

Variable	Total N = 71	Without LVDD N = 46	With LVDD N = 25	p Value
BMI, kg/m^2	29.7 (25–33)	29 (25–33)	29.7 (27–33)	0.572
Arterial hypertension	59 (83)	37 (80)	22 (88)	0.631
Stroke	5 (7)	2 (4)	3 (12)	0.472
Atrial fibrillation	4 (5)	3 (7)	1 (4)	0.921
Diabetic retinopathy	12 (17)	8 (17)	4 (16)	0.856
Diabetic neuropathy	7 (10)	4 (9)	3 (12)	0.977
Diabetic foot syndrome	3 (4)	1 (2)	2 (8)	0.583
Cardiovascular hospitalization	11 (15)	8 (17)	3 (12)	0.798
Family history of heart disease	35 (49)	24 (52)	11 (44)	0.511
Family history of diabetes mellitus	47 (66)	29 (63)	18 (72)	0.446
Current and former smokers	47 (66)	30 (65)	17 (68)	0.979
Nonsmokers	24 (34)	16 (35)	8 (32)	0.979

Note: Data are expressed as median (interquartile range) or number (%). Abbreviations: LVDD, left ventricular diastolic dysfunction; T2DM, type 2 diabetes mellitus; BMI, body mass index.

Table 2 demonstrates the laboratory test results according to an LV diastolic function status. In our study, we determined the concentration of FGF23, HbA1c, renal parameters, and a lipid profile.

Table 2. Laboratory test results.

Variable	Total N = 71	Without LVDD N = 46	With LVDD N = 25	p Value
FGF23, pg/mL	256 (214–567)	255 (206–567)	268 (232–380)	0.918
Cr, mg/dL	0.83 (0.73–0.96)	0.79 (0.7–0.92)	0.91 (0.79–1.04)	0.022
eGFR, mL/min/1.73 m^2	88 (75–102)	101 (76–102)	80 (64–101)	0.029
HbA1c, %	6.8 (6.4–7.4)	6.5 (6.3–7.2)	7 (6.7–7.7)	0.045
TC, mg/dL	155 (129–187)	157 (132–194)	140 (125–176)	0.327
HDL-C, mg/dL	51 (43–62)	51 (43–62)	51 (44–61)	0.764
LDL-C, mg/dL	73 (54–98)	80 (55–102)	71 (51–98)	0.489
non-HDL-C, mg/dL	102 (77–126)	104 (80–126)	98 (77–126)	0.381
TG, mg/dL	121 (90–169)	121 (93–169)	120 (90–166)	0.976

Note: Data are expressed as median (interquartile range). Abbreviations: LVDD, left ventricular diastolic dysfunction; FGF23, fibroblast growth factor 23; Cr, creatinine; eGFR, estimated glomerular filtration rate; HbA1c, hemoglobin A1c; TC, total cholesterol; HDL-C, high-density lipoprotein cholesterol; LDL-C, low-density lipoprotein cholesterol; TG, triglycerides.

FGF23 was elevated in all patients (256 pg/mL, IQR 214–567). Interestingly, there was no significant difference in its levels between patients with LVDD and normal LV diastolic function (255 pg/mL, IQR 206–567; 268 pg/mL, IQR 232–380; $p = 0.918$), as shown in Figure 3. Individuals with confirmed LVDD appeared to have significantly higher concentrations of HbA1c and lower levels of eGFR (7%, IQR 6.7–7.7; 80 mL/min/1.73 m^2, IQR 64–101) compared to subjects with normal diastolic function (6.5%, IQR 6.3–7.2; 101 mL/min/1.73 m^2, IQR 76–102). Furthermore, none of the lipid parameters correlated with either normal or abnormal LV diastolic function. A lipid profile included measurements of TC (155 mg/dL, IQR 129–187), HDL-C (51 mg/dL, IQR 43–62), LDL-C (73 mg/dL, IQR 54–98), non-HDL-C (102 mg/dL, IQR 77–126), and TG (121 mg/dL, IQR 90–169).

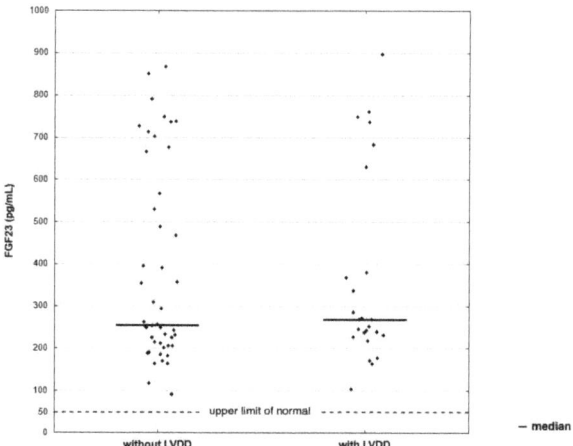

Figure 3. Scatter plot of FGF23 levels according to LV diastolic function status. Abbreviations: LVDD, left ventricular diastolic dysfunction; FGF23, fibroblast growth factor; LV, left ventricular.

All patients underwent TTE evaluation. The echocardiographic findings are summarized in Table 3. Individuals with LVDD had higher values of LVMI (109 g/m^2, IQR 100–121; p = 0.003), IVSs (17 mm, IQR 16–19; p = 0.014), and IVSd (13mm, IQR 11–13; p = 0.002). However, no correlation was found between either normal or abnormal LV diastolic function and the following variables: LVEF, LVESV (left ventricular end systolic volume), LVEDV (left ventricular end diastolic volume), left atrial volume, LAVI (left atrial volume index), TAPSE (tricuspid annular plane systolic excursion), and RVOT (right ventricular outflow tract) proximal diameter.

Table 3. Transthoracic echocardiographic parameters.

Variable	Total N = 71	Without LVDD N = 46	With LVDD N = 25	p Value
LVEF, %	56 (54–62)	56 (53–62)	56 (54–60)	0.827
LVESV, mL	31 (28–35)	31 (28–35)	33 (29–35)	0.353
LVEDV, mL	45 (43–48)	45 (43–48)	47 (45–49)	0.155
LVMI, g/m^2	98 (83–110)	92 (81–107)	109 (100–121)	0.003
LA volume, mL	50 (43–63)	49 (42–61)	56 (48–77)	0.166
LAVI, mL/m^2	27 (22–33)	27 (21–31)	30 (25–37)	0.158
TAPSE, mm	22 (20–25)	22 (21–25)	21 (19–24)	0.247
RVOT proximal diameter, mm	32 (30–34)	32 (31–34)	32 (30–35)	0.565
IVSs, mm	16 (15–17)	16 (15–16)	17 (16–19)	0.014
IVSd, mm	11 (10–12)	11 (10–12)	13 (11–13)	0.002
average E/e' ratio	9 (7–11)	8 (7–10)	11 (8–15)	0.002

Note: Data are expressed as median (interquartile range). Abbreviations: LVDD, left ventricular diastolic dysfunction; LVEF, left ventricular ejection fraction; LVESV, left ventricular end systolic volume; LVEDV, left ventricular end diastolic volume; LVMI, left ventricular mass index; LA, left atrium; LAVI, left atrial volume index; TAPSE, tricuspid annular plane systolic excursion; RVOT, right ventricular outflow tract; IVSs, interventricular septum thickness at end-systole; IVSd, interventricular septum thickness at end-diastole.

The parameters derived from 2DSTE are listed in Table 4. After considering age dependency, average GCS was diminished in the majority of patients. Average GCS was −16.4%, endocardial GCS was −24.8%, whereas epicardial GCS was considerably reduced and amounted to −9.2%. According to Nagata et al., the reference ranges for average, endocardial, and epicardial GCS are, respectively, as follows: $-21.2\% \pm 2.1$, $-29.3\% \pm 2.9$, and $-15.6\% \pm 1.9$ [28]. GLS was within the normal range, which is $-19.4\% \pm 1.7$ [28]. Contrary to our expectations, there were no significant differences in GLS and GCS between patients with LVDD and normal LV diastolic function. Even the analysis of a layer-specific GCS did not reveal any correlation with LV diastolic function. The examples of LV CS curves of endocardium, mid-wall, and epicardium from papillary muscles level are illustrated in Figure 4.

Table 4. Two-dimensional speckle-tracking echocardiography data.

	Variable	Total N = 71	Without LVDD N = 46	With LVDD N = 25	p Value
GLS, %	apical 4 chamber	−18.6 (−21.6, −16.5)	−19.5 (−21.6, −17.2)	−17.7 (−20.9, −15.6)	0.189
	apical 2 chamber	−19.4 (−22.5, −15.6)	−20.6 (−23.3, −16.9)	−18.4 (−19.6, −15.6)	0.060
	apical 3 chamber	−19.6 (−21.7, −14.1)	−19.9 (−21.5, −15.6)	−18.6 (−21.8, −13.2)	0.373
	average	−19.1 (−21.6, −16.1)	−19.9 (−22.0, −16.3)	−18.2 (−19.6, −16.1)	0.115
GCS, %	epicardial	−9.2 (−11.7, −9.2)	−8.8 (−11.2, −6.8)	−10.2 (−12.1, −7.6)	0.348
	mid-wall	−14.9 (−17.2, −11.1)	−15.1 (−17.1, −11.1)	−14.9 (−17.2, −11.8)	0.824
	endocardial	−24.8 (−29.0, −18.5)	−24.3 (−29.7, −18.8)	−25.3 (−27.6, −18.4)	1.000
	average	−16.4 (−18.8, −11.8)	−16.2 (−18.9, −11.8)	−16.4 (−18.4, −13.5)	0.962

Note: Data are expressed as median (interquartile range). Abbreviations: LVDD, left ventricular diastolic dysfunction; GLS, global longitudinal strain; GCS, global circumferential strain.

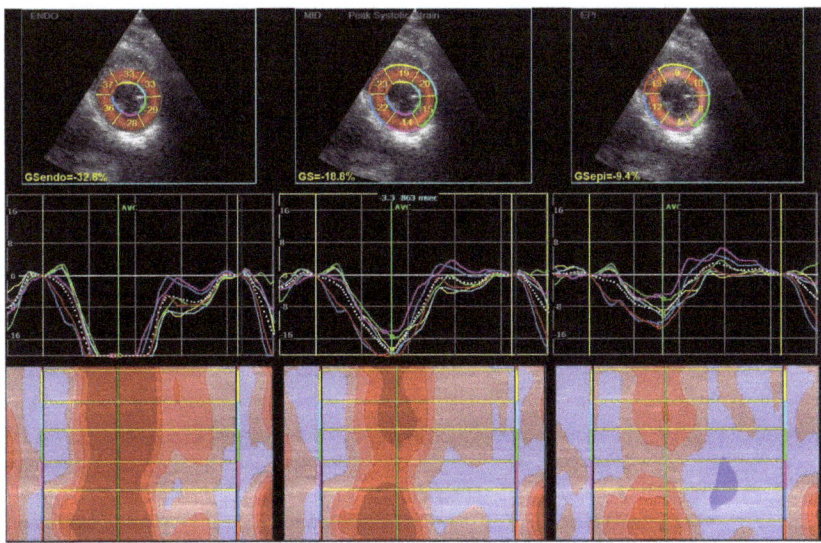

Figure 4. Layer–specific (endocardial, transmural, epicardial layer) circumferential global and segmental strain curves obtained from 2DSTE from papillary muscles level. Abbreviations: 2DSTE, two–dimensional speckle–tracking echocardiography.

This study also assessed the utility of FGF23 with reference to cardiac strain. It revealed that an epicardial GCS correlated with FGF23 level regardless of LV diastolic function status ($p = 0.041$), as shown in Figure 5. Such correlation was not found in the following subgroups, patients with LVDD and with normal diastolic function. None of the other strains correlated with the FGF23 levels either in the study population or in patients with LVDD or with normal diastolic function.

Distribution of GLS, endocardial and epicardial GCS values according to a LV diastolic function status are demonstrated in Figure 6A–C.

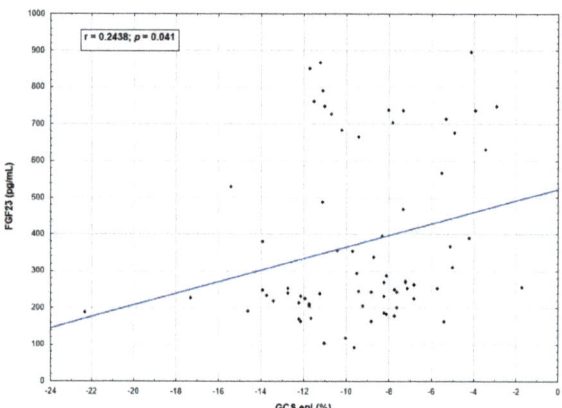

Figure 5. Spearman correlation between epicardial GCS values and FGF23 levels in patients with long–standing type 2 diabetes mellitus. Abbreviations: GCS, global circumferential strain; FGF23 fibroblast growth factor.

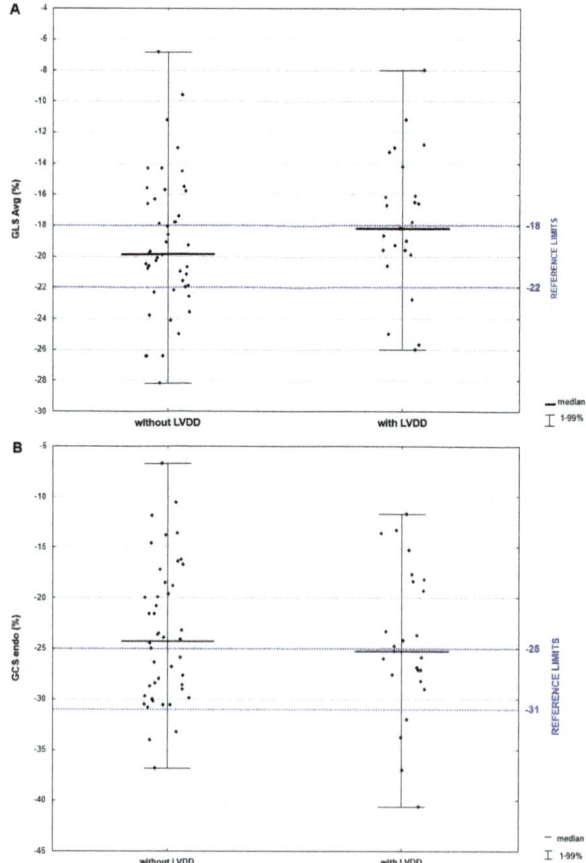

Figure 6. *Cont.*

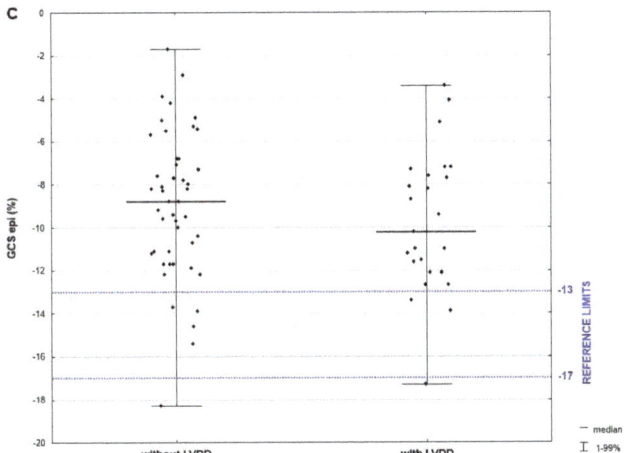

Figure 6. Scatter plot of average GLS (**A**), GCS endocardial (**B**), and GCS epicardial (**C**) levels according to LV diastolic function status. Abbreviations: LVDD, left ventricular diastolic dysfunction; GLS, global longitudinal strain; GCS, global circumferential.

4. Discussion

The overwhelming majority of publications indicate a significant correlation between an elevated level of FGF23 and increased CV risk in CKD. However, little is known about the relationship between FGF23 and CVDs in a diabetic population, particularly without kidney failure. Furthermore, most researchers have posited a clear association between FGF23 concentration and CV risk in the subjects with HF rather than IHD. Our study included patients with long-standing T2DM, relatively good glycemic control, preserved renal function, and no previous history of myocardial infarction. Due to a careful selection of the target group, the interference of confounding factors was reduced to a certain extent. The main goal of the research was to determine whether FGF23 may be used as an early marker of myocardial damage among patients with T2DM and no previous history of myocardial infarction. To the authors' best knowledge, this is the first study to investigate the correlation between FGF23 and a cardiac strain in a diabetic population. The study indicates that a cardiac strain is a reliable tool for a subtle myocardial damage assessment. We have proven that myocardial injury in patients with long-standing T2DM is layer-specific and starts from the epicardium. Furthermore, we performed an in-depth analysis showing that an elevated level of FGF23 is significantly associated with a reduced value of epicardial GCS among our patients. It is possible that FGF23 may become an early diagnostic marker of myocardial damage in patients with long-standing T2DM.

T2DM is a metabolic disease associated with a considerably higher risk of HF and CV mortality, even in the absence of IHD. Patients with T2DM and no previous history of IHD have an equal CV risk compared to a nondiabetic population with a prior MI. Pathophysiological links between T2DM and CVD have not been fully elucidated. It is known that DM has a profound effect on a CV system, causing extracellular matrix remodeling, increased oxidative stress, and endothelial cell dysfunction [29–32]. Over time, LV remodeling, myocardial fibrosis, and histological alterations lead to LVDD, which usually precedes systolic dysfunction. Eventually, one observes the development of overt HF. Concentric LV remodeling has been considered an adverse prognostic marker of CV events [33,34]. Some data also indicate that LV remodeling results from renin-angiotensin-aldosterone system activation, microangiopathy, inflammatory cytokines, or CV autonomic neuropathy [35,36]. Early myocardial injury among patients with T2DM is typically slow, insidious, and symptoms are not specific [37,38]. There is an increased risk of hospitalization and adverse outcomes.

Heart failure with preserved ejection fraction (HFpEF) is an urgent health and social problem. It is estimated that HFpEF accounts for nearly 50% of all HF cases [14]. It is possible that the high prevalence of HFpEF results from a greater awareness of physicians, but especially the ageing population and widely known risk factors, such as advanced age, HA, obesity, or metabolic syndrome. Its complex pathophysiology has not been fully elucidated; therefore, we may find multiple definitions in the literature. According to the earlier guidelines, LVDD was required to confirm HFpEF and responsible for HF manifestation. On the one hand, the CHARM echocardiographic substudy showed that LVDD was observed in 67% of patients, whereas only moderate and severe LVDD (44%) was a significant and independent predictor of adverse outcome [39]. On the other hand, a community-based study in Olmsted County (Minnesota, USA) demonstrated that among 2042 randomly selected residents, LVDD was confirmed in 28%, but only 2.2% were diagnosed with HF [40]. Diagnosis of HFpEF might be challenging, even for HF specialists. However, identification of patients, among LVDD cases, who will subsequently develop HF seems particularly difficult.

LVEF assessed in TTE is a cornerstone of cardiac function evaluation. Nonetheless, we must bear in mind that LVEF may remain preserved in the early stages of many heart diseases, despite actual impaired myocardial contractility. Many scientists suggest that the prognosis of patients with reduced and preserved LVEF is similar [14,41]. Myocardial strain is based on the speckle-tracking method and has been acknowledged as a more accurate tool for myocardial function assessment than conventional echocardiography. Park et al. conducted a study of 4172 patients with acute HF [42]. Approximately 40% of them died within 5 years. They demonstrated that GLS was a better prognostic marker than LVEF. No difference was observed in LVEF between still living individuals and those who had died, whereas GLS was reduced in deceased patients. The same researchers carried out a study, which included 355 patients with LVEF of $\geq$50% and without significant LVDD, to evaluate GLS value as a HF predictor [43]. Impaired GLS was defined as <16%. They showed that 28% of patients with acute HF and preserved LVEF as well as elevated levels of natriuretic peptides had no LVDD. The utility of conventional echocardiography appeared limited in this group of patients, because according to the contemporary definition of HFpEF, they would not have been classified as having HF [44]. The analysis of GLS during resting TTE indicated that the individuals with an impaired GLS had a worse prognosis. Data concerning GCS as a prognostic marker are rather poor. Collaborators from South Korea and Australia published an article implying that GCS is a better predictor of adverse cardiac events (readmission for HF or cardiac death) than LVEF and GLS [45]. They evaluated data of 201 subjects hospitalized for acute HF. Pezel et al. conducted a study of 1506 patients, of whom 122 were diagnosed with severe IHD and 91 had confirmed HF during follow-up (15.9 years [12.9–16.6]) [46]. They were the first to assess the prognostic value of layer-specific regional CS in the general population. Eventually, they proved that a layer-specific regional CS may be an independent predictor of incidental HF and severe IHD. Skaarup and colleagues demonstrated that endocardial GCS, rather than epicardial GCS, is independently related to incidental HF in the general population and may be used as a marker of early cardiac pathology [47]. Our study likewise indicates that a cardiac strain is a better tool for a subtle myocardial assessment than LVEF. In the literature, one may find rather inconsistent data regarding the best evaluated strain parameter. This issue clearly requires further research.

Interestingly, there are a few articles presenting the relationship between myocardial strain and DM; however, the great majority of them concern LV LS, while CS was not explored or did not show any difference in a diabetic population. Flores-Ramírez et al. conducted a study of 121 diabetic patients including: 14 individuals with mildly reduced LVEF, 76 diabetics with preserved LVEF, and 31 controls [48]. They showed that the diabetics had lower GLS than the controls; however, no difference was found in GLS in the diabetics with preserved LVEF compared to the controls. Chinese researchers analyzed the data of 247 patients with T2DM and no prior history of CV complications [49]. They concluded that impaired GLS in this population was an independent predictor of CV events, such as acute coronary syndrome, cerebrovascular stroke, CV death, and hospitalization for HF. A recent concept has been based on a multilayer analysis of myocardial deformation, which relates to an anatomical aspect. Tadic et al. evaluated 146 individuals (44 controls, 48 patients with DM, and 54 patients with DM and HA) who underwent 2DSTE [50]. The research led to the following conclusions: (1) GLS and GCS gradually worsened from controls, through patients with DM, to those with both DM and HA; (2) all layers of myocardium were affected by DM and HA; (3) progressive deterioration of impaired GLS and GCS in mid-wall and epicardial layers were observed; and (4) HA exerted an additional deleterious effect on LV deformation in patients with DM. Our findings unequivocally suggest that an epicardium is the first affected layer of myocardium in patients with T2DM. Apparently, large clinical trials are highly desired to dispel any doubts related to GLS or GCS as potential predictors of adverse outcomes in both the general and diabetic populations. It is possible that the multilayer analysis of myocardial deformation may prove beneficial for CV risk stratification as well.

Several publications indicate that the underlying pathophysiology of systolic and diastolic dysfunction is aberrant calcium homeostasis [51,52]. Adeniran et al. developed a biophysically detailed model of HFpEF to explore calcium mishandling in LVDD [53]. They demonstrated that HFpEF triggers systolic calcium level decline, which subsequently leads to reduction in contractile reserve. Simultaneously, they noted an increase in diastolic calcium concentration, which results in prolonged relaxation and increased filling pressure. Interestingly, mounting evidence pointed to FGF23 as a regulator of intracellular calcium and cardiac contractility. American scientists showed that an abrupt rise in FGF23 level affects primary cardiomyocytes causing a significant increase in intracellular calcium [54]. Furthermore, prolonged exposure to FGF23 triggered calcium overload. They suggested that calcium may appear to be a key link between increased FGF23 level, long-term cardiac remodeling, hypertrophy, and finally HF. Numerous publications demonstrated that elevations in a circulating FGF23 have a clear relationship with HF. For example, Robinson-Cohen et al. included 6413 participants without CVD, and found a significant correlation between FGF23 level and HF risk [23]. Another large study showed that an increased level of FGF23 was associated with subclinical cardiac disease, new HF, and a 14% greater risk of IHD [24]. Data concerning FGF23 level in a diabetic population are rather poor and inconsistent, especially in terms of patients with preserved renal function [55,56]. In the literature, there are a few hypotheses explaining the relationship between elevated FGF23 level and diabetes mellitus [57–64].

One of the questions that interested us concerned a relationship between FGF23 and myocardial strain in a diabetic population. Our results revealed that epicardial GCS correlated significantly with elevated FGF23 level in a T2DM population, with a preserved LVEF, but confirmed LVDD. It is noteworthy that patients enrolled in our study had relatively good glycemic control, despite long-standing T2DM, preserved kidney function, and no previous history of MI. To our knowledge, no studies have so far explored this issue. Patel et al. evaluated the relationships of baseline serum FGF23 with cardiac magnetic resonance (CMR) measurements at a 10-year follow-up [65]. They demonstrated that in a multi-ethnic, community-based cohort of 2276 participants, baseline FGF23 concentrations were independently associated with higher LV mass, reduced GCS, mid-wall CS, and lower left atrium function; GLS was not assessed. Belgian researchers prospectively analyzed the data of 143 patients with HFpEF and 31 controls of similar age and gender [66]. They showed that: (1) FGF23 level was significantly elevated in HFpEF patients compared to controls; (2) FGF23 correlated with fibrosis estimated by extracellular volume measured by CMR T1 mapping; and (3) higher FGF23 concentration was associated with some proinflammatory co-morbidities, such as CKD, DM, and AF.

According to the current state of the art findings and our findings, the incorporation of a new technique, such as 2DSTE in combination with FGF23, would increase the diagnostic sensitivity of subclinical myocardial dysfunction in asymptomatic patients with T2DM. The question arises whether GLS or GCS has better predictive value of adverse CV outcome in this population. Undoubtedly, GLS has become the most widely used strain parameter and has been considered a better risk predictor than LVEF. In the literature, one may find rather poor information about GCS as a tool for CV risk stratification, particularly in a diabetic population. FGF23 is another potent predictor of CV risk. Our results revealed that GLS and GCS were both diminished in all patients. However, only epicardial GCS correlated significantly with an elevated level of FGF23 in T2DM patients. Data from clinical trials are highly awaited in order to evaluate the role of GCS and FGF23 in patients with T2DM.

5. Study Limitations

The present investigation has certain limitations. Our study was limited by its sample size. Furthermore, FGF23 level might have been affected by numerous conditions. Moreover, its measurement might have been affected by technical problems. Finally, the normal range of FGF23 and GCS has not been established yet; therefore, their practical usefulness is limited.

6. Conclusions

Diabetes mellitus is a global epidemic, frequently associated with an increased CV risk, resulting in significant cardiac morbidity and mortality. Early detection of HF is of paramount importance to a preventive approach aimed at enhancing outcomes in this population. Our study indicates that a cardiac strain is a reliable tool for a subtle myocardial damage assessment. Interestingly, the myocardial injury in patients with T2DM was found to be layer-specific and started from the epicardium. Furthermore, we showed that an elevated level of FGF23 was significantly associated with a reduced value of epicardial GCS among patients with long-standing T2DM. It is possible that FGF23 may become an early diagnostic marker of myocardial damage in patients with long-standing T2DM Further larger investigations are essential to validate our findings. Estimation of calcium concentration would be a worthwhile subject of future research.

Author Contributions: Conceptualization, A.K. and M.Z.; methodology, A.K., K.S., P.W. and J.B.D.; validation, M.Z., J.B.D., K.S. and P.W.; formal analysis, M.Z.; investigation, A.K., M.Z. and J.B.D.; resources, A.K. and J.B.D.; data curation, M.Z. and A.K.; writing—original draft preparation, A.K.; writing—review and editing, M.Z.; visualization, M.Z.; supervision, M.Z.; project administration, M.Z. All authors have read and agreed to the published version of the manuscript.

Funding: The study was supported by a grant from the Medical University of Lodz for young scientists and doctoral candidates (No: MB 502-14-320).

Institutional Review Board Statement: The study was conducted in accordance with the Declaration of Helsinki and approved by the Institutional Review Board (or Ethics Committee) of the District Medical Chamber in Lodz (No. K.B.-10/18, 11 April 2018).

Informed Consent Statement: Informed consent was obtained from all subjects involved in the study

Data Availability Statement: The data presented in this study are available in the main article.

Conflicts of Interest: The authors declare no conflict of interest.

References

1. Magliano, D.J.; Boyko, E.J. Chapter 3, Global Picture. In *IDF Diabetes Atlas 10th Edition Scientific Committee*; International Diabetes Federation: Brussels, Belgium, 2021. Available online: https://www.ncbi.nlm.nih.gov/books/NBK581940/ (accessed on 10 January 2023).
2. Zheng, Y.; Ley, S.H.; Hu, F.B. Global aetiology and epidemiology of type 2 diabetes mellitus and its complications. *Nat. Rev. Endocrinol.* **2018**, *14*, 88–98. [CrossRef]
3. De Mattos Matheus, A.S.; Tannus, L.R.M.; Cobas, R.A.; Palma, C.C.S.; Negrato, C.A.; de Brito Gomes, M. Impact of diabetes on cardiovascular disease: An update. *Int. J. Hypertens.* **2013**, *2013*, 653789. [CrossRef]

1. Emerging Risk Factors Collaboration; Sarwar, N.; Gao, P.; Seshasai, S.R.; Gobin, R.; Kaptoge, S.; Di Angelantonio, E.; Ingelsson, E.; Lawlor, D.A.; Selvin, E.; et al. Diabetes mellitus, fasting blood glucose concentration, and risk of vascular disease: A collaborative meta-analysis of 102 prospective studies. *Lancet* **2010**, *375*, 2215–2222, Erratum in *Lancet* **2010**, *376*, 958. Hillage, H L [corrected to Hillege, H L]. [CrossRef]
2. Nichols, G.A.; Hillier, T.A.; Erbey, J.R.; Brown, J.B. Congestive heart failure in type 2 diabetes: Prevalence, incidence, and risk factors. *Diabetes Care* **2001**, *24*, 1614–1619. [CrossRef]
3. Dei Cas, A.; Khan, S.S.; Butler, J.; Mentz, R.J.; Bonow, R.O.; Avogaro, A.; Tschoepe, D.; Doehner, W.; Greene, S.J.; Senni, M.; et al. Impact of diabetes on epidemiology, treatment, and outcomes of patients with heart failure. *JACC Heart Fail.* **2015**, *3*, 136–145. [CrossRef]
4. Rubler, S.; Dlugash, J.; Yuceoglu, Y.Z.; Kumral, T.; Branwood, A.W.; Grishman, A. New type of cardiomyopathy associated with diabetic glomerulosclerosis. *Am. J. Cardiol.* **1972**, *30*, 595–602. [CrossRef]
5. Kannel, W.B.; Hjortland, M.; Castelli, W.P. Role of diabetes in congestive heart failure: The Framingham study. *Am. J. Cardiol.* **1974**, *34*, 29–34. [CrossRef]
6. Tan, Y.; Zhang, Z.; Zheng, C.; Wintergerst, K.A.; Keller, B.B.; Cai, L. Mechanisms of diabetic cardiomyopathy and potential therapeutic strategies: Preclinical and clinical evidence. *Nat. Rev. Cardiol.* **2020**, *17*, 585–607. [CrossRef]
10. Kakogawa, J.; Nako, T.; Igarashi, S.; Nakamura, S.; Tanaka, M. Peripartum heart failure caused by left ventricular diastolic dysfunction: A case report. *Acta. Obs. Gynecol. Scand.* **2014**, *93*, 835–838. [CrossRef]
11. Khalid, J.M.; Raluy-Callado, M.; Curtis, B.H.; Boye, K.S.; Maguire, A.; Reaney, M. Rates and risk of hospitalisation among patients with type 2 diabetes: Retrospective cohort study using the UK General Practice Research Database linked to English Hospital Episode Statistics. *Int. J. Clin. Pract.* **2014**, *68*, 40–48. [CrossRef]
12. Chen, S.; Shen, Y.; Liu, Y.H.; Dai, Y.; Wu, Z.M.; Wang, X.Q.; Yang, C.D.; Li, L.Y.; Liu, J.M.; Zhang, L.P.; et al. Impact of glycemic control on the association of endothelial dysfunction and coronary artery disease in patients with type 2 diabetes mellitus. *Cardiovasc. Diabetol.* **2021**, *20*, 64. [CrossRef] [PubMed]
13. Iribarren, C.; Karter, A.J.; Go, A.S.; Ferrara, A.; Liu, J.Y.; Sidney, S.; Selby, J.V. Glycemic control and heart failure among adult patients with diabetes. *Circulation* **2001**, *103*, 2668–2673. [CrossRef] [PubMed]
14. Owan, T.E.; Hodge, D.O.; Herges, R.M.; Jacobsen, S.J.; Roger, V.L.; Redfield, M.M. Trends in prevalence and outcome of heart failure with preserved ejection fraction. *N. Engl. J. Med.* **2006**, *355*, 251–259. [CrossRef] [PubMed]
15. Mirsky, I.; Parmley, W.W. Assessment of passive elastic stiffness for isolated heart muscle and the intact heart. *Circ. Res.* **1973**, *33*, 233–243. [CrossRef] [PubMed]
16. Brady, B.; King, G.; Murphy, R.T.; Walsh, D. Myocardial strain: A clinical review. *Ir. J. Med. Sci.* **2022**, 1–8. [CrossRef]
17. Cameli, M.; Sengupta, P.; Edvardsen, T. Deformation echocardiography. In *The EACVI Textbook of Echocardiography*, 2nd ed.; Lancellotti, P., Zamorano, J.L., Habib, G., Badano, L., Eds.; ESC Publications: Oxford, UK, 2016. [CrossRef]
18. Smith, E.R. The use of fibroblast growth factor 23 testing in patients with kidney disease. *Clin. J. Am. Soc. Nephrol.* **2014**, *9*, 1283–1303. [CrossRef]
19. Wolf, M. Update on fibroblast growth factor 23 in chronic kidney disease. *Kidney Int.* **2012**, *82*, 737–747. [CrossRef]
20. Faul, C.; Amaral, A.P.; Oskouei, B.; Hu, M.C.; Sloan, A.; Isakova, T.; Gutiérrez, O.M.; Aguillon-Prada, R.; Lincoln, J.; Hare, J.M.; et al. FGF23 induces left ventricular hypertrophy. *J. Clin. Investig.* **2011**, *121*, 4393–4408. [CrossRef]
21. Dai, B.; David, V.; Martin, A.; Huang, J.; Li, H.; Jiao, Y.; Gu, W.; Quarles, L.D. A comparative transcriptome analysis identifying FGF23 regulated genes in the kidney of a mouse CKD model. *PLoS ONE* **2012**, *7*, e44161. [CrossRef]
22. Yan, L.; Bowman, M.A. Chronic sustained inflammation links to left ventricular hypertrophy and aortic valve sclerosis: A new link between S100/RAGE and FGF23. *Inflamm. Cell Signal.* **2014**, *1*, e279. [CrossRef]
23. Robinson-Cohen, C.; Shlipak, M.; Sarnak, M.; Katz, R.; Peralta, C.; Young, B.; Hoofnagle, A.N.; Szklo, M.; Ix, J.H.; Psaty, B.M.; et al. Impact of Race on the Association of Mineral Metabolism with Heart Failure: The Multi-Ethnic Study of Atherosclerosis. *J. Clin. Endocrinol. Metab.* **2020**, *105*, e1144–e1151. [CrossRef] [PubMed]
24. Kestenbaum, B.; Sachs, M.C.; Hoofnagle, A.N.; Siscovick, D.S.; Ix, J.H.; Robinson-Cohen, C.; Lima, J.A.; Polak, J.F.; Blondon, M.; Ruzinski, J.; et al. Fibroblast growth factor-23 and cardiovascular disease in the general population: The Multi-Ethnic Study of Atherosclerosis. *Circ. Heart Fail.* **2014**, *7*, 409–417. [CrossRef] [PubMed]
25. Kurpas, A.; Supel, K.; Wieczorkiewicz, P.; Bodalska Duleba, J.; Zielinska, M. Fibroblast Growth Factor 23 and Cardiovascular Risk in Diabetes Patients-Cardiologists Be Aware. *Metabolites* **2022**, *12*, 498. [CrossRef] [PubMed]
26. Yamazaki, Y.; Okazaki, R.; Shibata, M.; Hasegawa, Y.; Satoh, K.; Tajima, T.; Takeuchi, Y.; Fujita, T.; Nakahara, K.; Yamashita, T.; et al. Increased circulatory level of biologically active full-length FGF-23 in patients with hypophosphatemic rickets/osteomalacia. *J. Clin. Endocrinol. Metab.* **2002**, *87*, 4957–4960. [CrossRef] [PubMed]
27. Nagueh, S.F.; Smiseth, O.A.; Appleton, C.P.; Byrd, B.F., 3rd; Dokainish, H.; Edvardsen, T.; Flachskampf, F.A.; Gillebert, T.C.; Klein, A.L.; Lancellotti, P.; et al. Recommendations for the Evaluation of Left Ventricular Diastolic Function by Echocardiography: An Update from the American Society of Echocardiography and the European Association of Cardiovascular Imaging. *J. Am. Soc. Echocardiogr.* **2016**, *29*, 277–314. [CrossRef]
28. Nagata, Y.; Wu, V.C.; Otsuji, Y.; Takeuchi, M. Normal range of myocardial layer-specific strain using two-dimensional speckle tracking echocardiography. *PLoS ONE* **2017**, *12*, e0180584. [CrossRef]

29. Frara, S.; Maffezzoni, F.; Mazziotti, G.; Giustina, A. Current and Emerging Aspects of Diabetes Mellitus in Acromegaly. *Trends Endocrinol. Metab.* **2016**, *27*, 470–483. [CrossRef]
30. Law, B.; Fowlkes, V.; Goldsmith, J.G.; Carver, W.; Goldsmith, E.C. Diabetes-induced alterations in the extracellular matrix and their impact on myocardial function. *Microsc. Microanal.* **2012**, *18*, 22–34. [CrossRef]
31. Storz, C.; Hetterich, H.; Lorbeer, R.; Heber, S.D.; Schafnitzel, A.; Patscheider, H.; Auweter, S.; Zitzelsberger, T.; Rathmann, W.; Nikolaou, K.; et al. Myocardial tissue characterization by contrast-enhanced cardiac magnetic resonance imaging in subjects with prediabetes, diabetes, and normal controls with preserved ejection fraction from the general population. *Eur. Heart J. Cardiovasc. Imaging* **2018**, *19*, 701–708. [CrossRef]
32. Levelt, E.; Mahmod, M.; Piechnik, S.K.; Ariga, R.; Francis, J.M.; Rodgers, C.T.; Clarke, W.T.; Sabharwal, N.; Schneider, J.E.; Karamitsos, T.D.; et al. Relationship Between Left Ventricular Structural and Metabolic Remodeling in Type 2 Diabetes. *Diabetes* **2016**, *65*, 44–52. [CrossRef]
33. Verdecchia, P.; Schillaci, G.; Borgioni, C.; Ciucci, A.; Gattobigio, R.; Zampi, I.; Santucci, A.; Santucci, C.; Reboldi, G.; Porcellati, C. Prognostic value of left ventricular mass and geometry in systemic hypertension with left ventricular hypertrophy. *Am. J. Cardiol.* **1996**, *78*, 197–202. [CrossRef] [PubMed]
34. Gilca, G.E.; Stefanescu, G.; Badulescu, O.; Tanase, D.M.; Bararu, I.; Ciocoiu, M. Diabetic Cardiomyopathy: Current Approach and Potential Diagnostic and Therapeutic Targets. *J. Diabetes Res.* **2017**, *2017*, 1310265. [CrossRef] [PubMed]
35. Jia, G.; Hill, M.A.; Sowers, J.R. Diabetic Cardiomyopathy: An Update of Mechanisms Contributing to This Clinical Entity. *Circ. Res.* **2018**, *122*, 624–638. [CrossRef] [PubMed]
36. Chong, C.R.; Clarke, K.; Levelt, E. Metabolic Remodeling in Diabetic Cardiomyopathy. *Cardiovasc. Res.* **2017**, *113*, 422–430. [CrossRef]
37. Lindman, B.R.; Dávila-Román, V.G.; Mann, D.L.; McNulty, S.; Semigran, M.J.; Lewis, G.D.; de las Fuentes, L.; Joseph, S.M.; Vader, J.; Hernandez, A.F.; et al. Cardiovascular phenotype in HFpEF patients with or without diabetes: A RELAX trial ancillary study. *J. Am. Coll. Cardiol.* **2014**, *64*, 541–549. [CrossRef]
38. Tribouilloy, C.; Rusinaru, D.; Mahjoub, H.; Soulière, V.; Lévy, F.; Peltier, M.; Slama, M.; Massy, Z. Prognosis of heart failure with preserved ejection fraction: A 5 year prospective population-based study. *Eur. Heart J.* **2008**, *29*, 339–347. [CrossRef]
39. Persson, H.; Lonn, E.; Edner, M.; Baruch, L.; Lang, C.C.; Morton, J.J.; Ostergren, J.; McKelvie, R.S.; Investigators of the CHARM Echocardiographic Substudy-CHARMES. Diastolic dysfunction in heart failure with preserved systolic function: Need for objective evidence: Results from the CHARM Echocardiographic Substudy-CHARMES. *J. Am. Coll. Cardiol.* **2007**, *49*, 687–694. [CrossRef]
40. Redfield, M.M.; Jacobsen, S.J.; Burnett, J.C., Jr.; Mahoney, D.W.; Bailey, K.R.; Rodeheffer, R.J. Burden of systolic and diastolic ventricular dysfunction in the community: Appreciating the scope of the heart failure epidemic. *JAMA* **2003**, *289*, 194–202. [CrossRef]
41. Kang, S.H.; Park, J.J.; Choi, D.J.; Yoon, C.H.; Oh, I.Y.; Kang, S.M.; Yoo, B.S.; Jeon, E.S.; Kim, J.J.; Cho, M.C.; et al. Prognostic value of NT-proBNP in heart failure with preserved versus reduced EF. *Heart* **2015**, *101*, 1881–1888. [CrossRef]
42. Park, J.J.; Park, J.B.; Park, J.H.; Cho, G.Y. Global Longitudinal Strain to Predict Mortality in Patients with Acute Heart Failure. *J. Am. Coll. Cardiol.* **2018**, *71*, 1947–1957. [CrossRef]
43. Park, J.J.; Hwang, I.C.; Kang, S.H.; Park, J.B.; Park, J.H.; Cho, G.Y. Myocardial strain for heart failure with preserved ejection fraction but without diastolic dysfunction. *ESC Heart Fail.* **2022**, *9*, 3308–3316. [CrossRef] [PubMed]
44. McDonagh, T.A.; Metra, M.; Adamo, M.; Gardner, R.S.; Baumbach, A.; Böhm, M.; Burri, H.; Butler, J.; Čelutkienė, J.; Chioncel, O.; et al. 2021 ESC Guidelines for the diagnosis and treatment of acute and chronic heart failure. *Eur. Heart J.* **2021**, *42*, 3599–3726, Erratum in *Eur. Heart J.* **2021**, *42*, 4901. [CrossRef] [PubMed]
45. Cho, G.-Y.; Marwick, T.H.; Kim, H.-S.; Kim, M.-K.; Hong, K.-S.; Oh, D.-J. Global 2-dimensional strain as a new prognosticator in patients with heart failure. *J. Am. Coll. Cardiol.* **2009**, *54*, 618–624. [CrossRef] [PubMed]
46. Pezel, T.; Bluemke, D.; Wu, C.; Lima, J.; Venkatesh, B.A. Layer-specific regional circumferential strain as prognostic marker of cardiovascular events. *Eur. Heart J.-Cardiovasc. Imaging* **2022**, *23*, jeab289.347. [CrossRef]
47. Skaarup, K.G.; Lassen, M.H.; Johansen, N.D.; Jensen, G.B.; Schnohr, P.; Mogelvang, R.; Biering-Srensen, T. Abstract 9893: The Associations Between Layer-Specific Global Circumferential Strain Parameters and Incident Heart Failure: The Copenhagen City Heart Study. *Circulation* **2022**, *146*, A9893. [CrossRef]
48. Flores-Ramírez, R.; Azpiri-López, J.R.; González-González, J.G.; Ordaz-Farías, A.; González-Carrillo, L.E.; Carrizales-Sepúlveda, E.F.; Vera-Pineda, R. Global longitudinal strain as a biomarker in diabetic cardiomyopathy. A comparative study with Gal-3 in patients with preserved ejection fraction. *Arch. Cardiol. Mex.* **2017**, *87*, 278–285. [CrossRef]
49. Liu, J.H.; Chen, Y.; Yuen, M.; Zhen, Z.; Chan, C.W.; Lam, K.S.; Tse, H.F.; Yiu, K.H. Incremental prognostic value of global longitudinal strain in patients with type 2 diabetes mellitus. *Cardiovasc. Diabetol.* **2016**, *15*, 22. [CrossRef]
50. Tadic, M.; Cuspidi, C.; Vukomanovic, V.; Ilic, S.; Obert, P.; Kocijancic, V.; Celic, V. Layer-specific deformation of the left ventricle in uncomplicated patients with type 2 diabetes and arterial hypertension. *Arch. Cardiovasc. Dis.* **2018**, *111*, 17–24. [CrossRef]
51. Kranias, E.G.; Hajjar, R.J. Modulation of cardiac contractility by the phospholamban/SERCA2a regulatome. *Circ. Res.* **2012**, *110*, 1646–1660. [CrossRef]
52. Eisner, D.A.; Caldwell, J.L.; Trafford, A.W.; Hutchings, D.C. The Control of Diastolic Calcium in the Heart: Basic Mechanisms and Functional Implications. *Circ. Res.* **2020**, *126*, 395–412. [CrossRef]

3. Adeniran, I.; MacIver, D.H.; Hancox, J.C.; Zhang, H. Abnormal calcium homeostasis in heart failure with preserved ejection fraction is related to both reduced contractile function and incomplete relaxation: An electromechanically detailed biophysical modeling study. *Front. Physiol.* **2015**, *6*, 78. [CrossRef] [PubMed]
4. Touchberry, C.D.; Green, T.M.; Tchikrizov, V.; Mannix, J.E.; Mao, T.F.; Carney, B.W.; Girgis, M.; Vincent, R.J.; Wetmore, L.A.; Dawn, B.; et al. FGF23 is a novel regulator of intracellular calcium and cardiac contractility in addition to cardiac hypertrophy. *Am. J. Physiol. Endocrinol. Metab.* **2013**, *304*, E863–E873. [CrossRef]
5. Tuñón, J.; Fernández-Fernández, B.; Carda, R.; Pello, A.M.; Cristóbal, C.; Tarín, N.; Aceña, Á.; González-Casaus, M.L.; Huelmos, A.; Alonso, J.; et al. Circulating fibroblast growth factor-23 plasma levels predict adverse cardiovascular outcomes in patients with diabetes mellitus with coronary artery disease. *Diabetes. Metab. Res. Rev.* **2016**, *32*, 685–693. [CrossRef] [PubMed]
6. Yeung, S.M.H.; Binnenmars, S.H.; Gant, C.M.; Navis, G.; Gansevoort, R.T.; Bakker, S.J.L.; de Borst, M.H.; Laverman, G.D. Fibroblast Growth Factor 23 and Mortality in Patients With Type 2 Diabetes and Normal or Mildly Impaired Kidney Function. *Diabetes Care* **2019**, *42*, 2151–2153. [CrossRef] [PubMed]
7. Simic, P.; Kim, W.; Zhou, W.; Pierce, K.A.; Chang, W.; Sykes, D.B.; Aziz, N.B.; Elmariah, S.; Ngo, D.; Pajevic, P.D.; et al. Glycerol-3-phosphate is an FGF23 regulator derived from the injured kidney. *J. Clin. Investig.* **2020**, *130*, 1513–1526. [CrossRef] [PubMed]
8. Giroix, M.H.; Rasschaert, J.; Bailbe, D.; Leclercq-Meyer, V.; Sener, A.; Portha, B.; Malaisse, W.J. Impairment of glycerol phosphate shuttle in islets from rats with diabetes induced by neonatal streptozocin. *Diabetes* **1991**, *40*, 227–232. [CrossRef]
9. Samadfam, R.; Richard, C.; Nguyen-Yamamoto, L.; Bolivar, I.; Goltzman, D. Bone formation regulates circulating concentrations of fibroblast growth factor 23. *Endocrinology* **2009**, *150*, 4835–4845. [CrossRef]
10. Anders, H.J.; Huber, T.B.; Isermann, B.; Schiffer, M. CKD in diabetes: Diabetic kidney disease versus nondiabetic kidney disease. *Nat. Rev. Nephrol.* **2018**, *14*, 361–377. [CrossRef]
11. Yamamoto, M.; Sugimoto, T. Advanced Glycation End Products, Diabetes, and Bone Strength. *Curr. Osteoporos. Rep.* **2016**, *14*, 320–326. [CrossRef]
12. Bär, L.; Wächter, K.; Wege, N.; Navarrete Santos, A.; Simm, A.; Föller, M. Advanced glycation end products stimulate gene expression of fibroblast growth factor 23. *Mol. Nutr. Food Res.* **2017**, *61*, 1601019. [CrossRef]
13. David, V.; Martin, A.; Isakova, T.; Spaulding, C.; Qi, L.; Ramirez, V.; Zumbrennen-Bullough, K.B.; Sun, C.C.; Lin, H.Y.; Babitt, J.L.; et al. Inflammation and functional iron deficiency regulate fibroblast growth factor 23 production. *Kidney Int.* **2016**, *89*, 135–146. [CrossRef] [PubMed]
14. Donath, M.Y.; Shoelson, S.E. Type 2 diabetes as an inflammatory disease. *Nat. Rev. Immunol.* **2011**, *11*, 98–107. [CrossRef] [PubMed]
15. Patel, R.B.; Ning, H.; de Boer, I.H.; Kestenbaum, B.; Lima JA, C.; Mehta, R.; Allen, N.B.; Shah, S.J.; Lloyd-Jones, D.M. Fibroblast Growth Factor 23 and Long-Term Cardiac Function: The Multi-Ethnic Study of Atherosclerosis. *Circ. Cardiovasc. Imaging* **2020**, *13*, e011925. [CrossRef] [PubMed]
16. Roy, C.; Lejeune, S.; Slimani, A.; de Meester, C.; Ahn As, S.A.; Rousseau, M.F.; Mihaela, A.; Ginion, A.; Ferracin, B.; Pasquet, A.; et al. Fibroblast growth factor 23: A biomarker of fibrosis and prognosis in heart failure with preserved ejection fraction. *ESC Heart Fail.* **2020**, *7*, 2494–2507. [CrossRef] [PubMed]

Disclaimer/Publisher's Note: The statements, opinions and data contained in all publications are solely those of the individual author(s) and contributor(s) and not of MDPI and/or the editor(s). MDPI and/or the editor(s) disclaim responsibility for any injury to people or property resulting from any ideas, methods, instructions or products referred to in the content.

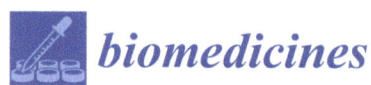

Article

Microbiota Metabolism Failure as a Risk Factor for Postoperative Complications after Aortic Prosthetics

Natalia Beloborodova [1,*], Alisa Pautova [1], Marina Grekova [2], Mikhail Yadgarov [1], Oksana Grin [2], Alexander Eremenko [2] and Maxim Babaev [2]

[1] Federal Research and Clinical Center of Intensive Care Medicine and Rehabilitology, 25-2 Petrovka Str., 107031 Moscow, Russia; alicepau@mail.ru (A.P.); mikhail.yadgarov@mail.ru (M.Y.)
[2] Petrovsky Russian Research Center of Surgery, 2 Abrikosovsky Pereulok, 119991 Moscow, Russia; levitskayams@yandex.ru (M.G.); grin_oksana@mail.ru (O.G.); aeremenko54@mail.ru (A.E.); maxbabaev@mail.ru (M.B.)
* Correspondence: nvbeloborodova@yandex.ru; Tel.: +7-(916)-131-74-54

Abstract: Postoperative complications in cardiovascular surgery remain an important unresolved problem, in particular in patients with aortic aneurysm. The role of the altered microbiota in such patients is of great interest. The aim of this pilot study was to determine whether the development of postoperative complications in patients with aortic aneurysm is related with initial or acquired disorders of microbiota metabolism by monitoring the level of some aromatic microbial metabolites (AMMs) circulating in the blood before the surgery and in the early postoperative period. The study comprised patients with aortic aneurysm ($n = 79$), including patients without complications ($n = 36$) and patients with all types of complications ($n = 43$). The serum samples from the patients were collected before and 6 h after the end of the surgery. The most significant results were obtained for the sum of three sepsis-associated AMMs. This level was higher before the surgery in comparison with that of healthy volunteers ($n = 48$), $p < 0.001$, and it was also higher in the early postoperative period in patients with all types of complications compared to those without complications, $p = 0.001$, the area under the ROC curve, the cut-off value, and the odds ratio were 0.7; 2.9 µmol/L, and 5.5, respectively. Impaired microbiota metabolism is important in the development of complications after complex reconstructive aortic surgery, which is the basis for the search for a new prevention strategy.

Keywords: cardiovascular surgery patients; aortic aneurism; aortic dissection; aromatic microbial metabolites; tyrosine metabolites; 4-hydroxyphenyllactic acid; infectious complications

Citation: Beloborodova, N.; Pautova, A.; Grekova, M.; Yadgarov, M.; Grin, O.; Eremenko, A.; Babaev, M. Microbiota Metabolism Failure as a Risk Factor for Postoperative Complications after Aortic Prosthetics. *Biomedicines* **2023**, *11*, 1335. https://doi.org/10.3390/biomedicines11051335

Academic Editor: Alfredo Caturano

Received: 3 April 2023
Revised: 25 April 2023
Accepted: 28 April 2023
Published: 30 April 2023

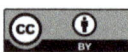

Copyright: © 2023 by the authors. Licensee MDPI, Basel, Switzerland. This article is an open access article distributed under the terms and conditions of the Creative Commons Attribution (CC BY) license (https://creativecommons.org/licenses/by/4.0/).

1. Introduction

With major reconstructive operations in cardiovascular surgery, the problem of the development of postoperative complications remains extremely relevant, since complications affect the short- and long-term results of surgical intervention, and also significantly increase financial costs. Aortic aneurysm is a severe life-threatening disease, which occurs with the involvement of almost all systems and organs in the pathological process, is characterized by hypoperfusion of organs, impaired tissue metabolism and progression of the inflammatory process, and is often accompanied by aortic dissection with the threat of fatal bleeding, etc. [1,2]. In modern cardiac surgery clinics, it is possible to minimize the adverse effect of a number of intraoperative factors during aortic prosthetics, namely to reduce the time of cardiopulmonary bypass and surgical intervention, the volume of blood loss, the degree of patient's cooling, etc. Excellent results have recently been achieved without lethal outcomes, even such large-scale operations as replacement of the entire aorta in patients with widespread aneurysmal dilatation of the aorta [3] or hybrid aortic repair in patients with type III aortic dissection and concomitant proximal aortic lesion [4]. Despite the fact that sterility is guaranteed in operating rooms and that perioperative antibiotic prophylaxis is widely used, the level of local and systemic infectious complications, including septic conditions, is still high. In a significant number of patients, complications develop not only in the early postoperative period, but also after discharge from the surgical clinic. For example, aortic endograft infection after endovascular aneurysm repair is one of the most dangerous infectious complications with the lethality of 16.9–39.2% [5].

The working hypothesis of this study is that microbiota disorders initially accompany aortic aneurysm and may subsequently cause the development of postoperative complications in conditions when preoperative preparation, surgery and early intensive therapy do not contribute to improvement, but, on the contrary, aggravate previous disorders.

In choosing research methods, the authors relied on a number of previous works. The fact of deep disturbances in the composition of the gut microbiota was revealed during the examination of patients in intensive care units using the 16S rRNA gene sequencing method. The authors point to the loss of biodiversity, a sharp reduction in the number of species of beneficial anaerobic bacteria inherent in the body of a healthy person, and excessive growth of potentially pathogenic microorganisms [6–9]. The mechanism for the development of complications associated with the altered microbiota of a cardiac surgery patient was also studied. It was reported that in planned heart operations (heart valve surgery, coronary artery bypass grafting, etc.), postoperative infectious complications were observed in 17% of cases, and the species composition of the microbiota in the group of patients with infectious complications was significantly changed initially in comparison with the group without complications [10].

Changes in the profile of microbiota metabolites in the gut and then in the blood are secondary to species dysbiosis. At the same time, the assessment of the degree of microbiota metabolism disorder may be clinically more significant than information about taxonomic disorders [11,12]. The chapter in the work by Beloborodova N.V., 2022 summarizes the results of the study of microbial metabolites of aromatic structure as markers for monitoring septic conditions in intensive care units [13]. Earlier, an explanation was offered describing an increase in serum concentrations of aromatic amino acid metabolites with its high diagnostic significance. The accumulation of intermediates of tyrosine and phenylalanine metabolism, namely phenyllactic, 4-hydroxyphenylacetic and 4-hydroxyphenyllactic acids, is a consequence of a violation of the microbiota, which loses the ability to biodegrade aromatic amino acids [14]. Later, the bacterial metabolic pathway of aromatic amino acids was studied in more detail and, using the model of gnotobiological mice, aromatic microbial metabolites was shown to affect intestinal permeability and systemic immunity [15]. Thus, the profile and levels of a number of aromatic amino acid metabolites circulating in the blood are associated with taxonomic and metabolic disorders of the gut microbiota, which can be used to assess the degree of metabolic dysfunction of the microbiota. In cardiac diseases, the study of microbiota metabolites is of interest both as markers of postoperative sepsis [16] and as participants in the genesis of myocardial infarction [17].

It is always difficult to compare groups of patients and the results of surgical treatment, especially in regard to such pathology as aortic aneurysm where different types of operations are used and much depends on the experience of surgeons and anesthesiologists. In order to avoid doubts about the results that could be related to the qualifications and experience of medical personnel, the ethics committee made a decision to include in this study patients operated on by one specific team of surgeons and treated by a specific team of specialists in anesthesia and intensive care.

The aim of this study was to determine whether the development of postoperative complications in patients with aortic aneurysm is related with initial or acquired disorders of microbiota metabolism by monitoring the level of aromatic microbial metabolites (AMMs) circulating in the blood before the surgery and in the early postoperative period (6 h).

2. Materials and Methods

2.1. Study Design

The present study was a single-center clinical study performed at the Petrovsky Russian Research Center of Surgery (Moscow, Russia). Patients with a diagnosis of aneurysm/aortic dissection were included in the study. In order to exclude the influence of individual qualities and skill of surgeons and anesthesiologists, all patients involved in the study were operated on by the same team of surgeons and anesthesiologists.

Inclusion criteria: patients aged from 18 to 75 years; reconstructive aortic surgery in 2021 performed by a team of surgeons under the guidance of Corresponding Member of the Russian Academy of Sciences, Professor, MD E.R. Charchyan; and a team of anesthesiologists under the guidance of Professor of the Russian Academy of Sciences, MD B.A. Axelrod; the presence of informed consent statement.

Exclusion criteria: age under 18 or over 75 years; aortic surgery performed by another surgical team; refusal of the patient to participate in the study at any stage; mental disorders that prevent obtaining informed consent statement; and patient's transfer to another hospital early after surgery.

2.2. Biological Samples

The total number of the serum samples was 206, including 158 samples from the patients and 48 samples from the healthy volunteers. The samples of blood serum from the patients ($n = 79$) before the surgery and 6 h after the end of the surgery were collected and frozen at $-30\ °C$ in Petrovsky Russian Research Center of Surgery (Moscow, Russia). The Local Ethic Committee approved the study (N7 from 15 February 2021) which was conducted in accordance with the ethical standards of the Declaration of Helsinki and formal consent for participation in this study was obtained from each patient or their legal representative. The samples of the blood serum from the healthy volunteers ($n = 48$) were collected in Federal State Budgetary Institution N.N. Burdenko Main Military Clinical Hospital (Moscow, Russia). The concentrations of aromatic acids (benzoic, phenylpropionic, phenyllactic, 4-hydroxybenzoic, 4-hydroxyphenylacetic, 4-hydroxyphenylpropionic, homovanillic, and 4-hydroxyphenyllactic acids) were measured using gas chromatography-mass spectrometry (Trace GC 1310 gas chromatograph and ISQ LT mass spectrometer, Thermo Electron Corporation, Waltham, MA, USA) in Federal Research and Clinical Center of Intensive Care Medicine and Rehabilitology (Moscow, Russia) as it was previously described [18]. The limit of quantitation for all aromatic acids is 0.5 μmol/L with relative standard deviation of 10–30%. The calibration curves were linear functions for all aromatic metabolites in the most clinically significant range of concentrations 0.5–7 μmol/L.

2.3. Statistical Analysis

The Shapiro–Wilk test was used to assess the normality of the data distribution. Continuous and categorial variables were described using median and interquartile ranges, frequency and percentages, respectively. Group differences were explored using Mann–Whitney U test for continuous variables; categorical baseline variables were analyzed using Chi-square test and Fisher's exact test. The cut-off value was chosen using the receiver operating characteristic (ROC) analysis with the assessment of area under the curve parameter and its 95% confidence intervals (CI) in order to achieve the optimal sensitivity/specificity ratio (Youden's J statistic). Additionally, odds ratio, sensitivity, specificity, positive and negative predictive values and accuracy were calculated. CI for sensitivity and specificity are "exact" Clopper–Pearson CI. Scatter plots with linear regression were used for visualization and modeling the relationship between metabolic status of the patients and anthropometric parameters. All analyses were conducted using IBM SPSS Statistics for Windows, Version 27.0. Armonk, NY, USA: IBM Corp. The differences were considered significant at $p < 0.05$.

3. Results

3.1. Patients

From 166 patients with thoraco-abdominal aorta surgeries performed in 2021, 81 patients met the protocol conditions because they were operated on by one specific team. Two patients were excluded from the analysis due to the positive test for COVID-19 infection and were transferred to another clinic. Finally, 79 patients were included in the study. The median age of patients was 57 (46–64) years, 57 (72%) men and 22 (28%) women. There were 15 (19%) patients with acute/subacute aortic dissection (Figure 1). All patients survived.

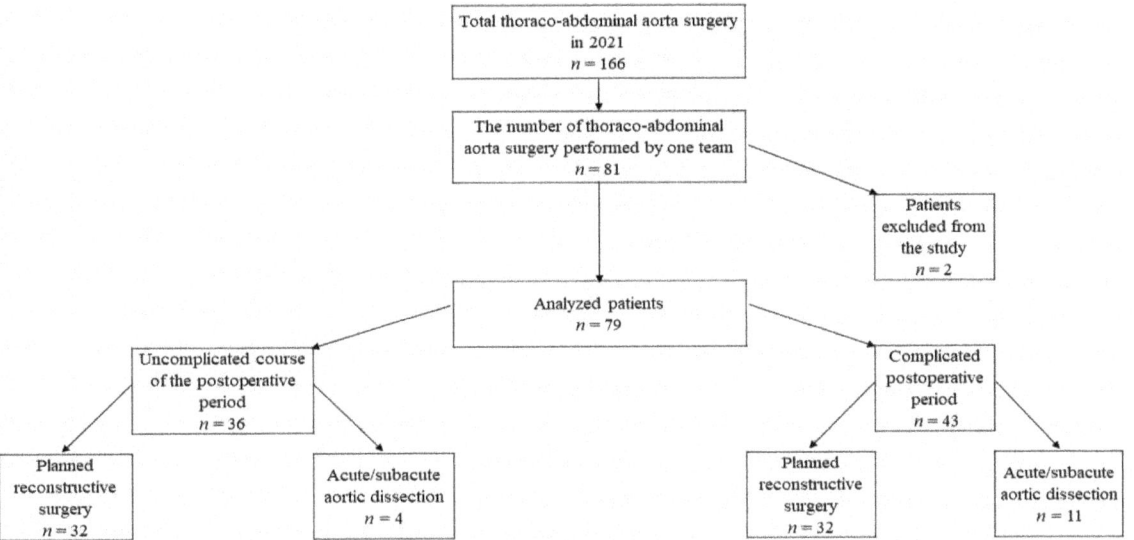

Figure 1. Scheme of the patients' recruitment in a prospective single-center study who were admitted during 2021 for thoracoabdominal aortic prosthetics surgery.

Several concomitant diseases were diagnosed in all patients participating in the study, including hypertension in 57 (72%) and heart defects in 55 (70%) patients, as well as various diseases of the gastrointestinal tract in 48 (61%) patients, multifocal atherosclerosis in 24 (30%) patients, ischemic heart disease in 20 (25%) patients, rhythm disturbances and cardiac conduction in 18 (22%) patients, and chronic kidney disease in 16 (20%) patients (Table S1). Prognostic comorbidity assessed by Charlson comorbidity index [19] was 4 (2; 5).

The patients underwent different types of reconstructive operations on the aorta, including

- Prosthetics of one or more parts of the thoracic aorta, $n = 21$ (27%);
- Hybrid surgery: stenting of the descending thoracic aorta with or without plastic surgery/prosthetics of the root and ascending aorta using Bentall–DeBono techniques or T. David, $n = 25$ (32%);
- Prosthetics of the aortic valve and ascending aorta using the Bentall–DeBono technique, $n = 14$ (18%);
- Prosthetics of the root and ascending aorta by the method of David, $n = 9$ (11%);
- Prosthetics of the thoracoabdominal aorta, $n = 5$ (6%).

Some patients underwent additional surgical interventions at the same time:

- Prosthetics/plastics of the aortic, mitral or tricuspid valve, $n = 19$ (24%);
- Myocardial revascularization (aorto-mammary coronary, prosthetic coronary bypass surgery), $n = 12$ (15%);
- Radiofrequency ablation, $n = 3$ (4%).

For perioperative antibiotic prophylaxis in 57 (72%) patients, cefazolin was standardly used (2 g once immediately before surgery), and then it was prescribed at a dosage of 2 g three times a day for two or three days. Other cephalosporins (cefuroxime, ceftazidime) or antimicrobials of other groups or their combinations with vancomycin, fluconazole, etc., were rarely used according to individual indications, taking into account the anamnesis.

When comparing indicators in groups of patients with and without complications who received different antimicrobials for antibiotic prophylaxis, no differences were detected.

3.2. Aromatic Metabolites in Patients and Healthy Volunteers

A number of tyrosine and phenylalanine metabolites was measured in the serum samples of the patients and healthy volunteers, and the limit of quantitation for all metabolites was 0.5 µmol/L (Table 1). The serum samples of all patients before the surgery ($n = 79$) were characterized by higher values of benzoic and 4-hydroxyphenyllactic acids compared to the healthy volunteers ($n = 48$). The parameter which describes the content of the diagnostically significant sepsis-associated microbial metabolites [20] includes the sum of phenyllactic, 4-hydroxyphenylacetic and 4-hydroxyphenyllactic acids (Σ3AMM). This parameter was also higher in the serum samples of the patients before the surgery. The concentration of other aromatic acids (phenylpropionic, phenyllactic, 4-hydroxybenzoic, 4-hydroxyphenylacetic, 4-hydroxyphenylpropionic, and homovanillic acids) was less than the limit of quantitation (0.5 µmol/L) in most cases.

Table 1. The concentrations of aromatic metabolites in the serum samples of the patients before the surgery ($n = 79$) and healthy volunteers ($n = 48$), and the results of the Mann–Whitney U test.

Aromatic Acid, µmol/L	Healthy Volunteers ($n = 48$)	Patients ($n = 79$)	p-Value
Benzoic	0.5 (0.5–0.6)	1.2 (0.9–1.5)	<0.001
Phenylpropionic	<0.5 (<0.5–0.5)	<0.5 (<0.5–<0.5)	-
Phenyllactic	<0.5 (<0.5–<0.5)	<0.5 (<0.5–0.5)	-
4-Hydroxybenzoic	<0.5 (<0.5–<0.5)	<0.5 (<0.5–<0.5)	-
4-Hydroxyphenylacetic	<0.5 (<0.5–<0.5)	<0.5 (<0.5–0.6)	-
4-Hydroxyphenylpropionic	<0.5 (<0.5–<0.5)	<0.5 (<0.5–0.7)	-
Homovanillic	<0.5 (<0.5–<0.5)	<0.5 (<0.5–<0.5)	-
4-Hydroxyphenyllactic	1.3 (1.0–1.6)	1.6 (1.2–1.9)	0.003
Σ3AMM	1.9 (1.4–2.3)	2.3 (1.9–3.1)	<0.001

3.3. Aromatic Metabolites in Different Groups of Patients

All patients ($n = 79$) were divided into groups according to the course of the postoperative period. There were patients without complications ($n = 36$) and patients with different types of complications ($n = 43$). More than half of patients with a complicated course of the postoperative period had infectious complications ($n = 26$) such as pneumonia or local infection of the skin and soft tissues in the area of surgery. Among other types of complications, there were the development of organ dysfunctions or surgical complications (bleeding, hematomas in the area of surgery), etc. Most often, patients with complications needed longer treatment in the ICU or were re-transferred from the specialized department to the intensive care at different times of the postoperative period, for example, due to the development of respiratory or cardiovascular insufficiency.

The serum samples from the patients were collected before the surgery (0 points) and 6 h after the end of the surgery (1 point). The characteristics of the patients, the intraoperative parameters, the length of stay, and the concentrations of aromatic metabolites are demonstrated in Table 2.

Table 2. The medical and demographic characteristics, the intraoperative parameters, the length of stay, and the concentrations of aromatic metabolites in the serum samples of the patients before the surgery (0 points), 6 h after the surgery (1 point) and the difference between these points (Δ 1–0) in all patients (n = 79), patients without complications (n = 36), patients with all types of complications (n = 43) including the patients with infectious complications (n = 26). The results of the Mann–Whitney U test for the patients without any complications (n = 36) and the patients with all types of complications (n = 43) are demonstrated as p-Value A; and for the patients without any complications (n = 36) and the patients with infectious complications (n = 26) are demonstrated as p-Value B. The statistically different data was highlighted with bold format.

Parameter	Patients (n = 79)	Patients without Complications (n = 36)	Patients with All Types of Complications (n = 43)	Patients with Infectious Complications (n = 26)	p-Value A	p-Value B
Medical and demographic characteristics						
Sex, male, %	57, 72.2%	25, 69.4%	32, 74.4%	22, 84.6%	0.6 *	0.2 *
Age, years	57 (46–64)	58 (45–63)	55 (48–66)	54 (48–66)	0.5	0.5
Body Mass Index (BMI), kg/m²	27.2 (24.2–30.7)	27.5 (23.9–31.2)	27.1 (24.1–30.0)	27.3 (24.8–30.4)	0.5	0.8
Charlson Comorbidity Index	4 (2–5)	3 (2–5)	4 (2–5)	4 (2–5)	0.3	0.3
Intraoperative parameters						
Acute/subacute aortic dissection	15, 81.0%	5, 13.9%	10, 23%	5, 19.2%	0.3 *	0.6 *
Cardiopulmonary Bypass, min	123 (101–162)	111 (73–140)	150 (116–188)	163 (138–217)	**<0.001**	**<0.001**
Myocardial Ischemia, min	91 (66–117)	82 (55–102)	99 (76–137)	119 (92–142)	**0.014**	**<0.001**
Intraoperative Blood Loss, mL	800 (700–1100)	800 (600–1000)	950 (700–1500)	1000 (800–2000)	**0.019**	**0.01**
Drainage, mL	250 (150–370)	190 (110–300)	300 (200–500)	325 (200–550)	**0.006**	**<0.001**
Total Blood Loss, mL	1100 (900–1500)	1000 (775–1300)	1250 (960–1750)	1475 (1020–2350)	**0.003**	**<0.001**
Length of stay						
Length of Stay in the ICU	2 (1–4)	1 (1–1)	3 (2–5)	4 (2–10)	**<0.001**	**<0.001**
Total Hospital Stay	10 (8–14)	8 (7–10)	13 (10–18)	15 (11–21)	**<0.001**	**<0.001**
Aromatic acids, μmol/L						
Benzoic (0)	1.2 (0.9–1.5)	1.1 (0.9–1.4)	1.2 (1.0–1.6)	1.3 (1.1–1.5)	0.2	0.3
Benzoic (1)	1.3 (1.1–1.8)	1.3 (1.1–1.7)	1.2 (1.1–2.0)	1.2 (1.1–1.6)	0.7	0.9
Δ Benzoic (1–0)	0.1 (−0.3–0.6)	0.2 (−0.1–0.4)	0.1 (−0.4–0.7)	0 (−0.4–0.6)	0.7	0.5
Phenylpropionic (0)	<0.5 (<0.5–<0.5)	<0.5 (<0.5–<0.5)	<0.5 (<0.5–<0.5)	<0.5 (<0.5–<0.5)	-	-
Phenylpropionic (1)	<0.5 (<0.5–<0.5)	<0.5 (<0.5–<0.5)	<0.5 (<0.5–<0.5)	<0.5 (<0.5–<0.5)	-	-
Δ Phenylpropionic (1–0)	0 (−0.1–0)	−0.1 (−0.2–[−0.1])	0 (−0.1–0)	0 (−0.1–0)	0.2	0.3
Phenyllactic (0)	<0.5 (<0.5–<0.5)	<0.5 (<0.5–<0.5)	<0.5 (<0.5–<0.5)	<0.5 (<0.5–<0.5)	-	-
Phenyllactic (1)	0.5 (<0.5–0.7)	0.5 (<0.5–0.6)	0.5 (<0.5–0.8)	0.6 (<0.5–0.8)	-	-
Δ Phenyllactic (1–0)	0.1 (0–0.3)	0.1 (0–0.2)	0.2 (0–0.3)	0.2 (0.1–0.3)	0.1	0.06

Table 2. Cont.

Parameter	Patients (n = 79)	Patients without Complications (n = 36)	Patients with All Types of Complications (n = 43)	Patients with Infectious Complications (n = 26)	p-Value A	p-Value B
4-Hydroxybenzoic (0)	<0.5 (<0.5–<0.5)	<0.5 (<0.5–<0.5)	<0.5 (<0.5–<0.5)	<0.5 (<0.5–<0.5)	-	-
4-Hydroxybenzoic (1)	<0.5 (<0.5–<0.5)	<0.5 (<0.5–<0.5)	<0.5 (<0.5–<0.5)	<0.5 (<0.5–<0.5)	-	-
Δ 4-Hydroxybenzoic (1–0)	0 (0–0)	0 (0–0)	0 (0–0)	0 (0–0)	-	-
4-Hydroxyphenylacetic (0)	<0.5 (<0.5–0.6)	<0.5 (<0.5–0.6)	0.5 (<0.5–0.7)	0.5 (<0.5–0.8)	-	-
4-Hydroxyphenylacetic (1)	<0.5 (<0.5–0.7)	<0.5 (<0.5–<0.5)	0.5 (<0.5–1.1)	0.5 (<0.5–1.2)	-	-
Δ 4-Hydroxyphenylacetic (1–0)	0 (−0.2–0.2)	−0.1 (−0.2–0)	0.1 (−0.1–0.4)	0.2 (−0.1–0.5)	0.001	0.003
4-Hydroxyphenylpropionic (0)	<0.5 (<0.5–0.7)	<0.5 (<0.5–0.7)	<0.5 (<0.5–0.5)	<0.5 (<0.5–0.5)	-	-
4-Hydroxyphenylpropionic (1)	<0.5 (<0.5–0.7)	<0.5 (<0.5–0.7)	<0.5 (<0.5–0.6)	<0.5 (<0.5–0.5)	-	-
Δ 4-Hydroxyphenylpropionic (1–0)	0 (0–0)	0 (0–0)	0 (0–0)	0 (0–0)	-	-
Homovanillic (0)	<0.5 (<0.5–<0.5)	<0.5 (<0.5–<0.5)	<0.5 (<0.5–<0.5)	<0.5 (<0.5–<0.5)	-	-
Homovanillic (1)	<0.5 (<0.5–<0.5)	<0.5 (<0.5–<0.5)	<0.5 (<0.5–0.8)	<0.5 (<0.5–<0.5)	-	-
Δ Homovanillic (1–0)	0 (0–0.3)	0 (0–0.1)	0.1 (0–0.6)	0 (0–0.3)	-	-
4-Hydroxyphenyllactic (0)	1.6 (1.2–1.9)	1.6 (1.2–1.9)	1.6 (1.2–1.9)	1.6 (1.2–1.9)	0.7	0.8
4-Hydroxyphenyllactic (1)	2.4 (1.8–3.2)	2.0 (1.6–2.9)	2.8 (2.0–3.5)	2.8 (2.0–3.7)	0.005	0.01
Δ 4-Hydroxyphenyllactic (1–0)	0.8 (0.3–1.3)	0.6 (0.3–0.9)	1.1 (0.6–1.7)	1.1 (0.6–1.8)	0.001	<0.001
Σ3AMM (0)	2.3 (1.9–3.1)	2.3 (1.8–3.1)	2.4 (1.9–3.1)	2.6 (1.9–3.3)	0.5	0.6
Σ3AMM (1)	3.4 (2.5–4.8)	2.7 (2.3–4.0)	4.1 (3.0–5.1)	4.3 (3.0–5.7)	0.001	0.002
Δ Σ3AMM (1–0)	0.9 (0.2–1.8)	0.6 (0.1–1.0)	1.3 (0.7–2.4)	1.4 (0.5–2.9)	0.001	0.004

* Chi-square test.

The intraoperative parameters (time of cardiopulmonary bypass and myocardial ischemia, drainage, intraoperative and total blood loss) and length of hospital stay were statistically different in the patients with all types of complications ($n = 43$) and without complications ($n = 36$). The concentration of one of the sepsis-associated metabolites 4-hydroxyphenyllactic acid in serum sample collected 6 h after the end of surgery (1 point) and the difference (Δ 1–0) was higher in patients with complications ($n = 43$). The same results were obtained for the sum of sepsis-associated microbial metabolites Σ3AMM.

The results for the comparison of the patients without complications ($n = 36$) and the patients with infectious complications ($n = 26$) were similar to those for patients with all types of complications ($n = 43$).

Age, gender, metabolic status of the patients (BMI), concomitant diseases and other initial factors of patients, as well as the general index of concomitant pathology of Charlson had no significant differences between the two groups of patients. We detected a trend towards an increase in Σ3AMM with increasing age that did not reach statistical significance ($p = 0.065$), and there was no significant relationship between BMI and Σ3AMM ($p = 0.892$) (Figure S1).

3.4. Aromatic Metabolites for the Assessment of the Risk of Postoperative Complications in Patients

The ROC-analysis (Figure 2, Table 3) was carried out for the 4-hydroxyphenyllactic acid and Σ3AMM concentrations in serum samples collected 6 h after the end of the surgery, which were significantly different in the patients with all types of complications ($n = 43$) and without complications ($n = 36$). The areas under the ROC curve for 4-hydroxyphenyllactic acid and Σ3AMM were 0.686 and 0.717, respectively. The optimal cut-off values for 4-hydroxyphenyl lactic acid (2.0 μmol/L) and Σ3AMM (2.9 μmol/L) were calculated. The risk of postoperative complications was 3.4 times greater (95% CI 1.3–9.0) and 5.5 times greater (95% CI 1.9–15.0) for 4-hydroxyphenyl lactic acid and Σ3AMM, respectively, when the cut-off value was exceeded.

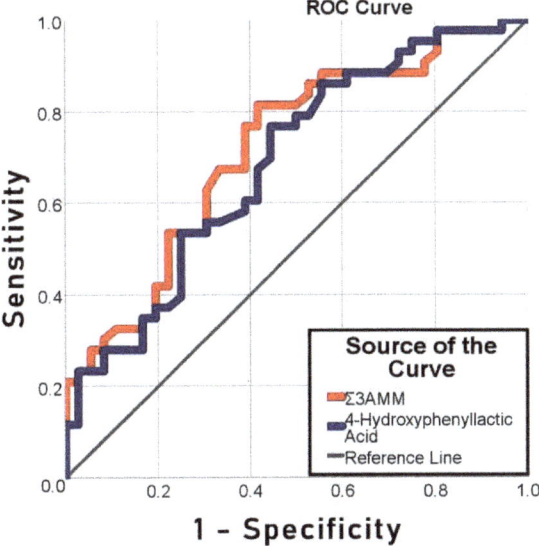

Figure 2. Prognostic value of 4-hydroxyphenyllactic acid and Σ3AMM in patients after cardiac surgery.

Table 3. The ROC analysis results for the 4-hydroxyphenyllactic acid and Σ3AMM concentrations in serum samples collected 6 h after the end of the surgery (1 point) as the predictors of the postoperative complications in cardiac surgery patients.

Parameter		4-Hydroxyphenyllactic Acid (1)	Σ3AMM (1)
Area Under the Curve		0.686	0.717
Standard Error		0.060	0.058
p-Value		0.005	0.001
Asymptotic 95% CI	Lower Bound	0.569	0.604
	Upper Bound	0.804	0.830
Cut-Off Value		2.0 µmol/L	2.9 µmol/L
Sensitivity (95% CI), %		79 (64–90)	81 (67–92)
Specificity (95% CI), %		47 (30–65)	56 (38–72)
Positive Predictive Value, %		64	69
Negative Predictive Value, %		65	71
Accuracy, %		65	70
Odds Ratio		3.4 (1.3–9.0)	5.5 (1.9–15.0)

4. Discussion

Despite the great progress in cardiovascular surgery, the percentage of postoperative complications, such as infections at the site of surgery, pneumonia, and others, does not decrease and, according to the literature, on average is registered to range from 12.6 to 21%. The studies on this topic provide analyses of the risk factors for complications, which most often include age, gender, chronic lung diseases, heart failure, duration of cardiopulmonary bypass [21–23]. In recent years, there has been a growing interest in studying the potential connection of human microbiota with cardiovascular diseases [24,25] and the role of the intestinal microbiota in the pathogenesis of heart failure [26,27]. Scientific data confirm the potential involvement of microbiota-related factors, for example, taxonomy features of gut microbiota in cardiosurgical intensive care patients [28] and increased risk of bacterial translocation followed by a pro-inflammatory condition [24,29]. The studies consider the possibilities of influencing the microbiota in order to improve the results of treatment of patients with heart diseases in the future [30–32]. However, we did not detect any studies describing the relationship between the metabolic activity of the microbiota though metabolites of tyrosine and phenylalanine and the development of cardiac surgical complications.

In this study, the authors took as a basis the postulate that "function is more important than systematics" [13] and assessed the state of the microbiota by the products of microbial metabolism of aromatic amino acids circulating in the blood. The obtained results confirmed the working hypothesis that patients with aortic aneurysm had deviations in the level of circulating AMMs at the stage of admission to the clinic, before surgery, in comparison with the healthy volunteers. This fact, on the one hand, is a manifestation of microbiota dysfunction as part of multiple organ disorders in conditions of atherosclerotic process, hypertensive and ischemic diseases, and genetically determined connective tissue dysplasia [33]. On the other hand, a disorder of the integrity of the vascular wall against the background of an inflammatory process of various etiologies may be due to active changes in microbial metabolism and bacterial translocation. Risk factors for the development of perioperative complications (surgical trauma, prolonged cardiopulmonary bypass, myocardial ischemia, massive blood loss) additionally disrupt the metabolic function of the microbiota, which was manifested by a statistically significant increase in serum AMMs 6 h after surgery (1 point) compared to those before surgery (0 points) in patients with complications (Table 2).

Age, gender, BMI, concomitant diseases and other initial factors of patients, as well as the general index of concomitant pathology of Charlson displayed no significant differences between the two groups of patients. At the same time, aromatic metabolites, such as 4-hydroxyphenylacetic and 4-hydroxyphenyllactic, and especially the sum of three AMMs, were significantly higher ($p < 0.05$). In the group of patients with complications, the median value of the difference of the sum of three AMMs (Δ 1–0) was more than two times higher than this level in the group without complications ($p = 0.001$), which can be used for monitoring and prognosis of complications in the future. It is noteworthy that 6 h after the surgery, the sum of three AMMs in patients with infectious complications ($n = 26$) was within 4.3 (3.0–5.7) μmol/L and did not reach high values (up to 10 μmol/L or more), as, for example, it was reported in patients with sepsis [20,34]. Moreover, all patients survived, and the average duration of stay of patients in the intensive care unit was 1 day for patients without complications in comparison with 4 days for patients with all types of complications ($p < 0.001$).

It is also interesting to note that not all patients at the highest risk with acute/subacute aortic dissection ($n = 15$) were in the group with complications after surgery. As can be seen from Figure 1, four patients (27%) had no postoperative complications. This fact once again indicates the high significance of microbiota metabolic disorders compared, for example, to the fact of the acute aortic dissection or the scope of surgical intervention.

Our study is a pilot single center study with obvious limitations. In the medical center where the study was conducted, 1087 different cardiac surgical interventions were performed in 2021, including 166 (15%) surgeries for aortic aneurysm/dissection. In accordance with the protocol of the study, patients ($n = 79$) which were operated on by one surgical team in 2021 were analyzed in our study. We purposefully selected operations on the aorta due to the greatest risk of postoperative complications, taking into account the severity of this pathology and a complex of concomitant diseases in every patient included in the study (Table S1). All patients with this pathology need individually selected options for reconstructive aortic surgery, differing in type, localization, duration, and volume, which are listed in Section 3.1. Despite the small number of patients, a disorder in metabolic function of the microbiota as an important risk factor for postoperative complications was identified, which was not previously taken into account. In addition, it was determined that this risk factor can be determined with a high degree of confidence early enough after surgery (6 h). The authors assume that this important result will be confirmed with other types of operations in further extensive studies.

It is important to consider that operations on the aorta in such patients with multiple risk factors are not performed in all cardiac surgery clinics, which makes it difficult to organize multicenter studies, and it is almost impossible to select a group of similar patients.

The authors believe that the results of this pilot study are extremely important for understanding the mechanisms of complications. Impaired microbiota metabolism is important in the development of complications after complex reconstructive aortic surgery, which is the basis for the search for a new prevention strategy. At the time of writing of this paper, a randomized clinical trial has already begun in the same cardiac surgery center to study the effectiveness of antimicrobial prevention based on the regulation of the metabolic activity of the microbiota.

5. Conclusions

The microbiota metabolism disruption is an important risk factor for postoperative complications in cardiovascular surgery, in particular, after aortic prosthetics. The degree of microbiota metabolism disruption can be assessed by monitoring the level of some AMMs circulating in the blood. It is necessary to look for the ways to adjust the metabolism of the microbiota to improve the results of surgical treatment in future by searching for replacement the compensation of its functions.

Supplementary Materials: The following supporting information can be downloaded at: https://www.mdpi.com/article/10.3390/biomedicines11051335/s1, Table S1: Frequency of concomitant diseases in patients with aortic aneurysm/dissection included in the study ($n = 79$); Figure S1: Scatter plot and linear regression for (A) Σ3AMM and age, (B) Σ3AMM and BMI.

Author Contributions: Conceptualization, M.B. and N.B.; methodology, M.B. and N.B.; formal analysis, M.Y.; investigation, A.P., M.G. and O.G.; resources, M.B. and N.B.; data curation, A.P., M.G. and O.G.; writing—original draft preparation, N.B. and A.P.; writing—review and editing, M.Y., M.B., M.G., O.G. and A.E.; visualization, A.P. and M.Y.; supervision, A.E.; project administration, M.B. and N.B.; funding acquisition, N.B. All authors have read and agreed to the published version of the manuscript.

Funding: This research received no external funding.

Institutional Review Board Statement: The study was conducted in accordance with the Declaration of Helsinki and approved by the Local Ethic Committee of Petrovsky Russian Research Center of Surgery, Moscow, Russia (protocol code N7 from 15 February 2021).

Informed Consent Statement: Informed consent was obtained from all subjects involved in the study.

Data Availability Statement: Not applicable.

Conflicts of Interest: The authors declare no conflict of interest.

References

1. Lindholm, E.; Seljeflot, I.; Aune, E.; Kirkeboen, K.A. Proinflammatory cytokines and complement activation in salvaged blood from abdominal aortic aneurism surgery and total hip replacement surgery. *Transfusion* **2012**, *52*, 1761–1769. [CrossRef] [PubMed]
2. Shukuzawa, K.; Ohki, T.; Maeda, K.; Kanaoka, Y. Risk factors and treatment outcomes for stent graft infection after endovascular aortic aneurysm repair. *J. Vasc. Surg.* **2019**, *70*, 181–192. [CrossRef] [PubMed]
3. Charchyan, E.R.; Chakal, D.A.; Belov, Y.V. Results of staged thoracoabdominal aorta replacement. *Kardiol. Serdechno-Sosud. Khirurgiya* **2019**, *12*, 281–285. [CrossRef]
4. Charchyan, E.R.; Breshenkov, D.G.; Belov, Y.V. Gibridnye operatsii u patsientov s rassloeniem aorty III tipa i porazheniem ee proksimal'nogo otdela. *Khirurgiia* **2020**, *9*, 28–37. [CrossRef]
5. Argyriou, C.; Georgiadis, G.S.; Lazarides, M.K.; Georgakarakos, E.; Antoniou, G.A. Endograft Infection after Endovascular Abdominal Aortic Aneurysm Repair: A Systematic Review and Meta-analysis. *J. Endovasc. Ther.* **2017**, *24*, 688–697. [CrossRef]
6. McDonald, D.; Ackermann, G.; Khailova, L.; Baird, C.; Heyland, D.; Kozar, R.; Lemieux, M.; Derenski, K.; King, J.; Vis-Kampen, C.; et al. Extreme Dysbiosis of the Microbiome in Critical Illness. *mSphere* **2016**, *1*, 199–215. [CrossRef] [PubMed]
7. Ojima, M.; Motooka, D.; Shimizu, K.; Gotoh, K.; Shintani, A.; Yoshiya, K.; Nakamura, S.; Ogura, H.; Iida, T.; Shimazu, T. Metagenomic Analysis Reveals Dynamic Changes of Whole Gut Microbiota in the Acute Phase of Intensive Care Unit Patients. *Dig. Dis. Sci.* **2016**, *61*, 1628–1634. [CrossRef]
8. Chernevskaya, E.; Beloborodova, N.; Klimenko, N.; Klimenko, N.; Pautova, A.; Shilkin, D.; Gusarov, V.; Tyakht, A.; Tyakht, A. Serum and fecal profiles of aromatic microbial metabolites reflect gut microbiota disruption in critically ill patients: A prospective observational pilot study. *Crit. Care* **2020**, *24*, 312. [CrossRef]
9. Iapichino, G.; Callegari, M.L.; Marzorati, S.; Cigada, M.; Corbella, D.; Ferrari, S.; Morelli, L. Impact of antibiotics on the gut microbiota of critically ill patients. *J. Med. Microbiol.* **2008**, *57*, 1007–1014. [CrossRef]
10. Chernevskaya, E.; Zuev, E.; Odintsova, V.; Meglei, A.; Beloborodova, N. Gut microbiota as early predictor of infectious complications before cardiac surgery: A prospective pilot study. *J. Pers. Med.* **2021**, *11*, 1113. [CrossRef]
11. Sitkin, S.I.; Vakhitov, T.Y.; Demyanova, E.V. Microbiome, gut dysbiosis and inflammatory bowel disease: That moment when the function is more important than taxonomy. *Alm. Clin. Med.* **2018**, *46*, 396–425. [CrossRef]
12. Huttenhower, C.; Gevers, D.; Knight, R.; Abubucker, S.; Badger, J.H.; Chinwalla, A.T.; Creasy, H.H.; Earl, A.M.; Fitzgerald, M.G.; Fulton, R.S.; et al. Structure, function and diversity of the healthy human microbiome. *Nature* **2012**, *486*, 207–214. [CrossRef]
13. Beloborodova, N.V. Serum Aromatic Microbial Metabolites as Biological Markers in Intensive Care. In *Biomarkers in Trauma, Injury and Critical Care. Biomarkers in Disease: Methods, Discoveries and Applications*; Rajendram, R., Preedy, V.R., Patel, V.B., Eds.; Springer: Cham, Switzerland, 2023; Chapter 13, pp. 245–268. [CrossRef]
14. Beloborodova, N.V.; Khodakova, A.S.; Bairamov, I.T.; Olenin, A.Y. Microbial origin of phenylcarboxylic acids in the human body. *Biochemistry* **2009**, *74*, 1350–1355. [CrossRef] [PubMed]
15. Dodd, D.; Spitzer, M.H.; Van Treuren, W.; Merrill, B.D.; Hryckowian, A.J.; Higginbottom, S.K.; Le, A.; Cowan, T.M.; Nolan, G.P.; Fischbach, M.A.; et al. A gut bacterial pathway metabolizes aromatic amino acids into nine circulating metabolites. *Nature* **2017**, *551*, 648–652. [CrossRef] [PubMed]
16. Natalia, V.; Olenin, A.Y.; Khodakova, A.S. Phenylcarboxylic acids as potential markers for diagnosis of sepsis in cardiac surgery patients. *ArchivEuromedica* **2011**, *1–2*, 20–26.
17. Lam, V.; Su, J.; Hsu, A.; Gross, G.J.; Salzman, N.H.; Baker, J.E. Intestinal microbial metabolites are linked to severity of myocardial infarction in rats. *PLoS ONE* **2016**, *11*, e0160840. [CrossRef]
18. Pautova, A.K.; Bedova, A.Y.; Sarshor, Y.N.; Beloborodova, N.V. Determination of Aromatic Microbial Metabolites in Blood Serum by Gas Chromatography–Mass Spectrometry. *J. Anal. Chem.* **2018**, *73*, 160–166. [CrossRef]

29. Charlson, M.E.; Pompei, P.; Ales, K.L.; MacKenzie, C.R. A new method of classifying prognostic comorbidity in longitudinal studies: Development and validation. *J. Chronic Dis.* **1987**, *40*, 373–383. [CrossRef]
30. Beloborodova, N.V.; Sarshor, Y.N.; Bedova, A.Y.; Chernevskaya, E.A.; Pautova, A.K. Involvement of aromatic metabolites in the pathogenesis of septic shock. *Shock* **2018**, *50*, 273–279. [CrossRef]
31. Gelijns, A.C.; Moskowitz, A.J.; Acker, M.A.; Argenziano, M.; Geller, N.L.; Puskas, J.D.; Perrault, L.P.; Smith, P.K.; Kron, I.L.; Michler, R.E.; et al. Management practices and major infections after cardiac surgery. *J. Am. Coll. Cardiol.* **2014**, *64*, 372–381. [CrossRef]
32. Dixon, L.K.; Di Tommaso, E.; Dimagli, A.; Sinha, S.; Sandhu, M.; Benedetto, U.; Angelini, G.D. Impact of sex on outcomes after cardiac surgery: A systematic review and meta-analysis. *Int. J. Cardiol.* **2021**, *343*, 27–34. [CrossRef] [PubMed]
33. O'Keefe, S.; Williams, K.; Legare, J.-F. Hospital-Acquired Infections After Cardiac Surgery and Current Physician Practices: A Retrospective Cohort Study. *J. Clin. Med. Res.* **2017**, *9*, 10–16. [CrossRef] [PubMed]
34. Tang, W.H.W.; Kitai, T.; Hazen, S.L. Gut microbiota in cardiovascular health and disease. *Circ. Res.* **2017**, *120*, 1183–1196. [CrossRef] [PubMed]
35. Yamashita, T.; Emoto, T.; Sasaki, N.; Hirata, K.I. Gut microbiota and coronary artery disease. *Int. Heart J.* **2016**, *57*, 663–671. [CrossRef]
36. Xu, H.; Wang, X.; Feng, W.; Liu, Q.; Zhou, S.; Liu, Q.; Cai, L. The gut microbiota and its interactions with cardiovascular disease. *Microb. Biotechnol.* **2020**, *13*, 637–656. [CrossRef]
37. Suslov, A.V.; Chairkina, E.; Shepetovskaya, M.D.; Suslova, I.S.; Khotina, V.A.; Kirichenko, T.V.; Postnov, A.Y. The neuroimmune role of intestinal microbiota in the pathogenesis of cardiovascular disease. *J. Clin. Med.* **2021**, *10*, 1995. [CrossRef]
38. Aardema, H.; Lisotto, P.; Kurilshikov, A.; Diepeveen, J.R.J.; Friedrich, A.W.; Sinha, B.; de Smet, A.M.G.A.; Harmsen, H.J.M. Marked Changes in Gut Microbiota in Cardio-Surgical Intensive Care Patients: A Longitudinal Cohort Study. *Front. Cell. Infect. Microbiol.* **2020**, *9*, 467. [CrossRef]
39. Piccioni, A.; Saviano, A.; Cicchinelli, S.; Franza, L.; Rosa, F.; Zanza, C.; Santoro, M.C.; Candelli, M.; Covino, M.; Nannini, G.; et al. Microbiota and myopericarditis: The new frontier in the cardiological field to prevent or treat inflammatory cardiomyopathies in COVID-19 outbreak. *Biomedicines* **2021**, *9*, 1234. [CrossRef]
40. Li, Q.; Gao, B.; Siqin, B.; He, Q.; Zhang, R.; Meng, X.; Zhang, N.; Zhang, N.; Li, M. Gut Microbiota: A Novel Regulator of Cardiovascular Disease and Key Factor in the Therapeutic Effects of Flavonoids. *Front. Pharmacol.* **2021**, *12*, 1093. [CrossRef]
41. Chen, X.; Li, H.Y.; Hu, X.M.; Zhang, Y.; Zhang, S.Y. Current understanding of gut microbiota alterations and related therapeutic intervention strategies in heart failure. *Chin. Med. J.* **2019**, *132*, 1843–1855. [CrossRef]
42. Jia, Q.; Li, H.; Zhou, H.; Zhang, X.; Zhang, A.; Xie, Y.; Li, Y.; Lv, S.; Zhang, J. Role and Effective Therapeutic Target of Gut Microbiota in Heart Failure. *Cardiovasc. Ther.* **2019**, *2019*, 5164298. [CrossRef] [PubMed]
43. Rumyantseva, V.A.; Charchyan, E.R.; Zaklyazminskaya, E.V.; Khovrin, V.V.; Rogozhina, Y.A.; Khachatryan, Z.R.; Yu, V.B. Marfan syndrome is caused by a nonsense mutation in the gene for fibrillin: Clinical application of DNA diagnostics in aortic surgery. *Clin. Exp. Surg. Petrovsk. J.* **2015**, *2*, 97–103.
44. Babaev, M.A.; Eremenko, A.A.; Grin, O.O.; Kostritca, N.S.; Dymova, O.V.; Beloborodova, N.V.; Pautova, A.K.; Zakharenkova, Y.S.; Levitskya, M.V. Successful therapy of endotoxin shock and multiple organ dysfunction using sequential targeted extracorporeal treatment in a patient after combined cardiac surgery. *Clin. Exp. Surg.* **2020**, *8*, 105–114. [CrossRef]

Disclaimer/Publisher's Note: The statements, opinions and data contained in all publications are solely those of the individual author(s) and contributor(s) and not of MDPI and/or the editor(s). MDPI and/or the editor(s) disclaim responsibility for any injury to people or property resulting from any ideas, methods, instructions or products referred to in the content.

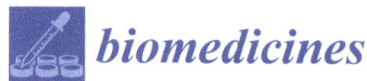

Article

Inflammation, Microcalcification, and Increased Expression of Osteopontin Are Histological Hallmarks of Plaque Vulnerability in Patients with Advanced Carotid Artery Stenosis

Ioan Alexandru Balmos [1,2,3,†], Emőke Horváth [4,5,†], Klara Brinzaniuc [2], Adrian Vasile Muresan [3,6], Peter Olah [7], Gyopár Beáta Molnár [5,8] and Előd Ernő Nagy [8,9,*]

1. Doctoral School of Medicine and Pharmacy, I.O.S.U.D., George Emil Palade University of Medicine, Pharmacy, Science, and Technology of Targu Mures, 540142 Targu Mures, Romania
2. Department of Anatomy, George Emil Palade University of Medicine, Pharmacy, Science, and Technology of Targu Mures, 540142 Targu Mures, Romania
3. Vascular Surgery Clinic, County Emergency Clinical Hospital of Targu Mures, 540136 Targu Mures, Romania
4. Department of Pathology, Faculty of Medicine, George Emil Palade University of Medicine, Pharmacy, Science, and Technology of Targu Mures, 38 Gheorghe Marinescu Street, 540142 Targu Mures, Romania
5. Pathology Service, County Emergency Clinical Hospital of Targu Mures, 50 Gheorghe Marinescu Street, 540136 Targu Mures, Romania
6. M3 Department of Surgery, George Emil Palade University of Medicine, Pharmacy, Science, and Technology of Targu Mures, 540142 Targu Mures, Romania
7. Department of Medical Informatics and Biostatistics, George Emil Palade University of Medicine, Pharmacy, Science, and Technology of Targu Mures, 540139 Targu Mures, Romania
8. Department of Biochemistry and Environmental Chemistry, George Emil Palade University of Medicine, Pharmacy, Sciences and Technology of Targu Mures, 540142 Targu Mures, Romania
9. Laboratory of Medical Analysis, Clinical County Hospital Mures, 540394 Targu Mures, Romania
* Correspondence: elod.nagy@umfst.ro
† These authors contributed equally to this work.

Abstract: Background: severe carotid artery stenosis is a major cause of ischemic stroke and consequent neurological deficits. The most important steps of atherosclerotic plaque development, leading to carotid stenosis, are well-known; however, their exact timeline and intricate causal relationships need to be more characterized. Methods: in a cohort of 119 patients, who underwent carotid endarterectomy, we studied the histological correlations between arterial calcification patterns and localization, the presence of the inflammatory infiltrate and osteopontin expression, with ulceration, thrombosis, and intra-plaque hemorrhage, as direct signs of vulnerability. Results: in patients with an inflammatory infiltrate, aphasia was more prevalent, and microcalcification, superficial calcification, and high-grade osteopontin expression were characteristic. Higher osteopontin expression was also correlated with the presence of a lipid core. Inflammation and microcalcification were significantly associated with plaque ulceration in logistic regression models; furthermore, ulceration and the inflammatory infiltrate were significant determinants of atherothrombosis. Conclusion: our results bring histological evidence for the critically important role of microcalcification and inflammatory cell invasion in the formation and destabilization of advanced carotid plaques. In addition, as a calcification organizer, high-grade osteopontin expression is associated with ulceration, the presence of a large lipid core, and may also have an intrinsic role in plaque progression.

Keywords: calcification; inflammation; osteopontin; carotid stenosis; carotid endarterectomy

Citation: Balmos, I.A.; Horváth, E.; Brinzaniuc, K.; Muresan, A.V.; Olah, P.; Molnár, G.B.; Nagy, E.E. Inflammation, Microcalcification, and Increased Expression of Osteopontin Are Histological Hallmarks of Plaque Vulnerability in Patients with Advanced Carotid Artery Stenosis. *Biomedicines* 2023, 11, 881. https://doi.org/10.3390/biomedicines11030881

Academic Editor: Alfredo Caturano

Received: 10 February 2023
Revised: 3 March 2023
Accepted: 7 March 2023
Published: 13 March 2023

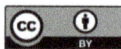

Copyright: © 2023 by the authors. Licensee MDPI, Basel, Switzerland. This article is an open access article distributed under the terms and conditions of the Creative Commons Attribution (CC BY) license (https://creativecommons.org/licenses/by/4.0/).

1. Introduction

Ischemic vascular brain disease, manifesting as brain infarction and white matter lesions (WMLs), is highly prevalent in the elderly, being the second leading cause of death globally, and can lead to permanent disability due to irreversible neurological and cognitive deficits [1]. It is most commonly caused by severe carotid stenosis or embolization from a high-risk carotid plaque resulting in a stroke. Atherosclerotic plaque development is driven by systemic and local factors that ultimately determine where plaques form and how they progress. Local susceptibility to plaque formation depends on the arterial microenvironment, including arterial mechanics, matrix remodeling, and lipid deposition through the regulation of vascular cell function [2].

The pathophysiology of atherosclerosis is well documented, considered a chronic, insidious lipid-driven inflammatory process with several potential contributors, which lead to ischemia of target tissues through narrowing of the large- and medium-sized arteries' lumen. This process is initiated by endothelial dysfunction, followed by a cascade of cellular, functional, and molecular events, which imply the activation of inflammatory pathways [3]. Lipid deposition in the arterial wall causes an influx of macrophages to remove the lipid deposits, but the continuous increase in plasma cholesterol and the ineffective removal result in extracellular lipid accumulations, along with macrophage necrosis, leading to the formation of a necrotic core. This intimal inflammatory response activates smooth muscle cells in the underlying medial layer, which shift their phenotype and migrate into the neointima. Through fibroproliferative remodeling, smooth muscle cells contribute to the growing plaque size and lumen occlusion. However, this fibroproliferative response also forms a protective fibrous cap, rich in smooth muscle cells and collagen, which ensures the mechanical stability of the plaque and prevents plaque rupture [3].

Before the era of the inflammatory theory, vascular calcification was thought to be a passive process and a late manifestation of atherosclerosis. In the coronaries, calcification is a predictor of future cardiovascular events [4]; less is known about its causal relationships in the case of carotids. Recent histological evidence from human cerebral artery specimens has demonstrated that calcification may affect two different layers of the wall: the intima and/or the media. Calcification of the media is often associated with diabetes and chronic kidney disease. Intimal calcification is a typical feature of advanced atherosclerosis and manifests as two sub-types: micro- or spotty, early-stage calcification or macro-, sheet-like, and late-stage calcification [5]. Evidence from histopathological analyses and clinical imaging studies has confirmed that intimal calcification is more associated with plaque vulnerability. In contrast, medial calcification, particularly of the inner elastic lamina, contributes to artery stiffness rather than lumen stenosis [6].

Microcalcification develops due to activated macrophages and smooth muscle cells, which first form matrix vesicles and then crystallizing mineral deposits [4]. These can be identified by PET-CT imaging or optical coherence tomography; functionally, they increase the mechanical stress between the fibrous cap and lipid core, resulting in plaque rupture [7]. Several analyses have associated the late-stage "macrocalcification" with the presence of more differentiated smooth muscle cells and a more organized extracellular matrix, conferring plaque stability [8,9]; however, other recent studies have suggested that superficial, multiple calcifications and ulceration are associated with intra-plaque hemorrhage, and may represent higher-risk lesions [10]. Conversely, intraplaque hemorrhage and erythrocyte extravasation may stimulate osteoblastic differentiation and intralesional calcium phosphate deposition [11]. Osteopontin (OPN), a phosphoglycoprotein expressed in many tissues, consistently co-localizes with ectopic calcification. The molecule is a pro-inflammatory cytokine and can be further induced by reactive oxygen species, interleukin-1β (IL-1β), and tumor necrosis factor α (TNFα) [12]. Due to the density of glutamic and aspartic acid residues, OPN can fix a significant amount of calcium [13]. It was suggested that acute increases in OPN might have a protective role because it reduce calcification and assist in wound healing and neovascularization. However, its sustained elevation confers a high cardiovascular risk [12]. According to these data, the risk of a cerebrovascular event due to a vulnerable atheromatous plaque depends on the severity of vascular stenosis and plaque morphology and composition.

Taking these considerations, we studied the relationships between calcification patterns, the presence of inflammatory cell infiltrates, and histological signs of vulnerability:

ulceration and thrombosis on arterial specimens of a cohort of patients who underwent carotid endarterectomy due to severe atherosclerosis.

2. Materials and Methods

2.1. Patients and Tissue Fragments

Carotid plaque specimens were collected by carotid endarterectomy from patients diagnosed with symptomatic carotid artery stenosis hospitalized between January 2020 and December 2022 in the Vascular Surgery Clinic—County Emergency Clinical Hospital and the Cardiovascular Surgery Clinic—Cardiovascular Disease and Transplantation Emergency Institute of Târgu Mureș (Romania).

A total of 119 cases were selected for the histopathology study (plaques collected during carotid endarterectomy from 82 males and 37 females, all of them with severe carotid stenosis) based on strict criteria: patients with complete clinical documentation and the written informed consent of enrollment in the study, and last but not least, tissue samples with adequate quantity and quality for histological evaluation (Figure 1). Indication for carotid endarterectomy (CEA) was made on the clinician's decision according to the European Society for Vascular Surgery and European Stroke Organization guidelines which recommend CEA for asymptomatic patients with carotid stenosis between 60–99% and for symptomatic patients with carotid stenosis between 50–99%. Prior to surgery, imaging tests (CT angiography and a Doppler ultrasonography) were performed to diagnose, localize, and grade the stenosis. The exclusion criteria consisted of patients with carotid near occlusion, which refers to severe carotid stenosis with distal vessel collapse and no significant improvement in stroke prevention within the first 5 years following endarterectomy [14,15], those who had experienced a major stroke, those with a second stenotic lesion in the intracranial segment of the internal carotid artery, and those who had previously undergone carotid endarterectomy on the same side [16]. Figure 1 shows the study flowchart with the main exclusion steps at the clinical and histopathological levels.

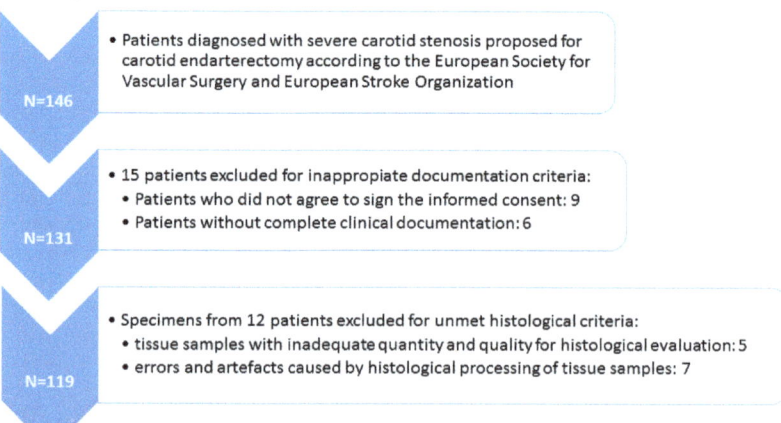

Figure 1. Flowchart of the study.

2.2. Patients Data Collection

Demographic information (age and sex) and clinical data (neurological symptoms at the time of admission, history of hypertension, diabetes mellitus, hypercholesterolemia, coronary heart disease, presence of atherosclerotic disease involving more than one vascular bed, current history of smoking, use of antiplatelet or anticoagulant, hypolipidemic, and anti-hypertensive drugs and previous stroke/transient ischemic attack history) were collected and checked against medical records. Hypertension, diabetes mellitus, and hypercholesterolemia have been defined according to recent guidelines [17–19]. A history of stroke was based on the definition in the World Health Organization criteria, including a syndrome of rapidly developing symptoms, with no apparent cause other than of vascular origin, of focal or global cerebral dysfunction lasting 24 h or longer, or leading to death [20]. From the laboratory examination results, we have noted recent data on absolute neutrophil and lymphocyte count and neutrophil/lymphocyte ratio. Our group's epidemiological, clinical imagistic, and laboratory characteristics are summarized in Table 1, which also shows the data broken down to subgroups with and without an inflammatory cellular infiltrate.

Table 1. Clinical variables of the 119 atheromatous plaques, with vs. without inflammatory infiltrate.

Variable	Median (Quartile Range)/Mean ± SE	INF+ Group (n = 75)	INF− Group (n = 44)	p Values
Demographic and lifestyle variables				
Age (years)	67 (61–72)	67 (60–73)	67.5 (63–71)	0.412
Gender (f/m)	37 (31.1)/82 (68.9)	23 (30.7)/52 (69.3)	14 (31.8)/30 (68.2)	1.000
Smoking (yes/no)	58 (48.7)/61 (51.3)	40 (53.3)/35 (46.7)	18 (40.9)/26 (59.1)	0.254
Disease characteristics and comorbidities				
Grade of stenosis * (%)	81.3 ± 0.7	80.3 ± 0.9	83.1 ± 1.2	0.062
Carotid atherosclerosis, uni- vs. bilateral (u/b)	84 (70.6)/35 (29.4)	50 (66.7)/25 (33.3)	34 (77.3)/10 (22.7)	0.297
Stroke history (y/n)	76 (63.9)/43 (36.1)	51 (68)/24 (32)	25 (56.8)/19 (43.2)	0.240
Occurrence of aphasia (yes/no)	17 (14.3)/102 (85.7)	15 (20)/60 (80)	2 (4.5)/42 (95.5)	0.027
Occurrence of paresis/plegia (yes/no)	13 (10.9)/106 (89.1)	11 (14.7)/64 (85.3)	2 (4.5)/42 (95.5)	0.128
Hypertension (y/n)	110 (92.4)/9 (7.6)	67 (89.3)/8 (10.7)	43 (97.7)/1 (2.3)	0.151
Diabetes (y/n)	33 (27.7)/86 (72.3)	18 (24)/57 (76)	15 (34.1)/29 (65.9)	0.471
Polyvascular disease (1/2/3 arterial beds affected)	80 (67.2)/28 (23.5)/11 (9.3)	58 (77.3)/15 (20)/2 (2.7)	22 (50)/13 (29.5)/9(20.5)	0.001
Plaque calcification				
Calcification extent (grade 3–4/grade 0–2)	54 (45.4)/65 (54.6)	30 (40)/45 (60)	24 (54.5)/19 (45.5)	0.142
Superficial/deep calcification	65 (54.6)/54 (45.4)	48 (64)/27 (36)	17(38.6)/27 (61.4)	0.008
Microcalcification (yes/no)	54 (45.4)/65 (54.6)	42 (56)/33 (44)	12 (27.3)/32 (72.7)	0.004
Nodular calcification (yes/no)	71 (59.7)/48 (40.3)	49 (65.3)/26 (34.7)	22 (50)/22 (50)	0.122
Extended/confluent calcification (yes/no)	41 (34.5)/78 (65.5)	20 (26.7)/55 (73.3)	21 (47.4)/23 (52.3)	0.027
Metaplasia (yes/no)	33 (27.7)/86 (72.3)	17 (22.6)/58 (77.3)	16 (40.9)/28 (59.1)	0.138
OPN expression (grade 1/2/3)	57(47.9)/36 (30.3)/26(21.8)	21(28)/29(38.7)/25(33.3)	36(81.8)/7(15.9)/1(2.3)	<0.001
Biological variables and medication				
Hypercholesterolemia (yes/no)	115 (96.6)/4 (3.4)	74 (98.7)/1 (1.3)	41 (93.2)/3 (6.8)	0.142
Abs. neutrophil count (10^9/L)	5.29 (4.05–6.66)	5.51 (4.04–6.8)	5.07 (4.05–6.38)	0.293
Abs. lymphocyte count (10^9/L)	1.95 (1.56–2.53)	1.95 (1.64–2.47)	1.93 (1.45–2.64)	0.686
Neutrophil/Lymphocyte ratio	2.70 (1.91–3.62)	2.8 (1.95–3.62)	2.55 (1.65–3.75)	0.338
Anti-hypertensive drugs (y/n)	110 (92.4)/9 (7.6)	67 (89.3)/8 (10.7)	43 (97.7)/1 (2.3)	0.151
Anticoagulant pre.op.(y/n)	7 (5.8)/112 (94.2)	0 (0)/ 75 (17.1)	37 (89.2)/7 (10.8)	0.077
Anti-aggregants pre.op.(y/n)	111 (93.2)/8 (6.8)	71 (94.6)/4 (5.4)	40 (90.9)/4 (9.1)	0.465
Anticoagulant post.op. (y/n)	95 (79.8)/24 (20.2)	62 (82.6)/13 (17.4)	33 (75)/11 (25)	0.349
Anti-aggregants post.op. (y/n)	119 (100)/0	75 (100)/0	44 (100)/0	-
Hypolipidemics (y/n)	116 (97.4)/3 (2.6)	73 (97.3)/2 (2.7)	43 (97.7)/1 (2.3)	1.000

Values of variables with normal distribution (marked with asterisk) are represented by the mean ± SE, whereas values of variables with abnormal distribution are shown as median (quartiles). Binomial variables are represented as absolute numbers and percentages (in brackets). Comparison of variables with discrete values was performed by the Fisher's exact test (2 × 2 groups) and the Pearson χ^2 test (3 × 2 groups). For the numeric variables, groups were compared with the Mann–Whitney U test. The level of statistical significance has been set to $p = 0.05$.

This study was conducted according to the principles of the Helsinki Declaration. It was approved by the Ethical Committee of the George Emil Palade University of Medicine Pharmacy, Science, and Technology of Targu Mures (no.906/2020) and the institutional review board of County Emergency Clinical Hospital of Targu Mures (no. 29496/2019) and of Cardiovascular Disease and Transplantation Emergency Institute of Târgu Mureș (no. 1680/2020). Written informed consent was obtained from each patient involved in this study.

2.3. Histological Processing

After surgery, the tissue samples were immediately fixed in 10% neutral buffered formalin and sent for histological analyses. Following decalcification in ethylene-diamine tetra-acetic acid (EDTA) solution pH 7, all fragments were processed according to the standard methodology. For immunohistochemistry, consecutive histological sections were prepared. Morphological features of carotid plaques were examined in 4–5 μm sections stained with hematoxylin and eosin (H&E) by a senior pathologist (EH) blinded to the patient's characteristics. Atherosclerotic plaques were classified accordingly to the Modified American Heart Association Classification in type IV-VII [21]. After establishing the grade based solely on visual estimation of histological features without quantitative measurements, detection of characteristic signs of plaque vulnerability for each case was proposed as follows: active mononuclear cells infiltration (macrophages and lymphocytes) within the atherosclerotic plaque, neovascularization within the lipid core, pattern of calcification (type, position, and extension), structure of lipid core (lipid-rich large necrotic core or hyaline rich core), intra-plaque hemorrhage, and fibrous cap damage (with or without parietal thrombus fragments) [22], each scored as being present or absent. Plaque rupture was identified by the presence of fibrous cap discontinuity with an endothelial defect of at least 1000 μm in width or a clear cavity formed inside the plaque [4], with or without thrombus, intra-plaque hemorrhage. The lipid core was categorized into large necrotic if cellular detritus predominated in its structure, along with macrophages with foamy cytoplasm and cholesterol crystals. In addition, we considered being fulfilled the criteria for an active mononuclear inflammatory infiltrate when macrophages and lymphocytes were observed around the core regardless of their quantity. The presence or absence of new vessels within the lipid core was also noted.

Focusing on their calcification type, plaques were included in four categories depending on the calcified patch distribution, size, and shape: (a) microcalcification (defined as a punctate pattern of numerous small micronodules/scattered small mineral foci) (b) nodular calcification (single/multiple stratified mineral deposits with a nodular aspect), (c) confluent/large calcification (a conglomerate of mineral material with irregular edges in collagen-rich plaque), and (d) osteoid metaplasia (mature bone with lamellar structure and bone marrow in a mineral mass of fibrocalcific plaque). Although there is no conventional standard of size, the consensus was taken into account that categorizes microcalcifications and macrocalcifications based on nodules of <50 and ≥50 μm, respectively [23]. Regarding position/location of calcification, we established two categories: superficial calcifications as calcified nodules located at the intimal–luminal interface or close to the lumen [10] and deep calcifications located in the thickness of the media or closer to the adventitia than to the lumen [4]. Extension of mineral mass was quantified depending on the occupied area from the total surface of the examined material and scored from 1 to 4, namely grade 1: less than 25%; grade 2: between 25–50%; grade 3: between 50–75% and grade 4: over 75%.

2.4. Investigation of the Osteopontin (OPN) Expression within the Atherosclerotic Plaque by Immunohistochemistry

Immunohistochemical staining was performed using Osteopontin (OPN) polyclonal antibody (pab73623) purchased from Covalab (Villeurbanne, France) in combination with EnVision FLEX/HRP (Agilent, Dako, Santa Clara, CA, USA) as secondary antibody and 3,3'-diaminobenzidine chromogen (DAB), respectively, according to the manufacturer's instructions. Nuclei were counterstained by hematoxylin. For negative control, normal serum was substituted for the primary antibody. According to the extension of the brown color reaction product, plaques were categorized in low-grade (score 1), mild-grade (score 2), and high-grade (score 3) OPN expression. Score 1 was considered as few positive cells (<25 cells in no more than two areas of the plaque examined with 20× magnification). Score 2 was represented by immunolabelled cells in slightly increased numbers, not exceeding 50 elements in no more than two areas of the plaque examined with 20× magnification. When the number of positive cells exceeded 50 in number in the examined areas, samples were labeled as score 3.

2.5. Statistical Analysis

Categorical variables and transformed continuous variables were assessed for absolute and relative distribution frequency. Analysis of 2 × 2 or 3 × 2 contingency tables has been performed with the Fisher's exact test and the Pearson χ^2 test. Nonlinear logistic regression models were set for the prediction of ulceration and atherothrombosis. In all tests, p-values < 0.05 were considered statistically significant. Data processing was performed using Microsoft Excel 2016 (Microsoft Corporation, Redmond, WA, USA) and GraphPad Prism 9.5.0 (GraphPad Software LLC., San Diego, CA, USA).

3. Results

3.1. Study Group Characteristics

A total of 119, out of which 82 were male and 37 female patients, were enrolled in the study group, with a median age of 67 (61–72). All patients had severe carotid artery stenosis over 70% (mean ± SE 81.3 ± 0.7). A total of 84 individuals showed unilaterally, and 35 possessed bilateral involvement of the carotids. Seventeen patients suffered from various forms of sensory or motor aphasia, and hemiparesis/hemiplegia occurred in 13 study group members. A previous stroke history was confirmed in 76 subjects. The vast majority of cases were hypertensive (92.4%), and 27.7% were diabetic (type 1 and type 2). Eighty of them showed only carotid atherosclerosis; in 28 patients, two arterial bed involvement (carotids and limbs or coronary), and in 11 cases, three arterial bed involvement (carotids, limbs, and coronary arteries) was established. A total of 48.7% of the cohort were smokers, and except for four subjects, the rest presented hypercholesterolemia. No significant differences in the absolute neutrophil count, the absolute leucocyte count, and the neutrophil/lymphocyte ratio were observed (Table 1).

3.2. Histopathogical Features of Carotid Atherosclerotic Plaques

First, we investigated the plaque architecture and histological features by light microscopy. These plaques, some unstable, others advanced, showed a varied histological composition. Characteristic signs of plaque vulnerability for each case were reported. A lipid-rich large necrotic core (Figure 2a) was detected in 58.8% of specimens. An active mononuclear cell component (macrophages and lymphocytes) was found in 63.02% of cases surrounding the necrotic core or extending to the hyalinised zones (Figure 2b). Accumulation of erythrocyte aggregates in the plaque structure (intra-plaque hemorrhage) (Figure 2c) was present in 32.8% of cases. Many plaques showed neovascularization by the proliferation of small, thin-walled microvessels with a collapsed lumen (66.4%), in most cases coexisting with inflammation and intra-plaque hemorrhage (Figure 2d). Ulcerated plaques with irregular and discontinuous fibrous caps (43.7%) led to thrombus formation in 16 cases (Figure 2e,f).

Because all examined plaques showed signs of calcification, the next step was to characterize the pattern, extent, and location of calcification. Regarding the intra-plaque calcification patterns, microcalcification, as numerous micronodules/scattered small mineral foci forming a calcification front within fibrosis (Figure 3a), was present by itself or in predominance in association with other types of calcification in 45.4% of cases. Seventy-one plaques (59.7%) showed a predominance of nodular calcification, as well-shaped single/multiple stratified mineral deposits with a nodular aspect (Figure 3b). Extensive (confluent) calcification (a conglomerate of mineral material with irregular edges (Figure 3c) dominated 34.5% of cases, and osteoid metaplasia (mature bone with lamellar structure and bone marrow (Figure 3d) was present in only 33 cases (27.7%). Depending on the location of the calcified foci in the thickness of the plaque, we observed a slight predominance in favor of superficial calcification over deep calcification 65 (54.6%) vs. 54 (45.4%). Mineral mass with grades 0–2 (54.6%) exceeded grades 3–4 (45.4%).

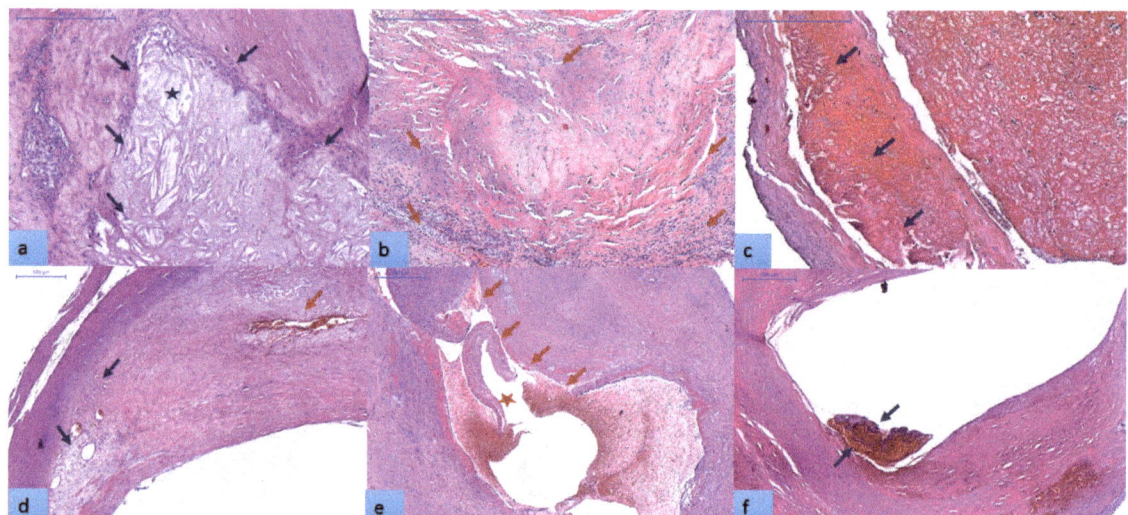

Figure 2. Representative sections of unstable carotid plaques from six different patients characterized by complex morphology and composition, H&E stain: (**a**). atherosclerotic plaque fragment with large necrotic lipid core (blue arrows; necrosis marked by star); (**b**). an abundant mononuclear inflammatory cell population (macrophages and lymphocytes) surrounds the lipid core and extends in the hyaline areas; (**c**). endarterectomy specimen shows erythrocyte aggregates in the plaque structure (intra- plaque hemorrhage) (blue arrows); (**d**). obvious intra-plaque neovascularization is seen both within and at the periphery of the plaque. The size of the neo-formed vessels varies between foci, some exceeding 10 μm (red arrow). (**e**). atheromatous plaque leading to narrowing and deformation of the lumen (blue arrows) shows fibrous cap discontinuity with an endothelial defect of at least 1000 μm in width (red arrows); (**f**). plaque ulceration in association with parietal thrombus represents a frequent cause of ischemic events. Bar represents 500 μm in all of the tissue sections.

3.3. Osteopontin Expression

After the characterization of carotid atherosclerotic plaque morphology, the ensuing investigation has focused on the role of OPN in plaque instability. We examined by immunohistochemical technique whether OPN expression is only cell-associated or is also present at the extracellular level in the plaque. In Figure 4, endothelial cells of the intima and neoformed vessels, macrophages, those transformed into foam cells, and fibroblasts are intensively cytoplasmic stained for OPN (Figure 4a). Vascular smooth muscle cells, other significant constituents of the atherosclerotic plaque and capable of transformation into foam cells, were also OPN positive (Figure 4b–d). In plaque structure without addition to the cells mentioned above, OPN staining of an extracellular component can also be observed. Details are shown on Figure 4.

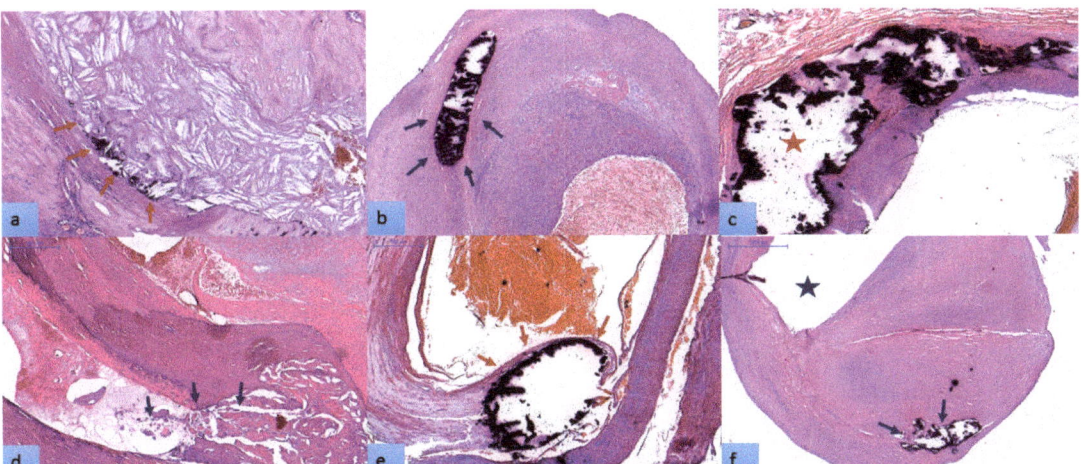

Figure 3. Calcification pattern in carotid plaques, H&E stain: Decalcified specimens from different cases show a various aspects and extension of mineral mass. (**a**). Large lipid core with sheet-like microcalcification forming a calcification front within fibrosis. (red arrows). Mononuclear inflammatory infiltrate is more abundant in the area around calcified foci; (**b**). nodular calcification with smooth rounded edges in the thickness of the fibrohyaline plaque (blue arrows); (**c**). plaque with heterogeneous structure, largely occupied by extensive calcification formed by conglomerated mineral nodules with irregular margins, extending towards the luminal surface of the plaque (red star); (**d**). plaque with large hyalinized areas in which osteoid metaplasia (trabecular bone and bone marrow foci) is also observed (blue arrows); (**e**). calcified nodule located at the intimal–luminal interface (red arrows), covered by thin fibrous cap (superficial calcification); (**f**). fibrous plaque with deep calcifications located in the thickness of the media (blue arrows, vascular lumen marked by star). Bar represents 500 µm in all of the tissue sections.

This result indicates that extracellular OPN is an active component of atherosclerotic plaque, but to clarify if it interacts with proteins involved in the plaque structure requires further immunohistochemical studies. Because the immunohistochemical results showed that osteopontin is produced by multiple cells, we hypothesized that the amount of OPN in situ influences plaque instability. Based on the scoring system applied to quantify the OPN expression, we found that a low-grade OPN expression (score 1) is significantly associated with the absence of an inflammatory infiltrate (63.1% vs. 36.9%). In contrast, in those with mid-grade (score 2) and high-grade (score 3) OPN expression, the incidence of the infiltrate was 80.5% and 96.1%, respectively ($p < 0.001$). The low-grade OPN expression was present in 59% of plaques without a lipid core, but the high-grade OPN was characteristic for 84.6% of plaques with a lipid core ($p < 0.001$). The OPN score 3 was also significantly correlated with plaque ulceration (53.8%), whereas the OPN score 1 case in 70.2% showed no ulcers ($p = 0.021$). Moreover, in patients with polyvascular atherosclerotic disease affecting 3 arterial beds, 10 had an OPN score of 1, and only 1 had an OPN score of 3. In cases with one arterial bed involvement, the expression of OPN was more equilibrated (41.2% OPN score one vs. 23.7%) ($p = 0.037$). No relationship was observed with age, gender, neovascularization, thrombosis, intra-plaque hemorrhage, hypertension, aphasia, hemiparesis/hemiplegia, or bilateral carotid involvement. Microcalcification strongly correlated with osteopontin expression: its absence was observed in 73.7% of the cases with an OPN score of 1. On the contrary, its presence was documented in 80.7% of those with an OPN score of 3 ($p < 0.001$). Out of 65 cases with calcification of the superficial vessel wall layers, 22 had an OPN score of 1, and 19 had an OPN score of 3. However, in those with deep layer (media and adventitia) calcification, the distribution was unequal: 35 cases showed low, whereas only 7 cases showed high OPN expression ($p = 0.003$).

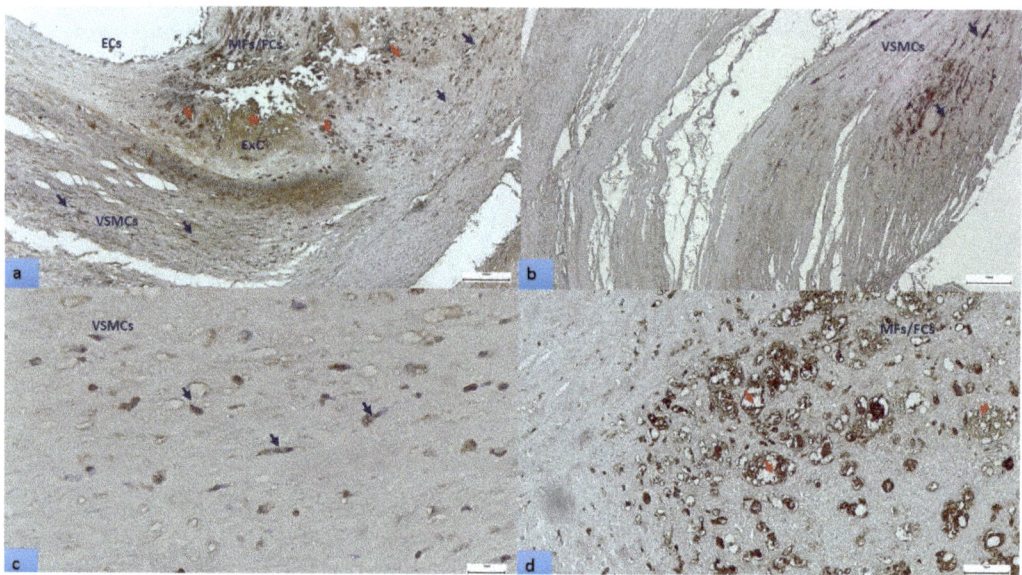

Figure 4. OPN-labelled cellular and extracellular structures in atherosclerotic plaque, immunohistochemical visualization (3,3′-diaminobenzidine chromogen): (**a**). OPN positive endothelial cells, macrophages (red arrows), fibroblasts (blue arrows). *OPN is also present extracellularly in the lipid core (star)*; bar represents 200 μm. (**b**,**c**). vascular smooth muscle cells are also OPN positive (blue arrows) bar represent 100 μm in (**b**), respectively, 20 μm in (**c**,**d**). OPN containing macrophages in the plaque at higher magnification. Many of these cells are foam cells with lipid droplets removed by organic solvents used for tissue processing, empty for OPN (red arrows); bar represents 50 μm.

The extent of calcification, the nodular, the extended/confluent patterns, metaplasia, and the cumulated calcification pattern did not have significant associations. The distribution of OPN expression scores is indicated in Supplementary Table S1.

3.4. Comparison of the Inflammatory Infiltrate Positive (INF+) and Negative (INF−) Groups

Seventy-five patients possessed atheromatous plaques with a significant inflammatory infiltrate (INF), whereas 44 showed no elements of inflammation. Table 1 synthesizes the distribution of different variables in these two groups. The demographic parameters were similar in the two groups. The occurrence of aphasia was significantly lower in the inflammatory infiltrate negative (INF−) subgroup: 4.5% compared to 20% in the positive (INF+) subgroup ($p = 0.027$). In addition, the frequency of hemiparesis/hemiplegia was lower (4.5% vs. 14.7%) but without significance. The grade of carotid stenosis showed a borderline difference between the groups ($p = 0.06$). There were no essential differences concerning the incidence of diabetes, hypertension, bilateral carotid involvement, or previous stroke history. Polyvascular atherosclerotic disease with three arterial beds involvement was represented in 20.5% of cases in the INF− group vs. 2.7% in the INF+ group, whereas solitaire carotid artery involvement equaled 50% in the INF− and 77.3% in the INF+ group ($p < 0.001$).

3.5. The Distribution of Atheroma Calcification Patterns

Fifty-four plaques presented extended calcification (grades 3 and 4), out of which 30 (40%) were classified in the INF+ and 24 (54.5%) in the INF− group. In addition, 54 specimens showed microcalcification from the overall group, with a significantly biased distribution between the groups: 42 (56%) in the INF+ group and only 12 (27.2%) in the INF−. Regarding the localization, the calcification was superficial in 54 and affected the deep layers in 65 cases. Superficial calcification characterized more (64%) INF⁺ plaques and less (38.4%) of those INF⁻ ($p = 0.008$). Among the calcification patterns, the nodular pattern was more frequent in the overall group than in the extended/confluent form (59.7% vs. 34.5%). The distribution of these patterns was significantly biased in the latter case: 26.7% of the INF⁺ group had extended/confluent calcification, compared to 47.4% of the INF⁻ cases ($p = 0.027$). Osteoid metaplasia was detected at 33 plaques in the entire group, being more frequent in those INF⁻ (40.9% vs. 22.6%), but this difference did not reach the significance threshold.

3.6. Treatment Correlations

Anti-hypertensive medication has been administered to all hypertensive patients ($n = 110$). A small subgroup was treated with anticoagulants ($n = 7$) preoperative (p.e.), and the majority of subjects received postoperative (p.o.) anti-coagulants ($n = 95$). Lipid-lowering treatment was administered to all, with the exception of three cases.

3.7. Correlations of Calcification Extent, Localization and Patterns with Ulceration, Thrombosis and Hemorrhagic Rupture of the Plaque

Ulceration occurred in a significantly higher proportion of plaques showing microcalcification: 34 of 54 vs. 18 of 65 ($p < 0.001$). Ulceration was relatively more frequent in those with superficial layer calcification than in plaques with deep layer involvement ($p = 0.064$). The nodular, the extended/confluent patterns, and the presence of metaplasia were not significantly associated with the ulcerative complication, neither as solitaire correlates nor in cumulative patterns (we classified in this group the occurrence of co-existing patterns, each component with a minimum weight of approximately 25%).

The presence of thrombosis was not correlated with calcification extent, localization, or patterns, as seen in Table 2.

Table 2. Occurence of ulceration, thrombosis and hemorrhage in subgroups with various calcification patterns.

		Ulceration				Thrombosis				Hemorrhage		
		No	Yes	p		No	Yes	p		No	Yes	p
Localization	superficial	32	33	0.064	superficial	57	8	0.789	superficial	38	27	0.031
	deep	36	18		deep	46	8		deep	42	12	
Microcalcification	No	47	18	<0.001	No	58	7	0.422	No	48	17	0.117
	Yes	20	34		Yes	45	9		Yes	32	22	
Nodular pattern	No	28	20	0.85	No	40	8	0.422	No	36	12	0.165
	Yes	39	32		Yes	63	8		Yes	44	27	
Extended/confluent pattern	No	40	38	0.173	No	67	11	1	No	47	31	0.019
	Yes	27	14		Yes	36	5		Yes	33	8	
Osteoid metaplasia	No	47	39	0.68	No	77	9	0.14	No	55	31	0.277
	Yes	20	13		Yes	26	7		Yes	25	8	
OPN expression	1+	40	17		1+	50	7		1+	42	15	
	2+	16	20	0.022	2+	31	5	0.924	2+	21	15	0.299
	3+	12	14		3+	22	4		3+	17	9	
Cumulative patterns: Nodular AND/OR extended/confluent AND/OR Osteoid metaplasia	No	47	39		No	76	10		No	55	31	
	Yes	21	12	0.493	Yes	27	6	0.47	Yes	25	8	0.46

Variables are represented as absolute numbers; comparisons were performed with the χ^2 test. The level of statistical significance has been set to $p = 0.05$.

The hemorrhagic rupture had a higher incidence in plaques with superficial calcification (27 of 65) than in those with deep layer calcification (12 of 54, $p = 0.031$). Further, the extended/confluent pattern was significantly associated with the lack of hemorrhagia ($p = 0.019$). No other calcification parameters or cumulative patterns correlated with the hemorrhagic rupture of the atheroma (Table 2).

3.8. Predictors of Plaque Ulceration

Univariate regression analysis revealed significant associations between plaque ulceration, the presence of single arterial bed involvement ($p = 0.042$), and morphological characteristics of the plaque: the lipid core ($p = 0.004$), micro-calcification ($p < 0.001$), and the presence of inflammatory infiltrate ($p < 0.001$). No significant relationships could be observed with diabetes, hypertension, a positive stroke history, unilateral vs. bilateral carotid involvement, age, gender, smoking, or hypercholesterolemia. A tendency for a lower odds ratio was registered in the presence of extended/confluent calcification pattern and in the highest vs. the lowest quartile of stenosis grade ($p = 0.079$ and $p = 0.091$). No other calcification patterns were correlated with ulceration (Table 3).

Table 3. Univariate logistic regression of variables associated with plaque ulceration.

Variables	Coefficient	SD	OR (95%CI)	p-Level
Age (Q4/Q1)	0.089	0.251	1.19 (0.45–3.18)	0.721
Gender (M/F)	0.182	0.408	0.83 (0.38–1.82)	0.656
Diabetes (Yes/No)	−0.044	0.227	0.82 (0.36–1.86)	0.846
Smoking (Yes/No)	−0.019	0.387	1.02 (0.49–2.11)	0.959
Hypertension (Yes/No)	−1.060	0.733	0.34 (0.08–1.45)	0.150
Carotid atherosclerosis, unilateral/bilateral (u/b)	−0.335	0.412	0.71 (0.32–1.60)	0.418
Stroke history (Yes/No)	−0.084	0.385	0.92 (0.43–1.90)	0.826
Polyvascular disease (≥2 a. beds/single bed)	−0.647	0.315	26.68 (1.52–468.19)	0.042
Stenosis grade (Q4/Q1)	−0.416	0.244	0.43 (0.16–1.14)	0.091
Hypercholesterolemia (Yes/No)	0.836	1.170	2.30 (0.23–22.85)	0.476
Revascularization (Yes/No)	−0.284	0.391	0.75 (0.35–1.62)	0.468
Calcification extent (High/Low)	−0.297	0.373	0.43 (0.15–1.21)	0.427
Nodular (Yes/No)	0.225	0.379	1.15 (0.55–2.41)	0.554
Extended/confluent (Yes/No)	−0.716	0.405	0.54 (0.25–1.19)	0.079
Osteoid metaplasia (Yes/No)	−0.197	0.417	0.78 (0.34–1.77)	0.637
Mixed calcification pattern (Yes/No)	−0.451	0.336	0.68 (0.30–1.57)	0.182
Microcalcification (Yes/No)	1.568	0.398	4.44 (2.04–9.63)	<0.001
Superficial/deep	−0.721	0.380	2.06 (0.98–4.35)	0.059
Lipid core (Yes/No)	1.190	0.402	3.28 (1.49–7.24)	0.004
Inflammatory infiltrate (INF⁺/INF⁻)	2.015	0.474	7.50 (2.96–19.00)	<0.001

We constructed non-linear multiple logistic regression models to predict the ulceration of the plaques. In a model adjusted for the absence of polyvascular disease, a greater stenosis extent, hypertension, the presence of superficial and an extended/confluent pattern of calcification, and the presence of a lipid core, microcalcification ($p = 0.003$), and the presence of an inflammatory infiltrate ($p = 0.007$) remained significant predictors (Table 4). However, when we also adjusted for osteopontin expression, this abolished the significant influence of microcalcification and lipid core.

Table 4. Summary of multiple logistic regression analysis of the factors correlated to atheromatous plaque ulceration in the overall patient group ($n = 119$).

Model 1. Variables	Estimate	SD	Odds Ratio (95% CI)	p Value
Microcalcification	1.470	0.491	4.44 (2.04–9.63)	0.003
Lipid core (Yes/No)	0.104	0.526	3.28 (1.49–7.24)	0.843
Superficial/deep	0.376	0.509	2.06 (0.98–4.35)	0.460
Extended/confluent calcification	−0.048	0.496	0.54 (0.25–1.19)	0.922
Inflammatory infiltrate (INF⁺/INF⁻)	1.575	0.574	7.50 (2.96–19.00)	0.007
Stenosis grade (Q4:Q1)	−0.376	0.300	0.43 (0.16–1.14)	0.212
Polyvascular disease (≥2 a. beds/single bed)	−0.390	0.409	26.68 (1.52–468.19)	0.342
Hypertension (Yes/No)	−0.042	0.880	0.34 (0.08–1.45)	0.961

3.9. Predictors of Atherothrombosis

In univariate regression models, ulceration proved to be a strong predictor of thrombosis ($p < 0.0001$). The inflammatory infiltrates were also significantly associated ($p = 0.046$), whereas revascularization and the lipid core showed a borderline significance ($p = 0.074$ and $p = 0.064$, respectively). The other factors did not correlate, as shown in Table 5.

Table 5. Univariate logistic regression of variables associated with thrombosis of the plaque.

Variables	Estimate	SD	OR (95%CI)	*p*-Level
Age (Q4/Q1)	0.150	0.364	1.60 (0.25–10.29)	0.681
Gender (M/F)	−1.284	0.408	1.44 (0.29–7.06)	0.656
Diabetes (Yes/No)	0.313	0.301	1.69 (0.56–5.09)	0.300
Smoking (Yes/No)	0.230	0.343	0.79 (0.27–2.29)	0.675
Hypertension (Yes/No)	0.233	1.095	1.26 (0.14–10.83)	0.821
Carotid atherosclerosis, unilateral/bilateral	−0.669	0.675	1.95 (0.52–7.33)	0.323
Stroke history (Yes/No)	0.603	0.612	1.82 (0.55–6.06)	0.326
Polyvascular disease (≥2 a. beds/single bed)	0.545	0.547	1.67 (0.57–4.88)	0.320
Stenosis grade (Q4/Q1)	−0.189	0.375	0.68 (0.15–2.98)	0.615
Revascularization (Yes/No)	1.409	0.783	4.09 (0.88–18.98)	0.074
Nodular (Yes/No)	−0.454	0.539	0.63 (0.22–1.82)	0.401
Extended/confluent (Yes/No)	−0.167	0.577	0.84 (0.27–2.62)	0.772
Osteoid metaplasia (Yes/No)	0.834	0.552	2.30 (0.78–6.80)	0.133
Mixed calcification pattern (Yes/No)	0.524	0.562	1.69 (0.56–5.09)	0.353
Microcalcification (Yes/No)	0.505	0.541	1.65 (0.57–4.79)	0.353
Superficial/deep	0.214	0.537	0.80 (0.28–2.31)	0.690
Lipid core (Yes/No)	1.252	0.670	3.49 (0.93–13.01)	0.064
Inflammatory infiltrate (INF$^+$/INF$^-$)	1.572	0.782	4.81 (1.04–22.33)	0.046
Ulceration (Yes/No)	23.78	-	61.02 (3.55–1046)	0.005

In univariate regression analysis, ulceration was strongly associated with plaque thrombosis ($p < 0.0001$). Further, the presence of inflammatory infiltrate was also significantly more frequent in those with thrombosis, ($p = 0.046$), whereas revascularization ($p = 0.074$) and the presence of the lipid core ($p = 0.064$) showed a tendency to significance. Age, gender, diabetes, hypertension, and smoking could not be associated, and no relationship has been revealed with the presence of polyvascular disease, unilateral involvement, and the grade of vascular stenosis. Furthermore, none of the calcification patterns could be correlated to the atherothrombotic complication (Table 6). In a multiple logistic regression model, ulceration and inflammation remained significant predictors, when adjusted for revascularization and the presence of the large lipid core ($p = 0.002$ and $p = 0.007$).

Table 6. Summary of multiple logistic regression analysis of the factors correlated to thrombotic complication in the overall patient group ($n = 119$). **Model 2.**

Variables	Estimate	SD	Odds Ratio (95% CI)	*p* Value
Lipid core (Yes/No)	0.609	0.823	3.28 (1.49–7.24)	0.843
Inflammatory infiltrate (INF$^+$/INF$^-$)	0.623	0.971	7.50 (2.96–19.00)	0.007
Revascularization (Yes/No)	2.021	0.832	0.43 (0.16–1.14)	0.212
Ulceration (Yes/No)	3.335	1.082	61.02 (0.08–1.45)	0.002

4. Discussion

Carotid endarterectomy and carotid stenting are two treatment modalities for patients with severe carotid stenosis. Histopathological processing of endarterectomy specimens provides useful information, which, together with clinical data and imaging investigation, contributes to the efficient secondary prevention of cerebrovascular events.

Carotid plaques have a complex morphology and composition, consisting of both extracellular (necrotic core, lipids, extracellular matrix proteins, lipids, and free cholesterol recognized as clefts) and cellular components dominated by inflammatory cells, smooth muscle cells, and fibrous tissue, which explains the existence of considerable differences in vulnerability between plaques with identical degrees of stenosis. In this context, histopathological assessment of plaque characteristics is one of the "gold standards" used to classify plaques as stable or unstable, first proposed by Lovett et al. in 2004 [22,24].

Although the precise sequence of lesion progression leading to plaque vulnerability is poorly elucidated, the morphological signs of instability as a potential indicator of stroke risk are well known. This hallmark includes a large lipid core, macrophage-mediated inflammatory changes, intraplaque neoangiogenesis/hemorrhage, ulceration, and microcalcification [25]. In this context, histological identification of these signs in endarterectomy specimens may provide valuable data concerning underlying plaque morphologies and should guide the treatment strategy to prevent further cerebral events.

Arterial plaques contain macrophages (MFs) involved in all steps of atherosclerosis. They are influenced by several cytokines and chemokines in the vessel wall and interact with local microenvironmental factors, which drive their differentiation into variable functional phenotypes. MFs can take up oxidized LDL and low-density lipoprotein (LDL)-derived cholesterol as lipid droplets and transform them into foam cells. These are significant players in the initiation and progression of atherosclerosis. The debris of macrophage-derived foam cells provides the major source of the necrotic core in the atherosclerotic plaque [26]. The liponecrotic tissue in atheroma with necrotic core appears to be developed by the structural collapse of the lipid core of atheroma due to the loss of elastic and collagen fibers; MFs are organically involved in this mechanism [27]. Matrix metalloproteinases synthesized by infiltrating macrophages are mainly responsible for their intra-plaque elastolytic and collagenolytic activity. Genetic deficiency of MMP-1a strongly suppresses atherogenesis in the aorta of apo E $-/-$ mice [28]. Interestingly collagen structure, along with synthesis, degradation, and remodeling of vascular wall elastin, proteoglycans, and glycosaminoglycans, modulate the phenotype of infiltrating inflammatory, but also of the resident cells [29].

In our case, histopathological examination of 119 endarterectomy specimens revealed the presence of a lipid-rich, large necrotic core (Figure 1a) in 58.8% of specimens. This core was associated with an active mononuclear cell component (macrophages and lymphocytes) that surrounded the necrotic core in 63% of cases. In patients without a high inflammatory component in their carotid plaques, the occurrence of cerebrovascular events such as aphasia, hemiparesis, or hemiplegia was significantly lower compared to the INF-positive subgroup. These results suggest that MF-mediated inflammation, initiated by the lipid content, destabilizes atherosclerotic plaques through the degradation of their cross-linked structural proteins. Increases in the size of the necrotic core may happen as a consequence of two factors, MF death, and impaired efferocytosis. In addition, necrosis contributes to forming an inflammatory microenvironment, enhanced oxidative stress, and thrombogenicity [3].

Fissuration and ulceration, landmarks of destabilization, are also the result of MF-released enzymatic activity. Tomas et al., in 159 carotid specimens obtained by endarterectomy, identified an altered metabolomic signature of unstable carotid plaques, comprising increased glycolysis and amino acid utilization along with low fatty-acid oxidation. A series of pro-inflammatory cytokines, like interleukins IL-1b, IL-6, IL-15, IL-17, and IL-18, are abundantly expressed in homogenates of the cluster characterized by the signature mentioned above [25,30]. Chemokines synthesized by MFs, like monocyte chemoattractant protein-1 (MCP-1) and MF inflammatory protein-1b (MIP-1b) were also up-regulated in unstable vs. stable plaques [30].

Our study defines ulceration, thrombosis, and intra-plaque hemorrhage as major morphological manifestations of atherosclerotic plaque vulnerability. Clinical findings support this assumption: the presence of ulceration, as the sole sign, is predictive of neurological symptoms and, together with advanced-grade stenosis, represents a high risk for stroke [31]. Sixty-one subjects were investigated by multi-detector computed tomography, and in 16 ulcerated plaques, no correlation was observed with the plaque volume. In contrast, ulcerative lesions were strongly associated with the presence of a lipid-rich content [31].

In univariate logistic regression models, we observed that the sizeable necrotic lipid core, but not hypercholesterolemia, was significantly associated with ulceration. However, this association was abolished in a multiple logistic regression model focused on ulceration, inflammation, revascularization and the lipid core. Regarding the infiltrating inflammatory elements of the atherosclerotic plaques and the circulating neutrophil count, or neutrophil/lymphocyte ratio, no correlation was found, even though several studies report higher neutrophil counts along the presence of microemboli detected by transcranial Doppler ultrasound in symptomatic patients [32]. Instead, the presence of the inflammatory cellular infiltrate, consisting predominantly of MFs, and microcalcification proved to be the strongest predictors of ulceration, which remained significant after adjustments for the stenosis grade, the presence of the lipid core, and superficial layer calcification. Further, ulceration and the inflammatory infiltrate, but not calcification extent or pattern, were defined as significant determinants of atherothrombosis, another important sign of plaque vulnerability.

An MF-rich inflammatory infiltrate was present in almost 2/3 of cases, so we investigated its histological correlates and compared it in INF+ and INF− groups. We showed that there were no essential differences between these groups in terms of the incidence of diabetes, hypertension, bilateral carotid involvement, or previous stroke history. In contrast, atheroma calcification patterns and location showed a significantly biased distribution of microcalcification and superficial calcification in favor of the INF+ group. Even though the effect of calcification is considered biphasic, from pro-inflammatory properties of "microcalcification" to anti-inflammatory properties of "macrocalcification," in our study, the distribution of extended/confluent pattern was almost twice less frequent in the case of the INF+ group (See Table 1). This result may suggest that extensive calcification, even if not a direct predictor of plaque ulceration and thrombosis, is less associated with inflammation and intra-plaque hemorrhage and might be considered a sign of plaque stability.

As reported in the literature, the calcification of atheromatous plaque is a remarkable feature of advanced atherosclerosis. It is triggered by inflammation, emerges as microcalcification, and develops through a spectrum of events to macrocalcification, with the formation of bone-like structures within the plaque. The release of matrix vesicles from macrophages and the death of VSMC initiates the calcification process of the plaque. Other factors are also involved in the process, including reduced levels of mineralization inhibitors or increased osteogenic transdifferentiation (VSMC pericytes) [3]. In our study, a part of the plaques showed mixed calcification patterns, containing foci with both microcalcification and different types of macrocalcification. In this case, the dominant patterns were considered, and for macrocalcification, cumulative patterns also were investigated. Our results demonstrated the presence of ulceration and intra-plaque hemorrhage in a significantly higher proportion of plaques with microcalcification. Furthermore, they showed dominance in plaques with superficial layer calcification compared to those with deep layer damage. No significant influence of the macrocalcification patterns was observed; no other single calcification parameters or cumulative patterns correlated with the hemorrhagic rupture of the plaque (See Table 2).

The role of calcification in the development of plaque progression is a controversial topic in the literature. The promoting role of microcalcification-induced stress on thin fibrous caps has been demonstrated in plaque rupture both by a three-dimensional blood-vessel modeling [33] and by imaging, histological and morphometric analysis [4,34]. Imagistic studies revealed some interesting aspects of calcification linkage with arterial wall inflammation: higher calcium scores appear along multiple sites in arteries in aging [35]. Carotid artery calcification was investigated in 130 patients included in the dal-PLAQUE study with 18F-labeled fluorodeoxyglucose positron emission tomography and computed tomography at entry and six months. The study revealed a poor overlap between vascular inflammation and calcification on multiple arterial beds. However, those with some calcification content at baseline showed more calcification progression than patients without. These arterial segments with progressive calcification showed a high [18F] FDG-PET signal, which highlights the putative causal role of inflammation in the progression of calcified lesions [35]. Macrocalcification is easily detected and quantified (calcium scores as predictive value for cardiovascular incidence) using the CT scan method. By contrast, microcalcification-the early stage of plaque calcification, is observed only with Positron Emission Tomography (PET)/CT Imaging and Optical Coherence Tomography (diagnostic methods that are not used in daily practice) [36]. However, the CT analysis of calcium subtypes is limited by the resolution and blooming artifacts. In this context, the histopathological examination of the endarterectomy specimens provides helpful information to the clinician to develop a treatment strategy. Molecular imaging of macrophages highlighted enhanced proteolytic activity via matrix metalloproteinases MMP-2, MMP-9, and MMP-13 [37]. MMP-9 is up-regulated by osteopontin, cleaves collagen and elastin substrates in the extracellular matrix, and determines hydroxyapatite crystal deposition [38]. In experimental conditions, the cysteine protease-activatable NIRF-imaging revealed that vascular calcification evolves parallel with bone osteolysis and might be driven by shared inflammatory driver mechanisms [37].

Several cytokine-type soluble regulators were described, which interact with different steps of calcification. For example, osteoprotegerin is elevated in the serum of patients with polyvascular atherosclerotic disease [39,40] and, in animal models, inhibits arterial calcification without affecting the development of the number and volume of atherosclerotic lesions [41]. Another regulator is osteopontin (OPN), a pro-inflammatory glycophosphoprotein involved in bone morphogenesis, a multi-faceted regulator of biomineralization, calcification, and tissue remodeling. Five isoforms of OPN may be expressed due to alternative splicing, which is a possible reason why it shows a diverse linkage with cardiovascular events in the population. OPN increases dramatically in acute stroke, and it is presumed that its early role is protective, attenuates vascular calcification, and promotes post-ischemic neovascularization. Paradigmatically, in chronic inflammatory pathways involving the vessel wall, OPN is probably harmful. It may be expressed in infiltrating macrophages, differentiating myofibroblasts, and endothelial cells of the vessel wall [42]. Wolak T. et al., in a study focusing on carotid atherosclerosis in hypertensive patients, demonstrated that none of the OPN "family members" have anti-inflammatory properties. OPN-N terminal fragment is associated with increased plaque inflammation [43].

In our tissue sections, a rather diverse cell population was stained for OPN. Morphologically, most of the OPN+ cells were macrophage-derived foam cells, VSMCs, and endothelial cells. We found that in our cohort, low-grade OPN expression was significantly associated with the absence of an inflammatory cell infiltrate. Furthermore, microcalcification was significantly correlated with OPN expression. Higher OPN scores were associated with plaque ulceration and the presence of a lipid core, and lower expression was observed in plaques without ulceration. Additionally, low OPN scores were observed in patients with polyvascular disease with three arterial bed involvement. These data converge with those obtained by Strobescu–Ciobanu in a recent study: the authors described in 49 carotid specimens a significant association of higher OPN with ulceration and inflammation of the atherosclerotic lesions [44]. However, no significant association could be defined with calcification; this discrepancy might lie in the applied methodology as calcium content was determined by carotid arteries' ultrasonography based on plaque echogenicity.

5. Limitations

The results from the histological processing of the 119 specimens characterize the CA plaques at a well-determined moment (the occurrence of neurological complications) without the possibility of following the disease progression.

We considered that the semi-quantitative evaluation of plaque complexity accurately characterizes the most important histological features of the plaque and may predict the behavior of the plaque at the time of examination. Although it has been based solely on visual estimation and might have been limited by subjectivity and variability between observers, we chose this method for the properties of the specimens; in contrast to autopsy and experimental study subjects, the fragmented aspect of the specimens does not allow the accurate evaluation of the components and their ratio by morphometric methods. It may have affected our sensitivity to detect relevant associations.

6. Conclusions

In a previous morphometric study, we demonstrated that femoral and carotid plaques show different morphology and the tendency for calcification, suggesting that the mechanism is site-specific and vessel wall structure dependent [45]. In the current study, we focused on the carotid plaque's intimate structure, with a particular emphasis on inflammation, as an important correlate and histological signs of vulnerability: ulceration, atherothrombosis, and hemorrhage.

Our results highlight the following critical issues related to carotid atherosclerotic plaques linked to severe carotid stenosis: (1) considerable differences in vulnerability signs between plaques with identical degrees of stenosis are due to complex morphology and composition; (2) in patients with carotid plaques with low/mild inflammatory components, the occurrence of cerebrovascular events (aphasia, hemiparesis/hemiplegia) is significantly lower compared to those with high degrees of inflammation, suggesting the role of pro-inflammatory MFs in atheroma vulnerability; (3) the presence of the inflammatory infiltrate and of the large necrotic lipid core increase the probability of ulceration; (4) ulceration and intra-plaque hemorrhage have appeared in a significantly higher proportion of specimens with microcalcification and dominated in plaques with superficial layer calcification compared to those with deep layer damage; and (5) our data suggest a potential role for OPN in the development of vulnerability: expression of OPN significantly correlated with microcalcification, and at the same time, higher OPN scores were associated with plaque ulceration and the presence of a sizeable necrotic lipid core.

Based on our results, we hypothesize that the lesions described are characteristic of advanced stages of atherogenesis; clarifying how plaque composition changes from apparent early lesion formation to clinically significant vascular stenosis require further longitudinal, multidisciplinary studies.

Supplementary Materials: The following supporting information can be downloaded at: https://www.mdpi.com/article/10.3390/biomedicines11030881/s1, Table S1: Associations of the OPN expression scores.

Author Contributions: Conceptualization, E.H., I.A.B. and E.E.N.; data curation, I.A.B., A.V.M. and E.H.; methodology, E.H., I.A.B., K.B., G.B.M. and E.E.N.; investigation, I.A.B., A.V.M., E.H. and G.B.M.; statistical analysis, E.E.N. and P.O.; writing—original draft preparation, E.H., I.A.B. and E.E.N.; supervision, P.O.; writing—review and editing, E.H., K.B. and E.E.N. All authors have read and agreed to the published version of the manuscript.

Funding: This research received no external funding.

Institutional Review Board Statement: Not applicable.

Informed Consent Statement: Written informed consent was obtained from each patient involved in this study.

Data Availability Statement: Data spreadsheets are available at https://data.mendeley.com/drafts/y6t5yxdsdd, doi: 10.17632/y6t5yxdsdd.2 (accessed on 9 February 2023).

Acknowledgments: The authors thank to Genoveva Rigmanyi (Center for Advanced Medical and Pharmaceutical Research, George Emil Palade University of Medicine, Pharmacy, Science, and Technology of Targu Mures) for expert technical assistance.

Conflicts of Interest: The authors declare no conflict of interest.

References

1. Katan, M.; Luft, A. Global Burden of Stroke. *Semin. Neurol.* **2018**, *38*, 208–211. [CrossRef]
2. Yurdagul, A.; Finney, A.C.; Woolard, M.D.; Orr, A.W. The arterial microenvironment: The where and why of atherosclerosis. *Biochem. J.* **2016**, *473*, 1281–1295. [CrossRef]
3. Jebari-Benslaiman, S.; Galicia-Garcia, U.; Larrea-Sebal, A.; Olaetxea, J.R.; Alloza, I.; Vandenbroeck, K.; Benito-Vicente, A.; Martin C. Pathophysiology of Atherosclerosis. *Int. J. Mol. Sci.* **2022**, *23*, 3346. [CrossRef]
4. Shi, X.; Gao, J.; Lv, Q.S.; Cai, H.D.; Wang, F.; Ye, R.D.; Liu, X.F. Calcification in Atherosclerotic Plaque Vulnerability: Friend or Foe? *Front. Physiol.* **2020**, *11*, 56. [CrossRef] [PubMed]
5. Akers, E.J.; Nicholls, S.J.; Di Bartolo, B.A. Plaque Calcification Do Lipoproteins Have a Role? *Arterioscler. Thromb. Vasc. Biol.* **2019**, *39*, 1902–1910. [CrossRef] [PubMed]
6. Du, H.; Yang, W.J.; Chen, X.Y. Histology-Verified Intracranial Artery Calcification and Its Clinical Relevance With Cerebrovascular Disease. *Front. Neurol.* **2022**, *12*, 789035. [CrossRef]
7. Rambhia, S.H.; Liang, X.; Xenos, M.; Alemu, Y.; Maldonado, N.; Kelly, A.; Chakraborti, S.; Weinbaum, S.; Cardoso, L.; Einav S.; et al. Microcalcifications Increase Coronary Vulnerable Plaque Rupture Potential: A Patient-Based Micro-CT Fluid-Structure Interaction Study. *Ann. Biomed. Eng.* **2012**, *40*, 1443–1454. [CrossRef]
8. Kwee, R.M. Systematic review on the association between calcification in carotid plaques and clinical ischemic symptoms. *J. Vasc Surg.* **2010**, *51*, 1015–1025. [CrossRef]
9. Seime, T.; van Wanrooij, M.; Karlof, E.; Kronqvist, M.; Johansson, S.; Matic, L.; Gasser, T.C.; Hedin, U. Biomechanical Assessment of Macro-Calcification in Human Carotid Atherosclerosis and Its Impact on Smooth Muscle Cell Phenotype. *Cells* **2022**, *11*, 3279. [CrossRef] [PubMed]
10. Yang, J.; Pan, X.J.; Zhang, B.; Yan, Y.H.; Huang, Y.B.; Woolf, A.K.; Gillard, J.H.; Teng, Z.Z.; Hui, P.J. Superficial and multiple calcifications and ulceration associate with intraplaque hemorrhage in the carotid atherosclerotic plaque. *Eur. Radiol.* **2018**, *28*, 4968–4977. [CrossRef] [PubMed]
11. Böhm, E.W.; Pavlaki, M.; Chalikias, G.; Mikroulis, D.; Georgiadis, G.S.; Tziakas, D.N.; Konstantinides, S.; Schäfer, K. Colocalization of Erythrocytes and Vascular Calcification in Human Atherosclerosis: A Systematic Histomorphometric Analysis. *TH Open* **2021**, *5*, e113–e124. [CrossRef] [PubMed]
12. Shirakawa, K.; Sano, M. Osteopontin in Cardiovascular Diseases. *Biomolecules* **2021**, *11*, 1047. [CrossRef] [PubMed]
13. Steitz, S.A.; Speer, M.Y.; McKee, M.D.; Liaw, L.; Almeida, M.; Yang, H.; Giachelli, C.M. Osteopontin inhibits mineral deposition and promotes regression of ectopic calcification. *Am. J. Pathol.* **2002**, *161*, 2035–2046. [CrossRef]
14. Naylor, R.; Rantner, B.; Ancetti, S.; de Borst, G.J.; De Carlo, M.; Halliday, A.; Kakkos, S.K.; Markus, H.S.; McCabe, D.J.H.; Sillesen H.; et al. European Society for Vascular Surgery (ESVS) 2023 Clinical Practice Guidelines on the Management of Atherosclerotic Carotid and Vertebral Artery Disease. *Eur. J. Vasc. Endovasc. Surg.* **2023**, *65*, 7–111. [CrossRef]
15. Bonati, L.H.; Kakkos, S.; Berkefeld, J.; de Borst, G.J.; Bulbulia, R.; Halliday, A.; van Herzeele, I.; Koncar, I.; McCabe, D.J.H.; Lal, A.; et al. European Stroke Organisation guideline on endarterectomy and stenting for carotid artery stenosis. *Eur. Stroke J.* **2021**, *6*, I–LXII. [CrossRef]
16. Orrapin, S.; Rerkasem, K. Carotid endarterectomy for symptomatic carotid stenosis. *Cochrane Database Syst. Rev.* **2017**, *6*, CD001081. [CrossRef]
17. Williams, B.; Mancia, G.; Spiering, W.; Rosei, E.A.; Azizi, M.; Burnier, M.; Clement, D.L.; Coca, A.; de Simone, G.; Dominiczak A.; et al. 2018 ESC/ESH Guidelines for the management of arterial hypertension. *Eur. Heart J.* **2018**, *39*, 3021–3104. [CrossRef] [PubMed]
18. Cosentino, F.; Grant, P.J.; Aboyans, V.; Bailey, C.J.; Ceriello, A.; Delgado, V.; Federici, M.; Filippatos, G.; Grobbee, D.E.; Hansen T.B.; et al. 2019 ESC Guidelines on diabetes, pre-diabetes, and cardiovascular diseases developed in collaboration with the EASD *Eur. Heart J.* **2020**, *41*, 255–323. [CrossRef]
19. Mach, F.; Baigent, C.; Catapano, A.L.; Koskinas, K.C.; Casula, M.; Badimon, L.; Chapman, M.J.; De Backer, G.G.; Delgado V.; Ference, B.A.; et al. 2019 ESC/EAS Guidelines for the management of dyslipidaemias: Lipid modification to reduce cardiovascular risk The Task Force for the management of dyslipidaemias of the European Society of Cardiology (ESC) and European Atherosclerosis Society (EAS). *Eur. Heart J.* **2020**, *41*, 111–188. [CrossRef]
20. Coupland, A.P.; Thapar, A.; Qureshi, M.I.; Jenkins, H.; Davies, A.H. The definition of stroke. *J. R. Soc. Med.* **2017**, *110*, 9–12. [CrossRef]
21. Stary, H.C. Natural history and histological classification of atherosclerotic lesions—An update. *Arterioscler. Thromb. Vasc. Biol.* **2000**, *20*, 1177–1178. [CrossRef] [PubMed]
22. Lovett, J.K.; Redgrave, J.N.E.; Gallagher, P.J.; Walton, J.; Hands, L.; Rothwell, P.M. Histological correlates of carotid plaque surface morphology on lumen contrast imaging. *Stroke* **2004**, *35*, E194.
23. Kelly-Arnold, A.; Maldonado, N.; Laudier, D.; Aikawa, E.; Cardoso, L.; Weinbaum, S. Revised microcalcification hypothesis for fibrous cap rupture in human coronary arteries. *Proc. Natl. Acad. Sci. USA* **2013**, *110*, 10741–10746. [CrossRef] [PubMed]
24. Zheng, H.E.; Gasbarrino, K.; Veinot, J.P.; Lai, C.; Daskalopoulou, S.S. New Quantitative Digital Image Analysis Method of Histological Features of Carotid Atherosclerotic Plaques. *Eur. J. Vasc. Endovasc. Surg.* **2019**, *58*, 654–663. [CrossRef]
25. Wang, Y.L.; Wang, T.; Luo, Y.M.; Jiao, L.Q. Identification Markers of Carotid Vulnerable Plaques: An Update. *Biomolecules* **2022**, *12*, 1192. [CrossRef]

26. Lee-Rueckert, M.; Lappalainen, J.; Kovanen, P.T.; Escola-Gil, J.C. Lipid-Laden Macrophages and Inflammation in Atherosclerosis and Cancer: An Integrative View. *Front. Cardiovasc. Med.* **2022**, *9*, 777822. [CrossRef]
27. Nakagawa, K.; Tanaka, M.; Hahm, T.H.; Nguyen, H.N.; Matsui, T.; Chen, Y.X.; Nakashima, Y. Accumulation of Plasma-Derived Lipids in the Lipid Core and Necrotic Core of Human Atheroma: Imaging Mass Spectrometry and Histopathological Analyses. *Arterioscler. Thromb. Vasc. Biol.* **2021**, *41*, E498–E511. [CrossRef]
28. Fletcher, E.K.; Wang, Y.L.; Flynn, L.K.; Turner, S.E.; Rade, J.J.; Kimmelstiel, C.D.; Gurbel, P.A.; Bliden, K.P.; Covic, L.; Kuliopulos, A. Deficiency of MMP1a (Matrix Metalloprotease 1a) Collagenase Suppresses Development of Atherosclerosis in Mice Translational Implications for Human Coronary Artery Disease. *Arterioscler. Thromb. Vasc. Biol.* **2021**, *41*, E265–E279. [CrossRef]
29. Gialeli, C.; Shami, A.; Goncalves, I. Extracellular matrix: Paving the way to the newest trends in atherosclerosis. *Curr. Opin. Lipidol.* **2021**, *32*, 277–285. [CrossRef]
30. Tomas, L.; Edsfeldt, A.; Mollet, I.G.; Matic, L.P.; Prehn, C.; Adamski, J.; Paulsson-Berne, G.; Hedin, U.; Nilsson, J.; Bengtsson, E.; et al. Altered metabolism distinguishes high-risk from stable carotid atherosclerotic plaques. *Eur. Heart J.* **2018**, *39*, 2301–2310. [CrossRef]
31. Saba, L.; Sanfilippo, R.; Sannia, S.; Anzidei, M.; Montisci, R.; Mallarini, G.; Suri, J.S. Association Between Carotid Artery Plaque Volume, Composition, and Ulceration: A Retrospective Assessment With MDCT. *Am. J. Roentgenol.* **2012**, *199*, 151–156. [CrossRef] [PubMed]
32. Poredos, P.; Gregoric, I.D.; Jezovnik, M.K. Inflammation of carotid plaques and risk of cerebrovascular events. *Ann. Transl. Med.* **2020**, *8*, 1281. [CrossRef] [PubMed]
33. Wong, K.K.L.; Thavornpattanapong, P.; Cheung, S.C.P.; Sun, Z.H.; Tu, J.Y. Effect of calcification on the mechanical stability of plaque based on a three-dimensional carotid bifurcation model. *BMC Cardiovasc. Disord.* **2012**, *12*, 7. [CrossRef] [PubMed]
34. Ahmed, M.; McPherson, R.; Abruzzo, A.; Thomas, S.E.; Gorantla, V.R. Carotid Artery Calcification: What We Know So Far. *Cureus* **2021**, *13*, e18938. [CrossRef] [PubMed]
35. Joshi, F.R.; Rajani, N.K.; Abt, M.; Woodward, M.; Bucerius, J.; Mani, V.; Tawakol, A.; Kallend, D.; Fayad, Z.A.; Rudd, J.H.F. Does Vascular Calcification Accelerate Inflammation? A Substudy of the dal-PLAQUE Trial. *J. Am. Coll. Cardiol.* **2016**, *67*, 69–78. [CrossRef] [PubMed]
36. Shioi, A.; Ikari, Y. Plaque Calcification During Atherosclerosis Progression and Regression. *J. Atheroscler. Thromb.* **2018**, *25*, 294–303. [CrossRef] [PubMed]
37. New, S.E.P.; Aikawa, E. Molecular Imaging Insights Into Early Inflammatory Stages of Arterial and Aortic Valve Calcification. *Circ. Res.* **2011**, *108*, 1381–1391. [CrossRef] [PubMed]
38. Lai, C.F.; Seshadri, V.; Huang, K.; Shao, J.S.; Cai, J.; Vattikuti, R.; Schumacher, A.; Loewy, A.P.; Denhardt, D.T.; Rittling, S.R.; et al. An osteopontin-NADPH oxidase signaling cascade promotes pro-matrix metalloproteinase 9 activation in aortic mesenchymal cells. *Circ. Res.* **2006**, *98*, 1479–1489. [CrossRef]
39. Fehervari, L.; Frigy, A.; Kocsis, L.; Szabo, I.A.; Szabo, T.M.; Urkon, M.; Jako, Z.; Nagy, E.E. Serum Osteoprotegerin and Carotid Intima-Media Thickness Are Related to High Arterial Stiffness in Heart Failure with Reduced Ejection Fraction. *Diagnostics* **2021**, *11*, 764. [CrossRef]
40. Nagy, E.E.; Varga-Fekete, T.; Puskas, A.; Kelemen, P.; Brassai, Z.; Szekeres-Csiki, K.; Gombos, T.; Csanyi, M.C.; Harsfalvi, J. High circulating osteoprotegerin levels are associated with non-zero blood groups. *BMC Cardiovasc. Disord.* **2016**, *16*, 106. [CrossRef]
41. Morony, S.; Tintut, Y.; Zhang, Z.; Cattley, R.C.; Van, G.; Dwyer, D.; Stolina, M.; Kostenuik, P.J.; Demer, L.L. Osteoprotegerin inhibits vascular calcification without affecting atherosclerosis in ldlr((-/-)) mice. *Circulation* **2008**, *117*, 411–420. [CrossRef] [PubMed]
42. Lok, Z.S.Y.; Lyle, A.N. Osteopontin in Vascular Disease Friend or Foe? *Arterioscler. Thromb. Vasc. Biol.* **2019**, *39*, 613–622. [CrossRef] [PubMed]
43. Wolak, T.; Sion-Vardi, N.; Novack, V.; Greenberg, G.; Szendro, G.; Tarnovscki, T.; Nov, O.; Shelef, I.; Paran, E.; Rudich, A. N-Terminal Rather Than Full-Length Osteopontin or Its C-Terminal Fragment Is Associated With Carotid-Plaque Inflammation in Hypertensive Patients. *Am. J. Hypertens.* **2013**, *26*, 326–333. [CrossRef]
44. Strobescu-Ciobanu, C.; Giusca, S.E.; Caruntu, I.D.; Amalinei, C.; Rusu, A.; Cojocaru, E.; Popa, R.F.; Lupascu, C.D. Osteopontin and osteoprotegerin in atherosclerotic plaque—Are they significant markers of plaque vulnerability? *Rom. J. Morphol. Embryol.* **2020**, *61*, 793–801. [CrossRef] [PubMed]
45. Cosarca, M.C.; Horvath, E.; Molnar, C.; Molnar, G.B.; Russu, E.; Muresan, V.A. Calcification patterns in femoral and carotid atheromatous plaques: A comparative morphometric study. *Exp. Ther. Med.* **2021**, *22*, 865. [CrossRef]

Disclaimer/Publisher's Note: The statements, opinions and data contained in all publications are solely those of the individual author(s) and contributor(s) and not of MDPI and/or the editor(s). MDPI and/or the editor(s) disclaim responsibility for any injury to people or property resulting from any ideas, methods, instructions or products referred to in the content.

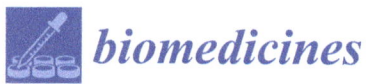

Brief Report

Impact of Previous Continuous Positive Airway Pressure Use on Noninvasive Ventilation Adherence and Quality in Obesity Hypoventilation Syndrome: A Pragmatic Single-Center Cross-Sectional Study in Martinique

Moustapha Agossou [1,*], Bérénice Awanou [1], Jocelyn Inamo [2], Mickael Rejaudry-Lacavalerie [3], Jean-Michel Arnal [4] and Moustapha Dramé [5,6]

1. Department of Respiratory Medicine, CHU of Martinique, 97261 Fort-de-France, France; sessito.awanou@chu-martinique.fr
2. Department of Cardiology, CHU of Martinique, 97261 Fort-de-France, France; jocelyn.inamo@chu-martinique.fr
3. Department of Neurophysiology, CHU of Martinique, 97261 Fort-de-France, France; mickael.lacavalerie@chu-martinique.fr
4. Intensive Care Unit, Hôpital Sainte Musse, 83100 Toulon, France; jean-michel@arnal.org
5. Department of Clinical Research and Innovation, CHU of Martinique, 97261 Fort-de-France, France; moustapha.drame@chu-martinique.fr
6. EpiCliV Research Unit, Faculty of Medicine, University of the French West Indies, 97261 Fort-de-France, France
* Correspondence: moustapha.agossou@chu-martinique.fr

Citation: Agossou, M.; Awanou, B.; Inamo, J.; Rejaudry-Lacavalerie, M.; Arnal, J.-M.; Dramé, M. Impact of Previous Continuous Positive Airway Pressure Use on Noninvasive Ventilation Adherence and Quality in Obesity Hypoventilation Syndrome: A Pragmatic Single-Center Cross-Sectional Study in Martinique. *Biomedicines* **2023**, *11*, 2753. https://doi.org/10.3390/biomedicines11102753

Academic Editor: Alice M Turner

Received: 9 September 2023
Revised: 5 October 2023
Accepted: 9 October 2023
Published: 11 October 2023

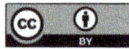

Copyright: © 2023 by the authors. Licensee MDPI, Basel, Switzerland. This article is an open access article distributed under the terms and conditions of the Creative Commons Attribution (CC BY) license (https://creativecommons.org/licenses/by/4.0/).

Abstract: There is a strong relationship between obstructive sleep apnea (OSA) and obesity hypoventilation syndrome (OHS). When OHS is combined with severe OSA, treatment consists of continuous positive airway pressure (CPAP), followed by noninvasive ventilation (NIV) in the case of CPAP failure. Currently, the impact of a previous use of CPAP on the quality of NIV is unknown. We conducted a cross-sectional study with OHS patients, to assess the quality of NIV according to previous CPAP use. We included 75 patients with OHS on NIV (65 women, 87%). Among these, 40 patients (53.3%) who had had prior CPAP (CPAP+ group) were compared to the remaining 35 patients (46.7%) (CPAP− group). Key characteristics were comparable between the CPAP+ and the CPAP− groups: age at diagnosis of OHS was 67 ± 3 vs. 66 ± 4 years (p = 0.8), age at inclusion was 73 ± 15 vs. 69 ± 15 years (p = 0.29), number of comorbidities was 3.7 ± 1.2 vs. 3.3 ± 1.5, the Charlson index was 5.1 ± 2 vs. 4.6 ± 1.8, and BMI was 41.6 ± 7.6 kg/m^2 vs. 41.2 ± 8.2, respectively, all p > 0.05. Follow-up length was greater in CPAP+ vs. CPAP− patients (5.6 ± 4.2 vs. 2.9 ± 2.9 years, p = 0.001). The quality of NIV based on daily adherence, pressure support, apnea–hypopnea index (AHI) and leaks was similar in both groups. Reduced adherence (less than 4 h daily) was found in 10 CPAP+ patients (25%) versus 7 CPAP− patients (20%), p = 0.80. NIV efficacy was also similar. This study found no difference in the quality of NIV or in adherence between patients who had had prior CPAP and those who had not. Previous CPAP does not appear to improve the quality of NIV.

Keywords: obesity hypoventilation syndrome; obstructive sleep apnea; CPAP; noninvasive ventilation; NIV adherence

1. Introduction

The worldwide prevalence of obesity is increasing. It is estimated by the World Health Organization (WHO) that approximately 4 million deaths each year are attributable to obesity globally [1]. Obesity hypoventilation syndrome (OHS) is a chronic respiratory failure that is related to obesity. It is defined as the simultaneous presence of obesity (namely, body mass index (BMI) of $\geq$30 kg/m^2) and daytime hypercapnia (pCO$_2$ > 45 mmHg) in the absence of other causes of alveolar hypoventilation [2]. Obstructive sleep apnea is frequently associated with OHS [2]. OHS carries substantial morbidity and mortality [2], with high consumption of healthcare in affected individuals [3,4]. The treatment of OHS has evolved over time and has long relied on noninvasive ventilation (NIV). Recent research has highlighted the role of continuous positive airway pressure (CPAP) therapy in the management of OHS in stable patients, notably when diagnosed in a sleep laboratory [5–8]. Accordingly, the latest recommendations from the American Thoracic society (ATS) proposed the introduction of first-line CPAP treatment in stable OHS, with a switch to NIV in the event of CPAP failure [9]. While NIV can be an effective treatment for OHS, its success depends on patient adherence, which improves efficacy and arterial blood gases, quality of life, and mortality [10]. Efficiency of the treatment also depends on the quality of the NIV in terms of leaks or obstructive events [11].

The clinician's task is to find strategies that will encourage the patient to adhere to a treatment regimen that may necessitate changes to their lifestyle. Thus, there is value in seeking all the possible levers that could be used to improve NIV compliance. Ennis et al. identified several factors that were associated with improved adherence to NIV in patients with nocturnal hypoventilation, including previous experiences with positive airway pressure therapy, subjective symptom improvement, familiarity with medical treatments, understanding of nocturnal hypoventilation and its consequences, support from family and healthcare providers, and early adaptation to treatments [12]. CPAP treatment uses similar equipment to NIV, and patients may thus feel familiar with the equipment and treatment. Because it also uses pressure to keep the airway open, one might imagine that CPAP creates a ventilation memory in the patient. In any case, there is little change in the patient's environment during the transition from CPAP to NIV. In daily practice, it is common to encounter patients already receiving CPAP for OSA, who then present hypercapnic respiratory insufficiency leading to a diagnosis of OHS. In this context, these patients are switched from CPAP to NIV.

We hypothesized that previous CPAP use would enhance the adherence to home nocturnal NIV in patients with OHS. Therefore, the aim of this study was to compare the adherence and quality of NIV in OHS patients who had previously received a CPAP device for OSA with those who had not. The primary outcome measure was NIV adherence, and secondary outcomes included NIV quality, assessed by leaks and the apnea–hypopnea index (AHI), and NIV efficacy, assessed by daytime partial pressure of carbon dioxide (pCO_2).

2. Patients and Methods

We performed an observational, cross-sectional, single-center study in a cohort of OHS patients from the Department of Respiratory Medicine at the University Hospital (CHU) of Martinique. All patients followed-up for OHS in our department are systematically entered into a database. The Respiratory Medicine Department is responsible for the management and care of all patients with chronic respiratory diseases on our island. Patients were adults (>18 years) diagnosed with OHS based on body mass index (BMI) > 30 kg/m^2, daytime hypercapnia, and the absence of another cause of hypoventilation. We excluded patients with a smoking history > 10 pack-years in women or 15 pack-years in men and patients associated with an obstructive pattern in spirometry (FEV1/FVC < 70%) in whom associated chronic obstructive pulmonary disease (COPD) cannot be ruled out [13,14].

At the time when OHS was diagnosed, patients systematically underwent screening for OSA (polygraphy or polysomnography, unless they already had documented and treated OSA) and (as far as possible) a pulmonary functional test and echocardiography. If pulmonary hypertension was suspected, exploratory right heart catheterization was performed to confirm or rule out the diagnosis. Polygraphy/polysomnography data were interpreted according to the International Classification of Sleep Diseases (ICSD-3 2023). Severity was defined based on AHI and classified as follows: absent if AHI < 5/h, mild OSA with AHI of 5 to <15, moderate with AHI of 15 to 29, and severe with AHI of $\geq$30. In the case of hypercapnic acute respiratory insufficiency, NIV was initiated during hospitalization.

Settings were fixed arbitrarily at the outset and adjusted during hospitalization. For patients who had previously been receiving CPAP, PAP was determined by subtracting 2 cmH$_2$O from the average pressure 90% of the time. For other patients, PAP was determined at the physician's discretion and then adjusted on the basis of the residual AHI. Support pressure was determined with a target tidal volume of 8 mL/kg of theoretical bodyweight calculated according to the Lorentz formula and optimized based on response to CO$_2$ and leaks. For initiation of CPAP, we started with three days of auto-adjusting CPAP and then set the device in fixed mode to the average pressure 90% of the time. Of note, patients who had previously received CPAP for OSA all had auto-adjusting devices, and they did not undergo screening for OHS.

All patients had regular follow-up in outpatient consultations, and at each follow-up we recorded mean adherence for the last 90 days, blood gases, ventilatory parameters, and data reflecting the quality of NIV (leaks and AHI). Patients included in the study were seen in consultation between 1 January 2022 and 31 October 2022. We collected sociodemographic data (age, age at diagnosis, sex, BMI), history of previous use of PAP devices for OSA at time of diagnosis, arterial blood gas at diagnosis, last blood gas in a stable state, and spirometry data at inclusion. Daily adherence, leaks, and AHI were measured for the last 90 days, and NIV parameters (IPAP, EPAP, and pressure support) were measured at inclusion, using stored data from the devices.

Functional tests were interpreted according to the EU Standard criteria, taking ethnicity into account [15–17].

The study was performed in accordance with the Declaration of Helsinki and received the approval of the Institutional Review Board of the University Hospitals of Martinique (under the number 2022/158).

We performed descriptive analysis. We describe quantitative variables as mean ± standard deviation (SD) and qualitative (categorical) variables as count and percentage. Continuous variables were compared using Student's t-test and proportions with the chi square or Fisher's exact test as appropriate. Normality of distributions was tested using the Shapiro–Wilk test. Bivariable analyses for the association between previous use of CPAP and daily adherence, quality of NIV, and efficacy were performed using binary logistic regression modeling. Statistical analyses were performed using SAS software version 9.4 (SAS Institute Inc., Cary, NC, USA). p-values < 0.05 were considered statistically significant.

3. Results

We included 75 patients with OHS using NIV, 65 (87%) of whom were women. Of the entire group, 40 (53%) had used CPAP previously (CPAP+ group), with the remaining 35 (47%) having gone directly onto NIV (CPAP− group). Key characteristics were comparable in the CPAP+ versus CPAP− groups as follows: mean age at diagnosis of OHS was 67 ± 3 vs. 66 ± 4 years, mean age at inclusion was 73 ± 15 versus 69 ± 15 years, mean number of comorbidities was 3.7 ± 1.2 versus 3.3 ± 1.5 (p = 0.3), mean Charlson index was 5.1 ± 2 versus 4.6 ± 1.8 (p = 0.3), and mean BMI was 41.6 ± 7.6 kg/m^2 versus 41.2 ± 8.2 (p = 0.8), respectively. The average length of follow-up was 5.6 ± 4.2 years in the CPAP+ group versus 2.9 ± 2.9 years in the CPAP− group (p = 0.001).

The comorbidities and therapeutic characteristics of the patients are detailed in Table 1

The spirometric data at inclusion are displayed in Table 1.

Adherence to NIV and quality of ventilation including ventilator settings, leaks, and residual AHI were similar in the two groups (Table 2).

Ten patients (25%) in the CPAP+ group and seven (20%) in the CPAP− group used NIV less than a mean of 4 h daily over 90 days (p = 0.8). There were also no differences in NIV efficacy between the two groups based on hypercapnia resolution (p = 0.3).

Table 1. Comorbidities, circumstances of diagnosis, and spirometry in patients undergoing noninvasive ventilation according to the previous use of continuous positive airway pressure (CPAP).

	CPAP+ N = 40	%	CPAP− N = 35	%	p
Age at diagnosis	67 ± 3		66 ± 4		0.8
Age at inclusion	75 ± 15		69 ± 15		0.29
Female sex	33	82.5	32	91.4	0.32
Body mass index (BMI) ≥ 40	20	36.7	19	44.4	0.6
Comorbidities					
Arterial hypertension	32	80.6	31	88.6	0.4
Diabetes mellitus	24	60	22	62.9	0.8
Asthma	17	42.5	8	22.9	0.09
Cardiac arrhythmia	5	12.5	7	20	0.5
Other heart diseases	7	17.5	7	20	1
Pulmonary hypertension	5	12.5	5	14.3	1
Lower limb arterial disease	4	10	1	2.9	0.4
Circumstances of OHS diagnosis					
Acute respiratory failure	25	52.5	31	88.6	0.02
Follow-up of sleep apnea	15	37.5	0	0	
Follow-up of another disease	0	0	1	2.9	
Unknown	0	0	3	8.6	
Pulmonary functional test at inclusion					
	CPAP+		CPAP−		p
FEV1 (%) *	58.7		56.1		0.5
FVC (%) *	63.2		58.1		0.3
FEV1/FVC (%) **	77		77.9		0.8
TLC (%) *	73.6		75.9		0.6
RV (%) *	90.8		109.9		0.09
ERV (%) *	80.3		71.4		0.6

* % of theoretical value ** RatioX100 FEV1: forced expiratory volume in 1 s. FVC: forced vital capacity. TLC: total lung capacity. RV: residual volume. ERV: expiratory reserve volume.

Table 2. Adherence, quality of NIV, and arterial blood gas at inclusion in OHS patients with and without previous CPAP.

Characteristics at Inclusion	CPAP+ N = 40	CPAP− N = 35	p
Daily adherence (Hours)	6.2 ± 3.2	6.1 ± 3.2	0.8
Adherence < 4 h	10	7	0.6
Median unintentional leaks (L/min)	13.8 ± 23.3	13.6 ± 21.3	0.9
AHI	5.2 ± 6.6	4 ± 5.9	0.4
Hypercapnia (>45 mmHg)	27	20	0.3
EPAP (cmH$_2$O)	8.7 ± 2.4	8.4 ± 2.7	0.9
IPAP (cmH$_2$O)	20.6 ± 3.2	20.3 ± 2.8	0.7
Support pressure (cmH$_2$O)	11.9 ± 2.6	11.9 ± 1.9	0.9
Arterial blood gas			
pH	7.38 ± 0.03	7.39 ± 0.03	0.4
pCO$_2$ (mmHg)	46 ± 5	47 ± 6	0.5
pO$_2$ (mmHg)	78 ± 17	71 ± 8	0.08
Bicarbonates (mmol/L)	27 ± 4	28 ± 4	0.4

CPAP: continuous positive airway pressure, AHI: apnea–hypopnea index, EPAP: expiratory positive airway pressure, IPAP: inspiratory positive airway pressure, pCO$_2$: partial pressure of carbon dioxide, pO$_2$: partial pressure of oxygen.

4. Discussion

In this study, we found that there was no significant difference in adherence to NIV between those individuals who were previously managed with CPAP and those who were prescribed NIV as an initial therapy. Similarly, no between-group differences in the quality of ventilation were reflected in residual AHI and leaks nor in the effectiveness of NIV measured by the resolution of hypercapnia among this population of patients with OHS. Because it is a pragmatic study, we were considering a calculation of power a posteriori. Because the averages are strictly the same (6.2 ± 3.2 versus 6.1 ± 3.2), this does not seem relevant.

Adherence to NIV is known to be an important predictor of treatment success in patients with hypercapnic chronic respiratory failure [10], and previous experience with therapy has been identified as a factor that can influence adherence in nocturnal hypoventilation [9]. While CPAP treatment is a viable alternative to NIV in stable OHS [6,8–10], it is important to note that the long-term effectiveness of CPAP may wane over time, leading to a transition to NIV in some cases [11]. In our cohort, 53% of patients had already received CPAP treatment for OSA before being diagnosed with OHS, and NIV treatment is recommended for those who continue to experience nocturnal hypoventilation despite using CPAP [6]. Adherence to NIV and correction of hypercapnia are critical to the effective management of nocturnal hypoventilation. A number of studies have demonstrated that persistent hypercapnia is linked to high mortality rates and significant healthcare utilization in affected individuals [1,2,18]. In this context, adherence to treatment is a key determinant of patient outcomes [7]. Molkhlesi et al. found that daily adherence to PAP of 5 to 7 h was associated with improved arterial blood gas parameters in patients with OHS [10]. Castro-Anon reported that NIV adherence of less than 4 h per day was linked to higher mortality in this patient population [19]. The quality of NIV has predominantly been studied in patients with hypercapnic chronic respiratory failure related to neuromuscular diseases. Morelot-Panzani et al. reported that the correction of leaks, management of OSA and adaptation to the patient's degree of ventilator dependence all improve the prognosis in amyotrophic lateral sclerosis (ALS) [11]. Georges et al. also reported that survival was reduced with upper obstructive events on NIV in ALS [20].

In this study, we hypothesized that patients who had previously received CPAP treatment might have better adherence to NIV and improved treatment outcomes, due to a possible "ventilation memory" effect. We hoped that this would lead to greater efficiency in the management of OHS. Our findings indicate that previous exposure to PAP devices does not seem to affect the quality of NIV via better adherence in patients with OHS. We observed in this study that patients were generally quite adherent overall, with an average of more than 4 h per day of use. Only a very small number of patients had daily use below 4 h during the study period. This was not evaluated at the time of NIV initiation, which may have occulted any effect of prior CPAP use over time.

We believe that patients on two-level pressure ventilation should receive the same attention and psychological support to improve adherence [16], regardless of whether they have previously used a PAP device or not.

Our study raises the question of the possible under-diagnosis of OHS. Indeed, patients being followed up in sleep clinics or by physicians specialized in sleep disorders do not undergo screening for OHS, and the diagnosis may come to be made in a context of acute respiratory insufficiency. We noted that patients who were already receiving CPAP less frequently had a diagnosis made in the context of acute respiratory failure, in line with a previous report [21]. There is clearly a need to implement systematic screening for OSA in persons with obesity, and a need of screening for OHS in those with OSA and obesity, with a view to initiating early management.

Furthermore, the patients in our study presented a predominantly restrictive syndrome, likely related to obesity. Restrictive syndrome may contribute to the occurrence of alveolar hypoventilation in obese patients. In a previous work, we already reported that the persistence of hypercapnia under NIV was more strongly associated with the severity of a restrictive syndrome than with the severity of obesity [22].

5. Study Strengths and Limitations

A strength of our study is that it presents data from a population of mainly Afro-Caribbean descent; a population that is markedly affected by both OSAS and obesity, but in whom OHS has not been widely investigated. This is also a population that is representative of real-life practice. The study question also has important public health implications, because CPAP is now recommended in first intention in OHS, with NIV used in case of CPAP failure, meaning that increasing numbers of patients may switch from CPAP to NIV in the future. It seems important to anticipate patient needs in terms of therapeutic education. There are a number of limitations of this study that need to be acknowledged. Firstly, it is a single-center, observational, retrospective study, which has the typical limitations associated with this design, such as the lack of knowledge about potential confounding biases, limited data availability, and a small number of patients. Additionally, we were unable to determine adherence to CPAP treatment before transitioning to NIV. Some patients had several years of NIV use, which may have allowed them time to adjust to their treatment. Due to the delay between diagnosis and study measurements, we cannot exclude the possibility that less compliant patients were no longer being followed up for various reasons (NIV discontinuation, death) and therefore could not be included in this study. Finally, we did not dispose of data regarding the initial polygraphy, which would have allowed us to compare polygraphy data between groups. The majority of patients were followed for OSA by specialists in respiratory medicine. We considered that their diagnosis, which had been made several years before, was reliable, and therefore, we did not re-conduct the examinations in view of the following factors:

- Difficulties and delays in accessing the required examinations.
- Most patients presented with acute respiratory insufficiency requiring immediate NIV or intubation.

Our results should be confirmed in prospective studies to better identify the factors that influence compliance in patients with OHS.

6. Conclusions

In current medical practice, it is common for patients with OHS to switch between continuous positive airway pressure (CPAP) and noninvasive ventilation (NIV) treatment. While the quality of NIV is a crucial element in its effectiveness as a treatment, our study did not find any effect of previous CPAP use on NIV quality, via improved adherence. Based on these findings, we recommend implementing the same therapeutic education procedure for all OHS patients, regardless of whether they have previously used CPAP therapy or not.

Author Contributions: M.A.: Conceived the study, collected data, analyzed and interpreted results, and wrote the manuscript. B.A.: Contributed to study conception and data collection. J.I.: Contributed to data analysis and writing the manuscript. M.R.-L.: Contributed to data analysis and writing the manuscript. J.-M.A.: Contributed to data analysis and interpretation and writing of the manuscript. M.D.: Contributed to study conception, analysis and interpretation of data, and writing of the manuscript. All authors have read and agreed to the published version of the manuscript.

Funding: This research received no specific grant from any funding agency in the public, commercial, or not-for-profit sectors.

Institutional Review Board Statement: Ethics approval and consent to participate: the study received the approval of the Institutional Review Board of the University Hospitals of Martinique, number 2022/158. Consent to participate: According to the French legislation, patients received information about the study. Patients who objected to the use of their data were excluded. All patients gave consent to participate in the study.

Informed Consent Statement: Not applicable.

Data Availability Statement: The datasets generated and/or analyzed during the current study are available from the corresponding author on reasonable request.

Conflicts of Interest: The authors declare no competing interests.

Abbreviations

BMI	Body mass index
CHU	University hospital center
CPAP	Continuous positive airway pressure
COPD	Chronic obstructive pulmonary disease
EPAP	Expiratory positive airway pressure
ERV	Expiratory reserve volume
FEV1	Forced expiratory volume in 1 s
FVC	Forced vital capacity
IPAP	Inspiratory positive airway pressure
mmHg	Millimeter of mercury
NIV	Noninvasive ventilation
pCO_2	Partial pressure of carbon dioxide
pO_2	Partial pressure of oxygen
PS	Pressure support
OHS	Obesity hypoventilation syndrome
OSA	Obstructive sleep apnea
RV	Residual volume
TLC	Total lung capacity

References

1. Obesity. Available online: https://www.who.int/health-topics/obesity (accessed on 27 February 2023).
2. Masa, J.F.; Pépin, J.L.; Borel, J.C.; Mokhlesi, B.; Murphy, P.B.; Sánchez-Quiroga, M.Á. Obesity hypoventilation syndrome. *Eur. Respir. Rev.* **2019**, *28*, 180097. [CrossRef] [PubMed]
3. Berg, G.; Delaive, K.; Manfreda, J.; Walld, R.; Kryger, M.H. The use of health-care resources in obesity-hypoventilation syndrome. *Chest* **2001**, *120*, 377–383. [CrossRef] [PubMed]
4. Wilson, M.W.; Labaki, W.W.; Choi, P.J. Mortality and Healthcare Utilization of Patients with Compensated Hypercapnia. *Ann. Am. Thorac. Soc.* **2021**, *18*, 2027–2032. [CrossRef] [PubMed]
5. Piper, A.J.; Wang, D.; Yee, B.J.; Barnes, D.J.; Grunstein, R.R. Randomised trial of CPAP vs bilevel support in the treatment of obesity hypoventilation syndrome without severe nocturnal desaturation. *Thorax* **2008**, *63*, 395–401. [CrossRef] [PubMed]
6. Soghier, I.; Brożek, J.L.; Afshar, M.; Kakazu, M.T.; Wilson, K.C.; Masa, J.F.; Mokhlesi, B. Noninvasive Ventilation versus CPAP as Initial Treatment of Obesity Hypoventilation Syndrome. *Ann. Am. Thorac. Soc.* **2019**, *16*, 1295–1303. [CrossRef] [PubMed]
7. Theerakittikul, T.; Ricaurte, B.; Aboussouan, L.S. Noninvasive positive pressure ventilation for stable outpatients: CPAP and beyond. *Cleve Clin. J. Med.* **2010**, *77*, 705–714. [CrossRef] [PubMed]
8. Masa, J.F.; Mokhlesi, B.; Benítez, I.; de Terreros, F.J.G.; Sánchez-Quiroga, M.Á.; Romero, A.; Caballero-Eraso, C.; Terán-Santos, J.; Alonso-Álvarez, M.L.; Troncoso, M.F.; et al. Long-term clinical effectiveness of continuous positive airway pressure therapy versus non-invasive ventilation therapy in patients with obesity hypoventilation syndrome: A multicentre, open-label, randomised controlled trial. *Lancet* **2019**, *393*, 1721–1732. [CrossRef] [PubMed]
9. Mokhlesi, B.; Masa, J.F.; Brozek, J.L.; Gurubhagavatula, I.; Murphy, P.B.; Piper, A.J.; Tulaimat, A.; Afshar, M.; Balachandran, J.S. Dweik, R.A.; et al. Evaluation and Management of Obesity Hypoventilation Syndrome. An Official American Thoracic Society Clinical Practice Guideline. *Am. J. Respir. Crit. Care Med.* **2019**, *200*, e6–e24. [CrossRef] [PubMed]
10. Mokhlesi, B.; Tulaimat, A.; Evans, A.T.; Wang, Y.; Itani, A.-A.; Hassaballa, H.A.; Herdegen, J.J.; Stepanski, E.J. Impact of Adherence with Positive Airway Pressure Therapy on Hypercapnia in Obstructive Sleep Apnea. *J. Clin. Sleep Med.* **2006**, *2*, 57–62. [CrossRef] [PubMed]
11. Morelot-Panzini, C.; Bruneteau, G.; Gonzalez-Bermejo, J. NIV in amyotrophic lateral sclerosis: The 'when' and 'how' of the matter. *Respirology* **2019**, *24*, 521–530. [CrossRef] [PubMed]
12. Ennis, J.; Rohde, K.; Chaput, J.P.; Buchholz, A.; Katz, S.L. Facilitators and Barriers to Noninvasive Ventilation Adherence in Youth with Nocturnal Hypoventilation Secondary to Obesity or Neuromuscular Disease. *J. Clin. Sleep. Med.* **2015**, *11*, 1409–1416. [CrossRef] [PubMed]
13. Referentiel_tabac.pdf. Available online: https://www.has-sante.fr/upload/docs/application/pdf/2016-06/referentiel_tabac.pdf (accessed on 24 September 2023).

4. Foreman, M.G.; Zhang, L.; Murphy, J.; Hansel, N.N.; Make, B.; Hokanson, J.E.; Washko, G.; Regan, E.A.; Crapo, J.D.; Silverman, E.K.; et al. Early-onset chronic obstructive pulmonary disease is associated with female sex, maternal factors, and African American race in the COPDGene Study. *Am. J. Respir. Crit. Care Med.* **2011**, *184*, 414–420. [CrossRef] [PubMed]
5. Quanjer, P.H.; Stanojevic, S.; Cole, T.J.; Baur, X.; Hall, G.L.; Culver, B.H.; Enright, P.L.; Hankinson, J.L.; Ip, M.S.M.; Zheng, J.; et al. Multi-ethnic reference values for spirometry for the 3-95-yr age range: The global lung function 2012 equations. *Eur. Respir. J.* **2012**, *40*, 1324–1343. [CrossRef] [PubMed]
6. Hall, G.L.; Filipow, N.; Ruppel, G.; Okitika, T.; Thompson, B.; Kirkby, J.; Steenbruggen, I.; Cooper, B.G.; Stanojevic, S. Official ERS technical standard: Global Lung Function Initiative reference values for static lung volumes in individuals of European ancestry. *Eur. Respir. J.* **2021**, *57*, 2000289. [CrossRef] [PubMed]
7. Stanojevic, S.; Graham, B.L.; Cooper, B.G.; Thompson, B.R.; Carter, K.W.; Francis, R.W.; Hall, G.L. Official ERS technical standards: Global Lung Function Initiative reference values for the carbon monoxide transfer factor for Caucasians. *Eur. Respir. J.* **2017**, *50*, 1700010. [CrossRef] [PubMed]
8. Budweiser, S.; Riedl, S.G.; Jörres, R.A.; Heinemann, F.; Pfeifer, M. Mortality and prognostic factors in patients with obesity-hypoventilation syndrome undergoing noninvasive ventilation. *J. Intern. Med.* **2007**, *261*, 375–383. [CrossRef] [PubMed]
9. Castro-Añón, O.; de Llano, L.A.P.; Sánchez, S.D.l.F.; Golpe, R.; Marote, L.M.; Castro-Castro, J.; Quintela, A.G. Obesity-Hypoventilation Syndrome: Increased Risk of Death over Sleep Apnea Syndrome. *PLoS ONE* **2015**, *10*, e0117808. [CrossRef] [PubMed]
10. Georges, M.; Attali, V.; Golmard, J.L.; Morélot-Panzini, C.; Crevier-Buchman, L.; Collet, J.-M.; Tintignac, A.; Morawiec, E.; Trosini-Desert, V.; Salachas, F.; et al. Reduced survival in patients with ALS with upper airway obstructive events on non-invasive ventilation. *J. Neurol. Neurosurg. Psychiatry* **2016**, *87*, 1045–1050. [CrossRef] [PubMed]
11. Agossou, M.; Awanou, B.; Inamo, J.; Dufeal, M.; Arnal, J.-M.; Dramé, M. Association between Previous CPAP and Comorbidities at Diagnosis of Obesity-Hypoventilation Syndrome Associated with Obstructive Sleep Apnea: A Comparative Retrospective Observational Study. *J. Clin. Med.* **2023**, *12*, 2448. [CrossRef] [PubMed]
12. Agossou, M.; Barzu, R.; Awanou, B.; Bellegarde-Joachim, J.; Arnal, J.-M.; Dramé, M. Factors Associated with the Efficiency of Home Non-Invasive Ventilation in Patients with Obesity-Hypoventilation Syndrome in Martinique. *J. Clin. Med.* **2023**, *12*, 3381. [CrossRef] [PubMed]

Disclaimer/Publisher's Note: The statements, opinions and data contained in all publications are solely those of the individual author(s) and contributor(s) and not of MDPI and/or the editor(s). MDPI and/or the editor(s) disclaim responsibility for any injury to people or property resulting from any ideas, methods, instructions or products referred to in the content.

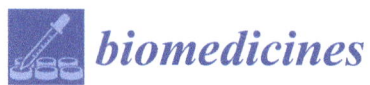

Review

Non-Conventional Risk Factors: "Fact" or "Fake" in Cardiovascular Disease Prevention?

Giovanni Cimmino [1,2,*], Francesco Natale [3], Roberta Alfieri [1,3], Luigi Cante [1,3], Simona Covino [1,3], Rosa Franzese [1,3], Mirella Limatola [1,3], Luigi Marotta [1,3], Riccardo Molinari [1,3], Noemi Mollo [1,3], Francesco S Loffredo [1,3] and Paolo Golino [1,3]

[1] Department of Translational Medical Sciences, Section of Cardiology, University of Campania Luigi Vanvitelli, 80131 Naples, Italy; francesco.loffredo@unicampania.it (F.S.L.)
[2] Cardiology Unit, Azienda Ospedaliera Universitaria Luigi Vanvitelli, 80138 Naples, Italy
[3] Vanvitelli Cardiology Unit, Monaldi Hospital, 80131 Naples, Italy
* Correspondence: giovanni.cimmino@unicampania.it; Tel.: +39-081-566-4269

Abstract: Cardiovascular diseases (CVDs), such as arterial hypertension, myocardial infarction, stroke, heart failure, atrial fibrillation, etc., still represent the main cause of morbidity and mortality worldwide. They significantly modify the patients' quality of life with a tremendous economic impact. It is well established that cardiovascular risk factors increase the probability of fatal and non-fatal cardiac events. These risk factors are classified into modifiable (smoking, arterial hypertension, hypercholesterolemia, low HDL cholesterol, diabetes, excessive alcohol consumption, high-fat and high-calorie diet, reduced physical activity) and non-modifiable (sex, age, family history, of previous cardiovascular disease). Hence, CVD prevention is based on early identification and management of modifiable risk factors whose impact on the CV outcome is now performed by the use of CV risk assessment models, such as the Framingham Risk Score, Pooled Cohort Equations, or the SCORE2. However, in recent years, emerging, non-traditional factors (metabolic and non-metabolic) seem to significantly affect this assessment. In this article, we aim at defining these emerging factors and describe the potential mechanisms by which they might contribute to the development of CVD.

Keywords: cardiovascular diseases; conventional risk factors; cardiovascular prevention; emerging risk factors

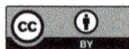

1. Introduction

Despite tremendous advancements in prevention and treatment, CVDs are still the leading causes of mortality and the major contributors to disability in industrialized countries, with a huge impact on social and economic systems. Since the first observations from the Framingham Heart Study started in 1948 [1], several other epidemiological studies have confirmed the impact of the so-called conventional CV risk factors, such as age, blood pressure, glucose blood levels, lipid profile, and smoking status, as major determinants of CV disease development and clinical outcome [2]. Based on all these data, the current guidelines on cardiovascular prevention using the SCORE algorithm define the risk of fatal and non-fatal events in a 10-year period [3]. The achievement of targets for all the modifiable risk factors is the *primum movens* in prevention [3]. However, despite the major effort in promoting a healthy lifestyle and keeping the cardiovascular risk factors at target, in 2019, an estimated 17.9 million people died from CVDs, representing 32% of all global deaths. Of these deaths, 85% were related to heart attack and stroke [4–7]. Thus, the optimistic expectation of cardiologists to reduce the CVD burden because of improved prevention strategies and treatment of the modifiable risk factors has been largely unmet. Several aspects should be taken into account to explain the reasons of such failure. In December 2022, the American College of Cardiology (ACC) announced the publication of "The Global Burden of Cardiovascular Diseases and Risk: A Compass for Future Health".

In this document, 18 specific CV conditions and 15 risk factors across 21 global regions were analyzed to provide an up-to-date overview of the global burden of CVD [8]. This document includes data from 204 countries, analyzing the major global modifiable CVD risk factors, how they contribute to disease burden, and recent strategies for prevention [8]. Based on this analysis, hypertension, hypercholesterolemia, dietary lifestyle, and air pollution were the leading causes of CVD worldwide. A total of 15 leading risks for CV diseases were included and divided in three categories: environmental (air pollution, household air pollution, low and high temperature); metabolic (systolic blood pressure, low-density lipoprotein cholesterol, body mass index, fasting plasma glucose, kidney dysfunction); and behavioral (dietary, smoking, alcohol use, physical activity). This report has also evaluated the disability-adjusted life years (DALYs), looking at the years of life lost because of premature mortality, and years lived with disability [8]. As a main result of this analysis, ischemic heart disease remains the major cause of CV death, with up to 9.44 million deaths in 2021 and 185 million DALYs. Hypertension remains the modifiable risk factor mainly associated with premature CV deaths, with up to 10.8 million CV deaths and 11.3 million deaths overall in 2021 [8]. A dietary lifestyle evaluation has considered under-consumed food, such as vegetables, fruits, fiber, vegetables, and over-consumed food, such as meats, sodium, and sugar-sweetened beverages. This analysis reveals an association of 6.58 million CV deaths and 8 million deaths overall in 2021 [8]. However, the conventional risk factors evaluated in this latest document may explain only part of the cardiovascular disease burden. In the last few years, several epidemiological and experimental studies have linked the development of CVDs to novel and emerging risk factors [9], such as homocysteine and vitamin D levels, gut microbiota, sleep apnea, sleep duration, uric acid plasma concentration over the air pollution, and climate change, as already stated by the ACC document [8]. In the present manuscript, we will evaluate how these emerging non-conventional risk factors are linked to CVDs and how they should be managed for cardiovascular prevention.

2. Literature Sources and Search Strategy

We performed a non-systematic review of the literature by applying the search strategy in different electronic databases (MEDLINE, EMBASE, Cochrane Register of Controlled Trials, and Web of Science). Original reports, meta-analyses, and review articles in peer-reviewed journals up to June 2023 evaluating the clinical role of non-conventional risk factors in determining CVD in the general population. Homocysteine, uric acid, vitamin D, gut microbiota, sleep apnea, air pollution, global temperature, and sleep duration were incorporated into the electronic databases for the search strategy. The references of all identified articles were reviewed to look for additional papers of interest to extrapolate the more recent available data on the link between non-traditional risk factors and CVD.

3. Metabolic Risk Factors

3.1. Homocysteine: The Never-Ending Debate in Cardiovascular Prevention

Homocysteine is a sulphur amino acid that originates from the metabolism of methionine. Methionine, an essential food-derived amino acid, plays a vital role in cellular processes through the donation of methyl groups [10]. The first metabolite originating from methyl transfer is S-adenosyl methionine, which is subsequently converted to S-adenosyl homocysteine, the immediate precursor of homocysteine. The latter can be 'recycled' by taking the methylation route, resulting in the regeneration of methionine, or alternatively, it can be eliminated renally via the transsulfuration route, leading to the formation of cysteine. Both processes are mediated by enzymes whose cofactors are vitamin B12, folic acid, and vitamin B6 [11,12]. Under physiological conditions, there is a balance between homocysteine formation and elimination [12]. If homocysteine can accumulate in the body, the biochemical transformation process fails, leading to a serum level increase [12]. Serum homocysteine values between 5 and 15 micromol/L are considered normal while mild hyperhomocysteinemia is defined as values between 15 and 30 micromol/L; moderate, between 30 and 100 micromol/L; and severe, if greater than 100 micromol/L [13]. In the healthy population, blood levels of homocysteine do not appear to be significantly influenced by dietary intake [14]. Hyperhomocysteinemia has many causes, with genetic profiles playing a dominant role: several genetic polymorphisms have been recognized [15] as responsible for the deficiency of enzymes involved in homocysteine metabolism [16] The most frequent polymorphisms involve the gene coding for methylenetetrahydrofolate reductase and the one coding for cystathionine beta synthase [17]. Other causes include vitamin B12, B6 and folic acid deficiency [18]; advanced age; male sex; menopause; lifestyle habits, such as alcohol abuse and smoking [19]; and certain diseases, including cancers [15] chronic kidney disease [20], hypothyroidism [21], and inflammatory bowel disease [22] Mention should be made of drugs that may interfere with the metabolism of homocysteine or its enzymatic cofactors: these include methotrexate, carbamazepine, nitrates, fibrates and metformin [23].

Over the past few decades, the correlation of homocysteine with the incidence of cardio- and cerebrovascular events as well as its potential role in the pathogenesis of atherosclerosis have been the subject of countless debates [24–26]. The first correlation between serum homocysteine levels and the incidence of coronary artery disease is dated 1956 [27] Numerous clinical studies and meta-analyses have subsequently supported this theory reporting a 20% increase in the risk of new coronary events for every 5 micromol/L increase above normal serum homocysteine levels [28] and an increased risk of fatal and non-fatal coronary [29–31] and cerebrovascular events [30,32]. Further analyses corroborate these data, showing a 25% reduction in homocysteine levels (approximately 3 micromol/L) correlates with a lower risk of cardiac ischemic events and stroke [32].

The relationship between hyperhomocysteinemia and mortality for coronary artery diseases or cardiovascular causes or all causes has been evaluated in a meta-analysis of 20 prospective studies reporting that elevated homocysteine levels were an independent predictor of cardiovascular events, mortality from cardiovascular causes, and mortality from all causes [33].

Other studies have correlated hyperhomocysteinemia with an increased risk for and recurrence of venous thromboembolic events [34–36], peripheral artery diseases [37], and congestive heart failure [38].

Based on this evidence, hyperhomocysteinemia has been proposed as an independent cardiovascular risk factor [38,39].

Several cellular mechanisms have been proposed to explain how hyperhomocysteinemia is implicated in the etiology of cardio- and cerebrovascular events. Endothelial dysfunction, increased arterial stiffness, and a prothrombotic state are common in patients with hyperhomosysteinemia [40]. The main pathways associated with this endothelial impairment are: a) increased oxidative stress [41]; b) a reduction in the expression of the endothelial isoform of nitric oxide synthetase (eNOS) and increase in the cellular expression of caveolin-1 that is an inhibitor of eNOS, thus leading to a reduced release of nitric oxide [42]; and c) the upregulation of cell adhesion molecules, resulting in an increased chemotaxis of monocytes on the endothelium and increased endothelial expression of IL-8, which favor inflammatory processes [43].

Hyperhomocysteinemia is also associated to collagen synthesis [44] and vessel smooth muscle cell proliferation [45], through activation of cyclin A, protein kinase C, and the proto-oncogenes c-myc and c-fos [45,46] as well as increased production of phospholipids [46] and increased expression of platelet growth factor [47]. This smooth muscle cells proliferation as well as increased collagen deposition and alterations in elastic tissue composition [48] is responsible for increased arterial wall stiffness [49–51]. This phenomenon is facilitated by the inactivation of eNOS and the reduced production of nitric oxide [52]. A schematic view of homocysteine pathways involved in CVD is provided in Figure 1.

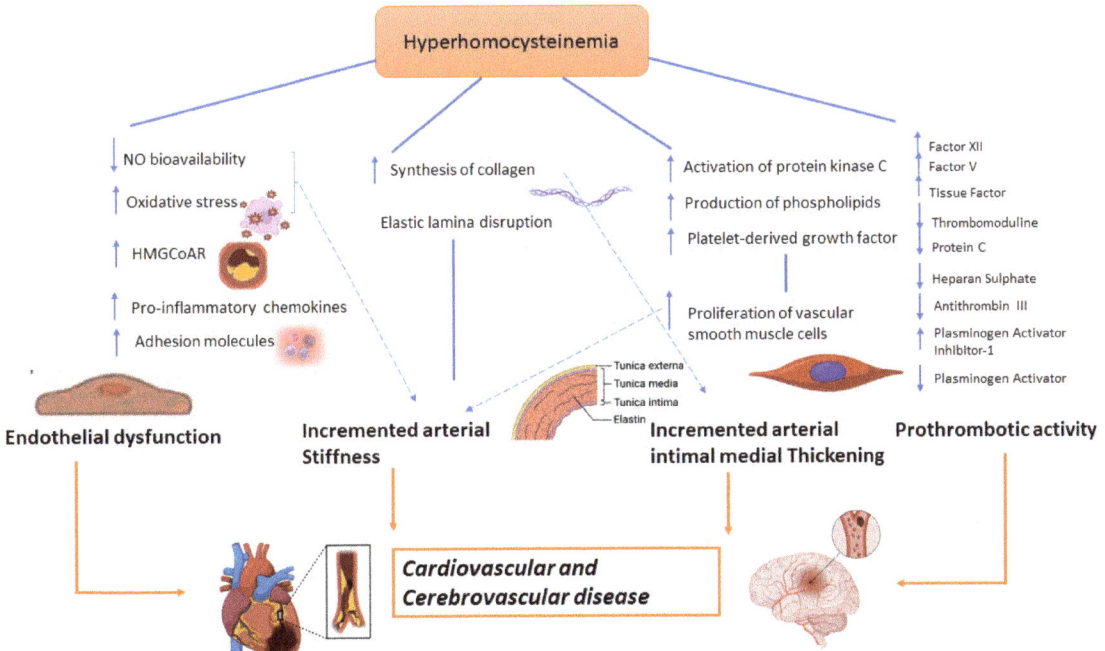

Figure 1. Possible role of homocysteine in CVD.

Moreover, several studies have also linked hyperhomocysteinemia to increased prothrombotic state [53]. This effect has been mainly related to: (a) factor XII and factor V activation [54]; (b) tissue factor expression [55]; (c) thrombomodulin inhibition [56] that results in a reduction of protein C activation [57]; (d) a reduction in the anticoagulant effect of antithrombin III, thus altering the binding capacity of endothelial heparan sulphate with the latter [58]; and (e) the reduction of plasminogen activator function and increased expression of its inhibitor [59].

In light of these basic findings, several clinical studies have investigated whether the treatment of hyperhomocysteinemia might result in cardiovascular benefits in terms of cardio- and cerebrovascular event reduction with conflicting results.

3.2. Uric Acid: Still a Controversial Cardiovascular Risk Factor?

Uric acid (UA) is the final product of purine metabolism. The increase in its blood levels may depend either on an increased production or on a reduced elimination [60]. If hyperuricemia develops, urate crystals accumulation may occurs in the joints leading to the clinical manifestations of gout, subsequently also affecting the renal parenchyma and the excretory tracts with the picture of gouty nephropathy and nephro/urolithiasis [61]. Beyond this known effect, several other clinical studies have also investigated the relationship between high blood levels of UA and the development of CVDs [62] and, as for homocysteine, with conflicting results. The Framingham Heart Study did not indicate hyperuricemia as an independent risk factor for coronary artery disease, cardiovascular death, and death from all causes [63,64]. Some epidemiological studies have described a J- or U-shaped relationship between UA levels and cardiovascular risk, meaning that patients with either very low or very high UA values have an increased cardiovascular risk [65]. More recently, clinical studies seem to support the role of hyperuricemia in atherosclerosis, systemic arterial hypertension, atrial fibrillation, and chronic kidney disease as the pathophysiological processes promoted by UA, such as oxidative stress and inflammation that are the basis of endothelial dysfunction, which may contribute to atherothrombotic events. An increase in the activity of the enzyme xanthine oxidase, which regulates the synthesis of UA and which uses molecular oxygen as an electron acceptor for its function determines the formation of reactive oxygen species (ROS) [66]. ROS are responsible for the lipid oxidation and the reduction of the nitric oxide concentration, which causes the loss of the physiological vasodilating effect of the endothelium and determines a prothrombotic phenotype. UA also favors an increase in the deposition of low-density lipoproteins at the endothelial level and their uptake by macrophages, which are transformed into foam cells thus starting the process of atherosclerosis [67]. More recently, it has been highlighted how endothelial cells (ECs) may acquire a prothrombotic phenotype by expressing functional tissue factor (TF) once exposed to increasing doses of UA that can be reversed by the preincubation with an uricosuric agent [68]. Moreover, the endothelial dysfunction induced by hyperuricemia also favors the expression on the cell surface of the adhesion molecules (CAMs) involved in the initiation of the atherosclerosis process. This mechanism appears to be regulated by a modulation of the NF-kappaB pathway, leading to the upregulation of TF on cell surface and downregulation of its natural inhibitor, the Tissue Factor Pathway inhibitor (TFPI) [69]. Furthermore, the inflammasome [70] seems also to be involved with an increase in caspase-1 function, which would promote a particular type of endothelial cell apoptosis, known as pyroptosis, and the release of TNF-alpha [71]. A summary of the possible mechanisms by which UA is involved in CVD is provided in Figure 2.

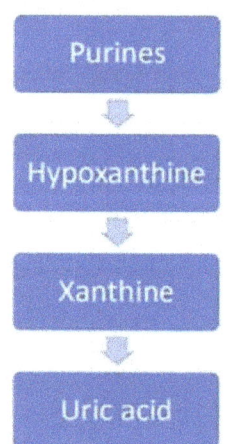
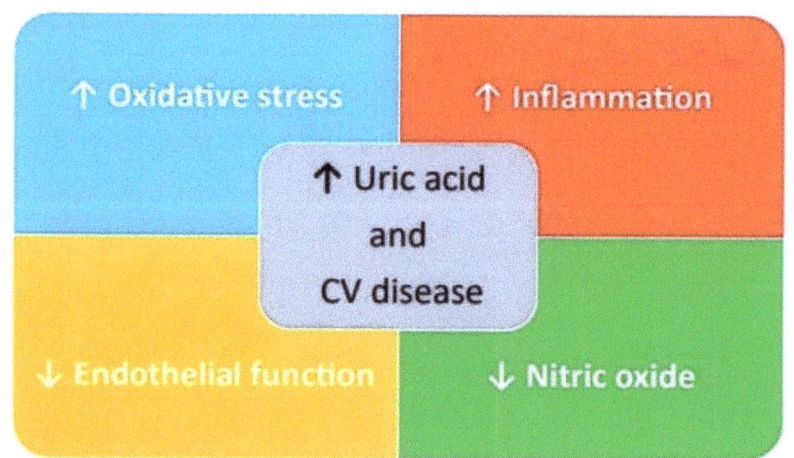

Figure 2. Major pathways UA related involved in pathogenesis of CVD.

These basic findings have been corroborated by a more recent clinical evaluation on patients with acute coronary syndrome (ACS) [72] by reporting that higher UA levels are associated with higher C-reactive protein (CRP) and troponin values. Additionally, ACS patients with high UA levels showed an angiographic picture of multivessel coronary artery disease and complex atherosclerosis according to the Ellis classification [72]. As regards the relationship between hyperuricemia and systemic arterial hypertension, several studies have shown an increase in blood pressure in patients with increased uric acid. A meta-analysis that studied 55,607 patients showed that for each 1 mg/dL increase in uric acid, the incidence of arterial hypertension increases by approximately 13% [73]. At the basis of this relationship, there would be the lower release of nitric acid and the activation of the renin–angiotensin–aldosterone system promoted by uric acid, which determine vasoconstriction and consequent increase in blood pressure. A relationship between hyperuricemia and increased onset of atrial fibrillation (AF) has been highlighted by the ARIC study, which shows a 1.16-fold increase in the risk of AF in subjects, mostly female and of African origin, with high UA values [74]. Atrial remodeling induced by the inflammatory effects and oxidative stress related to UA seems to be the underlying mechanism [75]. In light of the relationship between hyperuricemia and increased cardiovascular risk, the current therapeutic options mainly are represented by allopurinol and febuxostat, which inhibit the enzyme xanthine oxidase, and therefore, the UA production could have a role in reducing the incidence of cardiovascular events.

3.3. Vitamin D: Light and Shadow in Cardiovascular Prevention

Vitamin D, commonly known as the "sunshine vitamin", is an essential nutrient that plays a critical role in the absorption and regulation of calcium and phosphorus, essential minerals necessary for strong bones, teeth, and overall skeletal health [76]. Unlike other vitamins, the human body can produce vitamin D through exposure to sunlight [77]. The precursor form of vitamin D, indeed known as 7-dehydrocholesterol, is naturally present in the skin [78]. Upon exposure to UVB radiation emitted by sunlight, a photochemical reaction takes place, leading to the transformation of 7-dehydrocholesterol into pre-vitamin D3 [78]. Subsequently, through heat-induced isomerization, pre-vitamin D3 is converted into cholecalciferol, also known as vitamin D3. Another form of vitamin D, the Vitamin D2, also known as ergocalciferol, is primarily derived from plant-based sources and is commonly utilized in fortified food products and some dietary supplements. Vitamin D2 and D3 are fully activated through two consecutive hydroxylation reactions catalyzed by specific P450 isoenzymes. The First hydroxylation, which occurs on the carbon in position 25, takes place in the liver by vitamin D 25-hydroxylase (CYP2R1) to form the pro-hormone 25-hydroxyvitamin D. Due its solubility and BPD binding properties, the level of this metabolite better reflects the body's vitamin D status. The second hydroxylation occurs on the carbon in position 1 by 25-hydroxyvitamin D-1alpha-hydroxylase renal (CYP27B1) and is responsible for the synthesis of the biologically active metabolite, 1,25-dihydroxyvitamin D [78].

Beyond its well-known role in bone health, vitamin D has garnered increasing attention in relation to cardiovascular health. Numerous observational studies have investigated the link between vitamin D levels and CVDs. Although the results show some degree of variability, they consistently highlight an inverse association between vitamin D status and the risk of developing CVD [79–81]. The inverse correlation between vitamin D status and CVD seems to be particularly strong in older adults [82,83]. Meta-analyses of epidemiological studies support the inverse correlation between vitamin D levels and CVD [82,84]. The correlation between vitamin D levels and arterial hypertension holds significant importance. Blood pressure tends to exhibit geographical and racial disparities, whereby the risk of hypertension tends to rise from south to north in the Northern hemisphere. A suggested explanation for this latitude-based correlation is that sunlight exposure may offer protection, potentially due to the influence of ultraviolet B (UVB) radiation or vitamin D [85]. This association appears to be supported by animal studies. Mice that lack the vitamin D receptor (VDR) or have a genetic deficiency in the 1-alpha-hydroxylase gene, which is responsible for vitamin D activation, have been shown to develop high renin hypertension and cardiac hypertrophy [86,87]. In vitro studies highlight a favorable cardioprotective effect of 1,25-dihydroxyvitamin D. It has been reported that the pretreatment of ECs with vitamin D reduce the expression and activity of TF and CAMs induced by oxidized lipids [68] or interleukin-6 [88], possibly preserving endothelial function.

All the putative cardiovascular mechanisms associated with vitamin D are provided in Figure 3.

While in vitro studies and epidemiological studies have provided promising insights into the potential cardioprotective effects of vitamin D, the results from randomized controlled trials (RCTs) in this field have been inconclusive to date. The majority of trials conducted so far have primarily focused on investigating the impact of vitamin D supplementation on bone health. In many cases, vitamin D supplementation has been administered alongside calcium supplementation. Meta-analyses of randomized controlled trials (RCTs) have demonstrated non-significant reductions in CVD events with vitamin D supplementation [89–91]. According to a Cochrane review, vitamin D supplementation was found to significantly reduce all-cause mortality when compared to a placebo or no intervention. However, the review did not demonstrate a significant impact on cardiovascular mortality [92].

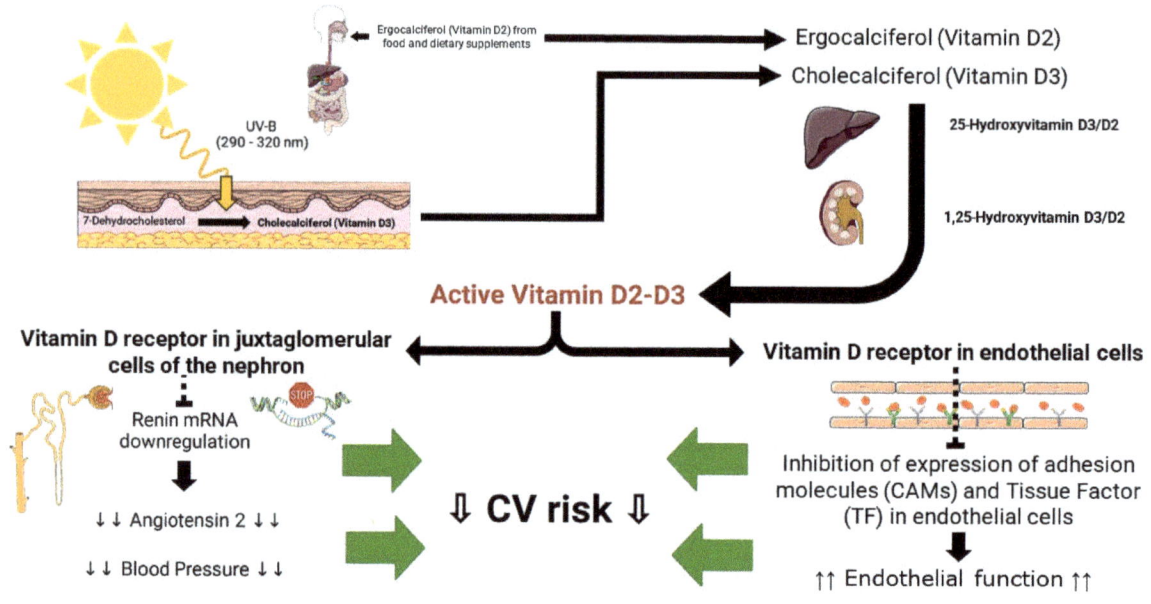

Figure 3. Putative cardiovascular pathways Vitamin D-related: see text for details.

3.4. Gut Microbiota: The Axis Heart–Intestine in CVDs Development

Gut microbiota is a community made up of 10^{14} microorganisms, in symbiosis with the host, with numerous functions, such as the fermentation of indigestible carbohydrates, synthesis of vitamin K and biotin, and promotion of mucosal immune system [93]. In recent years, emerging studies have considered gut microbiota as a "forgotten organ" with metabolic, endocrine, and immunological functions, relevant for human health [94] The balance of microbiota, in terms of number and diversification of species present, depends on various factors: presence of modulators (antibiotics, probiotics, and prebiotics), host's characteristics (genetic background, immune system, hormones), and environmental conditions (diet).

The imbalance of gut microbiota, defined intestinal dysbiosis, is involved in the pathogenesis of many diseases, including atherosclerotic CVDs [95].

A recent meta-analysis and systematic review [96] reported a decrease in Bacteroides and Lachnospira with an increase in Enterobacteria, Actinobacteria, and Verrucomicrobiota in patients affected by coronary artery disease (CAD).

Intestinal dysbiosis promotes atherosclerosis through various mechanisms: local infections with microbial translocation and systemic inflammatory state activation and the production of pro-atherogenic metabolites, acting on the cholesterol metabolism.

The formation of atherosclerotic plaque can be promoted by an infection of the arterial wall or a distant infection. Some studies report in the vascular wall the presence of DNA of the same bacteria found in human gut [97]. These data do not indicate that bacteria are a CAD etiological agent, but they suggest that these organisms can promote plaque formation or accelerate disease progression [98]. Moreover, even a distant infection can promote atherosclerosis. In fact, some bacteria can compromise the integrity of the intestinal barrier, favoring lipopolysaccharide (LPS) translocation to systemic circulation [99]. LPS interaction with Toll-like receptor 4 (TLR4) on immune cells' surface activates the NF-kappaB pathway with the production of pro-inflammatory cytokines that alter tissue homeostasis [100]. In fact, the pro-inflammatory state increases insulin resistance, which favors the development of diabetes mellitus and obesity and determines macrophage infiltration in the vascular wall, which initiates atherogenesis [101]. Certainly, microbial translocation, secondary to altered permeability of intestinal barrier, determinates a sub-acute or chronic low-grade inflammatory state, which induces metabolic syndrome development. The use of probiotics and prebiotics has been evaluated as a tool to reduce the systemic inflammatory response through the modulation of gut microbiota [102].

Furthermore, gut microbiota has a metabolic activity greater than the host's activity. Some microbial species are able to metabolize complex dietary carbohydrates, indigestible or partially digestible by humans, into short-chain fatty acids (SCFAs); Bacteroides are the principal producers of acetate and propionate, and Firmicutes are the principal producers of butyrate [103]. SCFAs may have anti-inflammatory effects [104]. Hence, the alteration of intestinal homeostasis correlates with systemic inflammation and, therefore, promotes atherogenesis [95]. Moreover, some substances (choline, carnitine, betaine), contained in some nutrients, such as red meat, are metabolized by gut microbiota into trimethylamine, subsequently oxidized by hepatic flavin monooxygenase (FMO) into trimethylamine N-oxide (TMAO) [105], a pro-atherogenic metabolite. At a systemic level, TMAO causes endothelial dysfunction, a crucial phase in the pathogenesis of atherosclerosis, and increases platelet calcium signaling with a pro-thrombotic effect [106,107]. TMAO blood levels are proportional to atherosclerotic plaque vulnerability and evaluated with optical coherence tomography (OCT). These data confirm TMAO's pathogenetic role in atherogenesis but also suggests its potential role as a biomarker of coronary plaque progression [108].

In addition, gut microbiota has important effects on cholesterol metabolism. In fact, there are bacteria that metabolize primary bile acids, produced in the liver from cholesterol, into secondary bile acids. These, through farnesoid X receptor (FXR) and G protein-coupled TGR5 receptor, have effects on the host's metabolic activity (hepatic accumulation of triglycerides) and on the inflammatory state [109]. Alterations in gut microbiota influence the type of secondary bile acids that are produced. Changes in the typology of bile acids correlate with metabolic disturbances. For example, an increase in 12α-hydroxylated bile acids (cholic acid, deoxycholic acid) correlate with insulin resistance development [110]. Recently, emerging data correlate blood cholesterol levels with different microbial species. In particular, Bacteroides reduce blood cholesterol levels through various mechanisms, mainly via the esterification of cholesterol into coprostanol that is not absorbed in the intestine and, therefore, eliminated with faeces and the inhibition of cholesterol synthesis [111].

Finally, a relationship between gut and thrombus microbiota in patients presenting with ACS has been also reported [112] with Prevotella coronary thrombus content remarkably increased and associated with higher thrombus burden, TMAO, CDL40, and vWF, especially in hyperglycemic ACS patients [112]. These data support the role of TMAO in increasing coagulation.

All the possible atherosclerotic mechanisms associated with gut microbiota are summarized in Figure 4.

Despite this growing evidence, the relationship between gut microbiota and CVDs is still under intensive investigation.

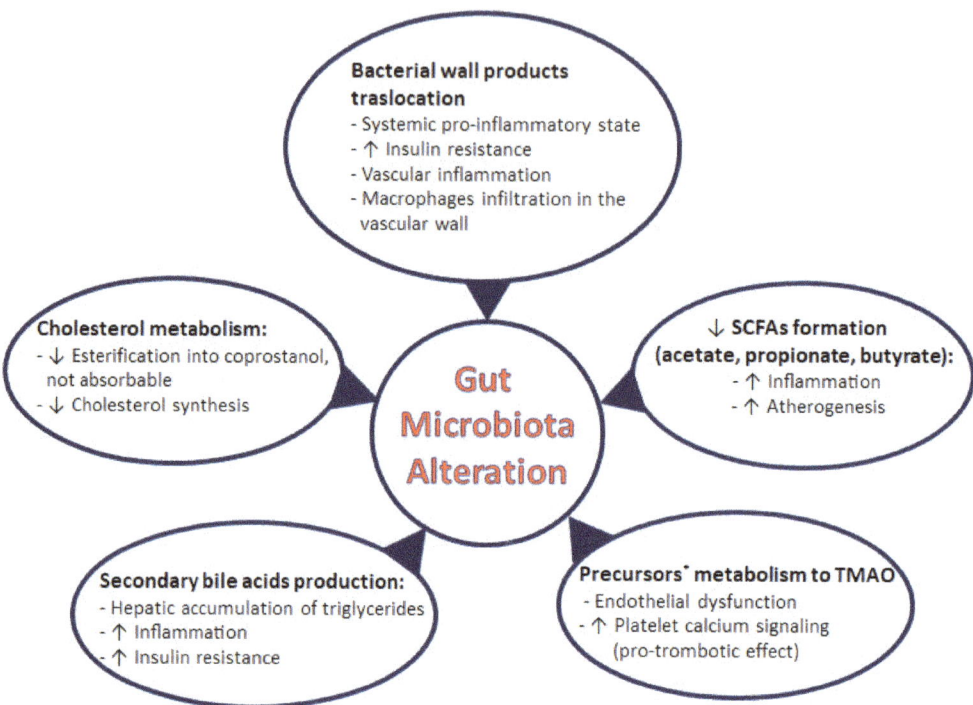

Figure 4. Summary of the main mechanisms by which gut microbiota, in condition of dysbiosis, influences the pathogenesis of atherosclerosis. * Precursors to TMAO: choline, L-carnitine and betaine. See text for details.

3.5. Lipoprotein(a): Unveiling the Enigmatic Lipid Particle

Lipoprotein(a), often abbreviated as Lp(a), is a lipoprotein particle that has garnered significant attention in the field of atherosclerotic CVD, becoming subject of intense research and debate in the last few decades [113]. The Lp(a) structure consists of a large and highly polymorphic glycoprotein referred to as apo(a) covalently bound to a molecule of apoB-100 [114]. In normotriglyceridemic individuals, apo(a) primarily associates with low-density lipoproteins (LDL). However, in dyslipidemic patients, apo(a) can also combine with apoB100 found in triglyceride-rich particles, specifically very low-density lipoproteins (VLDL) and intermediate-density lipoproteins (IDL) [115]. By the biochemical point of view, apo(a) is characterized by loop-like structures known as kringles, a structural motif also found in other coagulation factors, such as plasminogen (PLG), prothrombin, urokinase, and tissue-type PLG activators [114]. Elevated Lp(a) levels are thought to significantly contribute to atherosclerosis, primarily by interfering with macrophages [116]. Specifically, the macrophage's receptor for VLDL can engage with a high affinity to Lp(a), facilitating its breakdown via endocytosis within lysosomes, resulting in its degradation and prompting the formation of foam cells with the deposition of cholesterol in atherosclerotic plaques [116]. This hypothesis gains support from observations that Lp(a) is widely present in human coronary atheroma and is more abundant in tissue from culprit lesions of patients with unstable coronary disease when compared to those with stable disease [117]. Furthermore, oxidized phospholipids present on Lp(a) trigger inflammation through a TLR 2-mediated pathway, exacerbating endothelial dysfunction and contributing to increased inflammation within the arterial wall [118]. Lp(a) may also affect the coagulative homeostasis enhancing TF-mediated thrombosis and restrain the dissolution of clots [119], interfering with fibrinolysis competing with plasminogen [120,121]. However, therapeutic efforts to reduce Lp(a) levels using an mRNA inhibitor (Pelacarsen) did not result in changes to fibrinolysis, suggesting that negatively affecting fibrinolysis might not be a clinically significant characteristic of Lp(a) [122]. Large epidemiological studies support a strong correlation between Lp(a) levels and atherosclerotic CVD [113]. Pooled data derived from 36 prospective studies involving a total of 126,634 participants revealed that age and sex corrected risk ratio for CVD increases with each rise in standardized concentrations of Lp(a) [123]; elevated CVD risk persisted even after adjusting for conventional CV risk factors [123]. Lp(a) concentration shows consistent associations also with risk of stroke [123]. Recently, Lp(a) has been linked also to the inflammatory and calcification processes that underlie aortic valve degeneration and progression of aortic stenosis [124]. A summary of its putative mechanisms is provided in Figure 5.

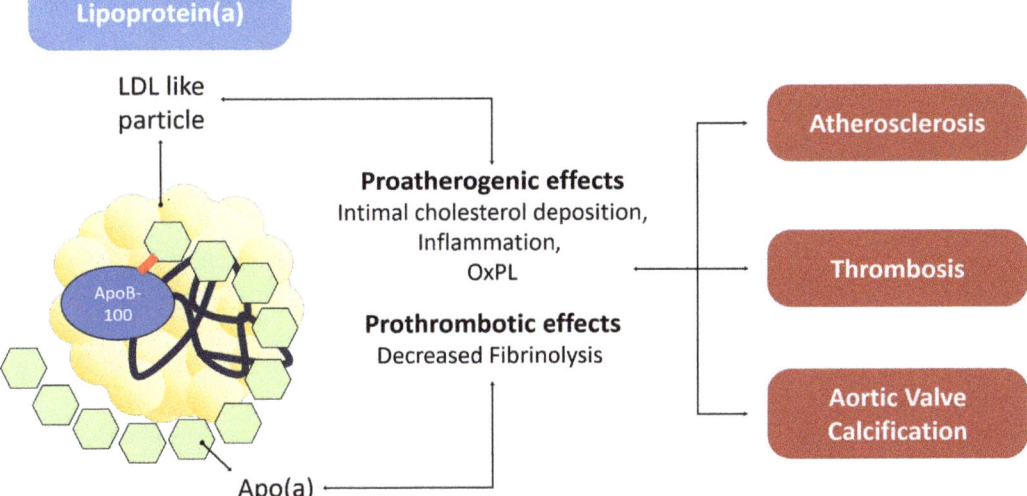

Figure 5. Lp(a) connection with CVD.

3.6. The Metabolic Syndrome: A Cocktail of Ingredients Interconnected with Cardiovascular Risk

Metabolic syndrome (MS) is defined as the presence of at least three diagnostic criteria (central obesity, hyperglycemia, HTN, hypertriglyceridemia, low high-density lipoprotein (HDL)) [125]. Its correlation with increased CV risk has been well characterized [125]. A multifactorial pathogenesis underlines this condition with inflammation and insulin resistance (IR) as key playmakers [125,126]. IR, characterized by a reduced cellular response to insulin, determines MS development through various pathways [127]. It is well established that IR is linked to obesity through several mechanisms (the alteration of glucose transport by down-regulation of GLUT4 and increased expression of protein tyrosine phosphatases, which dephosphorylate and interrupt intracellular signaling) [128]. Furthermore, hyperinsulinemia, secondary to IR, is also responsible for obesity [128]. IR determines development of HTN due to reduced NO production by ECs [129] and hyperactivation of the sympathetic system [129]. Lipid metabolism alterations are also induced by IR [130]. In particular, the increased release of fatty acids from adipocytes causes increased hepatic VLDL secretion and, therefore, hypertriglyceridemia. VLDL stimulates the exchange of cholesterol esters from HDL, reducing its bioavailability for reverse cholesterol transport [130]. A schematic view is provided in Figure 6.

Strict glycemic control has a cardioprotective action through anti-inflammatory, antioxidative mechanisms with a reduction in endothelial dysfunction [131,132]. However, despite the achievement of glycemic compensation, CVDs continue to develop. The improvement of insulin sensitivity, through drugs such as metformin, leads to a reduction in cardiovascular events [133]. This suggests that CV risk is more related to IR than to blood glucose levels [134]. Thus, a marker of IR should considered by the current guidelines to better evaluate CV risk [134]. On this regard, HOMA index is a well-established marker of IR [135] with a defined prognostic value in CV patients [136] and it should be add to the current score for CV risk estimation.

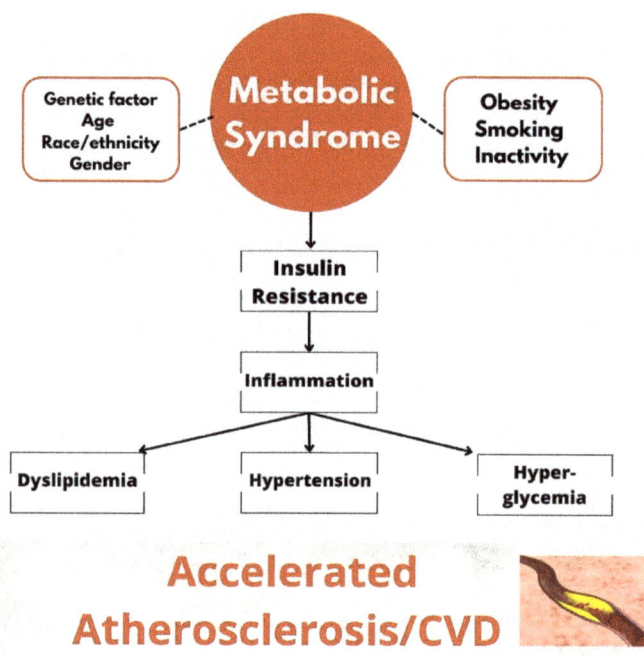

Figure 6. Schematic view of metabolic syndrome leading to CVD.

A summary of mechanisms involved in the relationship between non-metabolic risk factor and CVDs has provided in Table 1.

Table 1. Metabolic risk factors.

Risk Factor	Observed Effects/Impact on Conventional CV Risk Factors	Mechanisms
Homocysteine	- CHD - Stroke - peripheral arterial disease - venous thromboembolism	- Endotelial disfunction: oxidative stress; Reduced NO bioavailability; increased expression of HMGCoAR; increased expression of CAM and pro-inflammatory interleukin (IL-8) - Incremented arterial stiffness: elastic lamina disruption, proliferation of smooth muscle cells and incremented synthesis of collagen - Incremented arterial intimal-medial thickening: proliferation of smooth muscle cells; incremented synthesis of collagen. - Prothrombotic state: activation of pro-coagulant factor: factor XII, factor V, TF; plasminogen activator inhibitor-1 and reduced activity or expression of anti-coagulant factor: thrombomodulin; protein C, Heparan Sulfate; Antithrombin III; plasminogen activator

Table 1. Cont.

Risk Factor	Observed Effects/Impact on Conventional CV Risk Factors	Mechanisms
Uric Acid	- Increased Oxidative stress - Reduced NO - Endothelial disfunction - Inflammation	The synthesis of uric acid determines the formation of ROS. ROS are responsible for the lipid oxidation and the reduction of the NO concentration which causes the loss of the normal endothelial function and induces a pro-inflammatory and pro-trombotic state
Vitamin D	- CVD risk reduction. - Effects on blood pressure.	- Reduced expression and activity of TF and CAMs on ECs induced by oxidized lipids or interleukin-6, possibly preserving endothelial function. - Vitamin D regulation of renin synthesis
Gut Microbiota Alteration	- Cholesterol reduction - Insulin resistance - Systemic pro-inflammatory state - Endothelial dysfunction - Pro-trombotic state	- Reduction of cholesterol synthesis and absorption - Bacterial wall product translocation - Reduced SCFAs formation - TMAO production
Lipoprotein(a)	- Atherosclerotic CVD	- Intimal cholesterol deposition - Inflammation - Lipid oxidation - Hemostasis impairment
Metabolic Syndrome	- Hyperglicemia - Hypertension - Dyslipidemia	- alteration of glucose transport by down-regulation of GLUT4, increased expression of protein tyrosine phosphatases which dephosphorylate and interrupt intracellular signaling - reduced NO production and hyperactivation of the sympathetic system - increased release of fatty acids from adipocytes; increased hepatic VLDL secretion and therefore hypertriglyceridemia; stimulation exchange of cholesterol esters from HDL

4. Non-Metabolic Risk Factors and Surrogates

4.1. Obstructive Sleep Apnea Syndrome: The Diving Board to CVDs

Obstructive sleep apnea (OSA) syndrome is a clinical condition characterized by cyclical episodes of total (apnea) or partial (hypopnea) collapse of the upper airways, occurring during sleep, with the persistence of thoracoabdominal movements. At the end of the events, arousal occurs with transient hypoxemia, autonomic alterations, and sleep fragmentation [137].

Apnea is defined as a reduction in airflow of at least 90% compared to the basal one, lasting at least 10 s while hypopnea is defined as a reduction in airflow of at least 30%, for no less than 10 s, associated with a reduction of at least 3% in oxygen saturation (SaO_2) [138].

The severity of OSA is based on the number of events/hour, and it is defined as AHI index (apnea/hypopnea index). Specifically, <5 events/hour define a normal respiratory pattern, 5–14 events/hour a mild apnea, 15–29 events/hour a moderate apnea, and from 30 events/h a severe apnea [138]. The gold standard for the diagnosis of OSA is represented by polysomnography (PSG) [138].

A diagnosis of OSA is made based on nocturnal breathing disorders (snoring, breathing pauses in sleep, restless sleep, awakening choking) and/or daytime sleepiness symptoms associated with an AHI > 5; on the contrary, if the AHI index is greater than 15, OSA can be diagnosed in the absence of symptoms [139].

In general population, OSA prevalence is approximately 34% in men and 17% in women [137,140] while in CVD populations, it ranges from 40% to 60% [141,142].

During sleep, a failure of the neuromuscular reflex that preserves the patency of the airways occurs, resulting in hypoxemia and hypercapnia, determining an increase in the respiratory effort and an awakening of a few seconds, which restores patency of the upper airways, thanks to a series of reflex mechanisms. When sleep resumes, the cycle repeats [143].

OSA represents an independent risk factor for CVDs, such as HTN, AF and other arrhythmias, HF, CAD, stroke, pulmonary hypertension, metabolic syndrome, and diabetes as shown in Figure 7. The involved mechanisms are multiple and probably interconnected.

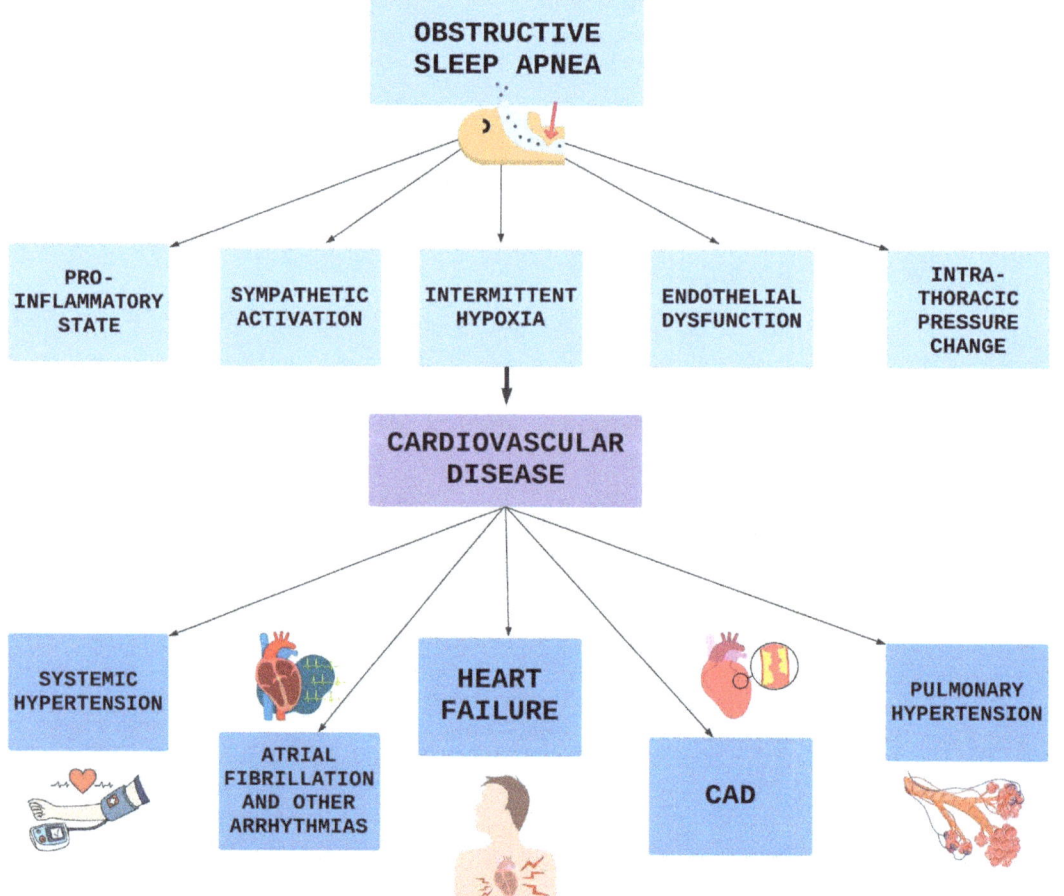

Figure 7. Pathophysiological pathways OSA related leading to CVD.

During the apneic phase, by stimulating peripheral and central chemoreceptors [144], hypoxia and hypercapnia determine the activation of the sympathetic nervous system with consequent peripheral vasoconstriction and an increase in vascular resistance and heart rate [145]. This results in an increase in left ventricular afterload and cardiac work. In addition, there is an overall increase in left ventricular transmural pressure (that is the difference between ventricular systolic pressure and intrathoracic pressure) with increased wall stress [146,147]. The cycle repeats many times every night; therefore, the cardiovascular system is chronically exposed to neuro-hormonal stress, and the hyperactivity of the autonomic nervous system also extends to the daytime hours over time [145,148].

Intermittent hypoxia is also responsible for an increase in oxidative stress [149]: during the hypoxic phase, the cells adapt to an environment with low oxygen content, and with the reoxygenation phase, there is a sudden increase of oxygen with ROS formation, leading to cellular damage in the ischemic tissue [150,151].

Furthermore, a reduction in the levels of circulating NO has also been highlighted during OSA [152], and this could be implicated in endothelial dysfunction [153].

OSA is present in up to 30–50% of HTN patients, and 80% of patients with resistant HTN have OSA [139,154], representing an independent risk factor [137]. In patients with OSA, due to the overactivity of the sympathetic nervous system, the physiological reduction in blood pressure during the night (which configures the "dipper" profile) does not occur [155,156]. Therefore, there seems to be a correlation between sleep apnea and the non-dipper profile of essential HTN [157,158]. Furthermore, several randomized trials and meta-analysis have shown a reduction in blood pressure in patients with sleep apnea treated with CPAP [137,159].

OSA is associated with heart rhythm disturbances and sudden death; pauses and bradycardia are common in patients with OSA [139].

OSA is also an independent risk factor for AF with several pathophysiological mechanisms implicated. In particular, sudden changes in intrathoracic pressure can cause atrial remodeling and atrial fibrosis with consequent electrophysiological alterations [160]. Moreover, the sudden increase in sympathetic activity during apneas can lead to the activation of catecholamine-sensitive atrial on channels, thus determining focal discharges from which AF can be originated [161]. OSA is also associated with an increase in systemic inflammation, which may contribute to the genesis of AF [162].

Sleep apnea also increases the risk of CAD by favoring atherosclerotic process via oxidative stress, endothelial dysfunction, inflammatory state, and autonomic dysfunction. It has been reported that in OSA patients, myocardial infarction occurs more frequently during the night hours [163], and a higher pro-inflammatory profile is present [164] with an effective reduction of the latter if CPAP therapy is used [164]. This study, therefore, suggests that OSA could activate vascular inflammation with non-traditional pathogenetic mechanisms.

OSA is also a risk factor for incident strokes, stroke recurrence [165], and functional and cognitive outcomes [166].

Pulmonary hypertension is closely related to OSA. Hypoxia and hypercapnia induce arteriolar vasoconstriction in the short term and vascular remodeling in the long term that could lead to an irreversible increase in pulmonary vascular resistance and the development of pulmonary hypertension [167].

Sleep apnea, mainly the central form (CSA), is highly prevalent in HF patients as well, ranging from 40% to 60% of symptomatic patients [168].

OSA is also linked to obesity and metabolic syndrome since chronic intermittent hypoxemia and sleep loss is associated to higher plasma leptin levels [169], glucose metabolism impairment, and insulin resistance [170].

At least, there is a reciprocal interaction between obesity and OSA where they both reinforce their progression and their severity in a vicious circle. It is believed that the deposition of fat in the upper airways and the functional alteration of the airways themselves are the mechanisms involved in the pathogenesis of OSA in the obese subjects [171]. On the other hand, daytime sleepiness and decreased physical activity together with hyperleptinemia are the mechanisms probably implicated in weight gain in OSA.

4.2. Air Pollution: Health Breath as Part of Prevention

Air pollution is the contamination of the environment, indoor or outdoor, by a mixture of chemical, physical, or biological agents that change the characteristics of the atmosphere and even at low concentrations cause damage to human health, other living organisms and the environment [172]. According to the Global Burden of Disease (GBD) report, air pollution was responsible for 6.7 million deaths in 2019 alone [172,173]. Globally, nearly 20% of CVD deaths are attributable to air pollution [173]. The main components of this mixture of pollutants are Total Suspended Particulate Matter (PM), gaseous compounds including ozone (O_3), nitrogen dioxide (NO_2), carbon monoxide (CO), sulfur dioxide (SO_2) and volatile organic compounds including benzene [172]. According to the World Health Organization, 99% of the world's population breathes air that contains annual average levels of air pollutants that exceed guideline recommendations. Particularly high exposures have been documented in cities in Asia, western sub-Saharan Africa, and Latin America [172]. The most consistent evidence on health damage is attributed to PM, i.e., the set of airborne particles, ranging in diameter from 0.1 to 100 mm, capable of remaining in suspension in the air even for long periods [174,175]. Short- and long-term exposure to PM is associated with increased morbidity and mortality, impacting the progression of atherosclerosis [176], ischemic heart disease [177–179], stroke [180], and lung disease as well as the course of pregnancy and the health of newborns [181]. PM_{10} (particles between 2.5 and 10 mm in diameter) and, largely, $PM_{2.5}$ (diameter < 2.5 mm), are the most linked to CVD and affecting global public health [182,183]. Lung inflammation and oxidative stress pathway is the primary response to air pollution exposure [184], contributing to the development of a systemic pro-inflammatory state and activation of secondary effector pathways that result in endothelial dysfunction, increased atherosclerotic plaque vulnerability, and the activation of a prothrombotic and proarrhythmic state [177,185,186]. Experimental animal models seem indeed to support this hypothesis [187]. Moreover, human exposure to pollutant nanoparticles causes their translocation into the systemic circulation through the alveolus-capillary membrane, interacting with the endothelium, accumulating at sites of vascular inflammation, thus favoring atherosclerotic process [188–190], with effects similar to those observed in the lungs [191] and thrombotic complications [192] A relevant change in platelet function toward increased prothrombotic tendency has been confirmed in diabetic patients after recent (within two hours) exposure to PM [193]. In addition to these mechanisms, short-term $PM_{2.5}$ exposure in animal models is associated with sympathetic nervous system activation and hypertension, probably mediated by neuroinflammation [194,195]. In a meta-analysis of 33 studies, short-term exposure to $PM_{2.5}$ was associated with a significant decrease in heart rate variability (HRV) [196]. Decreased HRV is an index of autonomic system dysfunction and predicts an increased risk of cardiovascular morbidity and mortality in patients with heart disease [197]. Increased blood pressure and decreased HRV suggest an autonomic imbalance in favor of sympathetic tone and could further explain the rapid cardiovascular responses associated with air pollution, such as the initiation of fatal tachyarrhythmias and increased myocardial infarctions [177], as confirmed by the available literature [198]. High short-term exposure to $PM_{2.5}$ is associated with an increased risk of acute coronary event, acutely destabilizing and rupturing atherosclerotic plaque, in patients with clinically significant pre-existing CAD but not in those with uninjured coronary arteries [199]. Moreover, short-term exposure to elevated levels of $PM_{2.5}$ and PM_{10} is also associated with increased daily hospitalizations for STEMI and increased incidence of STEMI-related ventricular arrhythmias and cardiac death [200] The effect of long-term exposure to major air pollutants was assessed by the ESCAPE study that have evaluated the incidence of acute coronary events in 11 European cohorts. At a mean follow-up of 11.5 years, exposure to annual mean levels of $PM_{2.5}$ > 5 µg/m^3 and PM_{10} > 10 µg/m^3 was associated with a 13% and 12% increase in the risk of nonfatal acute coronary events, respectively, with no evidence of heterogeneity between cohorts [201] Other observational studies and meta-analyses have reported a positive correlation between long-term exposure to air pollution and the development and progression of subclinical atherosclerosis and calcium accumulation [202] as well as increased carotid intima-media thickness [203]. Based on the published data, no more doubts should exist on the role of air pollutants in CVD development. A schematic view of the relationship between air pollution and CVD is provided in Figure 8.

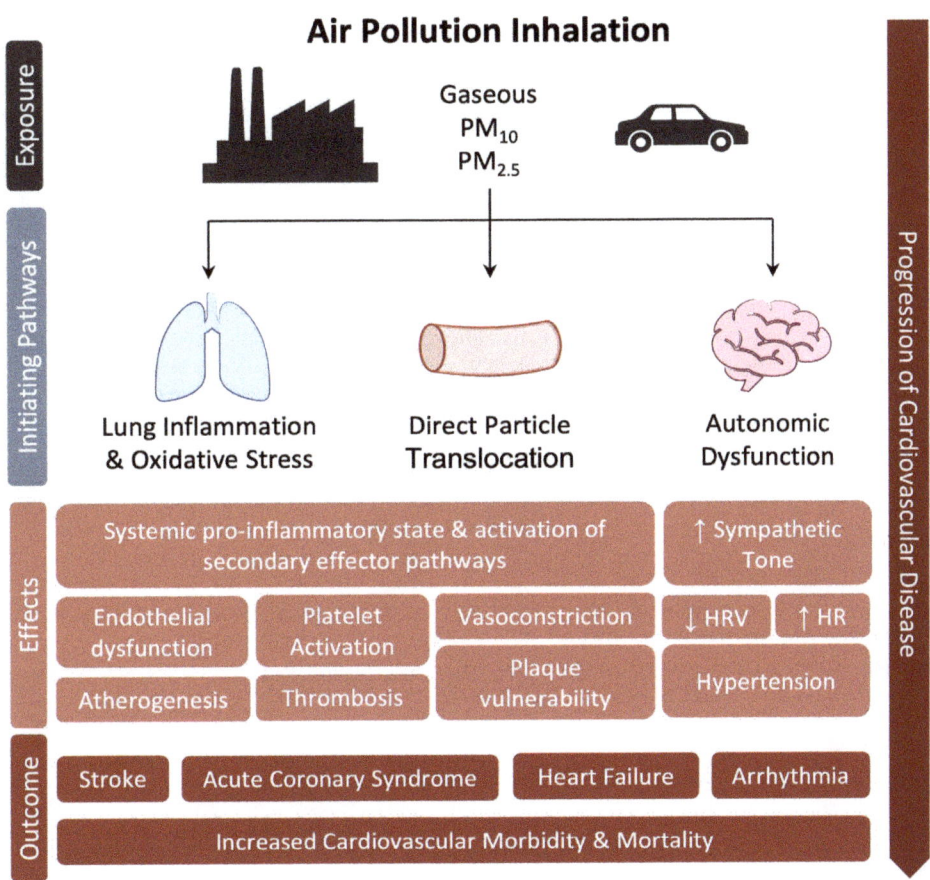

Figure 8. Molecular mechanisms linked air pollution to CVD.

4.3. Climate Change: The Impact of Temperature

Temperature and its extreme variation is now recognized as a cardiovascular risk factor [204–206]. A very recent analysis evaluating 32,000 cardiovascular deaths in 27 countries on 5 continents over 40 years support the role of extremely hot or cold temperatures in determining heart disease deaths [206]. Mortality and morbidity induced by climate change are not exclusively due to hypothermia or hyperthermia, but also to indirect causes, such as respiratory diseases and CVDs, which can be undetected when the human body tries to adapt to climate changes [207]. A relationship between mortality from CVD and temperature exists with a U-, V-, or J shaped curve [208–210]. While the correlation between temperature and CVD has been established, the role of diurnal temperature range (DTR), defined as the difference between the maximum and minimum temperatures recorded in one day, in determining CV events needs to be better evaluated. Extreme cold weather conditions associated to climate change contributes to an increase in temperature variability that might increase clinical cardiovascular events [205]. It is known that exposure to cold activates both the sympathetic nervous system (SNS) and the renin-angiotensin-aldosterone system (RAAS), which interact with each other, leading to HTN and myocardial damage [211]. Skin blood flow (SBF) is reduced in response to cold due to vasoconstriction and increased urine output, thus inducing dehydration, hemoconcentration, and hyperviscosity [212]. Furthermore, eNOS and adiponectin inhibition contributes to endothelial dysfunction and lipid deposition, thus favoring atherosclerosis and plaque instability. Cold exposure also triggers mitochondrial dysfunction with myocardial damage, cardiac hypertrophy, and cardiac dysfunction. The increase in cardiac work and peripheral resistance contributes to an increase in oxygen consumption and a reduction in the ischemic threshold [211], which is clinically relevant, especially when the coronary circulation is already compromised.

On the contrary, exposure to heat leads to increased blood flow and sweating with loss of fluids and dehydration. The resulting hemoconcentration and hyperviscosity may cause thromboembolism, leading to increased risk of ischemic stroke [213]. In the presence of heat stroke, the increase in core temperature redistributes the flow on the skin to facilitate heat loss. Intestinal blood flow is reduced, and this could cause increased permeability of the intestinal epithelium, allowing bacteria, their toxic cell wall component LPS, or HMBG1 to move from the intestinal lumen into the circulation. TLR4 recognizes these molecules, stimulating innate and adaptive immune responses and causing systemic inflammatory response syndrome (SIRS). Along with this, hyperthermia induces the occlusion of arterioles and capillaries (microcirculatory thrombosis) or excessive bleeding (consumptive coagulation), leading to multiorgan dysfunction. The putative mechanisms linking climate changes and CVD is provided in Figure 9.

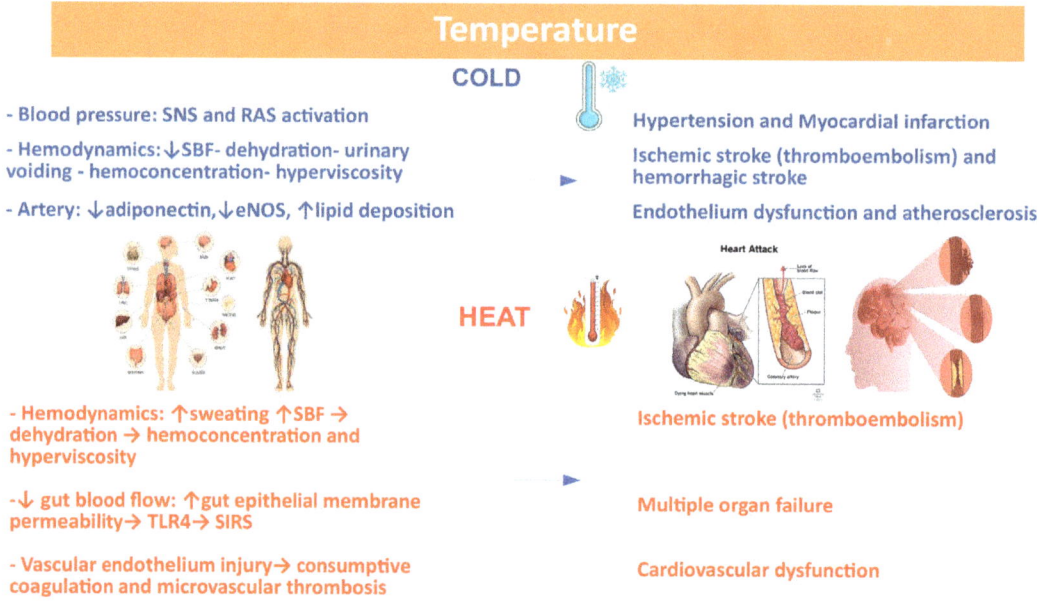

Figure 9. Correlation between climate changes and CVD: possible basic mechanisms. Several variables affect the response to temperature changes.

- Gender: historically, sex differences in thermoregulation were often assumed due to anthropometric factors. However, there is no evidence that women are at greater risk of heat illness when the usual risk-management techniques are in place regarding exercise intensity, clothing, and hydration [214]. It is still matter of debate whether the documented influences of reproductive hormones on thermoregulatory mechanisms in women result in quantifiable differences between the sexes in the capacity to dissipate heat [214]. In males, winter cold may play a role in the constriction of major epicardial vessels. In women, the greatest number of events occurs in the autumn and not in the winter, of which the mechanism remains unclear and should consider the different coronary anatomy (less elastic, smaller coronaries and fewer collateral circulations) [215]. In women in whom microvascular angina is more common, cold exposure could exacerbate its onset [216]. Furthermore, women have a higher temperature threshold beyond which the sweating mechanisms are activated and a lower production of sweat than men, which leads to less heat loss by evaporation and greater susceptibility to the effects of heat. Conversely, males had a greater reduction in core body temperature when exposed to cold, which could explain the higher cardiovascular risk and mortality in response to the cold [214]. Despite these pathophysiological difference, a recent meta-analysis indicates that gender did not affect the seasonal dynamics of myocardial infarction, with a trend of higher susceptibility in men than in women [217].

- Age: the elderly are more vulnerable to low temperatures, whose thermoregulatory capacity is often compromised (especially 65–75 or >75 years) [216,218], with exposure to heat, people > 60 years respond with less sweating, reduced blood flow to the skin, less increase in cardiac output, and less redistribution of splanchnic and renal blood flow than younger people. On the other hand, during exposure to the cold, elderly people respond with reduced peripheral vasoconstriction (implying greater heat loss) and reduced metabolic heat production.
- Regional differences: people living in metropolitan areas have greater socio-economic resources, medical resources, and a better ability to adapt, with lower mortality than people living in rural areas [219].
- Occupational exposure: heat exposure is an increasingly severe challenge, especially to those susceptible occupations (miners, farmers) [220].
- Diabetes: characterized by endothelial dysfunction and hypercoagulability. Several factors, such as oxidative stress and protein kinase C, could contribute to microvascular damage from hyperglycemia. The cold could affect diabetic patients more. The impaired thermoregulation and the reduced autonomic control could explain why diabetic patients are more vulnerable to warm temperatures [221].
- Cardiovascular diseases: patients with prior MI are more susceptible to extreme temperatures; endothelin 1, an indicator of vascular damage, is higher in these patients in response to cold than in the healthy population.
- Kidney disease: renal disorders are commonly associated with increased blood pressure, which is also an additional effect of extreme cold temperatures.
- Hypertension: among patients with a history of hypertension, increased urea/creatinine levels, a marker of dehydration, have been observed in response to climate change.

Traditional risk factors as well as hormones and environmental factors (air pollution and infections) have seasonal variability with a winter cluster [222,223].

A negative relationship has been also observed between cardiovascular events and humidity [224]. When the air has a high percentage of humidity, perspiration and thermal homeostasis processes could be impaired, which would increase respiratory fatigue and heart rate [224].

In recent years, the increased concentrations of greenhouse gases due to human activities have led to an increase in temperatures. Unfortunately, the modification of this risk factor requires a major effort worldwide with green political strategies able to reduce the impact of global warming in the next few decades.

4.4. Sleep Duration: Is There a Right Time for Cardiovascular Benefits?

The correlation between sleep duration (even napping) and CVD has been investigated in the last few decades. Some studies focused on "short sleep", defined as sleep time < 6 h/night, while others have focused on "long sleep", defined as sleep time > 9 h/night [225]. The most dated studies do not support this correlation [226]. However, recent evidence suggest a link between sleep duration and CVD development and outcome [227–230].

The MORGEN study (Sleep Duration and Sleep Quality in Relation to 12-Year Cardiovascular Disease Incidence) [231] has evaluated sleep length and quality in 20,432 subjects between 20–65-year-olds with no previous diagnosis of CVD during a follow-up period of 10–15 years. The population was stratified into short sleepers (<6 h), normal sleepers (7–8 h), and long sleepers (>9 h). Short sleepers showed a 15% higher risk of CVDs and 23% higher of CHD that increased up to 63% and 79% if a short sleep duration was associated with poor sleep quality. According to these data, a long sleep duration was not associated with increased risk of CVD or CHD. It has been reported that sleep restriction is associated with metabolic changes [232] with impaired fasting glucose (probably because of elevation in cortisol level) and higher energy intake due to altered production of hormones, such as leptin and ghrelin [233]. In addition, hyperactivation of the sympathetic branch of the autonomic nervous system, inflammation pathways (including secretion of IL-6 and TNF-alpha), and oxidative system proteins (such as myeloperoxidase) have been described [234]. Moreover, a higher risk of HTN and metabolic syndrome as well as higher arrhythmic risk (mainly AF) have also been linked to sleep deprivation [235–237]. More recent evidence has led researchers to reconsider the correlation between prolonged sleep duration (>9 h) and cardiovascular risk, such as stroke, CVD, CHD, obesity, and diabetes mellitus [238]. This risk is exponentially related with an increase in the hours of sleep. The PURE study, enrolling 116,632 subjects from seven different regions, showed a J-shaped correlation between sleep hours and mortality or major cardiovascular events, with an estimated minimum risk between 6–8 h/day of sleep, including both night and daytime rest (daytime naps) [230]. These findings were corroborated by other observations, too [239–241]. A more recent prospective study on 33,883 adults aged 20–74 years old also support this correlation, pointing out the driving role of underlying conditions (HTN and diabetes) [228]. This increased risk seems to be related to several factors, including inflammation markers and vascular diseases, a sense of fatigue and lethargy during the day and worsening of sleep fragmentation, which has been associated with atherosclerosis [242]. Moreover, long sleepers often have health issues, such as uncontrolled chronic diseases, OSAS or depression, or social discomfort due to low socioeconomic status, unemployment, or a low level of education [243,244], as shown in Figure 10.

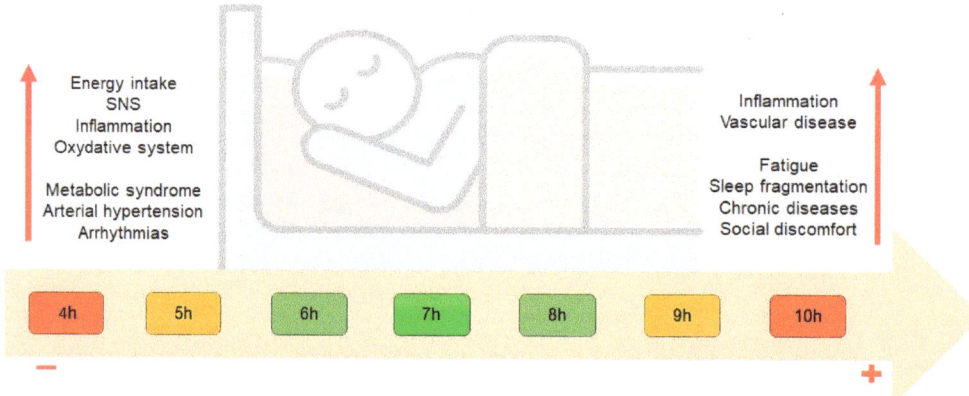

Figure 10. Association between Sleep duration and CVD.

A summary of mechanisms involved in the relationship between non-metabolic risk factor and CVDs has provided in Table 2.

Table 2. Non-metabolic risk factors.

Risk Factor	Observed Effects/Impact on Conventional CV Risk Factors	Mechanisms
Obstructive sleep apnea syndrome	HTN, AF and other arrhythmias, HF, CAD, stroke, pulmonary hypertension, metabolic syndrome and diabetes	Hyperactivation of SNS; systemic oxidative stress; endothelial dysfunction; systemic inflammation; atherosclerosis; higher plasma leptin levels; glucose metabolism impairment and insulin resistance

Table 2. *Cont.*

Risk Factor	Observed Effects/Impact on Conventional CV Risk Factors	Mechanisms
Air Pollution	HTN, endothelial dysfunction, increased atherosclerotic plaque vulnerability and activation of prothrombotic and proarrhythmic state	Systemic oxidative stress & Inflammation, autonomic imbalance in favor of sympathetic tone
Air temperature	-Cold: HTN, atherosclerosis, stroke -Heat: stroke, multiple organ failure, cardiovascular dysfunction	-Cold: SNS and RAAS activation; lipid deposition; dehydration, urinary voiding and hemoconcentration -Heat: dehydration and hemoconcentration; gut epithelial membrane permeability and SIRS; vascular endothelium injury
Sleep duration	Increased CVD risk and HTN in both short and long sleep duration	Short: metabolic changes, hyperactivation of ANS, inflammation and oxidative system protein. Long: increased inflammation, vascular disease, atherosclerosis. Association to uncontrolled chronic diseases and social discomfort.

5. Discussion

An evaluation of cardiovascular risk has evolved in the last few years. The optimistic expectations in managing traditional risk factors, such as HTN, hypercholesterolemia, hyperglycemia, and smoking, to reduce the burden of CVDs have been largely unmet. Clinicians and researchers have clearly realized that traditional risk factors may explain only part of the occurrence of acute events in the general population.

A risk factor is a factor associated with a greater probability of the onset of the disease. It must possess two fundamental characteristics: (1) constant (frequent) association and (2) plausible temporal sequence. An etiological or causal factor is a condition directly implicated in the determinism of the disease. It must meet the following requirements: biological plausibility, biological gradient of effects, strength of association, and specificity of the association. Starting from this statement, non-conventional risk factors are now emerging to better define cardiovascular risk profile. Several efforts have been made in exploring newer metabolic and non-metabolic risk factors and how they may affect cardiovascular outcome. The present article summarize the available evidence on these emerging factors and surrogates supporting the need for further researches to better address the controversial points.

On behalf of metabolic risk factors, homocysteine, UA and Vitamin D levels, gut microbiota status, Lp(a), and MS seem to be clearly linked to CVDs.

Although the role of homocysteine as a strong and independent cardiovascular risk factor is clear at present, conflicting data exist on the effect of the hyperhomocisteinamia lowering strategy and cardiovascular benefits. Observational studies and meta-analyses exploring the folic acid and vitamin B12 supplementation to reduce hyperhomocisteinemia seems to be beneficial in both primary and secondary prevention on the development of CAD and stroke and on the incidence of mortality from cardiovascular causes [245,246]. However, other prospective, randomized, case-controlled, and meta-analyses studies have shown no benefit of hyperhomocysteinemia treatment in the context of primary and secondary prevention of cardiovascular events (CAD, myocardial infarction, cardiovascular death, and all-cause mortality), except for a reduction in the risk of stroke, observed only in some of these meta-analyses [247–254]. Hence, current guidelines on cardiovascular prevention do not suggest serum homocysteine as standard practice in CVD prevention [3]. Better-designed clinical trials are needed to clarify the existing doubts on this regard.

Similarly, UA levels seem to offer a good picture of inflammatory status and coronary atherosclerosis in cardiovascular patients. Currently, the limit value for UA set by the Guidelines is <7 mg/dL in men and <6 mg/dL in women [255]. The URRAH observational study, which included 22,714 patients, defined the cutoff value > 5.6 mg/dL as associated with an increased risk of cardiovascular mortality [256]. Based on the available data correlating UA with the basic/clinical features of CVDs, the use of hypouricemic drugs even at an early age in patients with known CVD or other risk factors could represent a possible effective therapeutic strategy. However, current guidelines fail in defining a clear recommendation for this issue.

Vitamin D is another promising additional marker for cardiovascular evaluation, but the controversial findings from the clinical trial published to date have limited its predictive value. The primary challenge in investigating the relationship between vitamin D levels and CVD disease lies in distinguishing the cause–effect relationships from statistical correlations. While it is evident that vitamin D levels represent an unconventional cardiovascular risk factor, the existence of a direct causal relationship between vitamin D metabolism and CVD is still a subject of debate. The most controversial trial published to date is the VITAL study [257]. A total of 25,871 participants were enrolled to evaluate the effect of vitamin D supplementation on cardiovascular prevention [257]. However, only 15,787 vitamin D levels were available. Of these participants, only 12,7% (2005 subjects) were vitamin D deficient (with a value below 20 ng/dL), and 32,2% were insufficient (with a value between 20–30 ng/dL). Based on the available literature showing that cardiovascular risk increase for levels below 20 ng/dL [79,258], the number of deficient subjects in VITAL study seems to be too small for any conclusion. Taking into account the antithrombotic and anti-inflammatory properties reported in different experimental model, better-designed clinical trials are needed to finally clarify the role of vitamin D as a marker of CVD.

Gut microbiota is an organ with an important role in host's metabolism due to several systemic effects. Intestinal dysbiosis, through the mechanisms previously described, represents a non-traditional cardiovascular risk factor [259]. A greater knowledge of microbe-microbe and microbe-host relationships could be the prerequisite for targeted strategies for microbiota modulation with the purpose to modify host's immune-inflammatory and metabolic state in the desired direction.

Lp(a), with its distinctive composition, enigmatic functions, and substantial clinical implications, has ignited scientific interest and debate. As research progresses, a more profound comprehension of its pathophysiology could potentially unlock innovative diagnostic tools, therapeutic approaches, and preventive strategies, thereby enhancing our capacity to effectively manage and reduce risks linked to this intriguing lipid particle.

Several epidemiological and clinical studies have clearly shown the relationship between MS and CVD with an estimated risk up to 50–60% [125]. Taking into account that IR is the pathophysiological substrate of MS [127], its early detection by the available markers is of great importance. HOMA index is a reliable marker of IR [135]. It can be easily detected and should be considered by the current SCORE for CV definition.

Metabolic risk factors for CVDs are an evolving concept. Our understanding of their role in modulating cardiovascular pathways is increasing. A recent report has shown that even pre-menopausal breast fat density might predict cardiovascular outcome [260] because of its inflammatory, pro-apoptotic properties, and pleiotropic negative effects on the cardiovascular system [261]. This aspect is of great importance because despite the reported sex difference for incident and recurrent coronary events and all-cause mortality with lower risk in women [262], the presence of overweight and metabolic distress could cause major adverse cardiac events in women via over-inflammation [263] Thus, future researches should take into account most of these novel modulators to better define the metabolic CV risk of the general population.

Other non-metabolic risk factors with pathophysiological implications affect the cardiovascular system. Of these, OSA, air pollution, climate changes, and sleep duration may modify cardiovascular outcome; thus, they should be considered and quantify in defining cardiovascular risk.

OSA is clearly linked to any CVD, and because of its prevalence in general population, it should be added to the current score to define CV outcome. The chronic hypoxia and hypercapnia, induced by the mechanical collapse of the upper airways during sleep, leads to different functional and metabolic changes that, as discussed above, are responsible of the CVD pathogenesis. However, current studies have failed to show cardiovascular benefits from OSA treatment with CPAP [264]. These negative results seem to be related to the poor compliance of the patients to the treatment [264]. Hence, additional trials are needed to solve this issue.

On the contrary, the role of air pollution in CVD has been defined. Considering the evidence to date, the most recent guidelines of the European Society of Cardiology have identified air pollution as a major modifiable risk factor relevant to the prevention and management of CVD [3]. The APHEKOM project, conducted in 25 European cities, calculated that meeting the annual average $PM_{2.5}$ values recommended by the WHO guidelines (annual average 10 mg/m^3) would add up to 22 months of life expectancy at age 30, corresponding to a total of 19.000 delayed deaths [265]. A greater understanding of the mediators underlying the impact of air pollution on human health are needed to spur political forces to the implementation of targeted, effective, and enforceable legislation on global air pollution reduction in order to protect people at risk and reduce the effect on CVD.

Climate change is another well-defined non-conventional risk factor. The consequence of global warming is the exposure of the population to moderate to extremely hot temperatures and less exposure to the cold, with consequences for human health [266]. Several studies have suggested an increase in heat-related mortality. A reduction in risk is often considered a sign of adaptation, either as a result of a physiological acclimatization response to temperature changes (intrinsic adaptation) or through non-climatic factors that contribute to risk reduction (extrinsic adaptation), such as socioeconomic development or personal care [267]. Management of this risk factor should be part of a global strategy with green interventions able to reduce its impact in a close future.

Lastly, evaluation of sleep duration should become part of the medical examination since the available literature support its correlation with CVD [268]. Currently, the most important European and American associations for sleep and CVDs suggest a nocturnal sleep duration, preferably unfragmented, of about 7 h [269,270]. Daytime naps are discouraged, except for subjects who have a nocturnal sleep time below 6 h.

6. Conclusions

Management of CVD is evolving. Current evidence clearly indicates that beyond traditional risk factors, the medical community should start to consider different non-conventional factors and surrogates that may induce pathophysiological changes linked to CVD and outcome. The latest guidelines from international societies still fail to add these emerging factors and surrogates to the available SCORE for cardiovascular risk evaluation and better define the countries at risk taking into account their climate and air pollution status, too. Thus, a major effort should be made by researchers to generate a novel algorithm that by combining conventional and non-conventional risk factors might be more accurate for cardiovascular risk scoring.

Author Contributions: Conceptualization, G.C., F.N. and F.S.L.; software, R.A., L.C., S.C., R.F., M.L., L.M., R.M. and N.M.; formal analysis, R.A., L.C., S.C., R.F., M.L., L.M., R.M. and N.M.; resources, R.A., L.C., S.C., R.F., M.L., L.M., R.M. and N.M.; writing—original draft preparation, R.A., L.C., S.C., R.F., M.L., L.M., R.M. and N.M.; writing—review and editing, G.C., F.N. and F.S.L.; visualization, P.G.; supervision, P.G. All authors have read and agreed to the published version of the manuscript.

Funding: This research received no external funding.

Institutional Review Board Statement: Not applicable.

Informed Consent Statement: Not applicable.

Data Availability Statement: The data presented in this study are available on request from the corresponding author.

Conflicts of Interest: The authors declare no conflict of interest.

Abbreviations

ACC (American College of Cardiology); ACS (acute coronary syndrome); AF (atrial fibrillation); AHI (apnea-hypopnea index); ANS (autonomic nervous system); CAD (coronary artery disease); CAMs (cell adhesion molecules); CHD (congenital heart defects); CO (carbon monoxide); CPAP (continuous positive airway pressure); CRP (C-reactive protein); CSA (central sleep apnea); CV (cardiovascular); CVD (cardiovascular diseases); DALYs (disability-adjusted life years); DTR (diurnal temperature range); EC (endothelial cells); eNOS (endothelial nitric oxide synthetase); FMO (flavin monooxygenase); FXR (farnesoid X receptor); GBD (Global Burden of Disease); HDL (high-density lipoprotein); HF (heart failure); HMGB1 (high mobility group box 1); HRV (heart rate variability); HTN (hypertension); IDL (intermediate-density lipoproteins); IR (insulin resistance); LDL (low-density lipoprotein); Lp(a) (lipoprotein a); LPS (lipopolysaccharide); MS (metabolic syndrome); MI (myocardial infarction); NF-kappaB (nuclear factor kappa B); NO (nitric oxide); NO_2 (nitrogen dioxide); O_3 (ozone); OCT (optical coherence tomography); OSA (obstructive sleep apnea); PM (particulate matter); PLG (plasminogen); PSG (polysomnography); RAAS (renin-angiotensin-aldosterone system); RCTs (randomized controlled trials), ROS (reactive oxygen species); SaO_2 (oxygen saturation); SBF (skin blood flow); SCFAs (short-chain fatty acids); SCORE (Systematic COronary Risk Evaluation); SIRS (systemic inflammatory response syndrome); SNS (sympathetic nervous system); SO_2 (sulfur dioxide); STEMI (ST-elevation myocardial infarction); TF (tissue factor); TFPI (tissue factor pathway inhibitor); TLR (Toll-like receptor); TMAO (trimethylamine N-oxide); TNF-alpha (tumor necrosis factor alpha); UA (uric acid); UVB (ultraviolet B); VDR (vitamin D receptor); VLDL (very low-density lipoprotein); WHO (World Health Organization).

References

1. Mahmood, S.S.; Levy, D.; Vasan, R.S.; Wang, T.J. The Framingham Heart Study and the epidemiology of cardiovascular disease. A historical perspective. *Lancet* **2014**, *383*, 999–1008. [CrossRef]
2. Dzau, V.J.; Antman, E.M.; Black, H.R.; Hayes, D.L.; Manson, J.E.; Plutzky, J.; Popma, J.J.; Stevenson, W. The Cardiovascular Disease Continuum Validated: Clinical Evidence of Improved Patient Outcomes. *Circulation* **2006**, *114*, 2850–2870. [CrossRef]
3. Visseren, F.L.J.; Mach, F.; Smulders, Y.M.; Carballo, D.; Koskinas, K.C.; Back, M.; Benetos, A.; Biffi, A.; Boavida, J.M.; Capodanno, D.; et al. 2021 ESC Guidelines on cardiovascular disease prevention in clinical practice. *Eur. Heart J.* **2021**, *42*, 3227–3337 [CrossRef]
4. Townsend, N.; Kazakiewicz, D.; Wright, F.L.; Timmis, A.; Huculeci, R.; Torbica, A.; Gale, C.P.; Achenbach, S.; Weidinger, F.; Vardas, P. Epidemiology of cardiovascular disease in Europe. *Nat. Rev. Cardiol.* **2022**, *19*, 133–143. [CrossRef] [PubMed]
5. Virani, S.S.; Alonso, A.; Benjamin, E.J.; Bittencourt, M.S.; Callaway, C.W.; Carson, A.P.; Chamberlain, A.M.; Chang, A.R.; Cheng, S.; Delling, F.N.; et al. Heart Disease and Stroke Statistics-2020 Update: A Report From the American Heart Association. *Circulation* **2020**, *141*, e139–e596. [CrossRef]
6. Hackam, D.G. The Changing Epidemiology of Cardiovascular Disease: Two Steps Forward, One Step Back. *Can. J. Cardiol.* **2020**, *36*, 995–996. [CrossRef]
7. Noale, M.; Limongi, F.; Maggi, S. Epidemiology of Cardiovascular Diseases in the Elderly. *Frailty Cardiovasc. Dis. Res. Elder. Popul.* **2020**, *1216*, 29–38. [CrossRef]
8. Lindstrom, M.; DeCleene, N.; Dorsey, H.; Fuster, V.; Johnson, C.O.; LeGrand, K.E.; Mensah, G.A.; Razo, C.; Stark, B.; Varieur Turco, J.; et al. Global Burden of Cardiovascular Diseases and Risks Collaboration, 1990–2021. *J. Am. Coll. Cardiol.* **2022**, *80*, 2372–2425. [CrossRef]
9. Lacey, B.; Herrington, W.G.; Preiss, D.; Lewington, S.; Armitage, J. The Role of Emerging Risk Factors in Cardiovascular Outcomes. *Curr. Atheroscler. Rep.* **2017**, *19*, 28. [CrossRef]
10. Finkelstein, J.D.; Martin, J.J. Homocysteine. *Int. J. Biochem. Cell Biol.* **2000**, *32*, 385–389. [CrossRef]
11. Tchantchou, F. Homocysteine metabolism and various consequences of folate deficiency. *J. Alzheimer's Dis. JAD* **2006**, *9*, 421–427. [CrossRef] [PubMed]
12. Finkelstein, J.D. The metabolism of homocysteine: Pathways and regulation. *Eur. J. Pediatr.* **1998**, *157* (Suppl. S2), S40–S44. [CrossRef] [PubMed]
13. Kang, S.S.; Wong, P.W.; Malinow, M.R. Hyperhomocyst(e)inemia as a risk factor for occlusive vascular disease. *Annu. Rev. Nutr.* **1992**, *12*, 279–298. [CrossRef] [PubMed]
14. Ubbink, J.B.; Vermaak, W.J.; van der Merwe, A.; Becker, P.J. The effect of blood sample aging and food consumption on plasma total homocysteine levels. *Clin. Chim. Act Int. J. Clin. Chem.* **1992**, *207*, 119–128. [CrossRef]

5. Singal, R.; Ferdinand, L.; Das, P.M.; Reis, I.M.; Schlesselman, J.J. Polymorphisms in the methylenetetrahydrofolate reductase gene and prostate cancer risk. *Int. J. Oncol.* **2004**, *25*, 1465–1471. [CrossRef]
6. Sharma, P.; Senthilkumar, R.D.; Brahmachari, V.; Sundaramoorthy, E.; Mahajan, A.; Sharma, A.; Sengupta, S. Mining literature for a comprehensive pathway analysis: A case study for retrieval of homocysteine related genes for genetic and epigenetic studies. *Lipids Health Dis.* **2006**, *5*, 1. [CrossRef]
7. Summers, C.M.; Hammons, A.L.; Mitchell, L.E.; Woodside, J.V.; Yarnell, J.W.; Young, I.S.; Evans, A.; Whitehead, A.S. Influence of the cystathionine beta-synthase 844ins68 and methylenetetrahydrofolate reductase 677C>T polymorphisms on folate and homocysteine concentrations. *Eur. J. Hum. Genet. EJHG* **2008**, *16*, 1010–1013. [CrossRef]
8. Siri, P.W.; Verhoef, P.; Kok, F.J. Vitamins B6, B12, and folate: Association with plasma total homocysteine and risk of coronary atherosclerosis. *J. Am. Coll. Nutr.* **1998**, *17*, 435–441. [CrossRef]
9. Refsum, H.; Nurk, E.; Smith, A.D.; Ueland, P.M.; Gjesdal, C.G.; Bjelland, I.; Tverdal, A.; Tell, G.S.; Nygard, O.; Vollset, S.E. The Hordaland Homocysteine Study: A community-based study of homocysteine, its determinants, and associations with disease. *J. Nutr.* **2006**, *136*, 1731S–1740S. [CrossRef]
10. Bostom, A.G.; Lathrop, L. Hyperhomocysteinemia in end-stage renal disease: Prevalence, etiology, and potential relationship to arteriosclerotic outcomes. *Kidney Int.* **1997**, *52*, 10–20. [CrossRef]
11. Sengul, E.; Cetinarslan, B.; Tarkun, I.; Canturk, Z.; Turemen, E. Homocysteine concentrations in subclinical hypothyroidism. *Endocr. Res.* **2004**, *30*, 351–359. [CrossRef] [PubMed]
12. Papa, A.; De Stefano, V.; Danese, S.; Chiusolo, P.; Persichilli, S.; Casorelli, I.; Zappacosta, B.; Giardina, B.; Gasbarrini, A.; Leone, G.; et al. Hyperhomocysteinemia and prevalence of polymorphisms of homocysteine metabolism-related enzymes in patients with inflammatory bowel disease. *Am. J. Gastroenterol.* **2001**, *96*, 2677–2682. [CrossRef] [PubMed]
13. Desouza, C.; Keebler, M.; McNamara, D.B.; Fonseca, V. Drugs affecting homocysteine metabolism: Impact on cardiovascular risk. *Drugs* **2002**, *62*, 605–616. [CrossRef]
14. Cybulska, B.; Kłosiewicz-Latoszek, L. Homocysteine—Is it still an important risk factor for cardiovascular disease? *Kardiol. Pol.* **2015**, *73*, 1092–1096. [CrossRef]
15. Tripathi, P. Homocysteine- The Hidden Factor and Cardiovascular Disease: Cause or Effect? *Biochem. Anal. Biochem.* **2015**, *4*, 1000237. [CrossRef]
16. Brattstrom, L.; Wilcken, D.E. Homocysteine and cardiovascular disease: Cause or effect? *Am. J. Clin. Nutr.* **2000**, *72*, 315–323. [CrossRef]
17. Wilcken, D.E.; Wilcken, B. The pathogenesis of coronary artery disease. A possible role for methionine metabolism. *J. Clin. Investig.* **1976**, *57*, 1079–1082. [CrossRef]
18. Humphrey, L.L.; Fu, R.; Rogers, K.; Freeman, M.; Helfand, M. Homocysteine level and coronary heart disease incidence: A systematic review and meta-analysis. *Mayo Clin. Proc.* **2008**, *83*, 1203–1212. [CrossRef]
19. Drewes, Y.M.; Poortvliet, R.K.; Blom, J.W.; de Ruijter, W.; Westendorp, R.G.; Stott, D.J.; Blom, H.J.; Ford, I.; Sattar, N.; Wouter Jukema, J.; et al. Homocysteine levels and treatment effect in the PROspective Study of Pravastatin in the Elderly at Risk. *J. Am. Geriatr. Soc.* **2014**, *62*, 213–221. [CrossRef]
20. Boushey, C.J.; Beresford, S.A.; Omenn, G.S.; Motulsky, A.G. A quantitative assessment of plasma homocysteine as a risk factor for vascular disease. Probable benefits of increasing folic acid intakes. *JAMA* **1995**, *274*, 1049–1057. [CrossRef]
21. Nygard, O.; Nordrehaug, J.E.; Refsum, H.; Ueland, P.M.; Farstad, M.; Vollset, S.E. Plasma homocysteine levels and mortality in patients with coronary artery disease. *N. Engl. J. Med.* **1997**, *337*, 230–236. [CrossRef]
22. Homocysteine Studies, C. Homocysteine and risk of ischemic heart disease and stroke: A meta-analysis. *JAMA* **2002**, *288*, 2015–2022. [CrossRef]
23. Peng, H.Y.; Man, C.F.; Xu, J.; Fan, Y. Elevated homocysteine levels and risk of cardiovascular and all-cause mortality: A meta-analysis of prospective studies. *J. Zhejiang Univ. Sci. B* **2015**, *16*, 78–86. [CrossRef]
24. den Heijer, M.; Koster, T.; Blom, H.J.; Bos, G.M.; Briet, E.; Reitsma, P.H.; Vandenbroucke, J.P.; Rosendaal, F.R. Hyperhomocysteinemia as a risk factor for deep-vein thrombosis. *N. Engl. J. Med.* **1996**, *334*, 759–762. [CrossRef] [PubMed]
25. Ray, J.G. Meta-analysis of hyperhomocysteinemia as a risk factor for venous thromboembolic disease. *Arch. Intern. Med.* **1998**, *158*, 2101–2106. [CrossRef] [PubMed]
26. Ospina-Romero, M.; Cannegieter, S.C.; den Heijer, M.; Doggen, C.J.M.; Rosendaal, F.R.; Lijfering, W.M. Hyperhomocysteinemia and Risk of First Venous Thrombosis: The Influence of (Unmeasured) Confounding Factors. *Am. J. Epidemiol.* **2018**, *187*, 1392–1400. [CrossRef] [PubMed]
27. Cheng, S.W.; Ting, A.C.; Wong, J. Fasting total plasma homocysteine and atherosclerotic peripheral vascular disease. *Ann. Vasc. Surg.* **1997**, *11*, 217–223. [CrossRef] [PubMed]
28. Vasan, R.S.; Beiser, A.; D'Agostino, R.B.; Levy, D.; Selhub, J.; Jacques, P.F.; Rosenberg, I.H.; Wilson, P.W. Plasma homocysteine and risk for congestive heart failure in adults without prior myocardial infarction. *JAMA* **2003**, *289*, 1251–1257. [CrossRef]
29. Veeranna, V.; Zalawadiya, S.K.; Niraj, A.; Pradhan, J.; Ference, B.; Burack, R.C.; Jacob, S.; Afonso, L. Homocysteine and reclassification of cardiovascular disease risk. *J. Am. Coll. Cardiol.* **2011**, *58*, 1025–1033. [CrossRef]
30. Yuan, D.; Chu, J.; Lin, H.; Zhu, G.; Qian, J.; Yu, Y.; Yao, T.; Ping, F.; Chen, F.; Liu, X. Mechanism of homocysteine-mediated endothelial injury and its consequences for atherosclerosis. *Front. Cardiovasc. Med.* **2022**, *9*, 1109445. [CrossRef]

41. Cai, H.; Harrison, D.G. Endothelial dysfunction in cardiovascular diseases: The role of oxidant stress. *Circ. Res.* **2000**, *87*, 840–844. [CrossRef] [PubMed]
42. Nedvetsky, P.I.; Sessa, W.C.; Schmidt, H.H. There's NO binding like NOS binding: Protein-protein interactions in NO/cGMP signaling. *Proc. Natl. Acad. Sci. USA* **2002**, *99*, 16510–16512. [CrossRef] [PubMed]
43. Poddar, R.; Sivasubramanian, N.; DiBello, P.M.; Robinson, K.; Jacobsen, D.W. Homocysteine induces expression and secretion of monocyte chemoattractant protein-1 and interleukin-8 in human aortic endothelial cells: Implications for vascular disease. *Circulation* **2001**, *103*, 2717–2723. [CrossRef]
44. Lei, W.; Long, Y.; Li, S.; Liu, Z.; Zhu, F.; Hou, F.F.; Nie, J. Homocysteine Induces Collagen I Expression by Downregulating Histone Methyltransferase G9a. *PLoS ONE* **2015**, *10*, e0130421. [CrossRef] [PubMed]
45. Tsai, J.C.; Perrella, M.A.; Yoshizumi, M.; Hsieh, C.M.; Haber, E.; Schlegel, R.; Lee, M.E. Promotion of vascular smooth muscle cell growth by homocysteine: A link to atherosclerosis. *Proc. Natl. Acad. Sci. USA* **1994**, *91*, 6369–6373. [CrossRef] [PubMed]
46. Dalton, M.L.; Gadson, P.F., Jr.; Wrenn, R.W.; Rosenquist, T.H. Homocysteine signal cascade: Production of phospholipids, activation of protein kinase C, and the induction of c-fos and c-myb in smooth muscle cells. *FASEB J. Off. Publ. Fed. Am. Soc. Exp. Biol.* **1997**, *11*, 703–711. [CrossRef] [PubMed]
47. Nishio, E.; Watanabe, Y. Homocysteine as a modulator of platelet-derived growth factor action in vascular smooth muscle cells: A possible role for hydrogen peroxide. *Br. J. Pharmacol.* **1997**, *122*, 269–274. [CrossRef]
48. Rolland, P.H.; Friggi, A.; Barlatier, A.; Piquet, P.; Latrille, V.; Faye, M.M.; Guillou, J.; Charpiot, P.; Bodard, H.; Ghiringhelli, O.; et al. Hyperhomocysteinemia-induced vascular damage in the minipig. Captopril-hydrochlorothiazide combination prevents elastic alterations. *Circulation* **1995**, *91*, 1161–1174. [CrossRef]
49. Malinow, M.R.; Nieto, F.J.; Szklo, M.; Chambless, L.E.; Bond, G. Carotid artery intimal-medial wall thickening and plasma homocyst(e)ine in asymptomatic adults. The Atherosclerosis Risk in Communities Study. *Circulation* **1993**, *87*, 1107–1113. [CrossRef]
50. Voutilainen, S.; Alfthan, G.; Nyyssonen, K.; Salonen, R.; Salonen, J.T. Association between elevated plasma total homocysteine and increased common carotid artery wall thickness. *Ann. Med.* **1998**, *30*, 300–306. [CrossRef]
51. Arcaro, G.; Fava, C.; Dagradi, R.; Faccini, G.; Gaino, S.; Degan, M.; Lechi, C.; Lechi, A.; Minuz, P. Acute hyperhomocysteinemia induces a reduction in arterial distensibility and compliance. *J. Hypertens.* **2004**, *22*, 775–781. [CrossRef] [PubMed]
52. Upchurch, G.R., Jr.; Welch, G.N.; Fabian, A.J.; Freedman, J.E.; Johnson, J.L.; Keaney, J.F., Jr.; Loscalzo, J. Homocyst(e)ine decreases bioavailable nitric oxide by a mechanism involving glutathione peroxidase. *J. Biol. Chem.* **1997**, *272*, 17012–17017. [CrossRef] [PubMed]
53. Undas, A.; Brozek, J.; Szczeklik, A. Homocysteine and thrombosis: From basic science to clinical evidence. *Thromb. Haemost.* **2005**, *94*, 907–915. [CrossRef] [PubMed]
54. Coppola, A.; Davi, G.; De Stefano, V.; Mancini, F.P.; Cerbone, A.M.; Di Minno, G. Homocysteine, coagulation, platelet function, and thrombosis. *Semin. Thromb. Hemost.* **2000**, *26*, 243–254. [CrossRef]
55. Fryer, R.H.; Wilson, B.D.; Gubler, D.B.; Fitzgerald, L.A.; Rodgers, G.M. Homocysteine, a risk factor for premature vascular disease and thrombosis, induces tissue factor activity in endothelial cells. *Arterioscler. Thromb. A J. Vasc. Biol.* **1993**, *13*, 1327–1333. [CrossRef]
56. Lentz, S.R.; Sadler, J.E. Inhibition of thrombomodulin surface expression and protein C activation by the thrombogenic agent homocysteine. *J. Clin. Investig.* **1991**, *88*, 1906–1914. [CrossRef] [PubMed]
57. Rodgers, G.M.; Conn, M.T. Homocysteine, an atherogenic stimulus, reduces protein C activation by arterial and venous endothelial cells. *Blood* **1990**, *75*, 895–901. [CrossRef]
58. Nishinaga, M.; Ozawa, T.; Shimada, K. Homocysteine, a thrombogenic agent, suppresses anticoagulant heparan sulfate expression in cultured porcine aortic endothelial cells. *J. Clin. Investig.* **1993**, *92*, 1381–1386. [CrossRef]
59. Midorikawa, S.; Sanada, H.; Hashimoto, S.; Watanabe, T. Enhancement by homocysteine of plasminogen activator inhibitor-1 gene expression and secretion from vascular endothelial and smooth muscle cells. *Biochem. Biophys. Res. Commun.* **2000**, *272*, 182–185. [CrossRef]
60. Maiuolo, J.; Oppedisano, F.; Gratteri, S.; Muscoli, C.; Mollace, V. Regulation of uric acid metabolism and excretion. *Int. J. Cardiol.* **2016**, *213*, 8–14. [CrossRef]
61. Li, L.; Zhang, Y.; Zeng, C. Update on the epidemiology, genetics, and therapeutic options of hyperuricemia. *Am. J. Transl. Res.* **2020**, *12*, 3167–3181. [PubMed]
62. Tian, X.; Chen, S.; Zhang, Y.; Zhang, X.; Xu, Q.; Wang, P.; Wu, S.; Luo, Y.; Wang, A. Serum uric acid variation and the risk of cardiovascular disease: A prospective cohort study. *Eur. J. Intern. Med.* **2023**, *112*, 37–44. [CrossRef] [PubMed]
63. Yu, W.; Cheng, J.D. Uric Acid and Cardiovascular Disease: An Update from Molecular Mechanism to Clinical Perspective. *Front. Pharmacol.* **2020**, *11*, 582680. [CrossRef] [PubMed]
64. Kanbay, M.; Segal, M.; Afsar, B.; Kang, D.H.; Rodriguez-Iturbe, B.; Johnson, R.J. The role of uric acid in the pathogenesis of human cardiovascular disease. *Heart* **2013**, *99*, 759–766. [CrossRef] [PubMed]
65. Zhang, W.; Iso, H.; Murakami, Y.; Miura, K.; Nagai, M.; Sugiyama, D.; Ueshima, H.; Okamura, T.; Epoch-Japan, G. Serum Uric Acid and Mortality Form Cardiovascular Disease: EPOCH-JAPAN Study. *J. Atheroscler. Thromb.* **2016**, *23*, 692–703. [CrossRef] [PubMed]

5. Maruhashi, T.; Hisatome, I.; Kihara, Y.; Higashi, Y. Hyperuricemia and endothelial function: From molecular background to clinical perspectives. *Atherosclerosis* **2018**, *278*, 226–231. [CrossRef]
6. Kushiyama, A.; Okubo, H.; Sakoda, H.; Kikuchi, T.; Fujishiro, M.; Sato, H.; Kushiyama, S.; Iwashita, M.; Nishimura, F.; Fukushima, T.; et al. Xanthine oxidoreductase is involved in macrophage foam cell formation and atherosclerosis development. *Arterioscler. Thromb. Vasc. Biol.* **2012**, *32*, 291–298. [CrossRef]
7. Cimmino, G.; Morello, A.; Conte, S.; Pellegrino, G.; Marra, L.; Golino, P.; Cirillo, P. Vitamin D inhibits Tissue Factor and CAMs expression in oxidized low-density lipoproteins-treated human endothelial cells by modulating NF-kappaB pathway. *Eur. J. Pharmacol.* **2020**, *885*, 173422. [CrossRef]
8. Cimmino, G.; Conte, S.; Marra, L.; Morello, A.; Morello, M.; De Rosa, G.; Pepe, M.; Sugralyev, A.; Golino, P.; Cirillo, P. Uric Acid induces a pro-atherothrombotic phenotype in human endothelial cells by imbalancing TF/TFPI pathway. *Thromb. Haemost.* **2022**, *123*, 64–75. [CrossRef]
9. Wang, M.; Lin, X.; Yang, X.; Yang, Y. Research progress on related mechanisms of uric acid activating NLRP3 inflammasome in chronic kidney disease. *Ren. Fail.* **2022**, *44*, 615–624. [CrossRef]
10. Yu, P.; Zhang, X.; Liu, N.; Tang, L.; Peng, C.; Chen, X. Pyroptosis: Mechanisms and diseases. *Signal Transduct. Target. Ther.* **2021**, *6*, 128. [CrossRef] [PubMed]
11. Cimmino, G.; Gallinoro, E.; di Serafino, L.; De Rosa, G.; Sugraliyev, A.; Golino, P.; Cirillo, P. Uric acid plasma levels are associated with C-reactive protein concentrations and the extent of coronary artery lesions in patients with acute coronary syndromes. *Intern. Emerg. Med.* **2023**. [CrossRef] [PubMed]
12. Grayson, P.C.; Kim, S.Y.; LaValley, M.; Choi, H.K. Hyperuricemia and incident hypertension: A systematic review and meta-analysis. *Arthritis Care Res.* **2011**, *63*, 102–110. [CrossRef]
13. Tamariz, L.; Agarwal, S.; Soliman, E.Z.; Chamberlain, A.M.; Prineas, R.; Folsom, A.R.; Ambrose, M.; Alonso, A. Association of serum uric acid with incident atrial fibrillation (from the Atherosclerosis Risk in Communities [ARIC] study). *Am. J. Cardiol.* **2011**, *108*, 1272–1276. [CrossRef] [PubMed]
14. Maharani, N.; Kuwabara, M.; Hisatome, I. Hyperuricemia and Atrial Fibrillation. *Int. Heart J.* **2016**, *57*, 395–399. [CrossRef]
15. Holick, M.F. Vitamin D Deficiency. *N. Engl. J. Med.* **2007**, *357*, 266–281. [CrossRef]
16. Macdonald, H.M.; Mavroeidi, A.; Fraser, W.D.; Darling, A.L.; Black, A.J.; Aucott, L.; O'Neill, F.; Hart, K.; Berry, J.L.; Lanham-New, S.A.; et al. Sunlight and dietary contributions to the seasonal vitamin D status of cohorts of healthy postmenopausal women living at northerly latitudes: A major cause for concern? *Osteoporos. Int.* **2011**, *22*, 2461–2472. [CrossRef]
17. Dusso, A.S.; Brown, A.J.; Slatopolsky, E. Vitamin D. *Am. J. Physiol. Ren. Physiol.* **2005**, *289*, F8–F28. [CrossRef]
18. Melamed, M.L.; Michos, E.D.; Post, W.; Astor, B. 25-hydroxyvitamin D levels and the risk of mortality in the general population. *Arch. Intern. Med.* **2008**, *168*, 1629–1637. [CrossRef]
19. Kilkkinen, A.; Knekt, P.; Aro, A.; Rissanen, H.; Marniemi, J.; Heliovaara, M.; Impivaara, O.; Reunanen, A. Vitamin D status and the risk of cardiovascular disease death. *Am. J. Epidemiol.* **2009**, *170*, 1032–1039. [CrossRef]
20. Skaaby, T.; Thuesen, B.H.; Linneberg, A. Vitamin D, Cardiovascular Disease and Risk Factors. *Adv. Exp. Med. Biol.* **2017**, *996*, 221–230. [CrossRef] [PubMed]
21. Ginde, A.A.; Scragg, R.; Schwartz, R.S.; Camargo, C.A., Jr. Prospective study of serum 25-hydroxyvitamin D level, cardiovascular disease mortality, and all-cause mortality in older U.S. adults. *J. Am. Geriatr. Soc.* **2009**, *57*, 1595–1603. [CrossRef] [PubMed]
22. Pilz, S.; Dobnig, H.; Nijpels, G.; Heine, R.J.; Stehouwer, C.D.; Snijder, M.B.; van Dam, R.M.; Dekker, J.M. Vitamin D and mortality in older men and women. *Clin. Endocrinol.* **2009**, *71*, 666–672. [CrossRef] [PubMed]
23. Theodoratou, E.; Tzoulaki, I.; Zgaga, L.; Ioannidis, J.P. Vitamin D and multiple health outcomes: Umbrella review of systematic reviews and meta-analyses of observational studies and randomised trials. *BMJ* **2014**, *348*, g2035. [CrossRef]
24. Rostand, S.G. Ultraviolet light may contribute to geographic and racial blood pressure differences. *Hypertension* **1997**, *30*, 150–156. [CrossRef]
25. Bouillon, R.; Carmeliet, G.; Verlinden, L.; van Etten, E.; Verstuyf, A.; Luderer, H.F.; Lieben, L.; Mathieu, C.; Demay, M. Vitamin D and human health: Lessons from vitamin D receptor null mice. *Endocr. Rev.* **2008**, *29*, 726–776. [CrossRef]
26. Li, Y.C.; Kong, J.; Wei, M.; Chen, Z.F.; Liu, S.Q.; Cao, L.P. 1,25-Dihydroxyvitamin D(3) is a negative endocrine regulator of the renin-angiotensin system. *J. Clin. Investig.* **2002**, *110*, 229–238. [CrossRef]
27. Cimmino, G.; Conte, S.; Morello, M.; Pellegrino, G.; Marra, L.; Morello, A.; Nicoletti, G.; De Rosa, G.; Golino, P.; Cirillo, P. Vitamin D Inhibits IL-6 Pro-Atherothrombotic Effects in Human Endothelial Cells: A Potential Mechanism for Protection against COVID-19 Infection? *J. Cardiovasc. Dev. Dis.* **2022**, *9*, 27. [CrossRef]
28. Bolland, M.J.; Grey, A.; Gamble, G.D.; Reid, I.R. The effect of vitamin D supplementation on skeletal, vascular, or cancer outcomes: A trial sequential meta-analysis. *Lancet Diabetes Endocrinol.* **2014**, *2*, 307–320. [CrossRef]
29. Avenell, A.; MacLennan, G.S.; Jenkinson, D.J.; McPherson, G.C.; McDonald, A.M.; Pant, P.R.; Grant, A.M.; Campbell, M.K.; Anderson, F.H.; Cooper, C.; et al. Long-term follow-up for mortality and cancer in a randomized placebo-controlled trial of vitamin D(3) and/or calcium (RECORD trial). *J. Clin. Endocrinol. Metab.* **2012**, *97*, 614–622. [CrossRef]
30. Wang, T.J.; Pencina, M.J.; Booth, S.L.; Jacques, P.F.; Ingelsson, E.; Lanier, K.; Benjamin, E.J.; D'Agostino, R.B.; Wolf, M.; Vasan, R.S. Vitamin D deficiency and risk of cardiovascular disease. *Circulation* **2008**, *117*, 503–511. [CrossRef] [PubMed]
31. Bjelakovic, G.; Gluud, L.L.; Nikolova, D.; Whitfield, K.; Wetterslev, J.; Simonetti, R.G.; Bjelakovic, M.; Gluud, C. Vitamin D supplementation for prevention of mortality in adults. *Cochrane Database Syst. Rev.* **2014**, *1*, CD007470. [CrossRef]

93. Gerard, P. Metabolism of cholesterol and bile acids by the gut microbiota. *Pathogens* **2013**, *3*, 14–24. [CrossRef] [PubMed]
94. O'Hara, A.M.; Shanahan, F. The gut flora as a forgotten organ. *EMBO Rep.* **2006**, *7*, 688–693. [CrossRef] [PubMed]
95. Yoo, J.Y.; Sniffen, S.; McGill Percy, K.C.; Pallaval, V.B.; Chidipi, B. Gut Dysbiosis and Immune System in Atherosclerotic Cardiovascular Disease (ACVD). *Microorganisms* **2022**, *10*, 108. [CrossRef]
96. Choroszy, M.; Litwinowicz, K.; Bednarz, R.; Roleder, T.; Lerman, A.; Toya, T.; Kaminski, K.; Sawicka-Smiarowska, E.; Niemira, M.; Sobieszczanska, B. Human Gut Microbiota in Coronary Artery Disease: A Systematic Review and Meta-Analysis. *Metabolites* **2022**, *12*, 1165. [CrossRef]
97. Koren, O.; Spor, A.; Felin, J.; Fak, F.; Stombaugh, J.; Tremaroli, V.; Behre, C.J.; Knight, R.; Fagerberg, B.; Ley, R.E.; et al. Human oral, gut, and plaque microbiota in patients with atherosclerosis. *Proc. Natl. Acad. Sci. USA* **2011**, *108* (Suppl. S1), 4592–4598. [CrossRef]
98. Ott, S.J.; El Mokhtari, N.E.; Musfeldt, M.; Hellmig, S.; Freitag, S.; Rehman, A.; Kuhbacher, T.; Nikolaus, S.; Namsolleck, P.; Blaut, M.; et al. Detection of diverse bacterial signatures in atherosclerotic lesions of patients with coronary heart disease. *Circulation* **2006**, *113*, 929–937. [CrossRef]
99. Ghosh, S.S.; Wang, J.; Yannie, P.J.; Ghosh, S. Intestinal Barrier Dysfunction, LPS Translocation, and Disease Development. *J. Endocr. Soc.* **2020**, *4*, bvz039. [CrossRef]
100. Palsson-McDermott, E.M.; O'Neill, L.A. Signal transduction by the lipopolysaccharide receptor, Toll-like receptor-4. *Immunology* **2004**, *113*, 153–162. [CrossRef]
101. Cani, P.D.; Amar, J.; Iglesias, M.A.; Poggi, M.; Knauf, C.; Bastelica, D.; Neyrinck, A.M.; Fava, F.; Tuohy, K.M.; Chabo, C.; et al. Metabolic endotoxemia initiates obesity and insulin resistance. *Diabetes* **2007**, *56*, 1761–1772. [CrossRef] [PubMed]
102. McNaught, C.E.; Woodcock, N.P.; Anderson, A.D.; MacFie, J. A prospective randomised trial of probiotics in critically ill patients. *Clin. Nutr.* **2005**, *24*, 211–219. [CrossRef]
103. Feng, W.; Ao, H.; Peng, C. Gut Microbiota, Short-Chain Fatty Acids, and Herbal Medicines. *Front. Pharmacol.* **2018**, *9*, 1354. [CrossRef] [PubMed]
104. Tan, J.; McKenzie, C.; Potamitis, M.; Thorburn, A.N.; Mackay, C.R.; Macia, L. The role of short-chain fatty acids in health and disease. *Adv. Immunol.* **2014**, *121*, 91–119. [CrossRef] [PubMed]
105. Yu, Z.L.; Zhang, L.Y.; Jiang, X.M.; Xue, C.H.; Chi, N.; Zhang, T.T.; Wang, Y.M. Effects of dietary choline, betaine, and L-carnitine on the generation of trimethylamine-N-oxide in healthy mice. *J. Food Sci.* **2020**, *85*, 2207–2215. [CrossRef] [PubMed]
106. Janeiro, M.H.; Ramirez, M.J.; Milagro, F.I.; Martinez, J.A.; Solas, M. Implication of Trimethylamine N-Oxide (TMAO) in Disease: Potential Biomarker or New Therapeutic Target. *Nutrients* **2018**, *10*, 1398. [CrossRef]
107. Zhu, W.; Gregory, J.C.; Org, E.; Buffa, J.A.; Gupta, N.; Wang, Z.; Li, L.; Fu, X.; Wu, Y.; Mehrabian, M.; et al. Gut Microbial Metabolite TMAO Enhances Platelet Hyperreactivity and Thrombosis Risk. *Cell* **2016**, *165*, 111–124. [CrossRef]
108. Sacks, D.; Baxter, B.; Campbell, B.C.; Carpenter, J.S.; Cognard, C.; Dippel, D.; Eesa, M.; Fischer, U.; Hausegger, K.; Hirsch, J.A. Multisociety Consensus Quality Improvement Revised Consensus Statement for Endovascular Therapy of Acute Ischemic Stroke. *Int. J. Stroke Off. J. Int. Stroke Soc.* **2018**, *13*, 612–632. [CrossRef] [PubMed]
109. Just, S.; Mondot, S.; Ecker, J.; Wegner, K.; Rath, E.; Gau, L.; Streidl, T.; Hery-Arnaud, G.; Schmidt, S.; Lesker, T.R.; et al. The gut microbiota drives the impact of bile acids and fat source in diet on mouse metabolism. *Microbiome* **2018**, *6*, 134. [CrossRef]
110. Haeusler, R.A.; Astiarraga, B.; Camastra, S.; Accili, D.; Ferrannini, E. Human insulin resistance is associated with increased plasma levels of 12alpha-hydroxylated bile acids. *Diabetes* **2013**, *62*, 4184–4191. [CrossRef]
111. Kazemian, N.; Mahmoudi, M.; Halperin, F.; Wu, J.C.; Pakpour, S. Gut microbiota and cardiovascular disease: Opportunities and challenges. *Microbiome* **2020**, *8*, 36. [CrossRef] [PubMed]
112. Sardu, C.; Consiglia Trotta, M.; Santella, B.; D'Onofrio, N.; Barbieri, M.; Rizzo, M.R.; Sasso, F.C.; Scisciola, L.; Turriziani, F.; Torella, M.; et al. Microbiota thrombus colonization may influence athero-thrombosis in hyperglycemic patients with ST segment elevation myocardialinfarction (STEMI). Marianella study. *Diabetes Res. Clin. Pract.* **2021**, *173*, 108670. [CrossRef] [PubMed]
113. Nissen, S.E.; Wolski, K.; Cho, L.; Nicholls, S.J.; Kastelein, J.; Leitersdorf, E.; Landmesser, U.; Blaha, M.; Lincoff, A.M.; Morishita, R.; et al. Lipoprotein(a) levels in a global population with established atherosclerotic cardiovascular disease. *Open Heart* **2022**, *9*, e002060. [CrossRef] [PubMed]
114. Schmidt, K.; Noureen, A.; Kronenberg, F.; Utermann, G. Structure, function, and genetics of lipoprotein (a). *J. Lipid Res.* **2016**, *57*, 1339–1359. [CrossRef] [PubMed]
115. Scanu, A.M. Apolipoprotein(a): Structure and biology. *Front. Biosci.* **2001**, *6*, d546. [CrossRef]
116. Rehberger Likozar, A.; Zavrtanik, M.; Šebeštjen, M. Lipoprotein(a) in atherosclerosis: From pathophysiology to clinical relevance and treatment options. *Ann. Med.* **2020**, *52*, 162–177. [CrossRef]
117. Dangas, G.; Mehran, R.; Harpel, P.C.; Sharma, S.K.; Marcovina, S.M.; Dube, G.; Ambrose, J.A.; Fallon, J.T. Lipoprotein(a) and inflammation in human coronary atheroma: Association with the severity of clinical presentation. *J. Am. Coll. Cardiol.* **1998**, *32*, 2035–2042. [CrossRef]
118. Stiekema, L.C.A.; Prange, K.H.M.; Hoogeveen, R.M.; Verweij, S.L.; Kroon, J.; Schnitzler, J.G.; Dzobo, K.E.; Cupido, A.J.; Tsimikas, S.; Stroes, E.S.G.; et al. Potent lipoprotein(a) lowering following apolipoprotein(a) antisense treatment reduces the pro-inflammatory activation of circulating monocytes in patients with elevated lipoprotein(a). *Eur. Heart J.* **2020**, *41*, 2262–2271. [CrossRef]
119. Ferretti, G.; Bacchetti, T.; Johnston, T.P.; Banach, M.; Pirro, M.; Sahebkar, A. Lipoprotein(a): A missing culprit in the management of athero-thrombosis? *J. Cell. Physiol.* **2018**, *233*, 2966–2981. [CrossRef]

20. Loscalzo, J.; Weinfeld, M.; Fless, G.M.; Scanu, A.M. Lipoprotein(a), fibrin binding, and plasminogen activation. *Arterioscler. Off. J. Am. Heart Assoc. Inc.* **1990**, *10*, 240–245. [CrossRef]
21. Ugovšek, S.; Šebeštjen, M. Lipoprotein(a)—The Crossroads of Atherosclerosis, Atherothrombosis and Inflammation. *Biomolecules* **2021**, *12*, 26. [CrossRef]
22. Boffa, M.B.; Marar, T.T.; Yeang, C.; Viney, N.J.; Xia, S.; Witztum, J.L.; Koschinsky, M.L.; Tsimikas, S. Potent reduction of plasma lipoprotein (a) with an antisense oligonucleotide in human subjects does not affect ex vivo fibrinolysis. *J. Lipid Res.* **2019**, *60*, 2082–2089. [CrossRef]
23. The Emerging Risk Factors Collaboration. Lipoprotein(a) Concentration and the Risk of Coronary Heart Disease, Stroke, and Nonvascular Mortality. *JAMA* **2009**, *302*, 412. [CrossRef] [PubMed]
24. Hu, J.; Lei, H.; Liu, L.; Xu, D. Lipoprotein(a), a Lethal Player in Calcific Aortic Valve Disease. *Front. Cell Dev. Biol.* **2022**, *10*, 812368. [CrossRef] [PubMed]
25. Qiao, Q.; Gao, W.; Zhang, L.; Nyamdorj, R.; Tuomilehto, J. Metabolic syndrome and cardiovascular disease. *Ann. Clin. Biochem. Int. J. Lab. Med.* **2016**, *44*, 232–263. [CrossRef] [PubMed]
26. Wu, H.; Ballantyne, C.M. Metabolic Inflammation and Insulin Resistance in Obesity. *Circ. Res.* **2020**, *126*, 1549–1564. [CrossRef] [PubMed]
27. Zhao, X.; An, X.; Yang, C.; Sun, W.; Ji, H.; Lian, F. The crucial role and mechanism of insulin resistance in metabolic disease. *Front. Endocrinol.* **2023**, *14*, 1149239. [CrossRef]
28. Tong, Y.; Xu, S.; Huang, L.; Chen, C. Obesity and insulin resistance: Pathophysiology and treatment. *Drug Discov. Today* **2022**, *27*, 822–830. [CrossRef]
29. Sinha, S.; Haque, M. Insulin Resistance Is Cheerfully Hitched with Hypertension. *Life* **2022**, *12*, 564. [CrossRef]
30. Handy, R.M.; Holloway, G.P. Insights into the development of insulin resistance: Unraveling the interaction of physical inactivity, lipid metabolism and mitochondrial biology. *Front. Physiol.* **2023**, *14*, 1151389. [CrossRef]
31. Caturano, A.; Galiero, R.; Pafundi, P.C.; Cesaro, A.; Vetrano, E.; Palmiero, G.; Rinaldi, L.; Salvatore, T.; Marfella, R.; Sardu, C.; et al. Does a strict glycemic control during acute coronary syndrome play a cardioprotective effect? Pathophysiology and clinical evidence. *Diabetes Res. Clin. Pract.* **2021**, *178*, 108959. [CrossRef] [PubMed]
32. Salvatore, T.; Caturano, A.; Galiero, R.; Di Martino, A.; Albanese, G.; Vetrano, E.; Sardu, C.; Marfella, R.; Rinaldi, L.; Sasso, F.C. Cardiovascular Benefits from Gliflozins: Effects on Endothelial Function. *Biomedicines* **2021**, *9*, 1356. [CrossRef] [PubMed]
33. Salvatore, T.; Galiero, R.; Caturano, A.; Vetrano, E.; Rinaldi, L.; Coviello, F.; Di Martino, A.; Albanese, G.; Marfella, R.; Sardu, C.; et al. Effects of Metformin in Heart Failure: From Pathophysiological Rationale to Clinical Evidence. *Biomolecules* **2021**, *11*, 1834. [CrossRef] [PubMed]
34. Adeva-Andany, M.M.; Martínez-Rodríguez, J.; González-Lucán, M.; Fernández-Fernández, C.; Castro-Quintela, E. Insulin resistance is a cardiovascular risk factor in humans. *Diabetes Metab. Syndr. Clin. Res. Rev.* **2019**, *13*, 1449–1455. [CrossRef]
35. Singh, B.; Saxena, A. Surrogate markers of insulin resistance: A review. *World J. Diabetes* **2010**, *1*, 36–47. [CrossRef]
36. Hernandez, A.V.; Gast, K.B.; Tjeerdema, N.; Stijnen, T.; Smit, J.W.A.; Dekkers, O.M. Insulin Resistance and Risk of Incident Cardiovascular Events in Adults without Diabetes: Meta-Analysis. *PLoS ONE* **2012**, *7*, e52036. [CrossRef]
37. Tietjens, J.R.; Claman, D.; Kezirian, E.J.; De Marco, T.; Mirzayan, A.; Sadroonri, B.; Goldberg, A.N.; Long, C.; Gerstenfeld, E.P.; Yeghiazarians, Y. Obstructive Sleep Apnea in Cardiovascular Disease: A Review of the Literature and Proposed Multidisciplinary Clinical Management Strategy. *J. Am. Heart Assoc.* **2019**, *8*, e010440. [CrossRef]
38. Berry, R.B.; Budhiraja, R.; Gottlieb, D.J.; Gozal, D.; Iber, C.; Kapur, V.K.; Marcus, C.L.; Mehra, R.; Parthasarathy, S.; Quan, S.F.; et al. Rules for scoring respiratory events in sleep: Update of the 2007 AASM Manual for the Scoring of Sleep and Associated Events. Deliberations of the Sleep Apnea Definitions Task Force of the American Academy of Sleep Medicine. *J. Clin. Sleep Med. JCSM Off. Publ. Am. Acad. Sleep Med.* **2012**, *8*, 597–619. [CrossRef]
39. Yeghiazarians, Y.; Jneid, H.; Tietjens, J.R.; Redline, S.; Brown, D.L.; El-Sherif, N.; Mehra, R.; Bozkurt, B.; Ndumele, C.E.; Somers, V.K. Obstructive Sleep Apnea and Cardiovascular Disease: A Scientific Statement from the American Heart Association. *Circulation* **2021**, *144*, e56–e67. [CrossRef]
40. Peppard, P.E.; Young, T.; Barnet, J.H.; Palta, M.; Hagen, E.W.; Hla, K.M. Increased prevalence of sleep-disordered breathing in adults. *Am. J. Epidemiol.* **2013**, *177*, 1006–1014. [CrossRef]
41. Johnson, K.G.; Johnson, D.C. Frequency of sleep apnea in stroke and TIA patients: A meta-analysis. *J. Clin. Sleep Med. JCSM Off. Publ. Am. Acad. Sleep Med.* **2010**, *6*, 131–137. [CrossRef]
42. Worsnop, C.J.; Naughton, M.T.; Barter, C.E.; Morgan, T.O.; Anderson, A.I.; Pierce, R.J. The prevalence of obstructive sleep apnea in hypertensives. *Am. J. Respir. Crit. Care Med.* **1998**, *157*, 111–115. [CrossRef] [PubMed]
43. Fogel, R.B.; Malhotra, A.; White, D.P. Sleep. 2: Pathophysiology of obstructive sleep apnoea/hypopnoea syndrome. *Thorax* **2004**, *59*, 159–163. [CrossRef] [PubMed]
44. Somers, V.K.; Mark, A.L.; Zavala, D.C.; Abboud, F.M. Contrasting effects of hypoxia and hypercapnia on ventilation and sympathetic activity in humans. *J. Appl. Physiol.* **1989**, *67*, 2101–2106. [CrossRef] [PubMed]
45. Somers, V.K.; Dyken, M.E.; Clary, M.P.; Abboud, F.M. Sympathetic neural mechanisms in obstructive sleep apnea. *J. Clin. Investig.* **1995**, *96*, 1897–1904. [CrossRef]
46. Floras, J.S.; Bradley, T.D. Treating obstructive sleep apnea: Is there more to the story than 2 millimeters of mercury? *Hypertension* **2007**, *50*, 289–291. [CrossRef]

147. Hall, M.J.; Ando, S.; Floras, J.S.; Bradley, T.D. Magnitude and time course of hemodynamic responses to Mueller maneuvers in patients with congestive heart failure. *J. Appl. Physiol.* **1998**, *85*, 1476–1484. [CrossRef]
148. Peppard, P.E.; Young, T.; Palta, M.; Skatrud, J. Prospective study of the association between sleep-disordered breathing and hypertension. *N. Engl. J. Med.* **2000**, *342*, 1378–1384. [CrossRef]
149. Suzuki, Y.J.; Jain, V.; Park, A.M.; Day, R.M. Oxidative stress and oxidant signaling in obstructive sleep apnea and associated cardiovascular diseases. *Free Radic. Biol. Med.* **2006**, *40*, 1683–1692. [CrossRef]
150. Ambrosio, G.; Tritto, I. Reperfusion injury: Experimental evidence and clinical implications. *Am. Heart J.* **1999**, *138*, S69–S75. [CrossRef]
151. Ambrosio, G.; Zweier, J.L.; Duilio, C.; Kuppusamy, P.; Santoro, G.; Elia, P.P.; Tritto, I.; Cirillo, P.; Condorelli, M.; Chiariello, M. Evidence that mitochondrial respiration is a source of potentially toxic oxygen free radicals in intact rabbit hearts subjected to ischemia and reflow. *J. Biol. Chem.* **1993**, *268*, 18532–18541. [CrossRef]
152. Schulz, R.; Schmidt, D.; Blum, A.; Lopes-Ribeiro, X.; Lucke, C.; Mayer, K.; Olschewski, H.; Seeger, W.; Grimminger, F. Decreased plasma levels of nitric oxide derivatives in obstructive sleep apnoea: Response to CPAP therapy. *Thorax* **2000**, *55*, 1046–1051. [CrossRef]
153. Schulz, R.; Seeger, W.; Grimminger, F. Serum nitrite/nitrate levels in obstructive sleep apnea. *Am. J. Respir. Crit. Care Med.* **2001**, *164*, 1997–1998. [CrossRef]
154. Logan, A.G.; Perlikowski, S.M.; Mente, A.; Tisler, A.; Tkacova, R.; Niroumand, M.; Leung, R.S.; Bradley, T.D. High prevalence of unrecognized sleep apnoea in drug-resistant hypertension. *J. Hypertens.* **2001**, *19*, 2271–2277. [CrossRef] [PubMed]
155. Hoffstein, V.; Mateika, J. Evening-to-morning blood pressure variations in snoring patients with and without obstructive sleep apnea. *Chest* **1992**, *101*, 379–384. [CrossRef] [PubMed]
156. Leung, R.S.; Bradley, T.D. Sleep apnea and cardiovascular disease. *Am. J. Respir. Crit. Care Med.* **2001**, *164*, 2147–2165. [CrossRef] [PubMed]
157. Loredo, J.S.; Ancoli-Israel, S.; Dimsdale, J.E. Sleep quality and blood pressure dipping in obstructive sleep apnea. *Am. J. Hypertens.* **2001**, *14*, 887–892. [CrossRef] [PubMed]
158. Portaluppi, F.; Provini, F.; Cortelli, P.; Plazzi, G.; Bertozzi, N.; Manfredini, R.; Fersini, C.; Lugaresi, E. Undiagnosed sleep-disordered breathing among male nondippers with essential hypertension. *J. Hypertens.* **1997**, *15*, 1227–1233. [CrossRef]
159. Liu, L.; Cao, Q.; Guo, Z.; Dai, Q. Continuous Positive Airway Pressure in Patients with Obstructive Sleep Apnea and Resistant Hypertension: A Meta-Analysis of Randomized Controlled Trials. *J. Clin. Hypertens.* **2016**, *18*, 153–158. [CrossRef]
160. Patel, N.; Donahue, C.; Shenoy, A.; Patel, E.; El-Sherif, N. Obstructive sleep apnea and arrhythmia: A systemic review. *Int. J. Cardiol.* **2017**, *228*, 967–970. [CrossRef]
161. Roche, F.; Xuong, A.N.; Court-Fortune, I.; Costes, F.; Pichot, V.; Duverney, D.; Vergnon, J.M.; Gaspoz, J.M.; Barthelemy, J.C. Relationship among the severity of sleep apnea syndrome, cardiac arrhythmias, and autonomic imbalance. *Pacing Clin. Electrophysiol. PACE* **2003**, *26*, 669–677. [CrossRef]
162. Shamsuzzaman, A.S.; Winnicki, M.; Lanfranchi, P.; Wolk, R.; Kara, T.; Accurso, V.; Somers, V.K. Elevated C-reactive protein in patients with obstructive sleep apnea. *Circulation* **2002**, *105*, 2462–2464. [CrossRef] [PubMed]
163. Kuniyoshi, F.H.; Garcia-Touchard, A.; Gami, A.S.; Romero-Corral, A.; van der Walt, C.; Pusalavidyasagar, S.; Kara, T.; Caples, S.M.; Pressman, G.S.; Vasquez, E.C.; et al. Day-night variation of acute myocardial infarction in obstructive sleep apnea. *J. Am. Coll. Cardiol.* **2008**, *52*, 343–346. [CrossRef] [PubMed]
164. Zhao, Q.; Liu, Z.H.; Zhao, Z.H.; Luo, Q.; McEvoy, R.D.; Zhang, H.L.; Wang, Y. Effects of obstructive sleep apnea and its treatment on cardiovascular risk in CAD patients. *Respir. Med.* **2011**, *105*, 1557–1564. [CrossRef] [PubMed]
165. Brown, D.L.; Shafie-Khorassani, F.; Kim, S.; Chervin, R.D.; Case, E.; Morgenstern, L.B.; Yadollahi, A.; Tower, S.; Lisabeth, L.D. Sleep-Disordered Breathing Is Associated with Recurrent Ischemic Stroke. *Stroke* **2019**, *50*, 571–576. [CrossRef] [PubMed]
166. Lisabeth, L.D.; Sanchez, B.N.; Lim, D.; Chervin, R.D.; Case, E.; Morgenstern, L.B.; Tower, S.; Brown, D.L. Sleep-disordered breathing and poststroke outcomes. *Ann. Neurol.* **2019**, *86*, 241–250. [CrossRef]
167. Kholdani, C.; Fares, W.H.; Mohsenin, V. Pulmonary hypertension in obstructive sleep apnea: Is it clinically significant? A critical analysis of the association and pathophysiology. *Pulm. Circ.* **2015**, *5*, 220–227. [CrossRef]
168. Oldenburg, O.; Lamp, B.; Faber, L.; Teschler, H.; Horstkotte, D.; Topfer, V. Sleep-disordered breathing in patients with symptomatic heart failure: A contemporary study of prevalence in and characteristics of 700 patients. *Eur. J. Heart Fail.* **2007**, *9*, 251–257. [CrossRef]
169. Phillips, B.G.; Kato, M.; Narkiewicz, K.; Choe, I.; Somers, V.K. Increases in leptin levels, sympathetic drive, and weight gain in obstructive sleep apnea. *Am. J. Physiol. Heart Circ. Physiol.* **2000**, *279*, H234–H237. [CrossRef]
170. Wolk, R.; Somers, V.K. Sleep and the metabolic syndrome. *Exp. Physiol.* **2007**, *92*, 67–78. [CrossRef]
171. Vgontzas, A.N.; Papanicolaou, D.A.; Bixler, E.O.; Hopper, K.; Lotsikas, A.; Lin, H.M.; Kales, A.; Chrousos, G.P. Sleep apnea and daytime sleepiness and fatigue: Relation to visceral obesity, insulin resistance, and hypercytokinemia. *J. Clin. Endocrinol. Metab.* **2000**, *85*, 1151–1158. [CrossRef] [PubMed]
172. Perez Velasco, R.; Jarosinska, D. Update of the WHO global air quality guidelines: Systematic reviews—An introduction. *Environ. Int.* **2022**, *170*, 107556. [CrossRef] [PubMed]
173. Collaborators, G.B.D.R.F. Global burden of 87 risk factors in 204 countries and territories, 1990–2019: A systematic analysis for the Global Burden of Disease Study 2019. *Lancet* **2020**, *396*, 1223–1249. [CrossRef]

74. Liu, C.; Chen, R.; Sera, F.; Vicedo-Cabrera, A.M.; Guo, Y.; Tong, S.; Coelho, M.; Saldiva, P.H.N.; Lavigne, E.; Matus, P.; et al. Ambient Particulate Air Pollution and Daily Mortality in 652 Cities. *N. Engl. J. Med.* **2019**, *381*, 705–715. [CrossRef]
75. Yusuf, S.; Joseph, P.; Rangarajan, S.; Islam, S.; Mente, A.; Hystad, P.; Brauer, M.; Kutty, V.R.; Gupta, R.; Wielgosz, A.; et al. Modifiable risk factors, cardiovascular disease, and mortality in 155 722 individuals from 21 high-income, middle-income, and low-income countries (PURE): A prospective cohort study. *Lancet* **2020**, *395*, 795–808. [CrossRef]
76. Kaufman, J.D.; Adar, S.D.; Barr, R.G.; Budoff, M.; Burke, G.L.; Curl, C.L.; Daviglus, M.L.; Diez Roux, A.V.; Gassett, A.J.; Jacobs, D.R., Jr.; et al. Association between air pollution and coronary artery calcification within six metropolitan areas in the USA (the Multi-Ethnic Study of Atherosclerosis and Air Pollution): A longitudinal cohort study. *Lancet* **2016**, *388*, 696–704. [CrossRef]
77. Brook, R.D.; Rajagopalan, S.; Pope, C.A., 3rd; Brook, J.R.; Bhatnagar, A.; Diez-Roux, A.V.; Holguin, F.; Hong, Y.; Luepker, R.V.; Mittleman, M.A.; et al. Particulate matter air pollution and cardiovascular disease: An update to the scientific statement from the American Heart Association. *Circulation* **2010**, *121*, 2331–2378. [CrossRef]
78. Newby, D.E.; Mannucci, P.M.; Tell, G.S.; Baccarelli, A.A.; Brook, R.D.; Donaldson, K.; Forastiere, F.; Franchini, M.; Franco, O.H.; Graham, I.; et al. Expert position paper on air pollution and cardiovascular disease. *Eur. Heart J.* **2015**, *36*, 83–93. [CrossRef]
79. Rajagopalan, S.; Al-Kindi, S.G.; Brook, R.D. Air Pollution and Cardiovascular Disease: JACC State-of-the-Art Review. *J. Am. Coll. Cardiol.* **2018**, *72*, 2054–2070. [CrossRef]
80. Shah, A.S.; Lee, K.K.; McAllister, D.A.; Hunter, A.; Nair, H.; Whiteley, W.; Langrish, J.P.; Newby, D.E.; Mills, N.L. Short term exposure to air pollution and stroke: Systematic review and meta-analysis. *BMJ* **2015**, *350*, h1295. [CrossRef]
81. Schraufnagel, D.E.; Balmes, J.R.; Cowl, C.T.; De Matteis, S.; Jung, S.H.; Mortimer, K.; Perez-Padilla, R.; Rice, M.B.; Riojas-Rodriguez, H.; Sood, A.; et al. Air Pollution and Noncommunicable Diseases: A Review by the Forum of International Respiratory Societies' Environmental Committee, Part 2: Air Pollution and Organ Systems. *Chest* **2019**, *155*, 417–426. [CrossRef] [PubMed]
82. Stafoggia, M.; Cesaroni, G.; Peters, A.; Andersen, Z.J.; Badaloni, C.; Beelen, R.; Caracciolo, B.; Cyrys, J.; de Faire, U.; de Hoogh, K.; et al. Long-term exposure to ambient air pollution and incidence of cerebrovascular events: Results from 11 European cohorts within the ESCAPE project. *Environ. Health Perspect.* **2014**, *122*, 919–925. [CrossRef] [PubMed]
83. Baldauf, R.W.; Devlin, R.B.; Gehr, P.; Giannelli, R.; Hassett-Sipple, B.; Jung, H.; Martini, G.; McDonald, J.; Sacks, J.D.; Walker, K. Ultrafine Particle Metrics and Research Considerations: Review of the 2015 UFP Workshop. *Int. J. Environ. Res. Public Health* **2016**, *13*, 1054. [CrossRef] [PubMed]
84. Shukla, A.; Timblin, C.; BeruBe, K.; Gordon, T.; McKinney, W.; Driscoll, K.; Vacek, P.; Mossman, B.T. Inhaled particulate matter causes expression of nuclear factor (NF)-kappaB-related genes and oxidant-dependent NF-kappaB activation in vitro. *Am. J. Respir. Cell Mol. Biol.* **2000**, *23*, 182–187. [CrossRef] [PubMed]
85. Roy, A.; Gong, J.; Thomas, D.C.; Zhang, J.; Kipen, H.M.; Rich, D.Q.; Zhu, T.; Huang, W.; Hu, M.; Wang, G.; et al. The cardiopulmonary effects of ambient air pollution and mechanistic pathways: A comparative hierarchical pathway analysis. *PLoS ONE* **2014**, *9*, e114913. [CrossRef]
86. Daiber, A.; Oelze, M.; Steven, S.; Kroller-Schon, S.; Munzel, T. Taking up the cudgels for the traditional reactive oxygen and nitrogen species detection assays and their use in the cardiovascular system. *Redox Biol.* **2017**, *12*, 35–49. [CrossRef]
87. Haberzettl, P.; Lee, J.; Duggineni, D.; McCracken, J.; Bolanowski, D.; O'Toole, T.E.; Bhatnagar, A.; Conklin, D.J. Exposure to ambient air fine particulate matter prevents VEGF-induced mobilization of endothelial progenitor cells from the bone marrow. *Environ. Health Perspect.* **2012**, *120*, 848–856. [CrossRef]
88. Nemmar, A.; Vanbilloen, H.; Hoylaerts, M.F.; Hoet, P.H.; Verbruggen, A.; Nemery, B. Passage of intratracheally instilled ultrafine particles from the lung into the systemic circulation in hamster. *Am. J. Respir. Crit. Care Med.* **2001**, *164*, 1665–1668. [CrossRef]
89. Kreyling, W.G.; Semmler, M.; Erbe, F.; Mayer, P.; Takenaka, S.; Schulz, H.; Oberdorster, G.; Ziesenis, A. Translocation of ultrafine insoluble iridium particles from lung epithelium to extrapulmonary organs is size dependent but very low. *J. Toxicol. Environ. Health Part A* **2002**, *65*, 1513–1530. [CrossRef]
90. Oberdorster, G.; Sharp, Z.; Atudorei, V.; Elder, A.; Gelein, R.; Lunts, A.; Kreyling, W.; Cox, C. Extrapulmonary translocation of ultrafine carbon particles following whole-body inhalation exposure of rats. *J. Toxicol. Environ. Health Part A* **2002**, *65*, 1531–1543. [CrossRef]
91. Miller, M.R.; Raftis, J.B.; Langrish, J.P.; McLean, S.G.; Samutrtai, P.; Connell, S.P.; Wilson, S.; Vesey, A.T.; Fokkens, P.H.B.; Boere, A.J.F.; et al. Inhaled Nanoparticles Accumulate at Sites of Vascular Disease. *ACS Nano* **2017**, *11*, 4542–4552. [CrossRef] [PubMed]
92. Nemmar, A.; Hoet, P.H.; Dinsdale, D.; Vermylen, J.; Hoylaerts, M.F.; Nemery, B. Diesel exhaust particles in lung acutely enhance experimental peripheral thrombosis. *Circulation* **2003**, *107*, 1202–1208. [CrossRef] [PubMed]
93. Jacobs, L.; Emmerechts, J.; Mathieu, C.; Hoylaerts, M.F.; Fierens, F.; Hoet, P.H.; Nemery, B.; Nawrot, T.S. Air pollution related prothrombotic changes in persons with diabetes. *Environ. Health Perspect.* **2010**, *118*, 191–196. [CrossRef] [PubMed]
94. Ying, Z.; Xu, X.; Bai, Y.; Zhong, J.; Chen, M.; Liang, Y.; Zhao, J.; Liu, D.; Morishita, M.; Sun, Q.; et al. Long-term exposure to concentrated ambient PM2.5 increases mouse blood pressure through abnormal activation of the sympathetic nervous system: A role for hypothalamic inflammation. *Environ. Health Perspect.* **2014**, *122*, 79–86. [CrossRef] [PubMed]
95. Bartoli, C.R.; Wellenius, G.A.; Coull, B.A.; Akiyama, I.; Diaz, E.A.; Lawrence, J.; Okabe, K.; Verrier, R.L.; Godleski, J.J. Concentrated ambient particles alter myocardial blood flow during acute ischemia in conscious canines. *Environ. Health Perspect.* **2009**, *117*, 333–337. [CrossRef] [PubMed]

196. Niu, Z.; Liu, F.; Li, B.; Li, N.; Yu, H.; Wang, Y.; Tang, H.; Chen, X.; Lu, Y.; Cheng, Z.; et al. Acute effect of ambient fine particulate matter on heart rate variability: An updated systematic review and meta-analysis of panel studies. *Environ. Health Prev. Med.* **2020**, *25*, 77. [CrossRef] [PubMed]
197. Task Force of the European Society of Cardiology and the North American Society of Pacing and Electrophysiology. Heart rate variability: Standards of measurement, physiological interpretation and clinical use. *Circulation* **1996**, *93*, 1043–1065. [CrossRef]
198. Mustafic, H.; Jabre, P.; Caussin, C.; Murad, M.H.; Escolano, S.; Tafflet, M.; Perier, M.C.; Marijon, E.; Vernerey, D.; Empana, J.P.; et al. Main air pollutants and myocardial infarction: A systematic review and meta-analysis. *JAMA* **2012**, *307*, 713–721. [CrossRef]
199. Pope, C.A.; Muhlestein, J.B.; Anderson, J.L.; Cannon, J.B.; Hales, N.M.; Meredith, K.G.; Le, V.; Horne, B.D. Short-Term Exposure to Fine Particulate Matter Air Pollution Is Preferentially Associated with the Risk of ST-Segment Elevation Acute Coronary Events. *J. Am. Heart Assoc.* **2015**, *4*, e002506. [CrossRef]
200. Baneras, J.; Ferreira-Gonzalez, I.; Marsal, J.R.; Barrabes, J.A.; Ribera, A.; Lidon, R.M.; Domingo, E.; Marti, G.; Garcia-Dorado, D.; Codi, I.A.M.R.i. Short-term exposure to air pollutants increases the risk of ST elevation myocardial infarction and of infarct-related ventricular arrhythmias and mortality. *Int. J. Cardiol.* **2018**, *250*, 35–42. [CrossRef]
201. Cesaroni, G.; Forastiere, F.; Stafoggia, M.; Andersen, Z.J.; Badaloni, C.; Beelen, R.; Caracciolo, B.; de Faire, U.; Erbel, R.; Eriksen, K.T.; et al. Long term exposure to ambient air pollution and incidence of acute coronary events: Prospective cohort study and meta-analysis in 11 European cohorts from the ESCAPE Project. *BMJ* **2014**, *348*, f7412. [CrossRef] [PubMed]
202. Jilani, M.H.; Simon-Friedt, B.; Yahya, T.; Khan, A.Y.; Hassan, S.Z.; Kash, B.; Blankstein, R.; Blaha, M.J.; Virani, S.S.; Rajagopalan, S.; et al. Associations between particulate matter air pollution, presence and progression of subclinical coronary and carotid atherosclerosis: A systematic review. *Atherosclerosis* **2020**, *306*, 22–32. [CrossRef] [PubMed]
203. Provost, E.B.; Madhloum, N.; Int Panis, L.; De Boever, P.; Nawrot, T.S. Carotid intima-media thickness, a marker of subclinical atherosclerosis, and particulate air pollution exposure: The meta-analytical evidence. *PLoS ONE* **2015**, *10*, e0127014. [CrossRef] [PubMed]
204. Khraishah, H.; Alahmad, B.; Ostergard, R.L., Jr.; AlAshqar, A.; Albaghdadi, M.; Vellanki, N.; Chowdhury, M.M.; Al-Kindi, S.G.; Zanobetti, A.; Gasparrini, A.; et al. Climate change and cardiovascular disease: Implications for global health. *Nat. Rev. Cardiol.* **2022**, *19*, 798–812. [CrossRef] [PubMed]
205. Jacobsen, A.P.; Khiew, Y.C.; Duffy, E.; O'Connell, J.; Brown, E.; Auwaerter, P.G.; Blumenthal, R.S.; Schwartz, B.S.; McEvoy, J.W. Climate change and the prevention of cardiovascular disease. *Am. J. Prev. Cardiol.* **2022**, *12*, 100391. [CrossRef] [PubMed]
206. Alahmad, B.; Khraishah, H.; Royé, D.; Vicedo-Cabrera, A.M.; Guo, Y.; Papatheodorou, S.I.; Achilleos, S.; Acquaotta, F.; Armstrong, B.; Bell, M.L.; et al. Associations Between Extreme Temperatures and Cardiovascular Cause-Specific Mortality: Results From 27 Countries. *Circulation* **2023**, *147*, 35–46. [CrossRef]
207. Kysely, J.; Pokorna, L.; Kyncl, J.; Kriz, B. Excess cardiovascular mortality associated with cold spells in the Czech Republic. *BMC Public Health* **2009**, *9*, 19. [CrossRef]
208. Weerasinghe, D.P.; MacIntyre, C.R.; Rubin, G.L. Seasonality of coronary artery deaths in New South Wales, Australia. *Heart* **2002**, *88*, 30–34. [CrossRef]
209. Rogot, E.; Padgett, S.J. Associations of coronary and stroke mortality with temperature and snowfall in selected areas of the United States, 1962–1966. *Am. J. Epidemiol.* **1976**, *103*, 565–575. [CrossRef]
210. Kan, H.D.; Jia, J.; Chen, B.H. Temperature and daily mortality in Shanghai: A time-series study. *Biomed. Environ. Sci. BES* **2003**, *16*, 133–139.
211. De Lorenzo, F.; Kadziola, Z.; Mukherjee, M.; Saba, N.; Kakkar, V.V. Haemodynamic responses and changes of haemostatic risk factors in cold-adapted humans. *QJM Mon. J. Assoc. Physicians* **1999**, *92*, 509–513. [CrossRef] [PubMed]
212. Neild, P.J.; Syndercombe-Court, D.; Keatinge, W.R.; Donaldson, G.C.; Mattock, M.; Caunce, M. Cold-induced increases in erythrocyte count, plasma cholesterol and plasma fibrinogen of elderly people without a comparable rise in protein C or factor X. *Clin. Sci.* **1994**, *86*, 43–48. [CrossRef]
213. Gasparrini, A.; Guo, Y.; Hashizume, M.; Lavigne, E.; Zanobetti, A.; Schwartz, J.; Tobias, A.; Tong, S.; Rocklov, J.; Forsberg, B.; et al. Mortality risk attributable to high and low ambient temperature: A multicountry observational study. *Lancet* **2015**, *386*, 369–375. [CrossRef]
214. Yanovich, R.; Ketko, I.; Charkoudian, N. Sex Differences in Human Thermoregulation: Relevance for 2020 and beyond. *Physiology* **2020**, *35*, 177–184. [CrossRef] [PubMed]
215. Wolf, K.; Schneider, A.; Breitner, S.; von Klot, S.; Meisinger, C.; Cyrys, J.; Hymer, H.; Wichmann, H.E.; Peters, A.; Cooperative Health Research in the Region of Augsburg Study, G. Air temperature and the occurrence of myocardial infarction in Augsburg, Germany. *Circulation* **2009**, *120*, 735–742. [CrossRef] [PubMed]
216. Mosca, L.; Banka, C.L.; Benjamin, E.J.; Berra, K.; Bushnell, C.; Dolor, R.J.; Ganiats, T.G.; Gomes, A.S.; Gornik, H.L.; Gracia, C.; et al. Evidence-based guidelines for cardiovascular disease prevention in women: 2007 update. *Circulation* **2007**, *115*, 1481–1501. [CrossRef]
217. Kuzmenko, N.V.; Tsyrlin, V.A.; Pliss, M.G.; Galagudza, M.M. Seasonal dynamics of myocardial infarctions in regions with different types of a climate: A meta-analysis. *Egypt. Heart J.* **2022**, *74*, 84. [CrossRef]
218. Chan, E.Y.; Goggins, W.B.; Yue, J.S.; Lee, P. Hospital admissions as a function of temperature, other weather phenomena and pollution levels in an urban setting in China. *Bull. World Health Organ.* **2013**, *91*, 576–584. [CrossRef]

19. Conlon, K.C.; Rajkovich, N.B.; White-Newsome, J.L.; Larsen, L.; O'Neill, M.S. Preventing cold-related morbidity and mortality in a changing climate. *Maturitas* **2011**, *69*, 197–202. [CrossRef]
20. Petitti, D.B.; Harlan, S.L.; Chowell-Puente, G.; Ruddell, D. Occupation and environmental heat-associated deaths in Maricopa county, Arizona: A case-control study. *PLoS ONE* **2013**, *8*, e62596. [CrossRef]
21. Lavigne, E.; Gasparrini, A.; Wang, X.; Chen, H.; Yagouti, A.; Fleury, M.D.; Cakmak, S. Extreme ambient temperatures and cardiorespiratory emergency room visits: Assessing risk by comorbid health conditions in a time series study. *Environ. Health A Glob. Access Sci. Source* **2014**, *13*, 5. [CrossRef] [PubMed]
22. Crawford, V.L.; McNerlan, S.E.; Stout, R.W. Seasonal changes in platelets, fibrinogen and factor VII in elderly people. *Age Ageing* **2003**, *32*, 661–665. [CrossRef] [PubMed]
23. Ockene, I.S.; Chiriboga, D.E.; Stanek, E.J., 3rd; Harmatz, M.G.; Nicolosi, R.; Saperia, G.; Well, A.D.; Freedson, P.; Merriam, P.A.; Reed, G.; et al. Seasonal variation in serum cholesterol levels: Treatment implications and possible mechanisms. *Arch. Intern. Med.* **2004**, *164*, 863–870. [CrossRef] [PubMed]
24. Panagiotakos, D.B.; Chrysohoou, C.; Pitsavos, C.; Nastos, P.; Anadiotis, A.; Tentolouris, C.; Stefanadis, C.; Toutouzas, P.; Paliatsos, A. Climatological variations in daily hospital admissions for acute coronary syndromes. *Int. J. Cardiol.* **2004**, *94*, 229–233. [CrossRef]
25. Grandner, M.A.; Patel, N.P.; Gehrman, P.R.; Perlis, M.L.; Pack, A.I. Problems associated with short sleep: Bridging the gap between laboratory and epidemiological studies. *Sleep Med. Rev.* **2010**, *14*, 239–247. [CrossRef]
26. Cappuccio, F.P.; Cooper, D.; D'Elia, L.; Strazzullo, P.; Miller, M.A. Sleep duration predicts cardiovascular outcomes: A systematic review and meta-analysis of prospective studies. *Eur. Heart J.* **2011**, *32*, 1484–1492. [CrossRef]
27. Kuehn, B.M. Sleep Duration Linked to Cardiovascular Disease. *Circulation* **2019**, *139*, 2483–2484. [CrossRef]
28. Cui, H.; Xu, R.; Wan, Y.; Ling, Y.; Jiang, Y.; Wu, Y.; Guan, Y.; Zhao, Q.; Zhao, G.; Zaid, M. Relationship of sleep duration with incident cardiovascular outcomes: A prospective study of 33,883 adults in a general population. *BMC Public Health* **2023**, *23*, 124. [CrossRef]
29. Pan, Z.; Huang, M.; Huang, J.; Yao, Z. The association between napping and the risk of cardiovascular disease and all-cause mortality: A systematic review and dose-response meta-analysis. *Eur. Heart J.* **2020**, *41*, ehaa946-2818. [CrossRef]
30. Wang, C.; Bangdiwala, S.I.; Rangarajan, S.; Lear, S.A.; AlHabib, K.F.; Mohan, V.; Teo, K.; Poirier, P.; Tse, L.A.; Liu, Z.; et al. Association of estimated sleep duration and naps with mortality and cardiovascular events: A study of 116 632 people from 21 countries. *Eur. Heart J.* **2019**, *40*, 1620–1629. [CrossRef]
31. Hoevenaar-Blom, M.P.; Spijkerman, A.M.; Kromhout, D.; van den Berg, J.F.; Verschuren, W.M. Sleep duration and sleep quality in relation to 12-year cardiovascular disease incidence: The MORGEN study. *Sleep* **2011**, *34*, 1487–1492. [CrossRef] [PubMed]
32. Tobaldini, E.; Fiorelli, E.M.; Solbiati, M.; Costantino, G.; Nobili, L.; Montano, N. Short sleep duration and cardiometabolic risk: From pathophysiology to clinical evidence. *Nat. Rev. Cardiol.* **2019**, *16*, 213–224. [CrossRef] [PubMed]
33. St-Onge, M.P.; Grandner, M.A.; Brown, D.; Conroy, M.B.; Jean-Louis, G.; Coons, M.; Bhatt, D.L.; American Heart Association Obesity, Behavior Chage, Diabetes; Nutrition Committees of the Council on Lifestyle and Cardiometabolic Health; Council on Cardiovascular Disease in the Young; et al. Sleep Duration and Quality: Impact on Lifestyle Behaviors and Cardiometabolic Health: A Scientific Statement from the American Heart Association. *Circulation* **2016**, *134*, e367–e386. [CrossRef]
34. Faraut, B.; Boudjeltia, K.Z.; Vanhamme, L.; Kerkhofs, M. Immune, inflammatory and cardiovascular consequences of sleep restriction and recovery. *Sleep Med. Rev.* **2012**, *16*, 137–149. [CrossRef]
35. Bock, J.M.; Vungarala, S.; Covassin, N.; Somers, V.K. Sleep Duration and Hypertension: Epidemiological Evidence and Underlying Mechanisms. *Am. J. Hypertens.* **2022**, *35*, 3–11. [CrossRef]
36. Xi, B.; He, D.; Zhang, M.; Xue, J.; Zhou, D. Short sleep duration predicts risk of metabolic syndrome: A systematic review and meta-analysis. *Sleep Med. Rev.* **2014**, *18*, 293–297. [CrossRef] [PubMed]
37. Morovatdar, N.; Ebrahimi, N.; Rezaee, R.; Poorzand, H.; Bayat Tork, M.A.; Sahebkar, A. Sleep Duration and Risk of Atrial Fibrillation: A Systematic Review. *J. Atr. Fibrillation* **2019**, *11*, 2132. [CrossRef]
38. Jike, M.; Itani, O.; Watanabe, N.; Buysse, D.J.; Kaneita, Y. Long sleep duration and health outcomes: A systematic review, meta-analysis and meta-regression. *Sleep Med. Rev.* **2018**, *39*, 25–36. [CrossRef]
39. Yin, J.; Jin, X.; Shan, Z.; Li, S.; Huang, H.; Li, P.; Peng, X.; Peng, Z.; Yu, K.; Bao, W.; et al. Relationship of Sleep Duration with All-Cause Mortality and Cardiovascular Events: A Systematic Review and Dose-Response Meta-Analysis of Prospective Cohort Studies. *J. Am. Heart Assoc.* **2017**, *6*, e005947. [CrossRef]
40. Daghlas, I.; Dashti, H.S.; Lane, J.; Aragam, K.G.; Rutter, M.K.; Saxena, R.; Vetter, C. Sleep Duration and Myocardial Infarction. *J. Am. Coll. Cardiol.* **2019**, *74*, 1304–1314. [CrossRef]
41. Wang, D.; Li, W.; Cui, X.; Meng, Y.; Zhou, M.; Xiao, L.; Ma, J.; Yi, G.; Chen, W. Sleep duration and risk of coronary heart disease: A systematic review and meta-analysis of prospective cohort studies. *Int. J. Cardiol.* **2016**, *219*, 231–239. [CrossRef] [PubMed]
42. Huang, T.; Mariani, S.; Redline, S. Sleep Irregularity and Risk of Cardiovascular Events: The Multi-Ethnic Study of Atherosclerosis. *J. Am. Coll. Cardiol.* **2020**, *75*, 991–999. [CrossRef] [PubMed]
43. Basner, R.C. Cardiovascular morbidity and obstructive sleep apnea. *N. Engl. J. Med.* **2014**, *370*, 2339–2341. [CrossRef]
44. Patel, S.R.; Sotres-Alvarez, D.; Castaneda, S.F.; Dudley, K.A.; Gallo, L.C.; Hernandez, R.; Medeiros, E.A.; Penedo, F.J.; Mossavar-Rahmani, Y.; Ramos, A.R.; et al. Social and Health Correlates of Sleep Duration in a US Hispanic Population: Results from the Hispanic Community Health Study/Study of Latinos. *Sleep* **2015**, *38*, 1515–1522. [CrossRef]

245. Cui, R.; Iso, H.; Date, C.; Kikuchi, S.; Tamakoshi, A.; Japan Collaborative Cohort Study, G. Dietary folate and vitamin b6 and B12 intake in relation to mortality from cardiovascular diseases: Japan collaborative cohort study. *Stroke* **2010**, *41*, 1285–1289 [CrossRef] [PubMed]
246. Wang, Z.M.; Zhou, B.; Nie, Z.L.; Gao, W.; Wang, Y.S.; Zhao, H.; Zhu, J.; Yan, J.J.; Yang, Z.J.; Wang, L.S. Folate and risk of coronary heart disease: A meta-analysis of prospective studies. *Nutr. Metab. Cardiovasc. Dis. NMCD* **2012**, *22*, 890–899. [CrossRef] [PubMed]
247. Huang, T.; Chen, Y.; Yang, B.; Yang, J.; Wahlqvist, M.L.; Li, D. Meta-analysis of B vitamin supplementation on plasma homocysteine, cardiovascular and all-cause mortality. *Clin. Nutr.* **2012**, *31*, 448–454. [CrossRef]
248. Huo, Y.; Li, J.; Qin, X.; Huang, Y.; Wang, X.; Gottesman, R.F.; Tang, G.; Wang, B.; Chen, D.; He, M.; et al. Efficacy of folic acid therapy in primary prevention of stroke among adults with hypertension in China: The CSPPT randomized clinical trial. *JAMA* **2015**, *313*, 1325–1335. [CrossRef]
249. Li, Y.; Huang, T.; Zheng, Y.; Muka, T.; Troup, J.; Hu, F.B. Folic Acid Supplementation and the Risk of Cardiovascular Diseases: A Meta-Analysis of Randomized Controlled Trials. *J. Am. Heart Assoc.* **2016**, *5*, e003768. [CrossRef]
250. Park, J.H.; Saposnik, G.; Ovbiagele, B.; Markovic, D.; Towfighi, A. Effect of B-vitamins on stroke risk among individuals with vascular disease who are not on antiplatelets: A meta-analysis. *Int. J. Stroke Off. J. Int. Stroke Soc.* **2016**, *11*, 206–211. [CrossRef]
251. Tian, T.; Yang, K.Q.; Cui, J.G.; Zhou, L.L.; Zhou, X.L. Folic Acid Supplementation for Stroke Prevention in Patients with Cardiovascular Disease. *Am. J. Med. Sci.* **2017**, *354*, 379–387. [CrossRef] [PubMed]
252. Clarke, R.; Halsey, J.; Lewington, S.; Lonn, E.; Armitage, J.; Manson, J.E.; Bonaa, K.H.; Spence, J.D.; Nygard, O.; Jamison, R.; et al. Effects of lowering homocysteine levels with B vitamins on cardiovascular disease, cancer, and cause-specific mortality: Meta-analysis of 8 randomized trials involving 37 485 individuals. *Arch. Intern. Med.* **2010**, *170*, 1622–1631. [CrossRef] [PubMed]
253. Zhou, Y.H.; Tang, J.Y.; Wu, M.J.; Lu, J.; Wei, X.; Qin, Y.Y.; Wang, C.; Xu, J.F.; He, J. Effect of folic acid supplementation on cardiovascular outcomes: A systematic review and meta-analysis. *PLoS ONE* **2011**, *6*, e25142. [CrossRef] [PubMed]
254. Zhang, C.; Wang, Z.Y.; Qin, Y.Y.; Yu, F.F.; Zhou, Y.H. Association between B vitamins supplementation and risk of cardiovascular outcomes: A cumulative meta-analysis of randomized controlled trials. *PLoS ONE* **2014**, *9*, e107060. [CrossRef]
255. Richette, P.; Doherty, M.; Pascual, E.; Barskova, V.; Becce, F.; Castaneda-Sanabria, J.; Coyfish, M.; Guillo, S.; Jansen, T.L.; Janssens, H.; et al. 2016 updated EULAR evidence-based recommendations for the management of gout. *Ann. Rheum. Dis.* **2017**, *76*, 29–42. [CrossRef]
256. Virdis, A.; Masi, S.; Casiglia, E.; Tikhonoff, V.; Cicero, A.F.G.; Ungar, A.; Rivasi, G.; Salvetti, M.; Barbagallo, C.M.; Bombelli, M.; et al. Identification of the Uric Acid Thresholds Predicting an Increased Total and Cardiovascular Mortality Over 20 Years. *Hypertension* **2020**, *75*, 302–308. [CrossRef]
257. Manson, J.E.; Cook, N.R.; Lee, I.M.; Christen, W.; Bassuk, S.S.; Mora, S.; Gibson, H.; Gordon, D.; Copeland, T.; D'Agostino, D.; et al. Vitamin D Supplements and Prevention of Cancer and Cardiovascular Disease. *N. Engl. J. Med.* **2019**, *380*, 33–44. [CrossRef]
258. Wang, L.; Song, Y.; Manson, J.E.; Pilz, S.; Marz, W.; Michaelsson, K.; Lundqvist, A.; Jassal, S.K.; Barrett-Connor, E.; Zhang, C.; et al. Circulating 25-hydroxy-vitamin D and risk of cardiovascular disease: A meta-analysis of prospective studies. *Circ. Cardiovasc. Qual. Outcomes* **2012**, *5*, 819–829. [CrossRef]
259. Cimmino, G.; Muscoli, S.; De Rosa, S.; Cesaro, A.; Perrone, M.A.; Selvaggio, S.; Selvaggio, G.; Aimo, A.; Pedrinelli, R.; Mercuro, G.; et al. Evolving concepts in the pathophysiology of atherosclerosis: From endothelial dysfunction to thrombus formation through multiple shades of inflammation. *J. Cardiovasc. Med.* **2023**, *24*, e156–e167. [CrossRef]
260. Sardu, C.; Gatta, G.; Pieretti, G.; Viola, L.; Sacra, C.; Di Grezia, G.; Musto, L.; Minelli, S.; La Forgia, D.; Capodieci, M.; et al. Pre-Menopausal Breast Fat Density Might Predict MACE During 10 Years of Follow-Up. *JACC Cardiovasc. Imaging* **2021**, *14*, 426–438. [CrossRef]
261. Sardu, C.; Gatta, G.; Pieretti, G.; Onofrio, N.D.; Balestrieri, M.L.; Scisciola, L.; Cappabianca, S.; Ferraro, M.; Nicoletti, G.F.; Signoriello, G.; et al. SGLT2 breast expression could affect the cardiovascular performance in pre-menopausal women with fatty vs. non fatty breast via over-inflammation and sirtuins' down regulation. *Eur. J. Intern. Med.* **2023**, *113*, 57–68. [CrossRef] [PubMed]
262. Peters, S.A.E.; Colantonio, L.D.; Chen, L.; Bittner, V.; Farkouh, M.E.; Rosenson, R.S.; Jackson, E.A.; Dluzniewski, P.; Poudel, B.; Muntner, P.; et al. Sex Differences in Incident and Recurrent Coronary Events and All-Cause Mortality. *J. Am. Coll. Cardiol.* **2020**, *76*, 1751–1760. [CrossRef] [PubMed]
263. Sardu, C.; Paolisso, G.; Marfella, R. Impact of Sex Differences in Incident and Recurrent Coronary Events and All-Cause Mortality. *J. Am. Coll. Cardiol.* **2021**, *77*, 829–830. [CrossRef]
264. Faria, A.; Macedo, A.; Castro, C.; Valle, E.; Lacerda, R.; Ayas, N.; Laher, I. Impact of sleep apnea and treatments on cardiovascular disease. *Sleep Sci.* **2022**, *15*, 250–258. [CrossRef] [PubMed]
265. Pascal, M.; Corso, M.; Chanel, O.; Declercq, C.; Badaloni, C.; Cesaroni, G.; Henschel, S.; Meister, K.; Haluza, D.; Martin-Olmedo, P.; et al. Assessing the public health impacts of urban air pollution in 25 European cities: Results of the Aphekom project. *Sci. Total Environ.* **2013**, *449*, 390–400. [CrossRef]
266. Watts, N.; Amann, M.; Ayeb-Karlsson, S.; Belesova, K.; Bouley, T.; Boykoff, M.; Byass, P.; Cai, W.; Campbell-Lendrum, D.; Chambers, J.; et al. The Lancet Countdown on health and climate change: From 25 years of inaction to a global transformation for public health. *Lancet* **2018**, *391*, 581–630. [CrossRef]

67. McMichael, A.J.; Woodruff, R.E.; Hales, S. Climate change and human health: Present and future risks. *Lancet* **2006**, *367*, 859–869. [CrossRef]
68. Wang, S.; Li, Z.; Wang, X.; Guo, S.; Sun, Y.; Li, G.; Zhao, C.; Yuan, W.; Li, M.; Li, X.; et al. Associations between sleep duration and cardiovascular diseases: A meta-review and meta-analysis of observational and Mendelian randomization studies. *Front. Cardiovasc. Med.* **2022**, *9*, 930000. [CrossRef]
69. Arnett, D.K.; Blumenthal, R.S.; Albert, M.A.; Buroker, A.B.; Goldberger, Z.D.; Hahn, E.J.; Himmelfarb, C.D.; Khera, A.; Lloyd-Jones, D.; McEvoy, J.W.; et al. 2019 ACC/AHA Guideline on the Primary Prevention of Cardiovascular Disease: A Report of the American College of Cardiology/American Heart Association Task Force on Clinical Practice Guidelines. *Circulation* **2019**, *140*, e596–e646. [CrossRef]
70. Riemann, D.; Baglioni, C.; Bassetti, C.; Bjorvatn, B.; Dolenc Groselj, L.; Ellis, J.G.; Espie, C.A.; Garcia-Borreguero, D.; Gjerstad, M.; Goncalves, M.; et al. European guideline for the diagnosis and treatment of insomnia. *J. Sleep Res.* **2017**, *26*, 675–700. [CrossRef]

Disclaimer/Publisher's Note: The statements, opinions and data contained in all publications are solely those of the individual author(s) and contributor(s) and not of MDPI and/or the editor(s). MDPI and/or the editor(s) disclaim responsibility for any injury to people or property resulting from any ideas, methods, instructions or products referred to in the content.

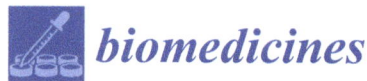

Review

Cardiovascular Diseases: Therapeutic Potential of SGLT-2 Inhibitors

Weronika Frąk, Joanna Hajdys, Ewa Radzioch, Magdalena Szlagor, Ewelina Młynarska *, Jacek Rysz and Beata Franczyk

Department of Nephrology, Hypertension and Family Medicine, Medical University of Lodz, ul. Żeromskiego 113, 90-549 Łódź, Poland; frweronika@gmail.com (W.F.); joanna.hajdys@gmail.com (J.H.); ewa.m.radzioch@gmail.com (E.R.); szlagor.magdalena@gmail.com (M.S.); jacek.rysz@umed.lodz.pl (J.R.); bfranczyk-skora@wp.pl (B.F.)
* Correspondence: emmlynarska@gmail.com; Tel.: +48-(042)-639-37-50

Abstract: Cardiovascular diseases (CVD) are a global health concern, affecting millions of patients worldwide and being the leading cause of global morbidity and mortality, thus creating a major public health concern. Sodium/glucose cotransporter 2 (SGLT2) inhibitors have emerged as a promising class of medications for managing CVD. Initially developed as antihyperglycemic agents for treating type 2 diabetes, these drugs have demonstrated significant cardiovascular benefits beyond glycemic control. In our paper, we discuss the role of empagliflozin, dapagliflozin, canagliflozin, ertugliflozin, and the relatively recently approved bexagliflozin, the class of SGLT-2 inhibitors, as potential therapeutic targets for cardiovascular diseases. All mentioned SGLT-2 inhibitors have demonstrated significant cardiovascular benefits and renal protection in clinical trials, in patients with or without type 2 diabetes. These novel therapeutic approaches aim to develop more effective treatments that improve patient outcomes and reduce the burden of these conditions. However, the major scientific achievements of recent years and the many new discoveries and mechanisms still require careful attention and additional studies.

Keywords: diabetes mellitus; heart failure; sodium/glucose cotransporter 2 (SGLT2) inhibitors; bexagliflozin

Citation: Frąk, W.; Hajdys, J.; Radzioch, E.; Szlagor, M.; Młynarska, E.; Rysz, J.; Franczyk, B. Cardiovascular Diseases: Therapeutic Potential of SGLT-2 Inhibitors. *Biomedicines* **2023**, *11*, 2085. https://doi.org/10.3390/biomedicines11072085

Academic Editors: Willibald Wonisch and Alfredo Caturano

Received: 28 May 2023
Revised: 21 June 2023
Accepted: 20 July 2023
Published: 24 July 2023

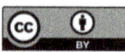

Copyright: © 2023 by the authors. Licensee MDPI, Basel, Switzerland. This article is an open access article distributed under the terms and conditions of the Creative Commons Attribution (CC BY) license (https://creativecommons.org/licenses/by/4.0/).

1. Introduction

Diabetes mellitus (DM) is a metabolic disease related to chronic hyperglycemia caused by impaired insulin secretion and/or action. It occurs mainly in the older population and is often undiagnosed. More than 400 million adults worldwide suffer from it, and it is estimated that this number will increase by more than 50% in the next 20 years [1].

Persistently increased levels of glucose in the blood result in symptoms such as polyuria, polydipsia, drowsiness, or weight loss. The consequences of uncontrolled diabetes are ketoacidosis or nonketotic hyperosmolar syndrome. Chronically elevated blood glucose levels are associated with the development of numerous complications, such as nephropathy, neuropathy, and retinopathy. However, the leading causes of morbidity and mortality in both type 1 and type 2 DM are heart failure and cardiovascular disorders [2].

DM and heart failure (HF) are among the most widespread diseases in the adult population, and their numbers are increasing with age. It is very common for the two illnesses to co-exist in the same patient, and in people over the age of 65, as many as 22% of people with type 2 diabetes have HF simultaneously [2–4]. The co-existence of these two diseases is complex and bidirectional. The risk of developing HF is over twice as high in patients with diabetes than in those without diabetes [5]. Furthermore, it increases the hospitalization rate and worsens cardiovascular outcomes. The prognosis in this group is far worse, and mortality from all causes is enhanced, but especially from cardiovascular causes [6]. Research shows that HF is also an independent predictor of clinical prognosis, both fatal and nonfatal, in patients with DM.

Diabetic cardiomyopathy is a state of ventricular dysfunction in the absence of other cardiac risk factors in diabetics [7]. There are various mechanisms that contribute to diabetic cardiomyopathy. This includes systemic metabolic disorders, subcellular component abnormalities, numerous molecular mechanisms, or dysfunction of the renin–angiotensin–aldosterone system [8].

Most current antidiabetic drugs have an adverse effect by exacerbating cardiovascular risk factors. Some antihyperglycemic therapies, such as the use of insulin or thiazolidinediones, cause weight gain and fluid retention [9], while saxagliptin, a dipeptidylpeptidase 4 (DDP4) inhibitor, is related to an increased risk of HF in comparison to standard treatment [10,11]. New classes of agents are proven to be beneficial for cardiovascular protection. They include glucagon-like peptide-1 receptor agonists (GLP-1 RAs) and sodium/glucose cotransporter 2 (SGLT2) inhibitors. SGLT-2 inhibitors have demonstrated cardiovascular benefits in large-scale clinical trials. The possible mechanisms of these profits are being widely investigated because there is a small likelihood that they are related to improved glycemic control. According to the Empagliflozin Cardiovascular Outcome Event Trial in Type 2 Diabetes Mellitus Patients–Removing Excess Glucose (EMPA-REG OUTCOME) study, treatment with one of the SGLT-2 inhibitors, empagliflozin, decreased the rate of cardiovascular death and hospitalization for HF in diabetic patients [12]. Empagliflozin is especially recommended for patients with prevalent cardiovascular diseases (CVD) to reduce the risk of death [13]. However, the choice of drug for CVD prevention should be based on the presence of risk factors and the co-existence of CVD.

SGLT-2 inhibitors that are nowadays available in the United States are empagliflozin, dapagliflozin, canagliflozin, and ertugliflozin. In the European Union, we also have sotagliflozin. Nevertheless, on 23 January 2023, the U.S. Food and Drug Administration (FDA) approved a new antihyperglycemic agent called bexagliflozin. It has been proven to significantly improve glycemic control with a single daily dose of 20 mg. Importantly, in addition to its hypoglycemic effect, it also shows a systolic blood pressure-lowering effect [14].

The aim of this review is to list, discuss, and compare each individual SGLT-2 inhibitor, with a focus on the recently approved bexagliflozin. We also want to outline the most important properties and side effects of this particular group of medications.

2. Empagliflozin

The SGLT-2 inhibitors, which include empagliflozin, are one of the more recent groups used in antihyperglycemic therapy. On the basis of numerous studies and comparative meta-analyses, it was noted that it significantly reduced HF hospitalizations in patients with both stable cardiovascular disease and acute HF. Empagliflozin reduced all-cause and cardiovascular mortality and reduced the risk of cardiovascular disease, regardless of the initial risk [6,15–17]. It also significantly improved myocardial function in patients, regardless of their ejection fraction levels [18–21]. The mechanisms by which SGLT-2 inhibitors both improve glycemic levels and improve parameters in cardiovascular disease are not fully understood. However, ongoing studies have noted that the use of empagliflozin reduces interstitial fibrosis of the ventricular myocardium, improves aortic stiffness, and induces anti-inflammatory effects [22–26]. As with other SGLT-2 inhibitors, it also reduces the amount of pericardial fat [27]. In addition, improvements in hematocrit and hemoglobin were found in patients, which, like the aforementioned findings, may have contributed to a reduction in HF hospitalizations and mortality in patients both with and without diabetes [18,19,22,28,29].

Preclinical studies report that the use of empagliflozin reverses the effect of glucotoxicity by lowering serum methylglyoxal levels and attenuating AGE/RAGE signaling [30,31]. It was also observed to inhibit NADPH oxidase and reduce reactive oxygen species (ROS) production, leading to a reduction in oxidative stress on endothelial cells. In addition, it led to increased NO production by improving endothelial nitric oxide synthase (eNOS) activity [30,32]. Empagliflozin was also responsible for decreasing the expression of inflammatory molecules such as adhesion molecules (ICAM-1, VCAM-1) and macrophage markers (MCP-1), contributing to the reduced induction of endothelial damage [32]. Empagliflozin also improved endothelial cell health by maintaining the integrity of the glycocalyx [33]. Moreover, the cardioprotective and anti-inflammatory effects of empagliflozin included a reduction in the concentrations of eicosanoids such as PGE2 and TXB2, which led to vascular wall damage and vessel lumen constriction [34]. Notably, empagliflozin contributed to the decline of atherosclerotic plaque by reducing the levels of circulating TNF alpha, IL-6, and MCP-1 in the blood [35].

The first study to evaluate the effect of SGLT-2 inhibitors on cardiovascular events was EMPA-REG OUTCOME [12]. The study was a randomized, double-blind, placebo-controlled trial, and its principal objective was to evaluate the effect of empagliflozin on the occurrence of cardiovascular events in adults with type 2 diabetes and established cardiovascular disease. The primary outcome was the occurrence of one of the events, such as death from cardiovascular causes, nonfatal myocardial infarction, or nonfatal stroke, while the key secondary outcome was the primary outcome along with hospitalization for unstable angina. After a mean follow-up of 3.1 years, it was noted that patients receiving empagliflozin had a significantly lower incidence of the primary outcome compared to the placebo group (10.5% and 12.1%, respectively). In contrast, given the similar incidence of hospitalization for unstable angina in both groups, there was no meaningful difference in the key secondary outcome. Furthermore, it was observed that empagliflozin markedly reduced cardiovascular mortality, any cause mortality, and hospitalization for HF [12]. During follow-up, a slight decrease in weight, systolic and diastolic blood pressure without an increase in heart rate, and elevated hematocrit and hemoglobin values were noted in patients. In a post-analysis of the EMPA-REG OUTCOME trial, it was concluded that an increase in hematocrit and hemoglobin levels was associated with a decreased risk of HF hospitalization and death from HF. This was related to enhanced myocardial function, improved oxygen supply, and reduced cardiac preload and afterload [36].

In the randomized EMPEROR-Reduced trial, 3730 patients with chronic HF (NYHA 2–4) and a left ventricular ejection fraction (LVEF) of 40% or less were screened to assess the effect of empagliflozin on the incidence of cardiovascular death or first HF hospitalization (the first outcome), as well as the rate of all HF hospitalizations (the first-second outcome) [37]. The primary composite outcome appeared in a distinct minority of those subjects who took empagliflozin in comparison to those who took a placebo, 19.4% and 24.7% (HR = 0.75, $p < 0.001$), respectively. The preceding effect was similar in both the diabetic and non-diabetic groups (hazard ratios of 0.72 and 0.78 in comparison with the placebo group, respectively). During the course of the trial, the number of all hospitalizations for HF in patients taking empagliflozin was lower as compared to the placebo group (HR = 0.70, $p < 0.001$). It should also be emphasized that patients experienced significant improvements in cardiovascular and renal outcomes regardless of their baseline diabetes status [21].

A subsequent study was EMPEROR-Preserved [20], enrolling patients with chronic HF (NYHA 2–4) and LVEF above 40%. Both the first outcome and secondary outcomes were similar to those of the EMPEROR-Reduced trial. The onset of the first outcome was lower in the empagliflozin group (13.8%) than in the placebo group (17.1%). Both hospitalizations for HF and deaths from cardiovascular causes decreased. Importantly, the observed changes were the same across subgroups, including patients with diabetes (16.3% vs. 19.8%, HR = 0.79) and without diabetes (11.5% vs. 14.5%, HR = 0.78), according to the placebo group. In the first-second outcome, the rate of hospitalization from HF was also lower in the empagliflozin group than in the placebo group (HR = 0.73, $p < 0.001$), and the time to first hospitalization was prolonged. In the post-analysis of the study, improvements in parameters were observed in the form of a decrease in glycated hemoglobin levels and body weight and an increase in hemoglobin levels [38]. In addition, a decrease in NT-proBNP levels was noted, which was initially similar in patients with and without diabetes. However, in the following weeks, a more pronounced decline was noted in patients with diabetes.

The EMPA-Tropism trial examined whether empagliflozin also had a positive effect on heart failure with reduced ejection fraction (HFrEF), exercise capacity, and quality of life in non-diabetic patients [22]. The first outcome was to determine whether empagliflozin attenuates adverse myocardial remodeling as assessed by improvements in left ventricular end-diastolic volume (LVEDV) and left ventricular end-systolic volume (LVESV). In the second outcome, among others, changes in peak oxygen consumption, left ventricular mass, LVEF, distance in the 6 min walk test (6MWT), and quality of life were assessed using the KCCQ-12 scale. After a 6-month follow-up, substantial improvement was noted in LVEDV in the empagliflozin versus placebo group (-25.1 ± 26.0 mL vs. -1.5 ± 25.4 mL; $p < 0.001$) compared to the beginning of the study [39]. Similar changes were observed for left ventricular end-systolic diameter (LVESD) (-26.6 ± 20.5 mL vs. -0.5 ± 21.9 mL, $p < 0.001$). In addition, the empagliflozin group had a significant reduction in left ventricular mass (-17.8 ± 31.9 g vs. 4.1 ± 13.4 g; $p < 0.001$) and a more pronounced increase in LVEF (6 ± 4.2 vs. -0.1 ± 3.9; $p < 0.001$) in comparison with placebo. There was a notable enhancement in peak oxygen consumption (1.1 ± 2.6 mL/min/kg) and distance extension in the 6MWT (81 ± 64 m) in the empagliflozin group [22,39]. All the above-mentioned elements contributed to a meaningful improvement in the patient's quality of life.

EMPULSE was a prominent trial that investigated empagliflozin's effects in people with acute HF [40]. The trial aimed to introduce empagliflozin into HF treatment while patients were still in the hospital. The developments observed during the trial provided clinically significant benefits to patients at the same time as providing no safety concerns about its use [41]. The main objective was to improve survival, reduce symptoms, and reduce the incidence of heart failure events. There were 11 deaths in the empagliflozin group (4.2%), while 22 patients (8.3%) died in the placebo group. Sixty-seven patients had at least one heart failure event (HFE) during the study, with twenty-eight patients in the empagliflozin group and thirty-nine in the placebo group (10.6% and 14.7%, respectively). Furthermore, there was a greater absolute change in the Kansas City Cardiomyopathy Questionnaire Total Symptom Score (KCCQ-TSS) from baseline to day 90 in patients in the empagliflozin group (HR = 4.45; 95% CI 0.32–8.59) and a significant reduction in NT-proBNP levels (HR = 0.90, 95% CI 0.82–0.98) [41].

The individual SGLT-2 inhibitors have a similar range of action; therefore, an important factor comparing them to one another will be cardiovascular events and the occurrence of adverse events [42]. In a meta-analysis conducted by Zelniker et al. [16] both empagliflozin, canagliflozin, and dapagliflozin were associated with reduced hospitalizations for HF and reduced progression of kidney disease. However, in patients with atherosclerotic CVD, the positive effect of empagliflozin on reducing cardiovascular death was more pronounced than with the other SGLT-2 inhibitors. A similar effect was observed for all-cause mortality [43,44]. In the retrospective trial conducted by Suzuki et al. [45], the incidence of subsequent cardiovascular risk in terms of HF, myocardial infarction, angina, stroke, and atrial fibrillation was compared in accordance with individual SGLT-2 inhibitors. It turned out that no significant differences in the risk of the above-mentioned cardiovascular events were observed between empagliflozin, dapagliflozin, canagliflozin, or other SGLT-2 inhibitors (ipragliflozin, tofogliflozin, and luseogliflozin). A comparable effect was observed in reducing HF progression [43]. Entirely different conclusions were reached in a study by Jing et al. [44], in which empagliflozin was associated with a more favorable effect on the occurrence of cardiovascular events than canagliflozin or dapagliflozin. Additionally, according to Tang et al. [46], it was more likely to reduce the risk of HF or HF requiring hospitalization compared to the other SGLT-2 inhibitors. The studies comparing empagliflozin with other SGLT-2 inhibitors are summarized in Table 1.

Table 1. A comparison of empagliflozin with other SGLT-2 inhibitors in patients with type 2 diabetes.

Study	Tang et al. [46]	Zelniker et al. [16]	Täger et al. [43]	Suzuki et al. [45]	Jiang et al. [44]
Year	2016	2019	2021	2022	2022
Study design	Meta-analysis	Meta-analysis	Meta-analysis	Retrospective cohort study	Meta-analysis
No of patients	28,859	34,322	74,874	25,315	70,574
Patient's characteristics	Patients > 18 years old with T2DM	Mean age 63.5 years, 60.2% patients with atherosclerotic CVD, 11.3% patients with history of HF, 14.9% patients with eGFR < 60 mL/min per 1.73 m^2	Patients 52–69 years old, HbA1c level between 7.2% and 9.3%	Median age 52 years, median HbA1c level 7.5%	Mean age 59.2 years old, mean HbA1c level 8.3%
SGLT2 inhibitors	Canagliflozin, dapagliflozin, or empagliflozin vs. placebo or other active anti-diabetic treatments	Empagliflozin 10 mg, 25 mg, canagliflozin 100 mg, 300 mg, dapagliflozin 10 mg	Canagliflozin, dapagliflozin, empagliflozin, ertugliflozin	Empagliflozin, dapagliflozin, canagliflozin, other SGLT2 inhibitors (ipragliflozin, tofogliflozin, luseogliflozin)	Empagliflozin 5 mg, 10 mg, 25 mg, 50 mg, canagliflozin 100 mg, 300 mg, dapagliflozin 2.5 mg, 5 mg, 10 mg, placebo
Comparison of SGLT2 inhibitors	Empagliflozin significantly lower the risk of MACE and any-cause mortality than placebo and other SGLT2 inhibitors. Furthermore, empagliflozin lower risk of HF and HF requiring hospitalization.	Empagliflozin has superior effect on reducing death from cardiovascular causes than canagliflozin or dapagliflozin. There is an increased risk of fractures and amputations with canagliflozin.	Empagliflozin is superior to canagliflozin and dapagliflozin in reducing all-cause mortality and cardiovascular mortality. However, all without significant differences reduce HF worsening.	There were no relevant differences in the risk of myocardial infarction, angina pectoris, heart failure, atrial fibrillation and stroke among individual SGLT2 inhibitors.	Empagliflozin is associated with significantly lower risk of all-cause mortality and cardiovascular events than canagliflozin and dapagliflozin.

T2DM, type 2 diabetes mellitus; MACE, major adverse cardiovascular events; HF, heart failure; CVD, cardiovascular disease; eGFR, estimated glomerular filtration rate.

3. Dapagliflozin

One example of a selective SGLT2 inhibitor is dapagliflozin, used under the trade name Forxiga® in Europe or Farxiga® in the US, in doses of 5 or 10 mg. It was approved in 2012 by the European Medicines Agency (EMA) and in 2014 by the Food and Drug Administration (FDA) [47,48]. As for the drug's pharmacokinetics, due to its approximately 14 h half-life, it can be used once daily, reaching maximum plasma concentrations after about 2 h, while its metabolites are excreted mainly in the urine and feces [47–49]. Dapagliflozin acts mainly in the proximal tubule of the kidney, and the mechanism involves reducing the reabsorption of glucose. This increases the excretion of glucose in the urine, which leads to the desired hypoglycemic effect. Indirectly, there is a partial reduction in body weight through negative energy balance and a reduction in blood pressure due to osmotic diuretic action—mild natriuresis [50,51]. The characteristics of the properties and actions of dapagliflozin are presented in Figure 1 [50,52].

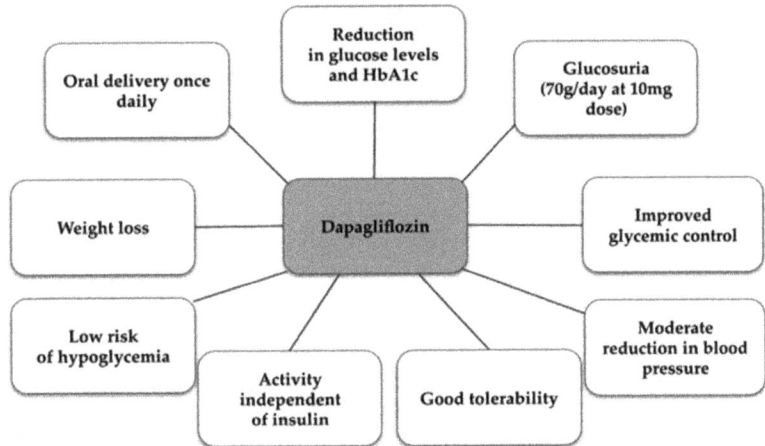

Figure 1. Characteristics of dapagliflozin [50,52].

In the European Union, it is used in monotherapy or combination therapy in T2DM when patients fail to achieve normal glycemic control despite lifestyle changes, i.e., diet and adequate exercise. Dapagliflozin has been shown in numerous studies to reduce hospital admissions for heart failure and the rate of death from cardiovascular causes in both patients with and without T2DM [49,53]. In patients with parenchymal CVD, it probably caused a reduction in renal disease progression [49]. Dapagliflozin also has a partial metabolic effect caused by increasing muscle insulin sensitivity [54]. Worthy of mention is the international, randomized Dapagliflozin Effect on Cardiovascular Events–Thrombolysis in Myocardial Infarction 58 (DECLARE–TIMI 58) study. It had a double-blind, placebo-controlled, phase 3 trial to evaluate the effect of dapagliflozin in patients with T2DM and established atherosclerotic cardiovascular disease or multiple atherosclerotic cardiovascular risk factors on cardiovascular events [1]. Positive effects on the kidneys, such as natriuresis and improved endothelial function, have also been observed [49]. The study included 17,160 patients diagnosed with T2DM. It showed that the use of dapagliflozin resulted in reduced cardiovascular deaths and hospitalizations for HF, regardless of ejection fraction [48,55,56]. In contrast, SGLT2 treatment did not lead to a statistically significant reduction in MACE [48,57,58]. Another study, Dapagliflozin and Prevention of Adverse Outcomes in Heart Failure (DAPA-HF), included 4744 patients with heart failure with or without T2DM, reduced EF ($\leq$40%), NYHA score II–IV, and elevated NT-proBNP. Patients were randomly assigned to take one 10 mg tablet of dapagliflozin daily. Less than 42% of the subjects had additional T2DM [59,60]. The characteristics of patients with T2DM participating in the DAPA-HF study are presented in Table 2.

Table 2. Characteristics of patients with T2DM participating in the DAPA-HF study [60].

Characteristics in Patients with T2DM
Higher body mass index
More obese individuals
More people with a history of myocardial infarction, ischemic disease, coronary artery disease
NYHA score II–IV
Higher serum NT-proBNP levels
Lower values of mean eGFR
More patients with hypertension

NYHA, New York Heart Association; eGFR, estimated glomerular filtration rate.

These studies indicated that HF and HFrEF, regardless of the presence or absence of T2DM, who were consuming dapagliflozin, had a lower risk of cardiovascular death [60] An important cardioprotective component of dapagliflozin is the reduction in cardiac preload and afterload through blood volume reduction caused by mild diuresis. Reducing oxidative stress in cells may improve the structure of damaged cardiac cells, which consequently improves long-term prognosis [56]. Studies in mice have shown a vasodilatory effect of dapagliflozin on the thoracic aorta, depending on the voltage of potassium channels [30]. This suggested a direct effect on vascular cells for both acute and chronic treatment. The vascular response resulted in a reduction in oxidative stress by reducing glycation [30,61]. The beneficial effect on the endothelium is due to several vasodilatory mechanisms, such as reduced infiltration of macrophages into the myocardium and activation of eNOS phosphorylation [61].

As for contraindications to the use of the drug, these are, of course, a history of hypersensitivity reactions, for example, angioedema or anaphylactic reaction, and patients on dialysis therapy [62]. Adverse reactions during dapagliflozin pharmacotherapy did occur, but they represented a small percentage.

Patients could experience rhinosinusitis, upper respiratory tract infections in general, headaches, back pain, or the occurrence of diarrhea [49]. The most well-known complication due to glucosuria is emerging urinary tract infections, including cases of urosepsis or pyelonephritis. There is also a risk of fungal genital infections or life-threatening Fournier gangrene [1,57,59]. The use of SGLT2 inhibitors has been linked to the occurrence of both hypoglycemia and cases of diabetic ketoacidosis, which have also led to deaths. Of course, these cases occurred only in patients with T2DM [1,49,58]. There were also transient decreases in renal creatinine clearance, and some patients presented clinical signs of hypotension [49,62]. When thinking about dapagliflozin, it is worth remembering a number of its systemic effects. In addition to its obvious and best-studied hypoglycemic and glycated hemoglobin-reducing effects, it also has cardioprotective and renoprotective properties [49]. The drug's mechanism of action also determines a positive effect on metabolic syndrome, which will indirectly contribute to the reduction of cardiovascular events in these patients [63]. What is important is that it is well tolerated by a wide range of patients, regardless of a history of CVD [49].

4. Canagliflozin

Canagliflozin is one of the SGLT2 inhibitors. Primarily used to treat type 2 diabetes, it has also been studied for its potential cardiovascular benefits. Principally, canagliflozin reduced the risk of cardiovascular events in people with type 2 diabetes, regardless of the coincidence of CVD [64–66]. Canagliflozin improves several cardiovascular risk factors, including lowering body weight and blood pressure, body composition, uric acid levels, vascular stiffness, pulse pressure, cardiac workload, and magnesium levels [67–70]. A growing body of literature points to the significant role of SGLT2 inhibitors in improving symptoms in patients with HF [71]. Canagliflozin improves patients' symptom burden, driven primarily by volume and hemodynamic effects. The protection provided may be a result of natriuresis-induced decreases in preload and afterload [72], systemic blood pressure lowering [73,74], modification of the intrarenal renin–angiotensin axis [75], and reduction in arterial stiffness [76]. In addition, it has shown beneficial solid effects on decreasing cardiovascular death rates and hospitalized HF, especially in those with a history of CVD [77–79]. Furthermore, according to this study, canagliflozin might reduce the progression of atherosclerosis, adhesion molecules, and markers of inflammation (i.e., vascular cell adhesion molecule-1 and monocyte chemotaxis protein-1). Additionally, canagliflozin enhances atherosclerotic plaque stability in mouse models [80]. Nevertheless, the characterization of cardiac function that would identify the patient groups that would benefit from the administration of canagliflozin has not been fully investigated, despite increasing proof of its positive effects on HF.

Canagliflozin demonstrates cardioprotective benefits independent of a glucose-lowering effect, including preservation of cardiac function during myocardial ischemia. Canagliflozin considerably attenuates the size of myocardial infarcts [81,82]. Sabe et al. found that canagliflozin therapy enhances myocardial function and perfusion to the ischemic region in a swine model of chronic myocardial ischemia. These outcomes may be mediated by antioxidant signaling, adenosine monophosphate-activated protein kinase activation, and attenuation of fibrosis via decreased Jak/STAT signaling [83]. Furthermore, according to this research, the intravenous administration of canagliflozin decreased the expression of apoptotic and nitro-oxidative stress markers while increasing the phosphorylation of cardioprotective signaling mediators, such as adenosine monophosphate-activated protein kinase, acetyl-CoA carboxylase, endothelial nitric-oxide synthase, and Akt, in non-diabetic rats. Additionally, canagliflozin has been linked to a slower increase in biomarkers of cardiac wall stress, such as high-sensitivity troponin I and NT-proBNP, as well as a rise in hematocrit [84]. Correspondingly, canagliflozin inhibited the onset of systolic and diastolic dysfunction after ischemia-reperfusion damage [85]. Table 3 provides a summary of canagliflozin's cardioprotective effects.

Table 3. Cardioprotective effects of canagliflozin on myocardial infarction.

Study	Year	Study Design	Participants	Findings
Januzzi, J.L.; Butler, J.; Jarolim, P. et al. [83]	2017	Randomized, double-blind, placebo-controlled	666 patients with DM type 2 and high cardiovascular risk	Canagliflozin had a favorable effect on cardiovascular biomarkers in older adults with DM type 2. In comparison to a placebo, the administration of canagliflozin in older patients with DM type 2 resulted in a significant delay in the increase of serum NT-proBNP and hsTnI levels
Huynh, K. [81]	2017	Randomized, controlled	10,142 patients with type 2 DM and high cardiovascular risk	Canagliflozin was associated with a lower risk of cardiovascular events in patients with DM type 2.
Lim, V.G.; Bell, R.M.; Arjun, S.; Kolatsi-Joannou, M.; Long, D.A.; Yellon, D.M. [80]	2019	Randomized, double-blind, placebo-controlled	Diabetic and non-diabetic rats	Canagliflozin attenuated myocardial infarction in both diabetic and non-diabetic mice. The observed effects were independent of glucose levels during the occurrence of ischemia/reperfusion injury.
Sayour, A.A.; Korkmaz-Icöz, S.; Loganathan, S. et al. [84]	2019	Randomized, controlled	Non-diabetic male rats	Acute canagliflozin treatment protected against in vivo myocardial ischemia-reperfusion injury in non-diabetic male rats and enhanced endothelium-dependent vasorelaxation.
Sabe, S.A.; Xu, C.M.; Sabra, M.; et al. [82]	2023	Randomized, controlled	Swine model of chronic myocardial ischemia	Canagliflozin improved myocardial perfusion, fibrosis, and function in a swine model of chronic myocardial ischemia.

DM, diabetes mellitus; NT-proBNP, N-terminal pro-B-type natriuretic peptide; hsTnI, high-sensitivity troponin I.

A remarkable cardioprotective effect against cardiac arrest and resuscitation-induced cardiac dysfunction was obtained by canagliflozin [85,86]. Interestingly, in comparison to control mice, animals pretreated with canagliflozin had better survival rates ($p < 0.05$), a faster return of spontaneous circulation ($p < 0.01$), and increased neurological scores ($p < 0.01$ or $p < 0.001$) following resuscitation. Canagliflozin may exert its effects through the STAT-3-dependent cell-survival signaling pathway, according to this study [85].

The possible benefit of canagliflozin use in the development and progression of atrial fibrillation (AF) has been suggested [87]. This study has demonstrated that the administration of canagliflozin reduces atrial electrical and structural remodeling, interstitial fibrosis, and oxidative stress levels in canine models [88]. On the contrary, this meta-analysis by Li et al. showed that SGLT2 inhibitor use is linked to a 19.33% lower risk of serious adverse events of AF and atrial flutter (AFL) when compared with placebo. However only dapagliflozin (1.02% vs. 1.49%; RR 0.73; 95% CI 0.59–0.89; p = 0.002; I^2 0%), but not canagliflozin (1.00% vs. 1.08%; RR 0.83; 95% CI 0.62–1.12; p = 0.23; I^2 0%), significantly reduced AF and AFL. Further studies are required to establish whether canagliflozin similarly exerts protective effects against AF/AFL development [89]. A summary of canagliflozin's effects on the cardiovascular system is shown in Table 4.

Table 4. Canagliflozin effects on cardiovascular system.

Cardiovascular Benefit	Effect on Cardiovascular Risk Factors	Mechanism of Action
Reduction in cardiovascular events	Lowered body weight and blood pressure, improved body composition, uric acid levels, vascular stiffness, pulse pressure, cardiac workload, and magnesium levels.	Not fully investigated.
Improvement in heart failure symptoms	Improvement in volume and hemodynamic effects, natriuresis-induced decreases in preload and afterload, systemic blood pressure lowering, modification of the intrarenal renin–angiotensin axis, and reduction in arterial stiffness.	Not fully investigated.
Reduction in cardiovascular death rates and hospitalization for heart failure	Decrease in atherosclerosis progression, adhesion molecules, and markers of inflammation.	Enhanced atherosclerotic plaque stability in mouse models.
Preservation of cardiac function during myocardial ischemia	Attenuation of myocardial infarct size.	Antioxidant signaling, adenosine monophosphate-activated protein kinase activation, and attenuation of fibrosis via decreased Jak/STAT signaling.
Slower increase in biomarkers of cardiac wall stress	Inhibition of onset of systolic and diastolic dysfunction after ischemia-reperfusion damage.	Not fully investigated.
Cardioprotective effect against cardiac arrest and resuscitation-induced cardiac dysfunction	Improved survival rates, shorter return of spontaneous circulation, and higher neurological scores following resuscitation.	STAT-3-dependent cell-survival signaling pathway.
Possible benefit in the development and progression of atrial fibrillation	Reduced atrial electrical and structural remodelling, interstitial fibrosis, and oxidative stress levels in canine models.	Not fully established; conflicting results in clinical studies.

5. Ertugliflozin

Ertugliflozin is an SGLT2 inhibitor that is used as an adjunct therapy for the treatment of DM. The cardioprotective effects of ertugliflozin among individuals with CVD have not been extensively investigated in clinical trials.

In preclinical models, ertugliflozin has been found to improve cardiac energy metabolism by increasing the availability of ketone bodies as an alternative energy source for the heart. This shift in substrate utilization may help preserve cardiac function in conditions such as HF. Furthermore, the drug has demonstrated the ability to attenuate cardiac remodeling, including left ventricular hypertrophy, fibrosis, and inflammation, pathological changes commonly observed in CVD [90,91].

The VERTIS CV trial assessed the impact of ertugliflozin in patients with type 2 diabetes and CVD, including those with a history of HF and known a pre-trial ejection fraction. The study demonstrated that treatment with ertugliflozin reduced the occurrence and total hospitalizations for HF events. This benefit was observed in patients with and without a history of HF, as well as in those with reduced or preserved ejection fraction [92].

The trial also revealed that the risk reduction for the first hospitalization for HF with ertugliflozin was consistent across most baseline subgroups. However, a greater benefit was observed in three specific populations: those with an estimated glomerular filtration rate (eGFR) less than 60 mL/min/1.73 m^2, albuminuria, and diuretic use. Additionally, ertugliflozin use was associated with decreased albuminuria and preservation of eGFR over time, indicating its potential for kidney protection in patients with type 2 diabetes and CVD [93,94].

Overall, these findings suggest that ertugliflozin may have additional cardiovascular positive effects, apart from its effects on lowering glucose levels. Thus, it might be a promising therapeutic method for those with HF and CVD. However, further research is needed to fully comprehend the underlying mechanisms responsible for these effects.

6. Bexagliflozin

Bexagliflozin is a novel agent approved by the FDA in 2023. This highly potent and selective inhibitor of SGLT2 is indicated for adults with type 2 DM with an eGFR greater than 30 mL/min/1.73 m^2. It is available as 20 mg oral tablets, recommended to be taken once daily, regardless of the meal. Patients with diabetes and mild to moderate kidney failure have fewer treatment options compared to those with preserved kidney function. Dosage modifications have been presented in Tables 5 and 6.

Table 5. Dosage modifications of bexagliflozin in renal impairment.

Renal Impairment	eGRF (mL/min/1.73 m^2)	Dosage Modifications
Mild-to-moderate	0–89	No dosage adjustment required.
Severe	<30	Not recommended owing to the decline of glucose-lowering effect and reduction in urine output.
Dialysis	-	Contraindicated.

eGFR, estimated glomerular filtration rate.

Table 6. Dosage modifications of bexagliflozin in hepatic impairment.

Hepatic Impairment	Child–Pugh Score	Dosage Modifications
Mild-to-moderate	A or B	No dosage adjustment required.
Severe	C	Not studied.

A 96-week phase 2 clinical study showed that bexagliflozin monotherapy led to a long-lasting, clinically relevant improvement in glycemic control, with a significant reduction in weight and blood pressure [14]. In a clinical study of patients with T2DM and co-existing chronic kidney disease (CKD) (at stage 3a/3b), bexagliflozin was well tolerated and demonstrated a decrease in hemoglobin A1c levels as well as body weight, systolic blood pressure, and albuminuria [95]. Allegretti et al. [95] have also revealed adverse events such as urinary tract infections and genital mycotic infections. However, those findings have been previously attributed to SGLT2 inhibition. A summary of side effects is shown in Table 7.

Table 7. Side effects of bexagliflozin [96].

Side Effects	Prevention
Ketoacidosis	Consideration of predisposing factors, discontinuing bexagliflozin for at least 3 days prior to surgery and clinical situations known to predispose to ketoacidosis.
Lower limb amputation	Consideration of predisposing factors, monitoring for signs and symptoms of infection, new pain or tenderness, sores or ulcers involving the lower limbs.
Volume depletion	Assessment of volume status and renal function, monitoring for signs and symptoms of volume depletion.
Urosepsis and pyelonephritis	Evaluation patients for signs and symptoms of urinary tract infections.
Hypoglycemia with concomitant use with insulin and insulin secretagogues	lower dose of insulin or insulin secretagogue.
Necrotizing fasciitis of the perineum (Fournier's gangrene)	Evaluation of patients for pain or tenderness, erythema, or swelling in the genital or perineal areas, along with fever or malaise.
Genital mycotic infections	Monitoring patients with a history of genital mycotic infections and those who are uncircumcised.

Bexagliflozin has been proven to be non-inferior to other SGLT2 inhibitors. Halvorsen et al. [97] revealed that its effects on body weight and blood pressure were even superior to commonly prescribed add-on therapy with the DPP-4 inhibitor, sitagliptin. It has also been non-inferior to glimepiride in lowering HbA1c [98]. Furthermore, it has achieved superiority over glimepiride in the reduction of body mass and systolic blood pressure (SBP) [5]. Another important finding was the demonstration of remarkably fewer hypoglycemic events than with glimepiride. Importantly, McMurray et al. [99] have shown bexagliflozin's non-inferiority for hard clinical outcomes in high-risk CVD cohorts.

7. SGLT-2 Inhibitors' Effects on the Kidney and Heart

The summary of SGLT2 inhibitors' effects on the kidney and heart is presented in Figures 2 and 3.

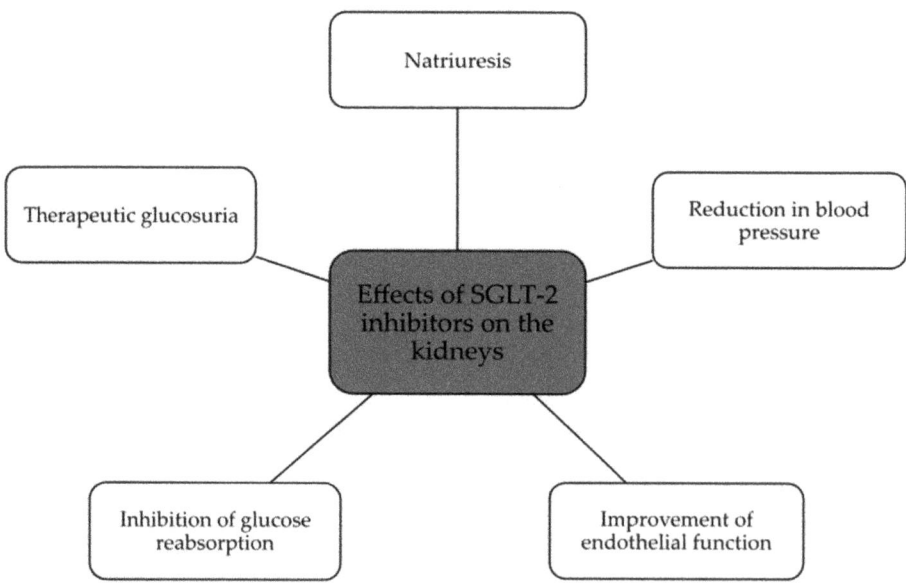

Figure 2. Beneficial effects of SGLT2 inhibitors on the kidney [47,49,51].

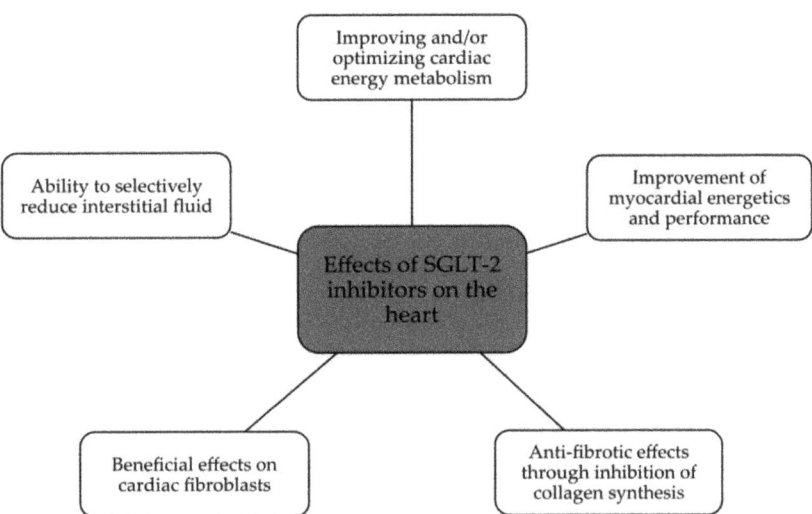

Figure 3. Beneficial effects of SGLT2 on the heart [26].

8. Conclusions

According to recent epidemiological data [100], type 2 DM is closely related to cardiovascular disease development. Heart failure, as a leading cause of morbidity and mortality in diabetics, is especially perilous among this group of patients [101]. Since 2008, the FDA has required proof of cardiovascular safety for new glucose-lowering therapies [102]. SGLT2 inhibitors have revealed a number of cardio-protective beneficial effects in both primary and secondary prevention [103]. Not only do they reduce cardiovascular events, improve HF symptoms, or decrease cardiovascular death rates and hospitalizations for HF, but they are also proven to preserve cardiac function during myocardial ischemia as well as slow the progression of AF. Evidence of the clinical benefits of this new anti-hyperglycemic therapy has led to a relevant change in the care paradigm across several high-risk populations.

Beyond their glucose-lowering effects, all of the mentioned SGLT2 inhibitors have been proven to have additional cardiovascular benefits and could be a promising treatment option for patients with CVD and HF. Empagliflozin has been proven to be the most effective SGLT2 inhibitor in lowering the risk of HF. It is also superior in reducing death from cardiovascular causes to canagliflozin or dapagliflozin. Undeniably, bexagliflozin has been actively awaited, mainly due to the ever-increasing prevalence of T2DM as well as increased morbidity and mortality from associated cardiovascular consequences. Studies have shown its non-inferiority for hard clinical outcomes in high-risk CVD cohorts [99]. Nowadays, it is also undergoing clinical development for the treatment of essential hypertension in the USA.

In conclusion, it has been proven that patients with HF and DM may benefit from SGLT2 inhibitors. The balance of profits and adverse impacts depends on the individual risk profiles.

Author Contributions: Conceptualization, B.F., E.M. and J.R.; methodology, W.F., J.H., E.R., M.S. and E.M.; software, E.M.; validation, B.F., E.M. and J.R.; formal analysis, W.F., J.H., E.R., M.S. and E.M.; investigation, W.F., J.H., E.R. and M.S.; resources, B.F., E.M. and J.R.; data curation, E.M.; writing—original draft preparation, E.M.; writing—review and editing, E.M.; visualization, W.F., J.H., E.R., M.S. and E.M.; supervision, B.F., E.M. and J.R.; project administration, B.F., E.M. and J.R.; funding acquisition, B.F. and J.R. All authors have read and agreed to the published version of the manuscript.

Funding: This research received no external funding.

Institutional Review Board Statement: Not applicable.

Informed Consent Statement: Not applicable.

Data Availability Statement: The data used in this article are sourced from materials mentioned in the References section.

Conflicts of Interest: The authors declare no conflict of interest.

Abbreviations

6MWT	6 min walk test
AF	Atrial fibrillation
AFL	Atrial flutter
CAD	Coronary artery disease
CKD	Chronic kidney disease
CVD	Cardiovascular disease
DAPA-HF	Dapagliflozin and Prevention of Adverse Outcomes in Heart Failure
DECLARE–TIMI 58	Dapagliflozin Effect on Cardiovascular Events–Thrombolysis in Myocardial Infarction 58
DM	Diabetes mellitus
DDP4	Dipeptidylpeptidase 4
eGFR	Estimated glomerular filtration rate
EMA	European Medicines Agency
EMPA-REG OUTCOME	Empagliflozin Cardiovascular Outcome Event Trial in Type 2 Diabetes Mellitus Patients–Removing Excess Glucose
FDA	Food and Drug Administration
GLP-1 RAs	Glucagon-like peptide-1 receptor agonists
HF	Heart failure
HFE	Heart failure event
HFrEF	Heart failure with reduced ejection fraction
LVEDV	Left ventricular end-diastolic volume
LVEF	Left ventricular ejection fraction
LVESD	Left ventricular end-systolic diameter
LVESV	Left ventricular end-systolic volume
MACE	Major adverse cardiovascular events
NYHA	New York Heart Association
SBP	Systolic blood pressure
SGLT2	Sodium/glucose cotransporter 2
T2DM	Type 2 diabetes mellitus

References

1. Wiviott, S.D.; Raz, I.; Bonaca, M.P.; Mosenzon, O.; Kato, E.T.; Cahn, A.; Silverman, M.G.; Zelniker, T.A.; Kuder, J.F.; Murphy, S.A.; et al. Dapagliflozin and Cardiovascular Outcomes in Type 2 Diabetes. *N. Engl. J. Med.* **2019**, *380*, 347–357. [CrossRef] [PubMed]
2. Bertoni, A.G.; Hundley, W.G.; Massing, M.W.; Bonds, D.E.; Burke, G.L.; Goff, D.C. Heart Failure Prevalence, Incidence, and Mortality in the Elderly with Diabetes. *Diabetes Care* **2004**, *27*, 699–703. [CrossRef] [PubMed]
3. Seferović, P.M.; Petrie, M.C.; Filippatos, G.S.; Anker, S.D.; Rosano, G.; Bauersachs, J.; Paulus, W.J.; Komajda, M.; Cosentino, F.; de Boer, R.A.; et al. Type 2 diabetes mellitus and heart failure: A position statement from the Heart Failure Association of the European Society of Cardiology. *Eur. J. Heart Fail.* **2018**, *20*, 853–872. [CrossRef]
4. Liang, B.; Zhao, Y.-X.; Zhang, X.-X.; Liao, H.-L.; Gu, N. Reappraisal on pharmacological and mechanical treatments of heart failure. *Cardiovasc. Diabetol.* **2020**, *19*, 55. [CrossRef]
5. Nichols, G.A.; Hillier, T.A.; Erbey, J.R.; Brown, J.B. Congestive heart failure in type 2 diabetes: Prevalence, incidence, and risk factors. Diabetes Care. *Diabetes Care* **2001**, *24*, 1614–1619. [CrossRef] [PubMed]
6. Liang, B.; Gu, N. Empagliflozin in the treatment of heart failure and type 2 diabetes mellitus: Evidence from several large clinical trials. *Int. J. Med. Sci.* **2022**, *19*, 1118–1121. [CrossRef] [PubMed]
7. Rubler, S.; Dlugash, J.; Yuceoglu, Y.Z.; Kumral, T.; Branwood, A.W.; Grishman, A. New type of cardiomyopathy associated with diabetic glomerulosclerosis. *Am. J. Cardiol.* **1972**, *30*, 595–602. [CrossRef]
8. Salvatore, T.; Pafundi, P.C.; Galiero, R.; Albanese, G.; Di Martino, A.; Caturano, A.; Vetrano, E.; Rinaldi, L.; Sasso, F.C. The Diabetic Cardiomyopathy: The Contributing Pathophysiological Mechanisms. *Front. Med.* **2021**, *8*, 695792. [CrossRef]

9. Lago, R.M.; Singh, P.P.; Nesto, R.W. Congestive heart failure and cardiovascular death in patients with prediabetes and type 2 diabetes given thiazolidinediones: A meta-analysis of randomised clinical trials. *Lancet* **2007**, *370*, 1129–1136. [CrossRef]
10. Scirica, B.M.; Braunwald, E.; Raz, I.; Cavender, M.A.; Morrow, D.A.; Jarolim, P.; Udell, J.A.; Mosenzon, O.; Im, K.; Umez-Eronini, A.A.; et al. Heart Failure, Saxagliptin, and Diabetes Mellitus: Observations from the SAVOR-TIMI 53 Randomized Trial. *Circulation* **2014**, *130*, 1579–1588, Erratum in *Circulation* 2015, *132*, e198. [CrossRef]
11. Pham, D.; Rocha, N.D.A.; McGuire, D.K.; Neeland, I.J. Impact of empagliflozin in patients with diabetes and heart failure. *Trends Cardiovasc. Med.* **2017**, *27*, 144–151. [CrossRef] [PubMed]
12. Zinman, B.; Wanner, C.; Lachin, J.M.; Fitchett, D.; Bluhmki, E.; Hantel, S.; Mattheus, M.; Devins, T.; Johansen, O.E.; Woerle, H.J.; et al. Empagliflozin, Cardiovascular Outcomes, and Mortality in Type 2 Diabetes. *N. Engl. J. Med.* **2015**, *373*, 2117–2128. [CrossRef] [PubMed]
13. Cosentino, F.; Grant, P.J.; Aboyans, V.; Bailey, C.J.; Ceriello, A.; Delgado, V.; Federici, M.; Filippatos, G.; Grobbee, D.E.; Hansen, T.B.; et al. 2019 ESC Guidelines on diabetes, pre-diabetes, and cardiovascular diseases developed in collaboration with the EASD. *Eur. Heart J.* **2020**, *41*, 255–323. [CrossRef]
14. Halvorsen, Y.C.; Walford, G.A.; Massaro, J.; Aftring, R.P.; Freeman, M.W. A 96-week, multinational, randomized, double-blind, parallel-group, clinical trial evaluating the safety and effectiveness of bexagliflozin as a monotherapy for adults with type 2 diabetes. *Diabetes Obes. Metab.* **2019**, *21*, 2496–2504. [CrossRef]
15. Odutayo, A.; da Costa, B.R.; Pereira, T.V.; Garg, V.; Iskander, S.; Roble, F.; Lalji, R.; Hincapié, C.A.; Akingbade, A.; Rodrigues, M.; et al. Sodium-Glucose Cotransporter 2 Inhibitors, All-Cause Mortality, and Cardiovascular Outcomes in Adults with Type 2 Diabetes: A Bayesian Meta-Analysis and Meta-Regression. *J. Am. Heart Assoc.* **2021**, *10*, e019918. [CrossRef]
16. Zelniker, T.A.; Wiviott, S.D.; Raz, I.; Im, K.; Goodrich, E.; Bonaca, M.P.; Mosenzon, O.; Kato, E.; Cahn, A.; Furtado, R.H.M.; et al. SGLT2 inhibitors for primary and secondary prevention of cardiovascular and renal outcomes in type 2 diabetes: A systematic review and meta-analysis of cardiovascular outcome trials. *Lancet* **2019**, *393*, 31–39, Erratum in *Lancet* 2019, *393*, 30. [CrossRef]
17. Muscoli, S.; Barillà, F.; Tajmir, R.; Meloni, M.; Della Morte, D.; Bellia, A.; Di Daniele, N.; Lauro, D.; Andreadi, A. The New Role of SGLT2 Inhibitors in the Management of Heart Failure: Current Evidence and Future Perspective. *Pharmaceutics* **2022**, *14*, 1730. [CrossRef]
18. Packer, M.; Butler, J.; Filippatos, G.S.; Jamal, W.; Salsali, A.; Schnee, J.; Kimura, K.; Zeller, C.; George, J.; Brueckmann, M.; et al. Evaluation of the effect of sodium–glucose co-transporter 2 inhibition with empagliflozin on morbidity and mortality of patients with chronic heart failure and a reduced ejection fraction: Rationale for and design of the EMPEROR-Reduced trial. *Eur. J. Heart Fail.* **2019**, *21*, 1270–1278. [CrossRef]
19. Anker, S.D.; Butler, J.; Filippatos, G.; Ferreira, J.P.; Bocchi, E.; Böhm, M.; Brunner–La Rocca, H.-P.; Choi, D.-J.; Chopra, V.; Chuquiure-Valenzuela, E.; et al. Empagliflozin in Heart Failure with a Preserved Ejection Fraction. *N. Engl. J. Med.* **2021**, *385*, 1451–1461. [CrossRef] [PubMed]
20. Butler, J.; Packer, M.; Filippatos, G.; Ferreira, J.P.; Zeller, C.; Schnee, J.; Brueckmann, M.; Pocock, S.J.; Zannad, F.; Anker, S.D. Effect of empagliflozin in patients with heart failure across the spectrum of left ventricular ejection fraction. *Eur. Heart J.* **2022**, *43*, 416–426. [CrossRef] [PubMed]
21. Anker, S.D.; Butler, J.; Filippatos, G.; Khan, M.S.; Marx, N.; Lam, C.S.; Schnaidt, S.; Ofstad, A.P.; Brueckmann, M.; Jamal, W.; et al. Effect of Empagliflozin on Cardiovascular and Renal Outcomes in Patients with Heart Failure by Baseline Diabetes Status: Results from the EMPEROR-Reduced Trial. *Circulation* **2021**, *143*, 337–349. [CrossRef] [PubMed]
22. Santos-Gallego, C.G.; Garcia-Ropero, A.; Mancini, D.; Pinney, S.P.; Contreras, J.P.; Fergus, I.; Abascal, V.; Moreno, P.; Atallah-Lajam, F.; Tamler, R.; et al. Rationale and Design of the EMPA-TROPISM Trial (ATRU-4): Are the "Cardiac Benefits" of Empagliflozin Independent of its Hypoglycemic Activity? *Cardiovasc. Drugs Ther.* **2019**, *33*, 87–95. [CrossRef] [PubMed]
23. Requena-Ibáñez, J.A.; Santos-Gallego, C.G.; Rodriguez-Cordero, A.; Vargas-Delgado, A.P.; Mancini, D.; Sartori, S.; Atallah-Lajam, F.; Giannarelli, C.; Macaluso, F.; Lala, A.; et al. Mechanistic Insights of Empagliflozin in Nondiabetic Patients With HFrEF: From the EMPA-TROPISM Study. *JACC Heart Fail.* **2021**, *9*, 578–589. [CrossRef] [PubMed]
24. Lee, M.M.Y.; Brooksbank, K.J.M.; Wetherall, K.; Mangion, K.; Roditi, G.; Campbell, R.T.; Berry, C.; Chong, V.; Coyle, L.; Docherty, K.F.; et al. Effect of Empagliflozin on Left Ventricular Volumes in Patients with Type 2 Diabetes, or Prediabetes, and Heart Failure with Reduced Ejection Fraction (SUGAR-DM-HF). *Circulation* **2021**, *143*, 516–525. [CrossRef] [PubMed]
25. Tan, Y.; Zhang, Z.; Zheng, C.; Wintergerst, K.A.; Keller, B.B.; Cai, L. Mechanisms of diabetic cardiomyopathy and potential therapeutic strategies: Preclinical and clinical evidence. *Nat. Rev. Cardiol.* **2020**, *17*, 585–607. [CrossRef]
26. Verma, S.; McMurray, J.J.V. SGLT2 inhibitors and mechanisms of cardiovascular benefit: A state-of-the-art review. *Diabetologia* **2018**, *61*, 2108–2117. [CrossRef]
27. Salvatore, T.; Galiero, R.; Caturano, A.; Vetrano, E.; Rinaldi, L.; Coviello, F.; Di Martino, A.; Albanese, G.; Colantuoni, S.; Medicamento, G.; et al. Dysregulated Epicardial Adipose Tissue as a Risk Factor and Potential Therapeutic Target of Heart Failure with Preserved Ejection Fraction in Diabetes. *Biomolecules* **2022**, *12*, 176. [CrossRef]
28. Zinman, B.; Inzucchi, S.E.; Lachin, J.M.; Wanner, C.; Ferrari, R.; Fitchett, D.; Bluhmki, E.; Hantel, S.; Kempthorne-Rawson, J.; Newman, J.; et al. Rationale, design, and baseline characteristics of a randomized, placebo-controlled cardiovascular outcome trial of empagliflozin (EMPA-REG OUTCOME™). *Cardiovasc. Diabetol.* **2014**, *13*, 102. [CrossRef]

29. Patorno, E.; Pawar, A.; Franklin, J.M.; Najafzadeh, M.; Déruaz-Luyet, A.; Brodovicz, K.G.; Sambevski, S.; Bessette, L.G.; Santiago Ortiz, A.J.; Kulldorff, M.; et al. Empagliflozin and the Risk of Heart Failure Hospitalization in Routine Clinical Care. *Circulation* **2019**, *139*, 2822–2830. [CrossRef]
30. Salvatore, T.; Caturano, A.; Galiero, R.; Di Martino, A.; Albanese, G.; Vetrano, E.; Sardu, C.; Marfella, R.; Rinaldi, L.; Sasso, F.C. Cardiovascular Benefits from Gliflozins: Effects on Endothelial Function. *Biomedicines* **2021**, *9*, 1356. [CrossRef]
31. Oelze, M.; Kröller-Schön, S.; Welschof, P.; Jansen, T.; Hausding, M.; Mikhed, Y.; Stamm, P.; Mader, M.; Zinßius, E.; Agdauletova, S.; et al. The Sodium-Glucose Co-Transporter 2 Inhibitor Empagliflozin Improves Diabetes-Induced Vascular Dysfunction in the Streptozotocin Diabetes Rat Model by Interfering with Oxidative Stress and Glucotoxicity. *PLoS ONE* **2014**, *9*, e112394. [CrossRef]
32. Juni, R.P.; Kuster, D.W.; Goebel, M.; Helmes, M.; Musters, R.J.; van der Velden, J.; Koolwijk, P.; Paulus, W.J.; van Hinsbergh, V.W. Cardiac Microvascular Endothelial Enhancement of Cardiomyocyte Function Is Impaired by Inflammation and Restored by Empagliflozin. *JACC: Basic Transl. Sci.* **2019**, *4*, 575–591. [CrossRef]
33. Cooper, S.; Teoh, H.; Campeau, M.A.; Verma, S.; Leask, R.L. Empagliflozin restores the integrity of the endothelial glycocalyx in vitro. *Mol. Cell. Biochem.* **2019**, *459*, 121–130. [CrossRef]
34. Suzuki, J.-I.; Ogawa, M.; Watanabe, R.; Takayama, K.; Hirata, Y.; Nagai, R.; Isobe, M. Roles of Prostaglandin E2 in Cardiovascular Diseases. *Int. Heart J.* **2011**, *52*, 266–269. [CrossRef] [PubMed]
35. Han, J.H.; Oh, T.J.; Lee, G.; Maeng, H.J.; Lee, D.H.; Kim, K.M.; Choi, S.H.; Jang, H.C.; Lee, H.S.; Park, K.S.; et al. The beneficial effects of empagliflozin, an SGLT2 inhibitor, on atherosclerosis in ApoE$^{-/-}$ mice fed a western diet. *Diabetologia* **2017**, *60*, 364–376. [CrossRef] [PubMed]
36. Fitchett, D.; Inzucchi, S.E.; Zinman, B.; Wanner, C.; Schumacher, M.; Schmoor, C.; Ohneberg, K.; Ofstad, A.P.; Salsali, A.; George, J.T.; et al. Mediators of the improvement in heart failure outcomes with empagliflozin in the EMPA-REG OUTCOME trial. *ESC Heart Fail.* **2021**, *8*, 4517–4527. [CrossRef]
37. Packer, M.; Anker, S.D.; Butler, J.; Filippatos, G.; Pocock, S.J.; Carson, P.; Januzzi, J.; Verma, S.; Tsutsui, H.; Brueckmann, M.; et al. Cardiovascular and Renal Outcomes with Empagliflozin in Heart Failure. *N. Engl. J. Med.* **2020**, *383*, 1413–1424. [CrossRef]
38. Filippatos, G.; Butler, J.; Farmakis, D.; Zannad, F.; Ofstad, A.P.; Ferreira, J.P.; Green, J.B.; Rosenstock, J.; Schnaidt, S.; Brueckmann, M.; et al. Empagliflozin for Heart Failure with Preserved Left Ventricular Ejection Fraction With and Without Diabetes. *Circulation* **2022**, *146*, 676–686. [CrossRef]
39. Santos-Gallego, C.G.; Vargas-Delgado, A.P.; Requena-Ibanez, J.A.; Garcia-Ropero, A.; Mancini, D.; Pinney, S.; Macaluso, F.; Sartori, S.; Roque, M.; Sabatel-Perez, F.; et al. Randomized Trial of Empagliflozin in Nondiabetic Patients With Heart Failure and Reduced Ejection Fraction. *J. Am. Coll. Cardiol.* **2020**, *77*, 243–255. [CrossRef] [PubMed]
40. Voors, A.A.; Angermann, C.E.; Teerlink, J.R.; Collins, S.P.; Kosiborod, M.; Biegus, J.; Ferreira, J.P.; Nassif, M.E.; Psotka, M.A.; Tromp, J.; et al. The SGLT2 inhibitor empagliflozin in patients hospitalized for acute heart failure: A multinational randomized trial. *Nat. Med.* **2022**, *28*, 568–574. [CrossRef]
41. Kosiborod, M.N.; Angermann, C.E.; Collins, S.P.; Teerlink, J.R.; Ponikowski, P.; Biegus, J.; Comin-Colet, J.; Ferreira, J.P.; Mentz, R.J.; Nassif, M.E.; et al. Effects of Empagliflozin on Symptoms, Physical Limitations, and Quality of Life in Patients Hospitalized for Acute Heart Failure: Results from the EMPULSE Trial. *Circulation* **2022**, *146*, 279–288. [CrossRef] [PubMed]
42. Forycka, J.; Hajdys, J.; Krzemińska, J.; Wilczopolski, P.; Wronka, M.; Młynarska, E.; Rysz, J.; Franczyk, B. New Insights into the Use of Empagliflozin—A Comprehensive Review. *Biomedicines* **2022**, *10*, 3294. [CrossRef] [PubMed]
43. Täger, T.; Atar, D.; Agewall, S.; Katus, H.A.; Grundtvig, M.; Cleland, J.G.F.; Clark, A.L.; Fröhlich, H.; Frankenstein, L. Comparative efficacy of sodium-glucose cotransporter-2 inhibitors (SGLT2i) for cardiovascular outcomes in type 2 diabetes: A systematic review and network meta-analysis of randomised controlled trials. *Heart Fail. Rev.* **2020**, *26*, 1421–1435. [CrossRef] [PubMed]
44. Jiang, Y.; Yang, P.; Fu, L.; Sun, L.; Shen, W.; Wu, Q. Comparative Cardiovascular Outcomes of SGLT2 Inhibitors in Type 2 Diabetes Mellitus: A Network Meta-Analysis of Randomized Controlled Trials. *Front. Endocrinol.* **2022**, *13*, 802992. [CrossRef] [PubMed]
45. Suzuki, Y.; Kaneko, H.; Okada, A.; Itoh, H.; Matsuoka, S.; Fujiu, K.; Michihata, N.; Jo, T.; Takeda, N.; Morita, H.; et al. Comparison of cardiovascular outcomes between SGLT2 inhibitors in diabetes mellitus. *Cardiovasc. Diabetol.* **2022**, *21*, 67. [CrossRef]
46. Tang, H.; Fang, Z.; Wang, T.; Cui, W.; Zhai, S.; Song, Y. Meta-Analysis of Effects of Sodium-Glucose Cotransporter 2 Inhibitors on Cardiovascular Outcomes and All-Cause Mortality Among Patients with Type 2 Diabetes Mellitus. *Am. J. Cardiol.* **2016**, *118*, 1774–1780. [CrossRef]
47. Vivian, E.M. Dapagliflozin: A new sodium–glucose cotransporter 2 inhibitor for treatment of type 2 diabetes. *Am. J. Heart Pharm.* **2015**, *72*, 361–372. [CrossRef]
48. Al-Bazz, D.Y.; Wilding, J.P. Dapagliflozin and cardiovascular outcomes in patients with Type 2 diabetes. *Futur. Cardiol.* **2020**, *16*, 77–88. [CrossRef]
49. Dhillon, S. Dapagliflozin: A Review in Type 2 Diabetes. *Drugs* **2019**, *79*, 1135–1146, Erratum in *Drugs* **2019**, *79*, 2013. [CrossRef]
50. Plosker, G.L. Dapagliflozin: A Review of Its Use in Patients with Type 2 Diabetes. *Drugs* **2014**, *74*, 2191–2209. [CrossRef]
51. Seufert, J.; Laubner, K. Outcome-Studien zu SGLT-2-Inhibitoren [Outcome studies on SGLT-2 inhibitors]. *Internist* **2019**, *60*, 903–911. [CrossRef] [PubMed]
52. Sposetti, G.; MacKinnon, I.; Barengo, N.C. Dapagliflozin: Drug profile and its role in individualized treatment. *Expert Rev. Cardiovasc. Ther.* **2015**, *13*, 129–139. [CrossRef] [PubMed]

3. Kato, E.T.; Silverman, M.G.; Mosenzon, O.; Zelniker, T.A.; Cahn, A.; Furtado, R.H.M.; Kuder, J.; Murphy, S.A.; Bhatt, D.L.; Leiter, L.A.; et al. Effect of Dapagliflozin on Heart Failure and Mortality in Type 2 Diabetes Mellitus. *Circulation* **2019**, *139*, 2528–2536. [CrossRef] [PubMed]
4. Scheen, A.J. Pharmacodynamics, Efficacy and Safety of Sodium–Glucose Co-Transporter Type 2 (SGLT2) Inhibitors for the Treatment of Type 2 Diabetes Mellitus. *Drugs* **2014**, *75*, 33–59. [CrossRef]
5. Gupta, M.; Rao, S.; Manek, G.; Fonarow, G.C.; Ghosh, R.K. The Role of Dapagliflozin in the Management of Heart Failure: An Update on the Emerging Evidence. *Ther. Clin. Risk Manag.* **2021**, *17*, 823–830. [CrossRef] [PubMed]
6. Dong, X.; Ren, L.; Liu, Y.; Yin, X.; Cui, S.; Gao, W.; Yu, L. Efficacy and safety of dapagliflozin in the treatment of chronic heart failure: A protocol for systematic review and meta-analysis. *Medicine* **2021**, *100*, e26420. [CrossRef]
7. Brust-Sisti, L.; Rudawsky, N.; Gonzalez, J.; Brunetti, L. The Role of Sodium-Glucose Cotransporter-2 Inhibition in Heart Failure with Preserved Ejection Fraction. *Pharmacy* **2022**, *10*, 166. [CrossRef]
8. Blair, H.A. Dapagliflozin: A Review in Symptomatic Heart Failure with Reduced Ejection Fraction. *Am. J. Cardiovasc. Drugs* **2021**, *21*, 701–710, Erratum in *Am. J. Cardiovasc. Drugs* **2022**, *22*, 109. [CrossRef]
9. Kosiborod, M.N.; Jhund, P.S.; Docherty, K.; Diez, M.; Petrie, M.C.; Verma, S.; Nicolau, J.; Merkely, B.; Kitakaze, M.; DeMets, D.L.; et al. Effects of Dapagliflozin on Symptoms, Function, and Quality of Life in Patients with Heart Failure and Reduced Ejection Fraction: Results from the DAPA-HF Trial. *Circulation* **2020**, *141*, 90–99. [CrossRef]
10. Kaplinsky, E. DAPA-HF trial: Dapagliflozin evolves from a glucose-lowering agent to a therapy for heart failure. *Drugs Context* **2020**, *9*, 2019-11-3. [CrossRef]
11. Alshnbari, A.S.; Millar, S.A.; O'sullivan, S.E.; Idris, I. Effect of Sodium-Glucose Cotransporter-2 Inhibitors on Endothelial Function: A Systematic Review of Preclinical Studies. *Diabetes Ther.* **2020**, *11*, 1947–1963. [CrossRef]
12. Palandurkar, G.; Kumar, S. Current Status of Dapagliflozin in Congestive Heart Failure. *Cureus* **2022**, *14*, e29413. [CrossRef]
13. Cheng, L.; Fu, Q.; Zhou, L.; Fan, Y.; Liu, F.; Fan, Y.; Zhang, X.; Lin, W.; Wu, X. Dapagliflozin, metformin, monotherapy or both in patients with metabolic syndrome. *Sci. Rep.* **2021**, *11*, 24263. [CrossRef]
14. Neal, B.; Perkovic, V.; Mahaffey, K.W.; de Zeeuw, D.; Fulcher, G.; Erondu, N.; Shaw, W.; Law, G.; Desai, M.; Matthews, D.R.; et al. Canagliflozin and Cardiovascular and Renal Events in Type 2 Diabetes. *N. Engl. J. Med.* **2017**, *377*, 644–657. [CrossRef] [PubMed]
15. Rådholm, K.; Figtree, G.; Perkovic, V.; Solomon, S.D.; Mahaffey, K.W.; de Zeeuw, D.; Fulcher, G.; Barrett, T.D.; Shaw, W.; Desai, M.; et al. Canagliflozin and heart failure in type 2 diabetes mellitus: Results from the CANVAS program. *Circulation* **2018**, *138*, 458–468. [CrossRef] [PubMed]
16. Davies, M.J.; Merton, K.; Vijapurkar, U.; Yee, J.; Qiu, R. Efficacy and safety of canagliflozin in patients with type 2 diabetes based on history of cardiovascular disease or cardiovascular risk factors: A post hoc analysis of pooled data. *Cardiovasc. Diabetol.* **2017**, *16*, 40. [CrossRef]
17. Blonde, L.; Stenlöf, K.; Fung, A.; Xie, J.; Canovatchel, W.; Meininger, G. Effects of canagliflozin on body weight and body composition in patients with type 2 diabetes over 104 weeks. *Postgrad. Med.* **2016**, *128*, 371–380. [CrossRef]
18. Davies, M.J.; Trujillo, A.; Vijapurkar, U.; Damaraju, C.V.; Meininger, G. Effect of canagliflozin on serum uric acid in patients with type 2 diabetes mellitus. *Diabetes, Obes. Metab.* **2015**, *17*, 426–429. [CrossRef]
19. Pfeifer, M.; Townsend, R.R.; Davies, M.J.; Vijapurkar, U.; Ren, J. Effects of canagliflozin, a sodium glucose co-transporter 2 inhibitor, on blood pressure and markers of arterial stiffness in patients with type 2 diabetes mellitus: A post hoc analysis. *Cardiovasc. Diabetol.* **2017**, *16*, 29. [CrossRef] [PubMed]
20. Gilbert, R.E.; Mende, C.; Vijapurkar, U.; Sha, S.; Davies, M.J.; Desai, M. Effects of Canagliflozin on Serum Magnesium in Patients with Type 2 Diabetes Mellitus: A Post Hoc Analysis of Randomized Controlled Trials. *Diabetes Ther.* **2017**, *8*, 451–458. [CrossRef] [PubMed]
21. Spertus, J.A.; Birmingham, M.C.; Nassif, M.; Damaraju, C.V.; Abbate, A.; Butler, J.; Lanfear, D.E.; Lingvay, I.; Kosiborod, M.N.; Januzzi, J.L. The SGLT2 inhibitor canagliflozin in heart failure: The CHIEF-HF remote, patient-centered randomized trial. *Nat. Med.* **2022**, *28*, 809–813. [CrossRef]
22. Fitchett, D.; Zinman, B.; Wanner, C.; Lachin, J.M.; Hantel, S.; Salsali, A.; Johansen, O.E.; Woerle, H.J.; Broedl, U.C.; Inzucchi, S.E. Heart failure outcomes with empagliflozin in patients with type 2 diabetes at high cardiovascular risk: Results of the EMPA-REG OUTCOME®trial. *Eur. Heart J.* **2016**, *37*, 1526–1534. [CrossRef]
23. Psaty, B.M.; Lumley, T.; Furberg, C.D.; Schellenbaum, G.; Pahor, M.; Alderman, M.H.; Weiss, N.S. Health Outcomes Associated with Various Antihypertensive Therapies Used as First-Line Agents. *JAMA* **2003**, *289*, 2534–2544. [CrossRef] [PubMed]
24. Staels, B. Cardiovascular Protection by Sodium Glucose Cotransporter 2 Inhibitors: Potential Mechanisms. *Am. J. Med.* **2017**, *130*, S30–S39. [CrossRef] [PubMed]
25. Marti, C.N.; Gheorghiade, M.; Kalogeropoulos, A.P.; Georgiopoulou, V.V.; Quyyumi, A.A.; Butler, J. Endothelial Dysfunction, Arterial Stiffness, and Heart Failure. *J. Am. Coll. Cardiol.* **2012**, *60*, 1455–1469. [CrossRef] [PubMed]
26. Tye, S.C.; Jongs, N.; Coca, S.G.; Sundström, J.; Arnott, C.; Neal, B.; Perkovic, V.; Mahaffey, K.W.; Vart, P.; Heerspink, H.J.L. Initiation of the SGLT2 inhibitor canagliflozin to prevent kidney and heart failure outcomes guided by HbA1c, albuminuria, and predicted risk of kidney failure. *Cardiovasc. Diabetol.* **2022**, *21*, 194. [CrossRef]
27. Vaduganathan, M.; Sattar, N.; Xu, J.; Butler, J.; Mahaffey, K.W.; Neal, B.; Shaw, W.; Rosenthal, N.; Pfeifer, M.; Hansen, M.K.; et al. Stress Cardiac Biomarkers, Cardiovascular and Renal Outcomes, and Response to Canagliflozin. *J. Am. Coll. Cardiol.* **2022**, *79*, 432–444. [CrossRef]

78. Figtree, G.A.; Rådholm, K.; Barrett, T.D.; Perkovic, V.; Mahaffey, K.W.; de Zeeuw, D.; Fulcher, G.; Matthews, D.R.; Shaw, W.; Neal, B. Effects of Canagliflozin on Heart Failure Outcomes Associated with Preserved and Reduced Ejection Fraction in Type 2 Diabetes Mellitus. *Circulation* **2019**, *139*, 2591–2593. [CrossRef]
79. Nasiri-Ansari, N.; Dimitriadis, G.K.; Agrogiannis, G.; Perrea, D.; Kostakis, I.D.; Kaltsas, G.; Papavassiliou, A.G.; Randeva, H.S.; Kassi, E. Canagliflozin attenuates the progression of atherosclerosis and inflammation process in APOE knockout mice. *Cardiovasc. Diabetol.* **2018**, *17*, 106. [CrossRef]
80. Lim, V.G.; Bell, R.M.; Arjun, S.; Kolatsi-Joannou, M.; Long, D.A.; Yellon, D.M. SGLT2 Inhibitor, Canagliflozin, Attenuates Myocardial Infarction in the Diabetic and Nondiabetic Heart. *JACC: Basic Transl. Sci.* **2019**, *4*, 15–26. [CrossRef]
81. Huynh, K. Diabetes: Lower risk of cardiovascular death with canagliflozin. *Nat. Rev. Cardiol.* **2017**, *14*, 442. [CrossRef]
82. Sabe, S.A.; Xu, C.M.; Sabra, M.; Harris, D.D.; Malhotra, A.; Aboulgheit, A.; Stanley, M.; Abid, M.R.; Sellke, F.W. Canagliflozin Improves Myocardial Perfusion, Fibrosis, and Function in a Swine Model of Chronic Myocardial Ischemia. *J. Am. Heart Assoc.* **2023**, *12*, e028623. [CrossRef]
83. Januzzi, J.L.; Butler, J.; Jarolim, P.; Sattar, N.; Vijapurkar, U.; Desai, M.; Davies, M.J. Effects of Canagliflozin on Cardiovascular Biomarkers in Older Adults with Type 2 Diabetes. *J. Am. Coll. Cardiol.* **2017**, *70*, 704–712. [CrossRef] [PubMed]
84. Sayour, A.A.; Korkmaz-Icöz, S.; Loganathan, S.; Ruppert, M.; Sayour, V.N.; Oláh, A.; Benke, K.; Brune, R.; Benkő, R.; Horváth, E.M.; et al. Acute canagliflozin treatment protects against in vivo myocardial ischemia–reperfusion injury in non-diabetic male rats and enhances endothelium-dependent vasorelaxation. *J. Transl. Med.* **2019**, *17*, 127. [CrossRef] [PubMed]
85. Ju, F.; Abbott, G.W.; Li, J.; Wang, Q.; Liu, T.; Liu, Q.; Hu, Z. Canagliflozin Pretreatment Attenuates Myocardial Dysfunction and Improves Postcardiac Arrest Outcomes After Cardiac Arrest and Cardiopulmonary Resuscitation in Mice. *Cardiovasc. Drugs Ther.* **2023**. [CrossRef] [PubMed]
86. Fernandes, G.C.; Fernandes, A.; Cardoso, R.; Penalver, J.; Knijnik, L.; Mitrani, R.D.; Myerburg, R.J.; Goldberger, J.J. Association of SGLT2 inhibitors with arrhythmias and sudden cardiac death in patients with type 2 diabetes or heart failure: A meta-analysis of 34 randomized controlled trials. *Heart Rhythm.* **2021**, *18*, 1098–1105. [CrossRef] [PubMed]
87. Engström, A.; Wintzell, V.; Melbye, M.; Hviid, A.; Eliasson, B.; Gudbjörnsdottir, S.; Hveem, K.; Jonasson, C.; Svanström, H.; Pasternak, B.; et al. Sodium–Glucose Cotransporter 2 Inhibitor Treatment and Risk of Atrial Fibrillation: Scandinavian Cohort Study. *Diabetes Care* **2022**, *46*, 351–360. [CrossRef]
88. Nishinarita, R.; Niwano, S.; Niwano, H.; Nakamura, H.; Saito, D.; Sato, T.; Matsuura, G.; Arakawa, Y.; Kobayashi, S.; Shirakawa, Y.; et al. Canagliflozin Suppresses Atrial Remodeling in a Canine Atrial Fibrillation Model. *J. Am. Heart Assoc.* **2021**, *10*, e017483. [CrossRef]
89. Li, D.; Liu, Y.; Hidru, T.H.; Yang, X.; Wang, Y.; Chen, C.; Li, K.H.C.; Tang, Y.; Wei, Y.; Tse, G.; et al. Protective Effects of Sodium-Glucose Transporter 2 Inhibitors on Atrial Fibrillation and Atrial Flutter: A Systematic Review and Meta-Analysis of Randomized Placebo-Controlled Trials. *Front. Endocrinol.* **2021**, *12*, 619586. [CrossRef]
90. Fediuk, D.J.; Nucci, G.; Dawra, V.K.; Cutler, D.L.; Amin, N.B.; Terra, S.G.; Boyd, R.A.; Krishna, R.; Sahasrabudhe, V. Overview of the Clinical Pharmacology of Ertugliflozin, a Novel Sodium-Glucose Cotransporter 2 (SGLT2) Inhibitor. *Clin. Pharmacokinet.* **2020**, *59*, 949–965. [CrossRef]
91. Cinti, F.; Moffa, S.; Impronta, F.; Cefalo, C.M.A.; Sun, V.A.; Sorice, G.P.; Mezza, T.; Giaccari, A. Spotlight on ertugliflozin and its potential in the treatment of type 2 diabetes: Evidence to date. *Drug Des. Dev. Ther.* **2017**, *11*, 2905–2919. [CrossRef] [PubMed]
92. Cosentino, F.; Cannon, C.P.; Cherney, D.Z.; Masiukiewicz, U.; Pratley, R.; Dagogo-Jack, S.; Frederich, R.; Charbonnel, B.; Mancuso, J.; Shih, W.J.; et al. Efficacy of Ertugliflozin on Heart Failure-Related Events in Patients With Type 2 Diabetes Mellitus and Established Atherosclerotic Cardiovascular Disease: Results of the VERTIS CV Trial. *Circulation* **2020**, *142*, 2205–2215. [CrossRef] [PubMed]
93. Cherney, D.Z.I.; Charbonnel, B.; Cosentino, F.; Dagogo-Jack, S.; McGuire, D.K.; Pratley, R.; Shih, W.J.; Frederich, R.; Maldonado, M.; Pong, A.; et al. Effects of ertugliflozin on kidney composite outcomes, renal function and albuminuria in patients with type 2 diabetes mellitus: An analysis from the randomised VERTIS CV trial. *Diabetologia* **2021**, *64*, 1256–1267. [CrossRef]
94. Cherney, D.Z.; Cosentino, F.; Dagogo-Jack, S.; McGuire, D.K.; Pratley, R.; Frederich, R.; Maldonado, M.; Liu, C.-C.; Liu, J.; Pong, A.; et al. Ertugliflozin and Slope of Chronic eGFR: Prespecified Analyses from the Randomized VERTIS CV Trial. *Clin. J. Am. Soc. Nephrol.* **2021**, *16*, 1345–1354. [CrossRef]
95. Allegretti, A.S.; Zhang, W.; Zhou, W.; Thurber, T.K.; Rigby, S.P.; Bowman-Stroud, C.; Trescoli, C.; Serusclat, P.; Freeman, M.W.; Halvorsen, Y.-D.C. Safety and Effectiveness of Bexagliflozin in Patients With Type 2 Diabetes Mellitus and Stage 3a/3b CKD. *Am. J. Kidney Dis.* **2019**, *74*, 328–337. [CrossRef] [PubMed]
96. Brenzavvy (Bexagliflozin) Dosing, Indications, Interactions, Adverse Effects, and More. 13 April 2023. Available online: https://reference.medscape.com/drug/brenzavvy-bexagliflozin-4000358#92 (accessed on 12 May 2023).
97. Halvorsen, Y.; Lock, J.P.; Zhou, W.; Zhu, F.; Freeman, M.W. A 24-week, randomized, double-blind, active-controlled clinical trial comparing bexagliflozin with sitagliptin as an adjunct to metformin for the treatment of type 2 diabetes in adults. *Diabetes Obes. Metab.* **2019**, *21*, 2248–2256. [CrossRef]
98. Halvorsen, Y.; Lock, J.P.; Frias, J.P.; Tinahones, F.J.; Dahl, D.; Conery, A.L.; Freeman, M.W. A 96-week, double-blind, randomized controlled trial comparing bexagliflozin with glimepiride as an adjunct to metformin for the treatment of type 2 diabetes in adults. *Diabetes, Obes. Metab.* **2022**, *25*, 293–301. [CrossRef]

99. Mcmurray, J.J.; Freeman, M.W.; Massaro, J.; Solomon, S.; Lock, P.; Riddle, M.C.; Lewis, E.; Halvorsen, Y.-D.C. 32-OR: The Bexagliflozin Efficacy and Safety Trial (BEST): A Randomized, Double-Blind, Placebo-Controlled, Phase IIII, Clinical Trial. *Diabetes* **2020**, *69* (Suppl. S1), 32-OR. [CrossRef]
100. Maan, A.; Heist, E.K.; Passeri, J.; Inglessis, I.; Baker, J.; Ptaszek, L.; Vlahakes, G.; Ruskin, J.N.; Palacios, I.; Sundt, T.; et al. Impact of Atrial Fibrillation on Outcomes in Patients Who Underwent Transcatheter Aortic Valve Replacement. *Am. J. Cardiol.* **2015**, *115*, 220–226. [CrossRef]
101. Khan, S.S.; Butler, J.; Gheorghiade, M. Management of Comorbid Diabetes Mellitus and Worsening Heart Failure. *JAMA* **2014**, *311*, 2379–2380. [CrossRef]
102. Food US and Admin Drug. Guidance for Industry on Diabetes Mellitus—Evaluating Cardiovascular Risk in New Antidiabetic Therapies to Treat Type 2 Diabetes; Availability. Fed. Regist 73. 2008. Available online: https://www.govinfo.gov/content/pkg/FR-2008-12-19/pdf/E8-30086.pdf (accessed on 14 May 2023).
103. Biviano, A.B.; Nazif, T.; Dizon, J.; Garan, H.; Fleitman, J.; Hassan, D.; Kapadia, S.; Babaliaros, V.; Xu, K.; Parvataneni, R.; et al. Atrial Fibrillation Is Associated With Increased Mortality in Patients Undergoing Transcatheter Aortic Valve Replacement: Insights From the Placement of Aortic Transcatheter Valve (PARTNER) Trial. *Circ. Cardiovasc. Interv.* **2016**, *9*, e002766. [CrossRef] [PubMed]

Disclaimer/Publisher's Note: The statements, opinions and data contained in all publications are solely those of the individual author(s) and contributor(s) and not of MDPI and/or the editor(s). MDPI and/or the editor(s) disclaim responsibility for any injury to people or property resulting from any ideas, methods, instructions or products referred to in the content.

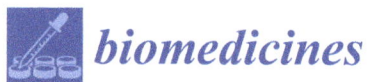

Review

TAVI in a Heart Transplant Recipient—Rare Case Report and Review of the Literature

Silvia Preda [1,2], Lucian Câlmâc [2], Claudia Nica [2], Mihai Cacoveanu [2,*], Robert Țigănașu [2], Aida Badea [2], Alexandru Zăman [2], Raluca Ciomag (Ianula) [1,3], Claudiu Nistor [1,4], Bogdan Severus Gașpar [1,3], Luminița Iliuță [1,5], Lucian Dorobanțu [6,7], Vlad Anton Iliescu [1,8] and Horațiu Moldovan [1,2,9,*]

1. Faculty of Medicine, Carol Davila University of Medicine and Pharmacy, 050474 Bucharest, Romania; dr.silvia.preda@gmail.com (S.P.); raluca.ianula@umfcd.ro (R.C.); ncd58@yahoo.com (C.N.); bogdan.gaspar@umfcd.ro (B.S.G.); luminitailiuta@yahoo.com (L.I.); vladanton.iliescu@gmail.com (V.A.I.)
2. Department of Cardiovascular Surgery, Bucharest Clinical Emergency Hospital, 014461 Bucharest, Romania; lcalmac@gmail.com (L.C.); bianca.nica@yahoo.com (C.N.); tiganasu.robert@yahoo.com (R.Ț.); aidafirtade@gmail.com (A.B.); alexandrusebastianzaman@gmail.com (A.Z.)
3. Department of Cardiology, "Bagdasar Arseni" Clinical Emergency Hospital, 041915 Bucharest, Romania
4. Department of Thoracic Surgery, Central Military Emergency University Hospital, 013058 Bucharest, Romania
5. Cardioclass Clinic for Cardiovascular Disease, 031125 Bucharest, Romania
6. Faculty of Medicine, Titu Maiorescu University, 040441 Bucharest, Romania; lucian.dorobantu@prof.utm.ro
7. Department of Cardiovascular Surgery, Monza Metropolitan Hospital, 040204 Bucharest, Romania
8. Department of Cardiovascular Surgery, Prof. Dr. C.C. Iliescu Emergency Institute for Cardiovascular Diseases, 022322 Bucharest, Romania
9. Academy of Romanian Scientists, 54, Spl. Independentei, 050711 Bucharest, Romania
* Correspondence: catalin.cacoveanu@gmail.com (M.C.); h_moldovan@hotmail.com (H.M.)

Citation: Preda, S.; Câlmâc, L.; Nica, C.; Cacoveanu, M.; Țigănașu, R.; Badea, A.; Zăman, A.; Ciomag, R.; Nistor, C.; Gașpar, B.S.; et al. TAVI in a Heart Transplant Recipient—Rare Case Report and Review of the Literature. *Biomedicines* **2023**, *11*, 2634. https://doi.org/10.3390/biomedicines11102634

Academic Editors: Shaker A. Mousa and Alfredo Caturano

Received: 29 June 2023
Revised: 18 August 2023
Accepted: 18 September 2023
Published: 26 September 2023

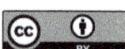

Copyright: © 2023 by the authors. Licensee MDPI, Basel, Switzerland. This article is an open access article distributed under the terms and conditions of the Creative Commons Attribution (CC BY) license (https://creativecommons.org/licenses/by/4.0/).

Abstract: The global demand for cardiac transplants continues to rise, even with advancements in assistive devices. Currently, the estimated annual mortality rate stands at 3–5%, and patients often face a waiting time of approximately four years on transplant waiting lists. Consequently, many transplant centers have started to consider heart transplants from donors who may be deemed "less than ideal" or marginal. However, the decision to accept such donors must be highly individualized, taking into consideration the risks associated with remaining on the waiting list versus those posed by the transplantation procedure itself. A potential solution lies in the creation of two distinct recipient lists, matched with donor criteria, allowing marginal donors to provide the lifeline that selected patients require. This paper follows a two-step approach. Firstly, it offers an overview of the current state of affairs regarding the topic of transcatheter aortic valve implantation (TAVI) in orthotopic heart transplant (OHT) patients. Secondly, it presents firsthand experience from our clinical center with a comprehensive case presentation of a patient in this unique medical context. The clinical case refers to a 62-year-old male patient, a smoker with a history of hypertension, dyslipidemia, and a prior OHT a decade earlier, who presented with fatigue during minimal physical exertion. The Heart Team carefully reviewed the case, considering the patient's immunosuppressed status and the heightened risk associated with a repeat intervention. In this instance, transcatheter aortic valve implantation (TAVI) was deemed the appropriate treatment. The TAVI procedure yielded successful results, leading to improved clinical status and enhanced cardiac function. The inclusion of marginal donors has introduced novel challenges related to the utilization of previously diseased marginal organs. TAVI has already demonstrated its efficacy and versatility in treating high-risk patients, including heart transplant recipients. Consequently, it emerges as a vital tool in addressing the unique challenges posed by the inclusion of marginal donors.

Keywords: orthotopic heart transplantation (OHT); transcatheter aortic valve implantation (TAVI); heart valve replacement; aortic valve

1. Background

In the present day, orthotopic heart transplantation (OHT) stands as one of the established approaches for managing advanced heart failure. Its legacy spans over 55 years, commencing with the controversial inaugural global human transplant in 1967 [1].

Much later, in 2002, the inaugural transcatheter aortic valve implantation (TAVI) procedure was successfully conducted by Professor Alain Cribier in France. The development of this technique began in 1980 due to an increasing demand for alternative treatments. In its early stages, the primary focus was on balloon aortic valvuloplasty for patients with high-risk aortic stenosis. Although this approach led to symptom improvement, it was associated with numerous complications and lacked favorable mid- to long-term outcomes. As a result, it is now considered only as a palliative measure when TAVI or surgical aortic valve replacement (SAVR) is not feasible.

In 1992, the first crimped biological valve prosthesis was patented, though it remained unused until further studies in 1994 demonstrated its ability to maintain its shape within a calcified annulus. Despite initial skepticism surrounding TAVI, multiple studies conducted between 1999 and 2002 affirmed its viability as a valuable treatment option [2].

Since its inception, OHT has witnessed significant advancements in patient survival, medical interventions, and the management of associated complications. Notably, the 5-year survival rate following OHT has increased from 62.7% in 1980 to 72.5% in 2014. Data from the registry of the International Society of Heart and Lung Transplantation (ISHLT) indicates that around 21% of patients remain alive at the 20-year mark, with select centers reporting an impressive 20-year survival rate of 55% of patients [3,4].

Complications that arise following OHT play a pivotal role in determining patient outcomes and their susceptibility to subsequent cardiac surgeries. Among the most commonly reported complications are chronic allograft vasculopathy (CAV), malignancies, infections, acute rejection, and renal insufficiency.

CAV is prevalent in approximately one third of patients within their initial five years post OHT, and this incidence surges to over 50% after a decade. Its significance is underscored by the fact that CAV contributes to approximately 10% of annual deaths among recipients. Ten years post OHT, malignancy diagnoses affect 35% of patients, with skin cancer being the most frequently reported type. After the first five years post OHT, malignancy-related mortality stands at approximately 22% annually.

Infections represent a critical complication, with a substantial mortality rate of up to 30% within the first year following OHT. However, this complication tends to decline in subsequent years, potentially attributable to a reduction in immunosuppressive therapy.

Acute rejection assumes particular importance, especially during the initial years post OHT, accounting for approximately 10% of deaths within the first three years.

The incidence of renal insufficiency escalates over time, reaching 30% at the ten-year mark following OHT [4,5].

Since the inception of OHT and TAVI, significant progress has been achieved in the field of cardiovascular surgery. These advancements have expanded the scope of indications, allowing for the application of these procedures even in cases that fall outside the established guidelines under specific circumstances.

Through consistently delivering positive outcomes and actively sharing experiences, the entire medical community can enhance their clinical practice and remain well-informed about the latest developments in this field. This collaborative approach ensures that patients benefit from the most current and effective treatments available [3].

Despite the remarkable advancements in cardiac surgery, it remains imperative to carefully consider patients with OHT and their unique set of risks and comorbidities. This thoughtful approach is essential for enhancing both their survival rates and overall quality of life. Through tailoring medical care and interventions to the specific needs and challenges of OHT patients, healthcare professionals can continue to improve patient outcomes and ensure a better quality of life for this distinct patient population.

2. Literature Review

This section delves into a thorough review of the existing literature, encompassing documented cases and studies related to OHT recipients facing aortic stenosis. It elucidates the challenges associated with this unique patient group and highlights instances where TAVI emerged as a viable intervention.

Currently, there is a noticeable absence of specific clinical guidelines for managing aortic stenosis in patients who have previously undergone OHT. The lack of such guidelines leaves clinicians with limited guidance on how to approach aortic stenosis in this unique patient population.

With the success of heart transplantations and the increasing number of OHT recipients, there is a growing need to address the specific medical conditions and complications that arise in this population. Aortic stenosis is not uncommon in this group, and as such, it necessitates specialized consideration.

Patients with a history of OHT present a clinical complexity that requires tailored approaches. Their immunosuppressive status, previous cardiac surgeries, and comorbidities need to be factored into treatment decisions. Aortic stenosis management in this context demands careful evaluation and a nuanced understanding of the associated risks and benefits of various interventions.

While the absence of established guidelines can be challenging, it also presents an opportunity for innovation in patient care. Exploring alternative procedures such as TAVI and evaluating their outcomes in OHT recipients can pave the way for the development of evidence-based protocols that improve patient outcomes and quality of life.

3. Objective

In this literature review, our primary aim was to identify previously published studies of individuals with a history of OHT who subsequently developed aortic valve disease necessitating aortic valve replacement. Our analysis focused on investigating the management strategies employed in such cases, specifically examining the choice of valve type (balloon-expandable or self-expandable) and the approach used (femoral artery or transapical). Additionally, we aimed to assess the clinical outcomes associated with these interventions.

4. Methods

4.1. Eligibility Criteria

For this literature review, we sought studies involving individuals who had previously undergone OHT and subsequently developed aortic valve disease necessitating aortic valve replacement. We conducted a comprehensive search for articles published in English In the selected articles, we examined demographic information, including population characteristics, sex, age at OHT, age at TAVI, the time elapsed between OHT and TAVI, the type of aortic valve prosthesis used, the procedural approach, and clinical outcomes.

4.2. Information Sources

Our search encompassed electronic databases, including Pubmed, Cochrane Library, and EMBASE. Additionally, we explored the PROSPERO registry for any relevant reviews, although none were identified.

4.3. Search Strategy

To identify pertinent studies, we conducted electronic searches using keywords such as heart transplant, OHT, heart transplant recipient aortic disease, aortic stenosis, TAVI, TAVR, and aortic valve replacement after heart transplant.

4.4. Study Records–Data Management

Upon selecting articles that described aortic valve replacement in OHT recipients, we sought data pertaining to patient characteristics, age at transplantation and at aortic valve

replacement, the duration between OHT and aortic valve replacement, prosthesis type and size, procedural approach, clinical status of patients at the time of OHT and/or aortic valve replacement, and outcomes.
- Selection process: Two independent reviewers selected studies adhering to the aforementioned eligibility criteria from the same electronic databases.
- Data collection process: Given the predominance of case reports in the literature, we independently extracted data from these reports.

We retrieved data related to population characteristics, including age at transplantation and aortic valve replacement, gender, and comorbidities. Additionally, we gathered information on the clinical status of patients at the time of OHT and aortic valve replacement, the type and size of the valve utilized, the procedural approach, and defined outcomes encompassing mortality, complications, the necessity for additional interventions, improvements in cardiac function, and post-procedural clinical status.

4.5. Outcomes and Prioritization

Our primary outcomes of interest were patient survival and procedure-related complications, including the need for reintervention, bleeding, tamponade, paravalvular leak, coronary complications associated with the procedure, the requirement for a pacemaker, and broader outcomes such as post-procedural contractility, clinical status enhancement, and hospital discharge.

4.6. Data Synthesis

Given the relatively small number of patients and their variability, a systematic representation of the targeted patient profile cannot be made.

Due to the incomplete data reported in the articles found and small population with this particular characteristic, we cannot have a statistical analysis of the cases found in the literature. So, we described each case published until the first draft of the manuscript was submitted and compared the data in a table to make it easier to observe.

5. Results

The current clinical guidelines do not provide specific recommendations for the management of individuals with aortic stenosis who have previously undergone OHT. Consequently, we recognized the significance of contributing a case study involving a patient who underwent a TAVI procedure following OHT.

While the medical literature contains an extensive body of research discussing OHT and TAVI as separate entities, there is a paucity of literature addressing the intersection of TAVI in OHT recipients. This knowledge gap has resulted in the absence of a consensus regarding the optimal management of this specific patient population. As a result, clinical decisions are typically made on a case-by-case basis by interdisciplinary Heart Teams [3].

Given the limited number of patients available for study and the inherent heterogeneity within this patient cohort, it is not feasible to construct a systematic representation of the typical characteristics of individuals undergoing TAVI after OHT.

Furthermore, due to the presence of incomplete data within the identified literature and the restricted size of the population possessing this unique clinical profile, we were unable to perform a robust statistical analysis of the cases reported in the literature. Consequently, we adopted a descriptive approach, summarizing each case published up to the submission of our initial manuscript draft and presenting this information in a tabular format to enhance ease of comprehension.

The inaugural case of TAVI in an OHT recipient was published in 2010 by Seiffert and colleagues. This case involved an 81-year-old patient, deemed high-risk, who had undergone OHT 15 years prior. The patient exhibited a reduced left ventricular ejection fraction (LVEF) of less than 30%, attributed to concomitant coronary artery disease (CAD). The choice of the transapical approach was made due to severe calcification of the entire aorta and kinking of the iliac arteries. A 26 mm Edward Sapien transcatheter heart valve

(THV) was utilized and successfully implanted, with minimal residual paravalvular regurgitation. Subsequently, the patient required a percutaneous coronary intervention (PCI) involving the placement of a drug-eluting stent (DES) in the left anterior descending (LAD) artery. Intraoperative transesophageal echocardiography (TEE) demonstrated improved contractility and an LVEF of 50%. Preoperative TTE had revealed a mean aortic gradient of 23 mm Hg and an effective orifice area of 0.6 cm^2, consistent with the characteristic findings of low-flow, low-gradient severe aortic stenosis [6].

The second documented case, reported in the same year by Bruschi et al., involved a 67-year-old male patient who underwent TAVI for severe aortic stenosis approximately nine years after receiving a heart transplant. Preoperative assessments revealed significant findings, including a peak gradient of 87 mmHg, an indexed aortic valve area (AVA) of 0.5 cm^2/m^2, and pronounced left ventricular (LV) systolic dysfunction, with a LVEF of 35%. The medical team opted for a 29 mm CoreValve prosthesis (Medtronic) for the TAVI procedure, which resulted in only mild paravalvular regurgitation [7].

TAVI has also been employed as a treatment option for heart transplant recipients presenting with aortic regurgitation and deemed at high surgical risk. The initial case report of such an intervention was published by Zanuttini et al., involving a 75-year-old individual who had OHT approximately 14 years after the original transplantation procedure. The patient's initial heart transplant had been necessitated by end-stage dilated cardiomyopathy (DCM) and had involved mitral and aortic valve replacements.

Preprocedural TTE revealed a mildly dilated left ventricle with moderate LVEF of 40% and thickening of the tricuspid aortic valve. The patient presented with severe aortic regurgitation characterized by a central jet, attributed to the deformation and retraction of the left coronary cusp. Given the patient's high surgical risk, as indicated by a EuroSCORE of 36%, the medical team elected to perform a TAVI procedure. A 29 mm CoreValve prosthesis was employed for this intervention. Post procedure, the patient developed a third-degree atrioventricular (AV) block, necessitating the placement of a permanent pacemaker. Subsequent TEE demonstrated normal prosthetic valve function, with peak and mean gradients measuring 16 and 10 mmHg, respectively, and a mild paravalvular leak [8].

In 2013, Praetere et al. reported the fourth case involving a 77-year-old male patient who underwent TAVI for the treatment of aortic stenosis. This intervention took place two decades after the patient had received an OHT. Initial assessment of the patient revealed an aortic valve area (AVA) of 1 cm^2, indicative of severe aortic stenosis. The patient also presented with a low-flow, low-gradient condition and severe left ventricular dysfunction, characterized by a left ventricular ejection fraction (LVEF) of less than 25%. Additionally, the patient had undergone multiple PCIs for CAD. Further diagnostic evaluation included low-dose dobutamine stress echocardiography (DSE), which was inconclusive in accurately assessing the true severity of aortic stenosis (AS). Consequently, a decision was made to perform a balloon aortic valvuloplasty (BAV) to reevaluate the patient's symptoms and LVEF. In the months following the BAV procedure, the patient experienced moderate symptom improvement and a subsequent increase in LVEF to 30%. However, after seven months, the patient experienced symptom relapse, prompting the medical team to consider TAVI as the next course of action. The TAVI procedure was carried out via the transapical approach, utilizing a 23 mm Edwards Sapien valve. Postprocedural evaluation demonstrated a 30% LVEF and the absence of paravalvular leak, with peak and mean gradients measuring 18 and 11 mmHg, respectively [9].

The fifth case, documented by Ahmad et al. In 2016, involves a 25-year-old female who underwent an urgent OHT at the age of 11 due to severe congestive heart failure. The patient had previously undergone corrective surgeries for ventricular septal defects at ages 1 and 3. It's worth noting that some cases of OHT lack comprehensive data regarding the dono's heart at the time of implantation. However, in this particular case, it was reported that the donor was a 62-year-old woman with preexisting moderate coronary artery disease and mild aortic stenosis. Approximately 14 years following the initial heart transplant, the recipient began experiencing NYHA III heart failure symptoms. TTE revealed a severely calcified tricuspid aortic valve with severe aortic stenosis, characterized by a peak gradient of 77 mmHg and a mean gradient of 44 mmHg. The AVA measured less than 1 cm^2, and severe aortic regurgitation was also present, despite normal LVEF. Subsequently, the patient underwent a TAVI procedure using a 23 mm Edwards Sapien 3 valve in a standard protocol. Following the TAVI intervention, the patien's clinical condition improved significantly. Postprocedural TTE demonstrated normal valve function with no evidence of paravalvular regurgitation. Additionally, peak and mean gradients were measured at 20 mmHg and 11 mmHg, respectively, indicating favorable hemodynamic outcomes [10].

In the same year, Herrmann et al. reported another case of TAVI in an OHT recipient. This case involved a 73-year-old male who had received a heart transplant 13 years earlier and subsequently developed severe aortic stenosis, with the additional finding of a bicuspid aortic valve. Preprocedural TTE revealed an AVA measuring 0.58 cm^2 and a mean gradient of 43 mmHg. Given the patient's high surgical risk, as indicated by a Society of Thoracic Surgeons (STS) score of 8.024%, the decision was made to proceed with the TAVI procedure. The intervention followed the standard approach, utilizing a 26 mm Edwards Sapien 3 valve and the transfemoral access route. Postprocedural TTE assessment demonstrated the normal functionality of the implanted valve. Furthermore, there was no evidence of paravalvular regurgitation, and the measured peak and mean gradients were 27 mmHg and 13 mmHg, respectively, reflecting successful hemodynamic outcomes [11].

In 2018, Akleh et al. reported a case involving TAVI in an OHT recipient. The patient was a 77-year-old male who had undergone heart transplantation 23 years earlier and presented with exertional dyspnea attributed to aortic stenosis. The original heart transplant had been conducted due to idiopathic dilated cardiomyopathy (DCM), although no records were available from the 1994 procedure. The patient's postoperative clinical course had been generally favorable, with the exception of paroxysmal atrial flutter, which necessitated the implantation of a single-chamber pacemaker in 2008. Subsequently, in 2010, the patient underwent atrial flutter ablation. TTE revealed progressive degeneration of a bicuspid aortic valve, indicated by a peak gradient of 65 mmHg, an AVA measuring 0.9 cm^2, and a preserved LVEF of 59%. Multidetector computer tomography (MDCT) confirmed significant calcification of the aortic valve and ruled out aortoiliac atherosclerosis, which was crucial in selecting the transfemoral approach for the TAVI procedure. Given the patient's high surgical risk, as denoted by a Society of Thoracic Surgeons (STS) score predicting a 7.035% mortality risk within 30 days, the Heart Team opted for TAVI as the preferred treatment strategy. The TAVI procedure adhered to established protocols and utilized a 29 mm Edwards Sapien 3 valve. Additionally, the patient's single-chamber pacemaker was upgraded to a dual-chamber system on the day following the TAVI. Postprocedural TTE revealed normal function of the aortic bioprosthesis, with peak and mean gradients measuring 14 mm Hg and 12 mm Hg, respectively. No paravalvular leak was observed, and the patient maintained a preserved LVEF. Following the procedure, the patient experienced symptomatic and hemodynamic improvement and was discharged 48 h post TAVI. He continued to receive immunosuppressive therapy as part of his ongoing post-transplant care [12].

In 2019, Avula S. et al. reported the eighth case of TAVI in an OHT recipient in the United States. This case involved a 73-year-old male who had undergone heart transplantation 19 years prior due to non-ischemic cardiomyopathy. Over the years following the transplant, a transthoracic echocardiogram revealed progressive sclerotic changes that began around 15 years post-transplantation and eventually led to the diagnosis of severe aortic stenosis in 2019. The patient's post-transplant medical history indicated the presence of non-occlusive CAD in addition to aortic stenosis. Given the patient's high surgical risk, as indicated by an STS score of 12.20%, the medical team opted for TAVI as the preferred treatment strategy. The TAVI procedure was conducted in a standard manner, utilizing a 29 mm Edwards Sapien 3 valve. Local anesthesia and sedation were employed for the procedure. Postprocedural TTE demonstrated the normal functioning of the implanted valve, with no evidence of valve leakage, and the patient exhibited a normal LVEF. Following the intervention, the patient's clinical course was favorable, and he was discharged on the second day after the procedure [13].

In 2020, Beale et al. reported the ninth case of TAVI in OHT recipients. This particular case involved a 45-year-old patient who had received a heart transplant 22 years earlier originally due to non-ischemic cardiomyopathy. The patient's medical history included several notable factors, such as a BAV in the transplanted heart, hypertension, hyperlipidemia and various transplantation-associated complications. Among the notable complications were squamous cell carcinoma of the hard palate, which had been treated with resection and grafting, as well as end-stage renal disease (ESRD) necessitating hemodialysis due to cyclosporine toxicity. Given the patient's complex medical history and high-risk status, the Heart Team elected to perform a TAVI procedure, which yielded optimal results [14].

The tenth case reported involved a 61-year-old patient who developed aortic stenosis a remarkable 34 years after undergoing an OHT. Unfortunately, there were no available details regarding the specific type of heart donor used in the transplantation. The patient's advanced aortic stenosis was treated with a self-expandable valve due to the presence of a significantly enlarged annulus and severe calcifications affecting both the mitral and aortic valves. The TAVI procedure yielded favorable outcomes, as evidenced by the absence of valve leakage and the preservation of a normal LVEF [15].

In Table 1, we have systematically summarized the findings to facilitate a comparative analysis of common characteristics between the case reports and the evidence found in the literature.

Table 1. Literature review summary of the TAVI procedure in OHT patients.

Authors	Year Published	Age at Transplant	Age at TAVI (Years)	Years from OHT to TAVI	LVEF (%)	TVG (mmHg)	TAVI Valve Size (mm)	Type of TAVI	Type of Implantation	Outcome
Seiffert et al. [6]	2010	66	81	15	<30	M23	26	Edward Sapien	TA	DES/LAD; LVEF 50%
Bruschi et al. [7]	2010	56	67	9	35	P87	29	CoreValve	TF	Mild paravalvular regurgitation
Zanuttini et al. [8]	2013	61	75	14	40	No data	29	CoreValve	TF	Mild paravalvular regurgitation 3rd-degree AV block, Permanent pacemaker
Praetere et al. [9]	2013	57	77	20	<25%	32/17	23	Edward Sapien	TA	LVEF 30%; no paravalvular leak
Ahmad et al. [10]	2016	11	25	14	Normal	77/44	23	Edward Sapien 3	TF	no paravalvular leak
Julien et al. [11]	2016	60	73	13	No data	M43	26	Edward Sapien 3	TF	no paravalvular leak
Akleh et al. [12]	2018	54	77	23	59	P65	29	Edward Sapien 3	TF	No paravalvular leak
Avula S. et al. [13]	2019	54	73	19	Normal		29	Edward Sapien 3	TF	No paravalvular leak
Beale et al. [14]	2020	23	45	22	Normal	M52	No data	No data	TF	complete heart block, trace paravalvular leak
Saad M. Ezad et al. [15]	2022	27	61	34	No data	No data	34	Evolut R	TF	No paravalvular leak

6. Case Presentation

We present the case of a 62-year-old male with a history of OHT a decade ago. He had a medical history that included a myocardial infarction with delayed admission, leading to refractory cardiogenic shock necessitating an intra-aortic balloon pump (IABP) and veno-arterial extracorporeal life support (V-A ECLS). Due to his critical condition, he underwent emergent OHT, resulting in a NYHA class II heart failure diagnosis and moderate aortic stenosis. Limited information was available about the donor, except that the allograft came from a marginal donor.

Upon discharge, the recipient had an aortic valve area of 1.1 cm^2, but no data were available regarding transvalvular gradients. The patient also had chronic kidney disease (creatinine 1.75 mg/dL), colonic diverticulosis, hyperuricemia, and a right bundle branch block. Several months before admission, the patient experienced flu-like symptoms, which were not confirmed as a COVID infection.

His current home treatment regimen included antiplatelet therapy, a low-dose diuretic, cholesterol-lowering medication, and immunosuppressive therapy (cyclosporine, prednisone, and mycophenolic acid). Unfortunately, the patient did not adhere to the mandatory follow-up plan for cardiac transplant recipients, and there had been no recent bloodwork or cardiac evaluations in the past five years.

Upon admission, TTE revealed a LVEF of 40% with mild diffuse hypokinesia. Additionally, there was evidence of degenerative aortic disease with severe stenosis and moderate aortic regurgitation, accompanied by substantial calcifications of the aortic leaflets. The AVA measured 0.4 cm^2, with a peak gradient of 100 mmHg, a mean gradient of 62 mmHg, and a 20 mm diameter aortic annulus. The patient exhibited moderate concentric hypertrophy, severe diastolic dysfunction with a restrictive pattern, and elevated filling pressures. Left atrium dilation was notable, with a volume of 140 mL. The evaluation of other valves indicated mild degenerative mitral regurgitation with posterior annulus calcifications, as well as moderate tricuspid and pulmonary regurgitations. The right ventricle displayed normal contractility, but the estimated pulmonary artery systolic pressure (PASP) was 69 mmHg. A further CT-angiography (CTA) scan indicated a dilated ascending aorta with a diameter of 41 mm.

The Heart Team reviewed the case, taking into account the patient's immunosuppressed status and the high risk associated with a redo intervention. The decision was made to proceed with TAVI. The patient underwent the necessary pre-procedural assessments, including coronary angiography, CTA scans, and bacteriology and viral screenings.

The CTA scan revealed a tricuspid aortic valve with an annulus area of 434 mm^2 and dimensions near the lower limit, measuring between 26 mm and 23 mm. Notably, calcium protrusions toward the left ventricular outflow tract (LVOT) were observed below the left coronary cusp (LCC) and non-coronary cusp (NCC), increasing the risk of disturbances. To determine sizing and assess calcium behavior, a balloon valvuloplasty was considered. The left coronary artery (LCA) was found to be at a distance of 15 mm from the aortic annulus, while the right coronary artery (RCA) was at a distance of 17.5 mm. The access vessels showed calcification, with borderline diameters for eSheath placement on both sides. CTA with 3D reconstruction—access vessels is presented in Figure 1. In Figure 2 can be observed aortography of aortic root and ascending aorta, and origins of coronary arteries (a) and CTA 3D reconstruction of aortic root with coronary arteries origin, ascending aorta (b). The lines in Figure 2a represent the plane of the aortic annulus (pink) and the position perpendicular to the aortic axis (yellow). Proper alignment for prosthesis implantation.

The TAVI procedure was performed under general anesthesia and standard monitoring protocols, with temporary rapid pacing achieved through an internal jugular vein catheter.

Percutaneous diagnosis was accomplished using a 6 French (F) sheath inserted via the left femoral artery. Subsequently, a Safari stiff guidewire was introduced, followed by the insertion of a specific eSheath through the right femoral artery. The hydrophilic guidewire, along with the AL 1 catheter, was navigated retrogradely across the aortic valve. Following this, the hydrophilic guidewire was exchanged for the stiff Safari guidewire, and the Sapien

3 valve, size 23 mm, was positioned at the level of the aortic annulus. Figure 3 presents a fluoroscopy image showing valve positioning. With the aid of rapid pacing, the valve was expanded (nominal volume +1 mL). During transesophageal echocardiography (TEE) assessment, a paravalvular leak was detected.

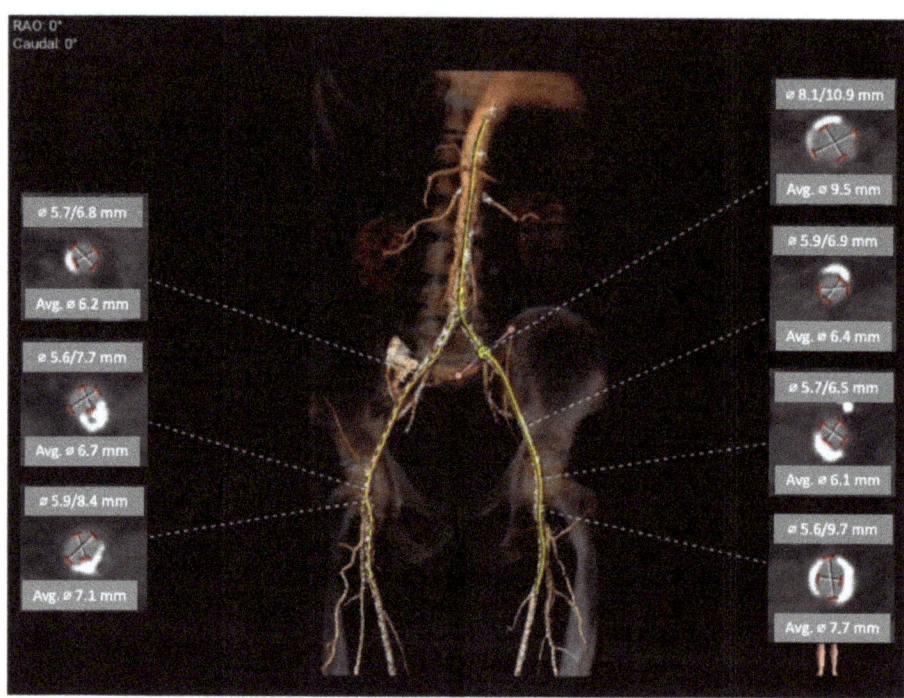

Figure 1. CTA with 3D reconstruction—access vessels.

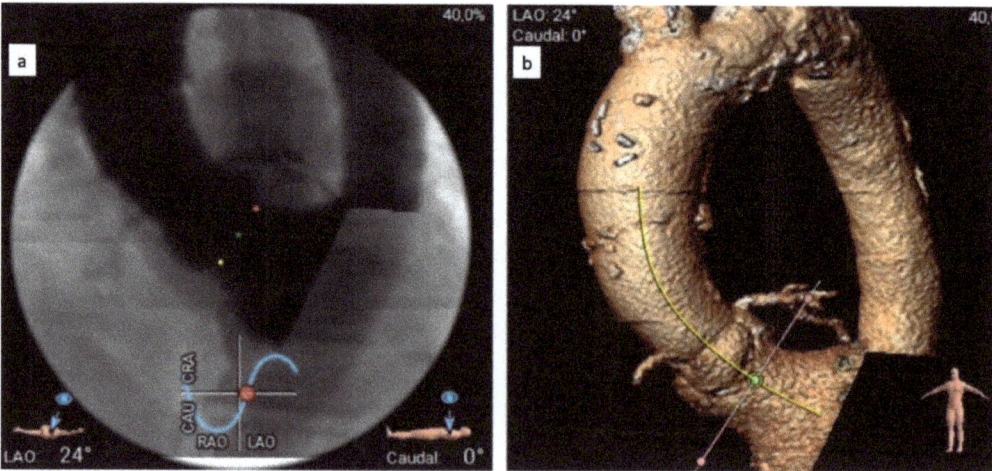

Figure 2. Investigative images: Aortography—aortic root and ascending aorta, and origins of coronary arteries (**a**) and CTA 3D reconstruction—aortic root with coronary arteries origin, ascending aorta (**b**).

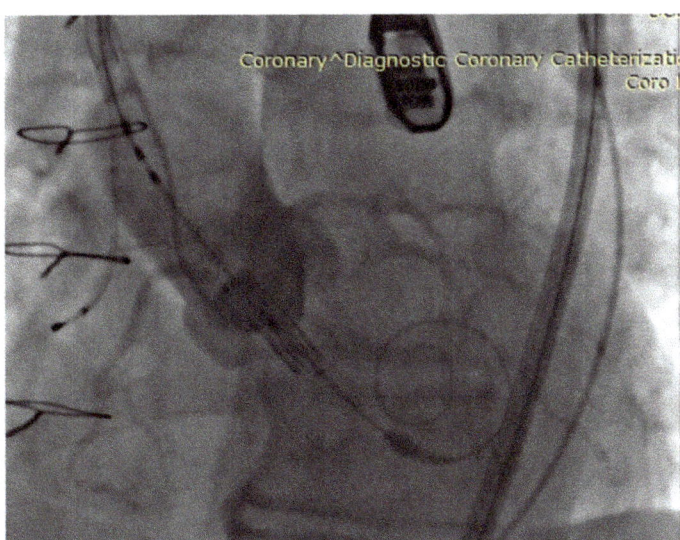

Figure 3. Fluoroscopy image—Valve positioning.

To address the paravalvular leak, a subsequent post-dilation was performed through inflating the valve's specific balloon with a nominal volume of +2 mL. Fluoroscopy image of aortic root showing baloon inflating in order to expand the aortic prosthesis is observed in Figure 4a, while Figure 4b presents a fluoroscopy image showing inflated baloon in the expanded prosthesis with coronary arteries visible. TEE examination following the post-dilation revealed minimal regurgitation. At the supravalvular aortic injection, only mild regurgitation was observed. Figure 5 presents a fluoroscopy image where checking the valve position and regurgitation can be observed. The guidewires were then carefully withdrawn, and another TEE confirmed minimal residual regurgitation. Hemostasis was achieved through the use of Proglide and Angioseal devices following the removal of guidewires and sheaths.

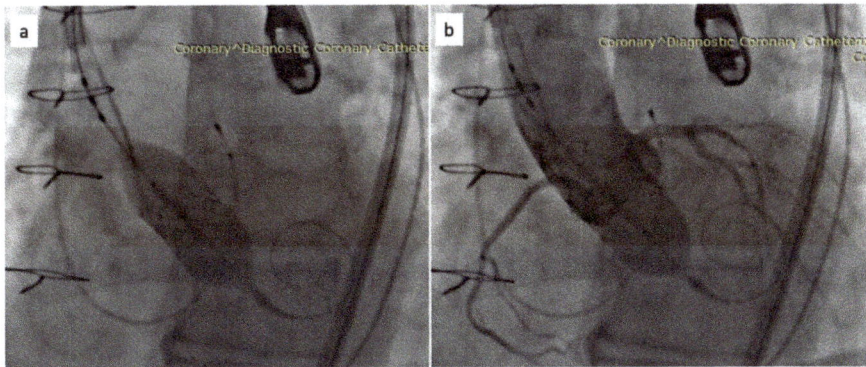

Figure 4. Fluoroscopy images of aortic root—baloon inflating in order to expand the aortic prosthesis (**a**) and inflated baloon in the expanded prosthesis with coronary arteries visible (**b**).

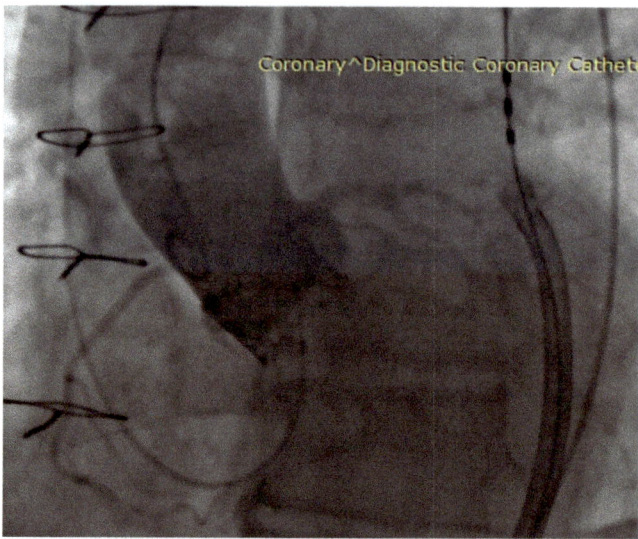

Figure 5. Fluoroscopy image—Checking the valve position and regurgitation.

The patient experienced an uneventful recovery, marked by extubation within one hour of the procedure. On the second day, the patient was transferred to the ward, and after one week, he was discharged. Upon discharge, the patient displayed no symptoms of heart failure and exhibited improved cardiac function. During the first follow-up appointment at one month post procedure, mild aortic regurgitation was detected, though it was not associated with significant symptoms.

At the time of discharge, the patient received the following medical treatment recommendations per day:

- 100 mg aspirin;
- 150 mg cyclosporine;
- 1440 mg mycophenolate;
- 5 mg prednisone;
- 150 mg allopurinol;
- 40 mg famotidine;
- 40 mg furosemide;
- 10 mg atorvastatin;
- 160 mg fenofibrate.

These medications were prescribed to optimize the patient's post-procedure care and management.

7. Discussion

The enhanced categorization of heart failure is imperative for optimizing the timing of surgical interventions, particularly in critical and emergent scenarios. A significant development in this regard occurred in 2009 with the publication of a study that introduced the INTERMACS classification (Interagency Registry for Mechanically Assisted Circulatory Support). This classification system delineates seven distinct clinical profiles of heart failure, offering a valuable framework for refining treatment strategies in advanced heart failure cases.

Of particular relevance are Classes 1 and 2 within the INTERMACS classification, as patients falling into these categories require urgent interventions such as assist device implantation or OHT. In these critical cases, there arises an opportunity to expand the pool of available donor organs through considering a supplementary list of marginal donors.

This approach aims to provide patients with a lifeline, thereby reducing the risk of mortality while awaiting transplantation [16]. Classes 1 to 3 encompass patients who are currently reliant on inotropic agents and are in pressing need of heart transplantation. It is noteworthy that a substantial majority, approximately 80%, of heart transplantations are conducted within this subset of heart failure patients. Furthermore, there is a burgeoning consensus within the medical community, particularly for patients falling under the INTERMACS Classes 1 and 2, in favor of considering hearts from marginal donors for transplantation. This shift in perspective acknowledges the critical urgency of addressing the needs of these high-risk patients and underscores the potential benefits of utilizing marginal donor organs to save lives in these challenging cases [17].

Given the rising demand for heart transplantation and the elevated mortality risk associated with patients classified under Class 1 and Class 2 heart failure, numerous transplant centers are confronted with the necessity of considering hearts that may not meet the traditional criteria for ideal transplantation candidates. This includes the potential acceptance of hearts from older donors with conditions such as moderate valvular disease, mild coronary artery disease, and comorbidities like hypertension, diabetes, and dyslipidemia. These deviations from the strict transplantation contraindications reflect the imperative to expand donor options in order to address the pressing need for life-saving heart transplants [3].

In select emergency cases, transplant centers may find it necessary to accept hearts from marginal donors, even if the results may be less than ideal. This decision may entail making certain annotations to the donor criteria. Notable considerations include:

- Increase in donor age: The acceptance of older donors, acknowledging that chronological age alone may not necessarily preclude organ suitability.
- Extended ischemic time: A willingness to tolerate longer periods of ischemia, recognizing that timely organ retrieval may not always be feasible.
- Acceptance of size mismatch: Being open to heart size variations between donor and recipient, as long as the functional compatibility is maintained.
- Atrioventricular valvular disease: The inclusion of donors with atrioventricular valvular disease, provided it does not compromise overall heart function.
- Left ventricular hypertrophy: The consideration of hearts with left ventricular hypertrophy, which may be compatible with transplantation in certain cases.
- Hepatitis B/C: The acceptance of hearts from donors with hepatitis B or C, while carefully evaluating the recipient's condition and risk factors.
- Significant coronary artery disease: The evaluation of donor hearts with significant coronary artery disease, taking into account the potential impact on transplantation success.
- Brain malignancies: The assessment of hearts from donors with brain malignancies, weighing the risks and benefits for recipients in critical need.
- Non-beating hearts: The consideration of non-beating hearts (donors who have experienced cardiac arrest), contingent upon the viability of the organ.
- Drug abuse/intoxication: The evaluation of hearts from donors with a history of drug abuse or intoxication, with careful consideration of the recipient's circumstances.

Each of these characteristics presents potential independent risk factors for the outcome of OHT. However, in cases involving terminally ill patients with no alternative treatment options, accepting hearts from donors with these characteristics may represent a viable solution, potentially leading to an extended lifespan and improved quality of life (QOL) for the recipient [3].

The concept of implementing alternative donor lists for marginal donors has arisen as a means to expand the pool of potential donor options. It is estimated that through increasing the age limit for donors to 55 years old and potentially even up to 65 years old, more than 15,000 patients could potentially benefit from OHT. In the case of the higher age limit, the number of potential beneficiaries could range from 50,000 to 70,000, assuming that the survival rates align with current research findings. The acceptance of alternative lists for marginal donors hinges on the condition that the survival rates achieved with these donors remain comparable to the existing standards. Similar to the strategies employed in kidney transplantation, where "old-to-old" donor–recipient pairings have been successful, embracing hearts from marginal donors could provide the opportunity to include older critically ill patients on the transplant waiting list. This approach seeks to maximize the utilization of available donor organs while prioritizing the well-being and survival of transplant recipients [3].

The International Thoracic Organ Transplant Registry of the International Society for Heart and Lung Transplantation (ISHLT) has compiled data from a total of 481 adult thoracic transplant centers across the globe. This dataset is estimated to encompass approximately 75% of all heart transplants performed worldwide. The ISHLT has leveraged this comprehensive data to analyze changes in recipient characteristics over recent decades According to the ISHLT's 2021 data publication, the landscape of heart transplant recipients has evolved significantly. This transformation can be attributed to advancements in mechanical circulatory support therapies, improved medical and surgical treatments, and modifications to the criteria for accepting candidates for heart transplantation. Consequently, older and sicker patients have been included in the transplant population and have benefited from appropriate medical care. The study conducted by the ISHLT spans a substantial timeframe, covering the years from 1992 to 2018, and includes data from three major regions: North America, Europe, and other countries, encompassing South America, Asia, the Middle East, Australia, and various other regions. This comprehensive analysis sheds light on the dynamic changes in heart transplant recipient demographics and highlights the evolving landscape of heart transplantation on a global scale [18–20].

To analyze the trend in recipient acceptance criteria, the study divided the data into three distinct periods: 1992–2000, 2001–2009, and 2010–2018, with a similar number of heart transplants performed in each period. Over this time frame, several noteworthy changes in recipient characteristics were observed:

- Increasing age: Recipient age has seen a steady rise, increasing from an average of 53 years in the first period to 57 years in the most recent period.
- Higher body mass index (BMI): The median BMI has also increased, with values rising from 25 kg/m^2 to 26.5 kg/m^2. This shift is attributed to a corresponding increase in median weight, from 75.7 kg to 80 kg.
- Kidney function trends: Surprisingly, there has been a declining trend in kidney dysfunction, as measured via glomerular filtration rate (GFR), across all three geographic regions. Several factors contribute to this trend, including an increased incidence of heart–kidney transplants for candidates with severe kidney disease, improved kidney function resulting from the use of ventricular assist devices before transplant, a decreasing incidence of recipients with ischemic cardiomyopathy (who are more prone to kidney disease due to cardiovascular risk factors), and a rising percentage of female recipients.
- Blood type compatibility: The blood type of recipients has remained relatively stable over time. This is attributed to the increase in transplantation of allo-sensitized patients, likely due to advances in managing patients before and after transplantation. These advances include therapies for pretransplant desensitization and posttransplant rejection, improved human leukocyte antigen (HLA) typing, enhanced antibody detection and quantification. Consequently, the percentage of patients with a pretransplant panel of reactive antibodies (PRA) exceeding 20% increased from 5.2% to 17.9%, and the percentage of highly sensitized patients (PRA > 80%) rose from 0.9% to 3.6% over the same period.
- Increased medical comorbidities: Heart transplant candidates have shown a greater burden of medical comorbidities over time. This includes a rising incidence of diabetes (from 16.7% to 27%), a history of malignancy (from 3.8% to 8.7%), previous cardiac surgery (from 37.8% to 50.1%), and dialysis (from 3% to 4.7%). The increase in dialysis cases is often associated with non-acute kidney failure and a higher likelihood of

recovery. Additionally, patients with chronic kidney disease on dialysis may be referred for simultaneous heart–kidney transplantation.

These trends highlight the evolving landscape of heart transplant recipient characteristics, reflecting changes in both the patient population and the criteria for heart transplant candidate acceptance over the decades [19].

During the same period from 1992 to 2018, Khush et al. conducted an analysis of donor data and observed several trends in how the donor profile has evolved. These trends include:

- Increased donor age: The median age of donors has seen a notable increase worldwide, rising from 31 years to 35 years. This trend is partly attributable to changes in transplant practices in Europe, where the median donor age has significantly increased from 31 to 45 years.
- Higher body mass index (BMI): Donor BMI has also experienced an increase, with the median BMI rising from 24.1 kg/m^2 to 26 kg/m^2. This change is likely associated with the growing prevalence of obesity, primarily observed in North America.
- Stable gender distribution: The distribution of donor genders has remained relatively stable over time, with approximately 70% of donors being male and 30% female.

These trends in donor characteristics provide insights into the shifting donor profile over the years, reflecting changes in both donor demographics and health-related factors [20].

An intriguing observation is that the cause of death among donors in the European region has shifted from predominantly head trauma to a higher incidence of cerebrovascular accidents (CVAs) or strokes. Conversely, in North America, head trauma remains the primary cause of donor death, but there is also an increase in deaths due to anoxia, which could be linked to a rise in opioid use and drug abuse.

The increasing age of donors in Europe may play a role in this change in the cause of death, as older donors are more likely to experience natural and age-related deaths. This shift in donor causes of death highlights the complex interplay of various factors, including medical conditions, lifestyle choices, and demographics, that can influence the donor pool and impact the availability and suitability of donor organs for transplantation [20].

Observations regarding substance use among donors have revealed notable trends over the years:

- Cigarette smoking: The percentage of donors with a history of cigarette smoking ($\geq$20 pack-years) has decreased significantly, dropping from 40% in 1995 to 15% in 2018. This decline likely reflects broader efforts to reduce smoking rates and improve public health.
- Alcohol use: Donor alcohol use ($\geq$2 alcoholic drinks per day) has remained relatively stable during this period, suggesting that alcohol consumption patterns among donors have not undergone significant changes.
- Cocaine use: There has been a troubling increase in cocaine use among donors, rising from 11% in 2000 to 27% in 2018. This increase in cocaine use raises concerns about the potential health implications for both donors and recipients.
- Use of other drugs: Donors reporting the use of other drugs, such as non-intravenous street drugs like crack, marijuana, prescription narcotics, sedatives, hypnotics, or stimulants, have seen a substantial increase.

This percentage surged from 25% to 57% over the same period. This significant rise in the use of other drugs underscores the need for careful donor screening and evaluation to ensure the safety and health of both donors and transplant recipients.

These trends in substance use among donors highlight the evolving landscape of donor health behaviors and underscore the importance of robust donor screening protocols to safeguard the well-being of transplant recipients [20].

Despite advancements in organ procurement and preservation, increased willingness to accept marginal donor hearts, and the utilization of hearts from donors with certain medical conditions (such as drug abuse or hepatitis C viremia) and after circulatory death the number of heart transplants has remained stable over this period. This stability in the number of heart transplants suggests that there may be limitations to increasing the rate of procedures, primarily due to a shortage of available donor organs [19,20].

The availability of suitable donor organs remains a critical factor in determining the number of heart transplants that can be performed. Efforts to address this limitation may include initiatives to increase organ donation rates, improve donor organ quality, and enhance organ preservation techniques. The stability in the number of heart transplants underscores the ongoing challenges in meeting the demand for life-saving heart transplan procedures [19–22].

8. Conclusions

Despite advancements in organ procurement and preservation, increased willingness to accept marginal donor hearts, and the utilization of hearts from donors with certain medical conditions (such as drug abuse or hepatitis C viremia) and after circulatory death the number of heart transplants has remained stable over this period. This stability in the number of heart transplants suggests that there may be limitations to increasing the rate of procedures, primarily due to a shortage of available donor organs.

The availability of suitable donor organs remains a critical factor in determining the number of heart transplants that can be performed. Efforts to address this limitation may include initiatives to increase organ donation rates, improve donor organ quality and enhance organ preservation techniques. The stability in the number of heart transplants underscores the ongoing challenges in meeting the demand for life-saving heart transplant procedures.

In conclusion, the growing need for improved treatment options in the medical field has driven physicians to explore innovative methods that were once considered unthinkable TAVI stands as a notable example of medical progress throughout history. Today, there is a rapid increase in the demand for effective treatments for end-stage heart failure, which has necessitated a reevaluation of the criteria for "ideal" donors.

Despite continuous advancements in assist devices, heart transplantation remains the ultimate solution for many patients. Expanding the donor pool has become imperative in addressing this increasing need. However, the inclusion of marginal donors presents new challenges in treating organs that may have previously been compromised.

TAVI has emerged as a proven and versatile treatment method, particularly for high risk patients like heart transplant recipients. It has become one of the primary tools in managing the complexities associated with the use of marginal donors. Our case presentation contributes to addressing the current gap in documentation regarding the use of TAVI in heart transplant recipients. Coupled with a brief literature review, it underscores the feasibility and reliability of TAVI as a valuable solution within this specific medical context

Author Contributions: Conceptualization, H.M.; Methodology, S.P., C.N. (Claudia Nica), M.C., R.C and V.A.I.; Software, L.C., R.Ț., A.B., A.Z. and C.N. (Claudiu Nistor); Validation, S.P., L.C., C.N (Claudia Nica), M.C., R.Ț., A.Z., R.C., C.N. (Claudiu Nistor), B.S.G., L.D., V.A.I. and H.M.; Formal analysis, C.N. (Claudia Nica), M.C., A.B., A.Z., C.N. (Claudiu Nistor), L.I. and V.A.I.; Investigation S.P., L.C., C.N. (Claudia Nica), R.Ț., A.Z., R.C., C.N. (Claudiu Nistor), L.I., L.D., V.A.I. and H.M. Resources, C.N. (Claudia Nica), M.C., R.Ț., A.B., A.Z. and B.S.G.; Data curation, L.C., A.B. and B.S.G.; Writing—original draft, S.P. and R.C.; Writing—review & editing, S.P., M.C., L.I. and L.D. Visualization, R.Ț. and H.M.; Supervision, L.I., V.A.I. and H.M.; Project administration, H.M. All authors have read and agreed to the published version of the manuscript.

Funding: The research received no external founding.

Informed Consent Statement: Written informed consent was obtained from the patient for the procedure and also for publishing this case report.

Conflicts of Interest: The authors declare no conflict of interest.

References

1. Stolf, N.A. History of Heart Transplantation: A hard and glorious journey. *Braz. J. Cardiovasc. Surg.* **2017**, *32*, 423–427. [CrossRef]
2. Cribier, A. The development of transcatheter aortic valve replacement (TAVR). *Glob. Cardiol. Sci. Pract.* **2016**, *2016*, e201632. [CrossRef] [PubMed]
3. Wittwer, T.; Wahlers, T. Marginal donor grafts in heart transplantation: Lessons learned from 25 years of experience. *Transpl. Int.* **2007**, *21*, 113–125. [CrossRef] [PubMed]
4. Wilhelm, M.J. Long-term outcome following heart transplantation: Current perspective. *J. Thorac. Dis.* **2015**, *7*, 549. [PubMed]
5. Lund, L.H.; Edwards, L.B.; Kucheryavaya, A.Y.; Benden, C.; Christie, J.D.; Dipchand, A.I.; Dobbels, F.; Goldfarb, S.B.; Levvey, B.J.; Meiser, B.; et al. The registry of the International Society for Heart and Lung Transplantation: Thirty-first official adult heart transplant report—2014; focus theme: Retransplantation. *J. Heart Lung Transpl.* **2014**, *33*, 996–1008. [CrossRef] [PubMed]
6. Seiffert, M.; Meyer, S.; Franzen, O.; Conradi, L.; Baldus, S.; Schirmer, J.; Deuse, T.; Costard-Jaeckle, A.; Reichenspurner, H.; Treede, H. Transcatheter Aortic Valve Implantation in a Heart Transplant Recipient: A Case Report. In *Transplantation Proceedings*; Elsevier: Amsterdam, The Netherlands, 2010. [CrossRef]
7. Bruschi, G.; De Marco, F.; Oreglia, J.; Colombo, P.; Moreo, A.; De Chiara, B.; Paino, R.; Frigerio, M.; Martinelli, L.; Klugmann, S. Transcatheter aortic valve implantation after heart transplantation. *Ann. Thorac. Surg.* **2010**, *90*, e66–e68. [CrossRef] [PubMed]
8. Zanuttini, D.; Armellini, I.; Bisceglia, T.; Spedicato, L.; Bernardi, G.; Muzzi, R.; Proclemer, A.; Livi, U. Transcatheter Aortic Valve Implantation for Degenerative Aortic Valve Regurgitation Long After Heart Transplantation. *Ann. Thorac. Surg.* **2013**, *96*, 1864–1866. [CrossRef] [PubMed]
9. De Praetere, H.; Ciarka, A.; Dubois, C.; Herijgers, P. Transapical transcatheter aortic valve implantation in a heart transplant recipient with severely depressed left ventricular function. *Interact. CardioVascular Thorac. Surg.* **2013**, *16*, 906–908. [CrossRef] [PubMed]
10. Ahmad, K.; Terkelsen, C.J.; Terp, K.A.; Mathiassen, O.N.; Nørgaard, B.L.; Andersen, H.R.; Poulsen, S.H. Transcatheter aortic valve implantation in a young heart transplant recipient crossing the traditional boundaries. *J. Thorac. Dis.* **2016**, *8*, E711. [CrossRef] [PubMed]
11. Julien, M.B.; Desai, N.; Brozena, S.; Herrmann, H.C. Transcatheter aortic valve replacement for bicuspid aortic stenosis. *Cardiovasc. Revascularization Med.* **2016**, *18*, 32–33. [CrossRef] [PubMed]
12. Akleh, S.I.; Bandali, A.; Edwards, R. Transcatheter aortic valve implantation in an orthotopic heart transplant recipient with bicuspid aortic valve. *Clin. Case Rep.* **2018**, *6*, 2262. [CrossRef] [PubMed]
13. Avula, S.; Mungee, S.; Barzallo, M.A. Successful minimal approach transcatheter aortic valve replacement in an allograft heart recipient 19 years post transplantation for severe aortic stenosis: A case report. *World J. Cardiol.* **2019**, *11*, 209. [CrossRef] [PubMed]
14. Beale, R.; Beale, C.; DeNofrio, D.; Gordon, P.; Levine, D.; Sodha, N.; Yousefzai, R.; Apostolidou, E. Transcatheter Aortic Valve Replacement of a Bicuspid Aortic Valve in a Heart Transplant Recipient. *Case Rep.* **2020**, *2*, 716–720.
15. Ezad, S.M.; Curzen, N.; Abbas, A.; Rawlins, J. TAVI Between a Rock and a Hard Place in a Transplanted Heart. *J. Invasive Cardiol.* **2022**, *34*, E576–E577, ISSN 1557-2501. [PubMed]
16. Stevenson, L.W.; Pagani, F.D.; Young, J.B. INTERMACS Profiles of Advanced Heart Failure. *J. Heart Lung Transpl.* **2009**, *28*, 28. [CrossRef] [PubMed]
17. Elliott, A.M.; Lampert, B.C. Patient Selection for Long-Term Mechanical Circulatory Support: Is It Ever too Early for the NYHA Class III Patient? *Curr. Heart Fail. Rep.* **2016**, *13*, 13–19. [CrossRef] [PubMed]
18. Laks, H.; Marelli, D.; Fonarow, G.C.; Hamilton, M.A.; Ardehali, A.; Moriguchi, J.D.; Bresson, J.; Gjertson, D.; Kobashigawa, J.A. Use of two recipient lists for adults requiring heart transplantation. *J. Thorac. Cardiovasc. Surg.* **2003**, *125*, 49–59. [CrossRef]
19. Khush, K.K.; Hsich, E.; Potena, L.; Cherikh, W.S.; Chambers, D.C.; Harhay, M.O.; Hayes, D.; Perch, M.; Sadavarte, A.; Toll, A.; et al. The International Thoracic Organ Transplant Registry of the International Society for Heart and Lung Transplantation: Thirty-Eighth Adult Heart Transplantation Report—2021; Focus on Recipient Characteristics; Elsevier: Amsterdam, The Netherlands, 2021. [CrossRef]
20. Khush, K.K.; Potena, L.; Cherikh, W.S.; Chambers, D.C.; Harhay, M.O.; Hayes, D.; Hsich, E.; Sadavarte, A.; Singh, T.P.; Zuckermann, A.; et al. The International Thoracic Organ Transplant Registry of the International Society for Heart and Lung Transplantation: 37th adult heart transplantation report—2020; focus on deceased donor characteristics. *J. Heart Lung Transpl.* **2020**, *39*, 1003–1015. [CrossRef] [PubMed]
21. Iosifescu, A.G.; Moldovan, H.; Iliescu, V.A. Aortic prosthesis-patient mismatch strongly affects early results of double valve replacement. *J Heart Valve Dis.* **2014**, *23*, 149–157. [PubMed]
22. Joshi, S.; Mosleh, W.; Amer, M.R.; Tawayha, M.; Mather, J.F.; Kiernan, F.J.; McKay, R.G.; Piccirillo, B. Outcomes of Transcatheter Aortic Valve Replacement in Patients Treated With Systemic Steroids. *J. Invasive Cardiol.* **2022**, *34*, E49–E54, ISSN 1557-2501. [PubMed]

Disclaimer/Publisher's Note: The statements, opinions and data contained in all publications are solely those of the individual author(s) and contributor(s) and not of MDPI and/or the editor(s). MDPI and/or the editor(s) disclaim responsibility for any injury to people or property resulting from any ideas, methods, instructions or products referred to in the content.

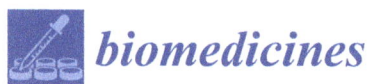

Review

Cardiovascular Remodeling Post-Ischemia: Herbs, Diet, and Drug Interventions

Ayodeji A. Olabiyi * and Lisandra E. de Castro Brás

Department of Physiology, Brody School of Medicine, East Carolina University, Greenville, NC 27858, USA; decastrobrasl14@ecu.edu
* Correspondence: olabiyia22@ecu.edu

Abstract: Cardiovascular disease (CVD) is a serious health burden with increasing prevalence, and CVD continues to be the principal global source of illness and mortality. For several disorders, including CVD, the use of dietary and medicinal herbs instead of pharmaceutical drugs continues to be an alternate therapy strategy. Despite the prevalent use of synthetic pharmaceutical medications, there is currently an unprecedented push for the use of diet and herbal preparations in contemporary medical systems. This urge is fueled by a number of factors, the two most important being the common perception that they are safe and more cost-effective than modern pharmaceutical medicines. However, there is a lack of research focused on novel treatment targets that combine all these strategies—pharmaceuticals, diet, and herbs. In this review, we looked at the reported effects of pharmaceutical drugs and diet, as well as medicinal herbs, and propose a combination of these approaches to target independent pathways that could synergistically be efficacious in treating cardiovascular disease.

Keywords: cardiovascular disease; diet; herbs; pharmaceutical drugs; remodeling

Citation: Olabiyi, A.A.; de Castro Brás, L.E. Cardiovascular Remodeling Post-Ischemia: Herbs, Diet, and Drug Interventions. *Biomedicines* **2023**, *11*, 1697. https://doi.org/10.3390/biomedicines11061697

Academic Editor: Alfredo Caturano

Received: 18 May 2023
Revised: 8 June 2023
Accepted: 9 June 2023
Published: 13 June 2023

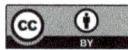

Copyright: © 2023 by the authors. Licensee MDPI, Basel, Switzerland. This article is an open access article distributed under the terms and conditions of the Creative Commons Attribution (CC BY) license (https://creativecommons.org/licenses/by/4.0/).

1. Introduction

According to the World Health Organization, each year 17.9 million people worldwide die from cardiovascular disease (CVD), accounting for 31% of all mortality [1]. The American Heart Association reports that roughly half of all Americans have a type of CVD [2]. Of these, heart attacks (i.e., myocardial infarction, MI) and strokes account for 80% of CVD fatalities [2]. An MI occurs when an artery to the heart is clogged, and the heart does not receive enough blood or oxygen for a significant amount of time leading to ischemia/infarction of the tissue downstream of the obstruction. Upon infarction, if reperfusion does not occur in a timely manner, cardiac cells will become ischemic and metabolically compromised.

Cardiac cells (including cardiomyocytes), capillaries, and extracellular matrix (ECM), which is made up of various collagen fiber types and ensures structural integrity, are the three crucial components of heart muscle that enable effective contraction and pumping of the blood to the whole body. When cells die due to ischemia, a cascade of events is triggered to clear and replace the damaged cells and tissues. These events are dynamic and are broadly divided into three stages: inflammation/necrosis to remove dead cells/tissue; proliferation/fibrosis to replace cells, ECM, and set up tissue vascularization; and long-term remodeling/maturation to regenerate the tissue and/or mature the scar and provide tissue integrity and function [3]. Different risk cues, either exogenous or endogenous, may start the inflammatory response. Microorganism invasion is considered exogenous, whereas tissue injury is considered endogenous. Pathogen-associated molecular patterns (PAMPs) and damage-associated molecular patterns (DAMPs) are the names given to the external and endogenous signaling molecules that are released, respectively, by pathogens or necrotic cells [4]. Toll-like receptors (TLRs), nucleotide-binding oligomerization domain

(NOD)-like receptors (NLRs), C-type lectins, and receptors for advanced glycation end-products (RAGE) are just a few of the pattern recognition receptors (PRRs) that may detect PAMPs and DAMPs. A described genus of specific pro-resolving mediators (SPMs) including lipoxins, resolvins, protectins, and maresins is activated during the resolution phase of inflammation [5]. These mediators have strong, direct anti-inflammatory and pro-resolution properties that limit the recruitment of inflammatory leukocytes while encouraging macrophage clearance of apoptotic neutrophils. By controlling ventricular size, shape, and function, left ventricular (LV) remodeling defines the heart's (mal)adaptation to injury and/or mechanical, neurohormonal, and hereditary alterations. While the increased microcirculatory blood supply provided during the proliferation phase will support any live cardiomyocytes, continual LV remodeling (due to uncontrolled inflammation) leads to cardiomyocyte loss, expansion of the ischemic area, persistent collagenase activity, and degradation of high-tensile collagens; this in turn leads to LV dilation, with wall thinning and fibrosis [6]. This "adverse" or "pathological" remodeling following MI is maladaptive, carries a disproportionate risk of heart failure (HF), and dramatically lowers survival [7]. Over the last twenty years, the prevalence of HF has increased [8]. Despite immediate revascularization and subsequent treatment options that significantly lower the mortality of acute MI, ischemic heart disease remains the main cause of HF [8,9]. Comorbidities foretell the severity and progression of HF [10,11]; in fact, more than 50% of HF patients have more than seven comorbidities, with age and sex being the two main predictors of HF [12]. Men have a larger heart mass and a higher incidence of subclinical coronary artery disease than women [13,14]. Women show less severe incidence than men in terms of atherosclerosis, left ventricular hypertrophy, and cardiomyocyte apoptosis [15,16]. Similarly, mortality post-MI correlates with advancing age, regardless of infarct size [17], which may be related to a higher prevalence of ventricular hypertrophy but also to a decreased immunological response, scarring, and autophagy [18].

Medications that have been effective in treating HF include neurohormonal antagonists (beta blockers, angiotensin receptor blockers, and aldosterone antagonists), which can prevent or reverse remodeling and have been shown to lower mortality and morbidity [19]. The use of medications has been practiced over the years for the prevention of HF. However, some of these medications produce adverse effects and due to high cost are not easily available to every patient. Over the past three decades, there has been a significant rise in the use of herbal supplements to prevent, avoid, and/or treat different conditions, including CVD; this rise results from a perceived safety (natural, non-toxic sources), efficiency with few or no adverse effects (unlike synthetic/chemical medications), and low cost [20]. The US Dietary Supplement Health and Education Act (DSHEA) of 1994 categorizes herbal products as dietary supplements. In addition to herbal supplements, epidemiological research showed that consuming fruits, vegetables, olive oil, wine, legumes, and whole grains, as found in the Mediterranean diet, has a cardioprotective effect [21]. Foods high in polyphenols, such as berries and olive oil, have been demonstrated to have cardioprotective benefits that enhance endothelial function and plasma lipid profiles while preventing aberrant platelet aggregation and decreasing inflammation [22]. Thus, diet and dietary supplements have important roles in maintaining homeostasis and reducing CVD and warrant further investigation. Preload, afterload, and molecular mechanisms of remodeling have been targeted using synthetic drug therapy to date; can this also be achieved through diet and natural supplements? This review focuses on the use of prescription drugs, herbal products, and diet modification on cardiovascular remodeling.

2. Cardiovascular Health and Drugs Treatment

Over the past two centuries, the pathways of discovery, innovation, and therapeutic improvement in cardiovascular science and medicine have been really astounding. Nabel and Braunwald [23] discussed the remarkable decrease in cardiovascular disease deaths due to scientific advancements from 1950, when it was over 450 deaths per 100,000 of the population, to approximately 100 deaths per 100,000 by 2010. Even though many clinical advancements have contributed to this impressive decline, they emphasized the significance of β-blocking therapy and 3-hydroxy-3-methyl-glutaryl coenzyme A (HMG Co-A) reductase inhibition, as well as the introduction of novel antihypertensive agents in the context of the national high blood pressure education program. Nevertheless, notwithstanding these medical advances, concurrent disorders such as diabetes mellitus, obesity, and congestive HF contribute to the consistently high prevalence of CVD. Additionally, because of the remarkable decline in MI mortality rates, affected individuals live longer but nearly 40% develop HF, which has a worse prognosis than acute MI. Despite prior advancements in pharmacological therapy, such as oral diuretics and medication treatment for hypertension, progress is still being made in the management of cardiovascular disorders such as HF and cardiac arrhythmias.

HF patients with systolic LV dysfunction treated with angiotensin-converting enzyme (ACE) inhibitors present reduced mortality and morbidity [24]. ACE inhibitors act as vasodilators and their effectiveness in reducing remodeling is supported by both experimental and clinical studies, particularly in the post-infarction setting [20–22,25–27]. However, with ACE inhibitors, reverse remodeling has infrequently been observed in sizable patient cohorts. One of the aspects of this therapy that may limit its ability to provide long-term benefit is protection without reversion of remodeling. In clinical studies with ACE inhibitors, the survival curves of patients assigned to either the active treatment or the placebo groups typically show an early divergence of the curves followed by a parallel trend through time [28,29]. This shows that these medications more often delay the onset of the disease than stop it [30].

Angiotensin receptor blockers (ARBs) are also used in HF treatment, instead of or in combination with ACE inhibitors. ARBs selectively reduce the activity of type 2 receptors (AT2R), which mediate vasodilation and may prevent myocardial fibrosis, without affecting type 1 receptors (AT1R), which primarily mediate cardiac hypertrophy, aldosterone production, fibrosis, and vasoconstriction [31].

Matrix metalloproteinase (MMP) activation and maladaptive LV remodeling have a clear cause-and-effect relationship, as shown by experimental research [32–34]. Thus, MMPs have long been recognized as an attractive target to decrease or prevent maladaptive cardiac remodeling. MMP inhibitors have been suggested as a treatment for several illnesses in order to lessen matrix deterioration, blunt inflammation, and enhance tissue regeneration. However, difficulties in producing MMP specific inhibitors and the many functions of MMPS (both beneficial and detrimental) have led to little progress in clinical trials and still need further investigation [35–37].

3. Cardiovascular Health and Diet

According to data from the Centers for Disease Control (CDC) and Prevention, some of the most common health problems in the United States are chronic diseases such as cancer, diabetes, heart disease, and stroke. Many of these chronic illnesses can be prevented, though, as they are linked to unhealthy eating and lifestyle choices. Dietary intervention allows for a better blending of various diets and nutrients. Healthy eating practices therefore encourage a greater magnitude of favorable impacts than the potential effects of a single nutrient supplementation because of the synergistic health effects among them. Research has shown that a high intake of fiber, antioxidants, vitamins, minerals, polyphenols, monounsaturated fatty acids (MUFA), and polyunsaturated fatty acids (PUFA), low intakes of salt, saturated fats, and trans fats, and a high intake of carbohydrates with low glycemic loads are all indicators of healthy eating habits [38].

Although some cardiovascular diseases are congenital, years of investigation into the relationship between diet and heart disease concentrated on specific vitamins and minerals, types of fats, and individual nutrients such as cholesterol (and foods high in dietary cholesterol, such eggs). This has been eye-opening, but it has also led to some dead ends and perpetuated misconceptions about what a heart-healthy diet is. People eat food, not nutrition, which explains this [38]. A growing heart need nutritious grains, vegetables, and fruits, as well as a mineral balance (sodium and potassium) and body weight maintenance, as well as sufficient sleep. People who follow this eating pattern have a 31% lower risk of heart disease, a 33% lower risk of diabetes, and a 20% lower risk of stroke [39]. Neonatal malnutrition, inflammation, and growth retardation are linked to a lifelong decrease in cardiomyocyte number, systolic and diastolic dysfunction, ischemia sensitivity, and hypertension [40–43]. A significant body of scientific research supports nutrition as one of the most effective ways to avoid CVD associated mortality [44] and may even be able to reverse heart disease [45]. Even more, the management of other risk factors, such as excess weight, hypertension, diabetes, or dyslipidemia, appears to depend heavily on nutrition and exercise [45]. In this regard, foods or dietary habits that can improve CVD prevention have been identified and categorized.

3.1. Mediterranean Diet

The Mediterranean diet (MeDiet), known as a mainly plant-based diet, characterized by a high consumption of fruits, vegetables, and whole grains as well as fish, nuts, and legumes, unsaturated fatty acids, and low to moderate intake of alcohol (consumed with a meal) has been reported to have a great impact on the arterial wall, which could account for the association between MeDiet and low CVD prevalence [46]. Intriguingly, MeDiet appears to modulate the expression of pro-atherogenic genes like cyclooxygenase-2 (COX-2), monocyte chemoattractant protein-1 (MCP-1), and low-density lipoprotein receptor-related protein (LRP1), while decreasing plasmatic levels of molecules negatively linked to plaque stability and rupture, such as MMP-9 and interleukins (IL-10, IL-13, or IL-18) [47,48]. Furthermore, in order to reduce the risk of CVD, the American Heart Association Nutrition Committee and the European Society of Cardiology both strongly recommend daily consumption of several portions of both fruits and vegetables [49,50], hallmarks of the MeDiet. These recommendations are mostly supported by epidemiological studies and meta-analyses [49–53]. According to a meta-analysis [52] of 83 studies, an increase in the consumption of fruits and vegetables was significantly inversely related to C-reactive protein (CRP) and tumor necrosis factor (TNF) levels and directly related to an increase in the proliferation of T-cell populations (71 clinical trials and 12 observational studies). The main component of the MeDiet, extra virgin olive oil (EVOO), has bioactive components shown to improve endothelial dysfunction, oxidative stress, and overall inflammatory state [54]. A meta-analysis by Schwingshackl et al. [55] found that, compared to controls, daily ingestion of 1 mg and 50 mg of olive oil significantly reduced CRP in 30 randomized control studies with a total of 3106 participants. Additionally, those who consumed the most olive oil had a substantially higher flow-mediated dilatation score (0.6%, $p < 0.002$). Similar to EVOO, nuts contain monosaturated fats; numerous sizable studies have shown that nuts significantly lower CVD morbidity and death [56–59]. Hence, a MeDiet rich in nuts had been linked to better weight reduction, lower low-density lipoprotein-cholesterol (LDL-c) levels [60–62], lower risk of developing hypertension [61,63], and lower levels of inflammatory and oxidative mediators [64,65].

3.2. Paleo Diet

Another eating plan based on foods popular during the Old Stone Age is the Paleolithic diet (Paleo), which primarily consists of lean meat, fish, eggs, fruits, vegetables, roots, and nuts while avoiding grains, dairy products, processed foods, added sugars, and salts [66]. This eating plan has less salt but more protein, several micronutrients such as vitamins C and E, carotenes, and fiber [67]. It also has fewer calories from refined carbohydrates and fat [67–69]. According to a meta-analysis of 8 studies, a Paleo diet significantly improved circulating concentrations of total cholesterol, triglycerides, LDL-c, and CRP while also significantly lowering body weight, waist circumference, body mass index, body fat percentage, and systolic and diastolic blood pressure. It was also reported to significantly increase HDL cholesterol [70]. Another meta-analysis of four randomized control trials

(RCTs) suggested short-term improvements in metabolic syndrome components following adoption of a Paleo diet, as reported by Manheimer et al. [71].

3.3. Keto Diet

Diets low in carbohydrates, but usually high in fats and/or proteins, have also become increasingly popular, referred to as ketogenic diets (keto diet). A keto diet restricts carbohydrate intake to less than 25 to 50 g per day, in an attempt to induce tissues to use fat or ketones as fuel during caloric restriction. As a result, the liver begins to produce ketone bodies, which are then utilized as an alternative energy source, particularly by the central nervous system [62]. From several reports, the keto diet may be linked to some improvements in various cardiovascular risk factors, such as obesity, type 2 diabetes, and HDL cholesterol levels [72–77]. On the other hand, a recent report describes keto diet causing cardiac fibrosis and inhibiting mitochondrial biogenesis [78]. According to their study, keto diet or repeated deep fasting impaired mitochondrial biogenesis, decreased cell respiration, and enhanced cardiac fibrosis and death in cardiomyocytes. As revealed by the research, increased levels of the histone deacetylase 2 (HDAC2) and inhibitor ketone body -hydroxybutyrate (-OHB), which promotes histone acetylation of the Sirt7 promoter and activates Sirt7 transcription, caused an increase in cardiac fibrosis and cardiomyocyte apoptosis [75]. Sirt7 transcription also prevents the transcription of mitochondrial ribosome-encoding genes. According to Xu and colleagues, consuming a keto diet over an extended period or accumulating -OHB may raise the chance of developing cardiovascular disease. In another population-based study, a low-carbohydrate diet, similar to keto, resulted in deleterious effects on the coronary artery [79]. In contrast, a research study in 2020 showed a keto diet was beneficial in diabetic patients by promoting cardiomyocyte survival and reducing interstitial fibrosis [79]. Although it is not clear what the reason(s) are for the discrepancies observed within these studies, it could result from differences between the animal models.

3.4. DASH

In 1990, dietary approaches to stop hypertension (DASH) were initiated; these approaches have received attention and several grants from the National Institute of Health (NIH) to see if specific dietary interventions were useful in treating hypertension. Some of the individuals enrolled showed a 6 to 11 mm Hg reduction in systolic blood pressure from the food intervention alone [80]. Both hypertensive and normotensive individuals experienced this effect, and as a result, DASH has occasionally been recommended as the first-line pharmacologic therapy in conjunction with lifestyle modifications. DASH encourages the eating of fresh produce, lean meat, low-fat dairy products, and foods rich in micronutrients. Additionally, it encourages limiting daily sodium intake to 1500 mg. DASH places a strong emphasis on eating fresh, minimally processed foods. The DASH diet is very similar to other dietary styles that are supported for cardiovascular health. The DASH diet is a synthesis of the old and new [81–83].

4. Cardiovascular Health and Herbal Medicine

Traditional herbal remedies have been used for decades and are typically regarded as safer than synthetic pharmaceuticals [84–86]. Approaches influenced by traditional medicine are still crucial, particularly for the management of chronic illnesses and to speed up the development of natural product drugs [87,88]. When administered with contemporary synthetic treatments, combinations of herbal medications or phytochemical active ingredients have been demonstrated to be useful in treating several disorders [89]. While the market for dietary botanical supplements is expanding, it is strongly recommended that more thorough clinical and scientific research be conducted on herbal and traditional medicines to increase their acceptance and visibility. Moreover, it is necessary to increase control on the quality of the materials used for formulation of the herbal/dietary supplements to ensure efficacy and safety.

In plants, certain polyphenols are present with adequate bioavailability singly or in combination with others (acting additively or synergistically). According to laboratory data gathered over the years, medicinal herbs can affect several CVD risks factors and, therefore, may have therapeutic utility in treating CVDs (Table 1). To effectively use herbs in CVD therapy, there have been numerous initiatives to shift studies on medicinal herbs from the bench to the bedside [90,91]. Natural products' biological activity and structural variety outperform any existing synthetic drug screening library, which is another factor leading to a return of interest in them [90].

The herbs *ginseng, ginkgo biloba, ganoderma lucidum,* and *gynostemma pentaphyllum* have been reported to prevent CVDs [92,93]. These herbs are becoming more and more well-known due to their presence in commercial commodities in numerous markets around the world and their established therapeutic potential in a variety of settings, including cardiovascular conditions [92]. These organic compounds profoundly alter important cellular, molecular, and metabolic processes that regulate the etiology and pathogenesis of CVDs [94]. Recent research shows that these herbal remedies have strong therapeutic effects and can improve pathological diseases linked to CVDs [92,93]. Clear clinical therapeutic advantages have not, however, been established. Rafacho et al. [95] demonstrated rosemary supplementation (*Rosmarinus oficinallis* L.) to cause reduced myocardial damage and blood pressure in hypertensive rats fed a high-fructose diet and protected the heart against cardiac dysfunction and fibrosis after MI in rats. From their findings, it was concluded that the mechanism could involve improved energy metabolism and reduced oxidative stress. In general, herbs could prevent or treat more than one disease since they have several therapeutic properties. As an illustration, the herb *Crocus sativus* L. was discovered to contain therapeutic properties that may be used to treat five different types of heart illness, including hypertension, heart attacks, blood fat reduction, antioxidants, and cardiac tonics [96–98]. This herb's role in preventing cardiovascular disorders was reportedly attributed to its anti-inflammatory and antioxidant properties [84,99].

In another study, due to strong antioxidant and free radical-scavenging activity, *Citrus medica* L. has also been reported to have cardioprotective potential [100]. In addition, a *Crataegus* species was observed to be a safe, nontoxic therapy option for ischemic heart disease and cardiovascular disease [101]. For example, the fruit or, alternatively, the leaves and flowers of *Crataegus monogyna*, which are high in polyphenols, are used medicinally. Direct scavenging of reactive oxygen species (ROS), increased catalase and superoxide dismutase activities, antioxidant activity, and downregulation of the caspase 3 gene are some of the known mechanisms of action of the *Crataegus* species [101]. Hawthorns are frequently utilized in a holistic approach to treat circulatory problems and congestive heart failure [102]. Moreover, stage 1 hypertension individuals who consume *Elettaria cardamom* have significantly lower blood pressure, increased fibrinolysis, and improved antioxidant status [103]. A recent study investigated the ability of cardamom oil to reestablish lipid homeostasis in the presence of hypercholesterolemia [104]. This study reduced atherogenicity index with dietary intervention with cardamom powder and oil, demonstrating the cardioprotective benefit of cardamom [104]. Researchers have also discovered two major methods through which the bark of *Terminalia arjuna* demonstrates cardioprotective advantages against induced cardiotoxicity which includes increased coronary artery flow and protection of the myocardium from ischemic damage [105].

Table 1. List of herbal remedies traditionally used for the treatment of different forms of CVDs.

Herbs	Forms of CVDs	Reference
Ginseng	Oxidative stress, hypertension, cardiac disease, hyperlipidemia and ion regulation	[93,106]
Ginkgo biloba	Cardiac activity, vasorelaxant and vasoconstriction activity, hypertension	[93]
Ganoderma lucidum	Atherosclerosis, hyperlipidemia	[107]
Gnostemma pentaphyllum	Hyperlipidemia	[92]
Rosemary oficinalis L.	Cardiac dysfunction and fibrosis	[95]
Cocus sativus L.	Systolic hypertension, oxidative stress, inflammation	[86,92]
Citrus medica L.	Ischemia heart disease	[100]
Crataegus monogyna	Congestive heart failure	[101]
Elettaria cardamom	Hypercholesterolemia	[104]
Terminalia arjuna	Cardiotoxicity	[105]
Punica granatum L.	Blood pressure, inflammation	[108,109]
Apple (Malus pumila)	Blood lipid levels	[110,111]
Watermelon (Citrullus lanatus)	Heart attacks, ischemic strokes, atherosclerosis	[112–114]
Berries	Myocardial infarction, oxidative stress, inflammation, platelet aggregation	[115–117]
Grapes (Vitis vinifera L.)	Cardiac fibrosis, hyperlipidemia	[118,119]
Garlic (Allium satinum L.)	Hypertension, hypercholesterolemia	[120]
Cinnamon (Cinnamomum verum)	Oxidative stress, inflammation, artherosclerosis	[121]

5. Polyphenols and Cardiovascular Health

Plants and plant products have been documented to have over 8000 known polyphenols [122]. Human health and wellness have been shown to directly be affected by a polyphenol-rich diet. According to Quideau et al. [123], polyphenols are substances with several phenolic units and no nitrogen-based functionalities that are generated from the polyketide and/or shikimate/phenyl propanoid pathways. After being metabolized, most polyphenols are glycosylated and either can bind to other phenols or conjugate with glucuronic acid, galacturonic acid, or glutathione [124]. Polyphenols are categorized into four main types: phenolic acids, stilbenes, lignans, and flavonoids (Figure 1).

5.1. Phenolic Acids

Phenolic acids include caffeic acid, which can be found in almost all fruits; chlorogenic acid, found in strawberries, pineapple, and other foods; and p-coumaric acid, present in cereal grains. The two families of phenolic acids—derivatives of benzoic acid and derivatives of cinnamic acid—are widely present in foods. Except for some red fruits, black radishes, and onions, which can have concentrations of many tens of milligrams per kilogram fresh weight of hydroxybenzoic acid, the hydroxybenzoic acid content of food plants are often modest [125].

5.2. Stilbenes

Stilbenes are phenolic substances with two phenyl groups joined by a bridge made of two carbon atoms in the methylene ring. Most stilbenes in plants function as phytoalexins, which are substances that are often only produced as a result of infection or injury. Resveratrol is one of the most thoroughly investigated stilbenes. Red wines, red grape juice, and peanuts all contain stilbenes [126,127].

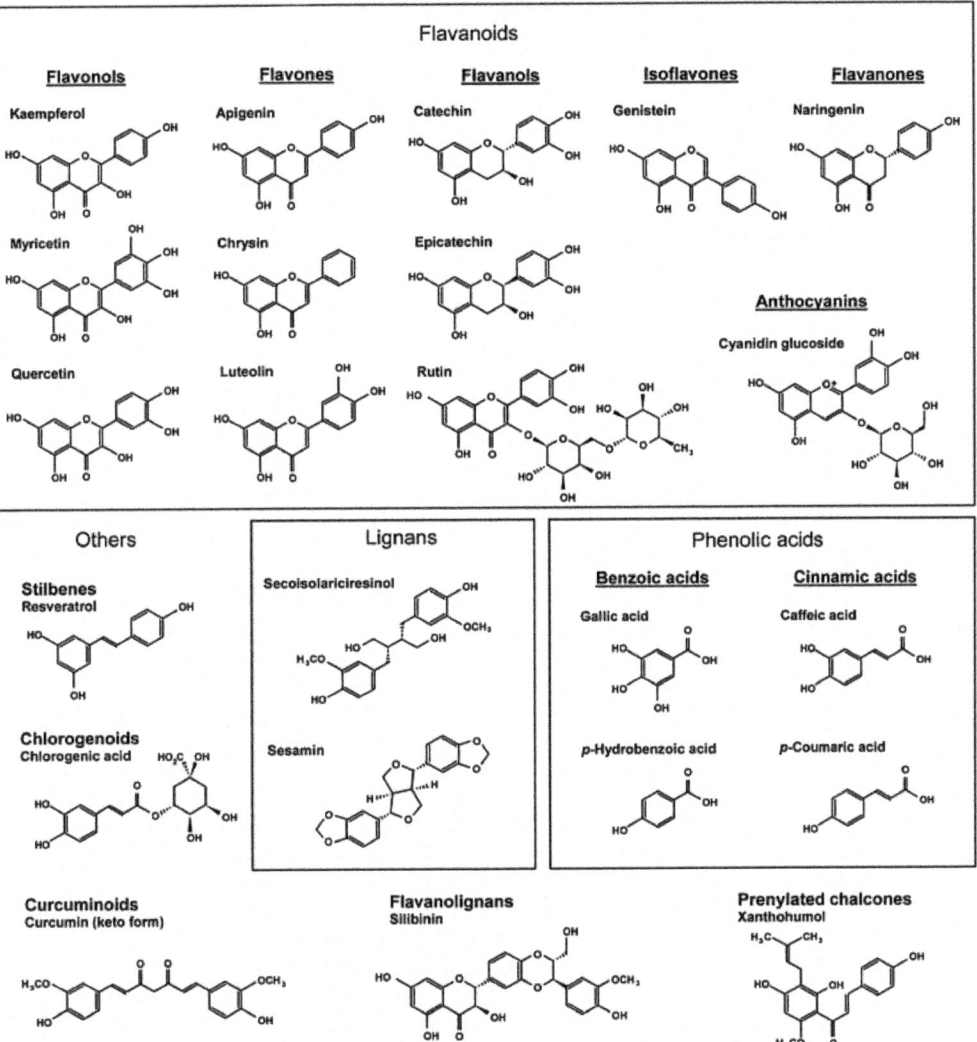

Figure 1. Chemical compositions of the various polyphenol classes. The amount of phenol rings a polyphenol contains and the structural components that hold these rings together are used to categorize polyphenols. They can be generally divided into four classes: stilbenes, lignans, phenolic acids, and flavonoids. Hydroxyl benzoic and hydroxyl cinnamic acids are two more subgroups of phenolic acids. Phenolic acids, which are present in all plant material but are more prevalent in fruits with an acidic flavor, make up around one-third of the polyphenolic substances in our diet. Some common phenolic acids include ferulic acid, gallic acid, and caffeic acid. The most prevalent polyphenols in the human diet are flavonoids, which have a basic structure that consists of two aromatic rings connected by three carbon atoms to create an oxygenated heterocycle. Biogenetically, one ring typically develops from a resorcinol molecule, while the other ring develops from the shikimate route. Two phenyl moieties are joined by a two-carbon methylene bridge in stilbenes. The majority of stilbenes in plants function as phytoalexins, which are substances that are only produced in reaction to infection or damage. Resveratrol has been the stilbene that has been investigated the most. The 2,3-dibenzylbutane structure of lignans, which are diphenolic substances, is created when two cinnamic acid residues dimerize.

5.3. Lignans

A wide class of low molecular weight polyphenols called lignans is present in many types of plants, especially seeds, whole grains, and vegetables. The word "wood" in Latin is the source of the name. Phytoestrogens' predecessors are lignans [128]. They might act as antifeedants to protect seeds and plants from herbivores [129]. Secoisolariciresinol from flaxseed [130] and sesamin from sesame seed [131] are two major examples of lignans.

5.4. Flavonoids

Fruits, vegetables, legumes, red wine, and green tea all contain flavonoids. They are further divided into chalcones, anthocyanins, proanthocyanidins, flavanols, flavonols, flavones, isoflavones, and flavanones [97]. Green and black tea include flavanols, such as epigallocatechin gallate [132]. Onions, broccoli, and blueberries all contain flavonols, such as kaempferol and quercetin [133]. In strongly colored fruit, anthocyanins can be discovered (cyanin glucoside is one of the examples) as reported by Ly et al. [124]. Parsley and celery both contain flavones, such as apigenin, chrysin, and luteolin [124]. Soya and its processed derivatives contain isoflavones, such as daidzein and genistein [134]. Grapefruit contains flavanones, such as naringenin [124]. Chalcones are primarily plentiful in hops used in beer making. They are also plentiful in numerous plants and spices, as well as in several vegetables and fruits, such as shallots, tomatoes, potatoes, and bean sprouts (as well as licorice and cardamom). The primary prenylated chalcone is xanthohumol, which is mostly present in hops and hence in beer [135]. Condensed flavan-3-ols known as proanthocyanidins are present in numerous plants, including apples, grape seeds, grape skin, and cocoa beans (the main source) [136]. Another group of polyphenols is the curcuminoids which includes turmeric or the compound curcumin.

Generally, the most prevalent polyphenols among these several types are phenolic acids and flavonoids [137]. Various protective properties of natural polyphenols against cardiovascular illnesses have been reported [59,88,138,139]. It has been noted that polyphenols belonging to various subclasses can reduce heart fibrosis and dysfunction after a cardiac injury. Quercetin with its glycoside derivative, rutin, or solitary quercetin reduced cardiac dysfunction and myocardial damage brought on by isoproterenol, prevented cardiac fibrosis, and inhibited the synthesis of connective tissue growth factor (CTGF), transforming growth factor-β (TGF-β1), and ECM components [140]. Panchal et al. [141] reported that by blocking the NF-κB signaling pathway and promoting nuclear factor erythroid 2-related factor 2 (Nrf-2) and its downstream components, heart remodeling was prevented in an obese rat model fed a Western diet supplemented with quercetin.

The most common and powerful catechin in green tea is epigallocatechin-3-gallate (EGCG) [142]. In rats, EGCG has been reported to reduce heart hypertrophy and the proliferation of cardiac fibroblasts (CFs) [143]. Other findings revealed EGCG inhibited oxidative stress, which slowed heart hypertrophy both in vivo and in vitro [144]. In the meantime, it reduced the activation of rat CFs induced by AngII through the involvement of β-arrestin1 [145]. By blocking the NF-κB signaling pathway during hypertrophic stimulation, Cai et al. [146] discovered that EGCG might inhibit the expression of fibronectin and collagen formation in rat CFs brought on by AngII. It also significantly improved excessive CTGF expression and cardiac fibrosis [146]. An appropriate dose is necessary for EGCG to play its protective effect in reducing heart fibrosis, though. In contrast, a high dose of EGCG causes the creation of cardiac collagen and worsens cardiac fibrosis in mice [147].

NADPH oxidases (NOXs), a class of enzymes linked to the production of ROS, were found to contribute to the advancement of myocardial fibrosis and HF [148]. The myocardium expresses all forms of NOX, but NOX2 and NOX4 are predominant. In disease, the human heart's end-stage failure exhibits enhanced NOX expression, and cardiac hypertrophy is evidently a significant source of elevated cardiac ROS. According to Wang et al. [149], luteolin inhibits CFs proliferation by reducing oxidative stress in vitro. The mechanism underlying this effect is dependent on the regulation of NOX2 and NOX4 in cardiac hypertrophy, which reduces the production of c-Jun N-terminal kinase (JNK) and TGF-1 β and lowers cardiac fibrosis [150]. Additionally, the anthocyanins found in grape skins, such as malvidin-3-glucoside, delphinidin-3-glucoside (Dp3G), cyanidin-3-glucoside (Cy3G), petunidin-3-glucoside (Pg3G), and peonidin-3-glucoside, guard against problems from ischemia/reperfusion and diabetic mellitus [151]. Dp3G and Cy3G, but not Pg3G, were able to restore complex I of the mitochondrial respiratory chain to its original condition and increase ischemia-depleted ATP levels via promoting oxidative phosphorylation [152]. Because of its high potential to decrease cytosolic cytochrome c, Cy3G, but not Pg3G, protects the rat heart against ischemia/reperfusion-induced apoptosis and necrosis [153]. Administration of Cy3G improves cardiac dysfunction and cardiac inflammation in STZ-induced diabetic cardiomyopathy by activating MMP-9 and lowering the level of tissue inhibitor of MMP-9 (TIMP-1) found in diabetic rat hearts [154].

Curcumin, a natural inhibitor of p300-specific histone acetyltransferase, has been demonstrated to prevent HF [155]. Curcumin alone or in combination with enalapril reduces severe perivascular fibrosis in rats after MI and enhances left ventricular systolic function via reducing nuclear expression of p300 [155,156]. According to a different study, curcumin prevents unfavorable cardiac repair and lessens the fibrotic response to ischemia and reperfusion by slowing the breakdown of the extracellular matrix and preventing the synthesis of collagens through the TGF-β/Smad pathway [157]. Curcumin dramatically reduced collagen buildup in vivo, as well as CF proliferation, migration, and MMP production, according to another line of study [158]. According to Zeng et al. [159], curcumin's ability to up-regulate Nrf-2 expression and suppress NF-κB activation was directly related to its protective role. Resveratrol administration has been shown to prevent and/or slow down the progression of cardiac remodeling in an animal model of HF [160].

Due to their biological actions as an antioxidant, an anti-inflammatory, and an anticancer agent, polyphenols are commonly present in many foods and have received significant attention. Polyphenols are chemicals with a benzene ring structure with two or more phenolic hydroxyl groups and, depending on their structural properties, they can be divided into flavonoids and phenolic acids. Several positive impacts of polyphenols on health have been documented [161–166]. They are endowed with special functional capabilities to exercise their good effects on human health and are added to meals owing to their remarkable biological activities, such as antioxidant and antibacterial effects, as well as their natural availability and biocompatibility. In the prevention of numerous chronic diseases such as diabetes, hypertension, and cancer, the potential significance of functional foods containing polyphenolic chemicals is of importance.

Flavonoids are divided into six main subclasses based on the variety in the type of heterocycle involved: flavonols, flavanones, flavanols, flavones, anthocyanins, and isoflavones. Individual variances within each group are caused by differences in the quantity, arrangement, alkylation, and/or glycosylation levels of the hydroxyl groups. The C ring of flavonols (such as quercetin and kaempferol) has a 3-hydroxy pyran-4-one group. The C ring of flavanones (such as naringenin and taxifolin) contains an unsaturated carbon-carbon bond. The 4-one structure in the C ring and the 3-hydroxyl group are absent from flavanols (such as the catechins). There is no hydroxyl group in the 3-position on the C ring of flavones (such as luteolin). Isoflavones, such as genistein, have the B ring connected to the C ring in the 3-position rather than the 2-position as is the case with other flavonoids. Anthocyanins, such as cyanidin, are characterized by the presence of an oxonium ion on the C ring and are strongly colored as a result.

6. Food-Drug and Herb-Drug Interactions

Drug release, absorption, distribution, metabolism, and/or elimination can be significantly impacted by the concurrent consumption of food or herbs and medications, which can also have a negative/positive impact on the efficacy and safety of pharmacotherapy. Food and herb consumption alters the human gastrointestinal (GI) tract's physiological environment in a number of ways that can influence a drug's release, absorption, distribution, metabolism, and/or elimination. These interactions between food, herbs, and drugs are general, thus they will apply to any oral formulation [167]. Their applicability, however depends on the drug's formulation and physical characteristics. It is possible to lessen negative drug reactions and iatrogenic disorders by increasing understanding of interindividual variation in drug breakdown capability and results regarding the influence of drugs, nutrition, and herbal items. Medical care needs to be increasingly individually adjusted to each patient, and when diet and herbal treatments are administered in conjunction with medications, this can boost therapeutic efficacy and reduce drug toxicity. Designing a patient's ideal personal regimen can be aided by understanding how dietary components might increase or decrease pharmacological efficacy. Understanding all the variables can aid in creating individualized medicine, nutrition, and herbal remedy plans for patients, preventing negative side effects, and fostering healing and health [168]. The synergistic impact of some herbs with some drugs to lessen xenobiotic inputs may be intriguing in that situation. Herbs/foods that boost a prescription drug's effectiveness may allow for lower drug doses when taken concurrently—a potentially advantageous interaction.

7. Conclusions

Numerous epidemiological studies have found a link between consuming natural polyphenols and a lower risk of developing chronic diseases. The risk of developing major cardiovascular illnesses, MI, and cardiovascular mortality is inversely correlated with higher fruit and vegetable consumption [169]. Synthetic medications, herbal medicine, and diets have been utilized in the management of CVDs for decades. It is important to note that though many reports establish that the molecular mechanisms of cardiac remodeling have been improved using these therapies individually and not as combinations medication of HF, little research has investigated new therapeutic targets that incorporate all three tactics. While their possible interactions should be considered, a combination of treatments that target independent pathways could proof very efficacious in the treatment of CVD (Figure 2).

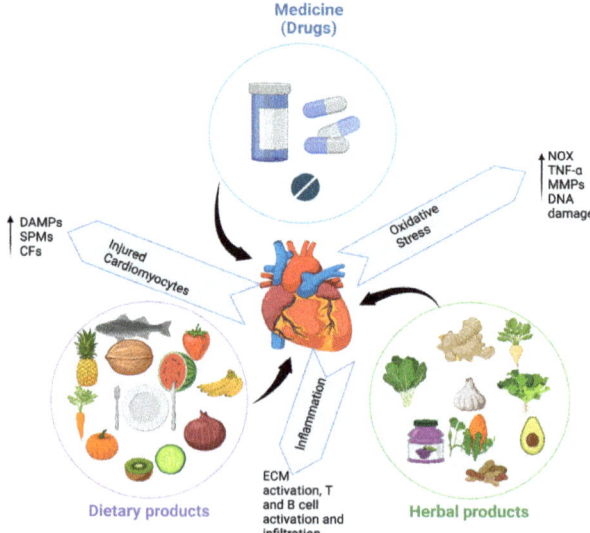

Figure 2. Diagrammatic representation of the influence of synthetic pharmaceutical medications, dietary and herbal products in CVD management, with emphasis in common pathways that are targeted by each intervention. DAMPs = damage-associated molecular patterns, SPMs = specific pro-resolving mediators, CFs = cardiac fibroblasts, NOX = NADPH oxidases, TNF-α = tumor necrosis factor, MMPs = metalloproteinases, DNA = deoxyribonucleic acid, ECM = extracellular matrix. Figure created with Biorender.com.

Author Contributions: Conceptualization, A.A.O. and L.E.d.C.B.; writing—original draft preparation, A.A.O.; writing—review and editing, A.A.O. and L.E.d.C.B.; supervision and project leader, L.E.d.C.B. All authors have read and agreed to the published version of the manuscript.

Funding: This work was supported by the NIH/NHLBI (grant HL152297).

Institutional Review Board Statement: Not applicable.

Informed Consent Statement: Not applicable.

Data Availability Statement: Not applicable.

Conflicts of Interest: The authors declare no conflict of interest.

References

1. World Health Organization. Cardiovascular Diseases (CVDs) (World Health Organization). 2017. Available online: https://www.who.int/news-room/factsheets/detail/cardiovascular-diseases-(cvds) (accessed on 18 October 2020).
2. Benjamin, E.J.; Blaha, M.J.; Chiuve, S.E.; Cushman, M.; Das, S.R.; Deo, R.; De Ferranti, S.D.; Floyd, J.; Fornage, M.; Gillespie, C.; et al. Heart disease and stroke statistics—2017 update: A report from the American Heart Association. *Circulation* **2017**, *135*, e146–e603. [CrossRef]
3. Frangogiannis, N.G. The inflammatory response in myocardial injury, repair, and remodelling. *Nat. Rev. Cardiol.* **2014**, *11*, 255–265. [CrossRef]
4. Lugrin, J.; Rosenblatt-Velin, N.; Parapanov, R.; Liaudet, L. The role of oxidative stress during inflammatory processes. *Biol. Chem.* **2014**, *395*, 203–230. [CrossRef] [PubMed]
5. Serhan CN Novel lipid mediators and resolution mechanisms in acute inflammation: To resolve or not? *Am. J. Pathol.* **2010**, *177*, 1576–1591. [CrossRef] [PubMed]
6. Janicki, J.S.; Brower, G.L.; Henegar, J.R.; Wang, L. Ventricular remodeling in heart failure: The role of myocardial collagen. *Adv. Exp. Med. Biol.* **1995**, *382*, 239–245. [CrossRef] [PubMed]
7. Bolognese, L.; Neskovic, A.N.; Parodi, G.; Cerisano, G.; Buonamici, P.; Santoro, G.M.; Antoniucci, D. Left ventricular remodeling after primary coronary angioplasty: Patterns of left ventricular dilation and long-term prognostic implications. *Circulation* **2002**, *106*, 2351–2357. [CrossRef]
8. Virani, S.S.; Alonso, A.; Benjamin, E.J.; Bittencourt, M.S.; Callaway, C.W.; Carson, A.P.; Chamberlain, A.M.; Chang, A.R.; Cheng, S.; Delling, F.N.; et al. Heart disease and stroke statistics—2020 update: A report from the American Heart Association. *Circulation* **2020**, *141*, e139–e596. [CrossRef] [PubMed]
9. Conrad, N.; Judge, A.; Tran, J.; Mohseni, H.; Hedgecott, D.; Crespillo, A.P.; Allison, M.; Hemingway, H.; Cleland, J.G.; McMurray, J.J.; et al. Temporal trends and patterns in heart failure incidence: A population-based study of 4 million individuals. *Lancet* **2018**, *391*, 572–580. [CrossRef]
10. Störk, S.; Hense, H.W.; Zentgraf, C.; Uebelacker, I.; Jahns, R.; Ertl, G.; Angermann, C.E. Pharmacotherapy according to treatment guidelines is associated with lower mortality in a community-based sample of patients with chronic heart failure A prospective cohort study. *Eur. J. Heart Fail.* **2008**, *10*, 1236–1245. [CrossRef]
11. Desta, L.; Jernberg, T.; Spaak, J.; Hofman-Bang, C.; Persson, H. Risk and predictors of readmission for heart failure following a myocardial infarction between 2004 and 2013: A Swedish nationwide observational study. *Int. J. Cardiol.* **2017**, *248*, 221–226. [CrossRef]
12. Romiti, G.F.; Recchia, F.; Zito, A.; Visioli, G.; Basili, S.; Raparelli, V. Sex and Gender-Related Issues in Heart Failure. *Cardiol. Clin.* **2022**, *40*, 259–268. [CrossRef] [PubMed]
13. Salton, C.J.; Chuang, M.L.; O'Donnell, C.J.; Kupka, M.J.; Larson, M.G.; Kissinger, K.V.; Edelman, R.R.; Levy, D.; Manning, W.J. Gender differences and normal left ventricular anatomy in an adult population free of hypertension: A cardiovascular magnetic resonance study of the Framingham Heart Study Offspring cohort. *J. Am. Coll. Cardiol.* **2002**, *39*, 1055–1060. [CrossRef] [PubMed]
14. Laufer, E.M.; Mingels, A.M.; Winkens, M.H.; Joosen, I.A.; Schellings, M.W.; Leiner, T.; Wildberger, J.E.; Narula, J.; Van Dieijen-Visser, M.P. and Hofstra, L. The extent of coronary atherosclerosis is associated with increasing circulating levels of high sensitive cardiac troponin T. *Arterioscler. Thromb. Vasc. Biol.* **2010**, *30*, 1269–1275. [CrossRef] [PubMed]
15. Piro, M.; Della Bona, R.; Abbate, A.; Biasucci, L.M.; Crea, F. Sex-related differences in myocardial remodeling. *J. Am. Coll. Cardiol.* **2010**, *55*, 1057–1065. [CrossRef]
16. Westerman, S.; Wenger, N.K. Women and heart disease, the underrecognized burden: Sex differences, biases, and unmet clinical and research challenges. *Clin. Sci.* **2016**, *130*, 551–563. [CrossRef]
17. Maggioni, A.A.; Maseri, A.; Fresco, C.; Franzosi, M.G.; Mauri, F.; Santoro, E.; Tognoni, G. Age-related increase in mortality among patients with first myocardial infarctions treated with thrombolysis. *N. Engl. J. Med.* **1993**, *329*, 1442–1448. [CrossRef]
18. Bujak, M.; Kweon, H.J.; Chatila, K.; Li, N.; Taffet, G.; Frangogiannis, N.G. Aging-related defects are associated with adverse cardiac remodeling in a mouse model of reperfused myocardial infarction. *J. Am. Coll. Cardiol.* **2008**, *51*, 1384–1392. [CrossRef]
19. Koitabashi, N.; Kass, D.A. Reverse remodeling in heart failure--mechanisms and therapeutic opportunities. *Nat. Rev. Cardiol.* **2011**, *9*, 147–157. [CrossRef]

20. Nisar, B.; Sultan, A.; Rubab, S.L. Comparison of medicinally important natural products versus synthetic drugs-a short commentary. *Nat. Prod. Chem. Res.* **2018**, *6*, 308. [CrossRef]
21. Martinez-Gonzalez, M.A.; Fernández-Jarne, E.; Serrano-Martínez, M.; Wright, M.; Gomez-Gracia, E. Development of a short dietary intake questionnaire for the quantitative estimation of adherence to a cardioprotective Mediterranean diet. *Eur. J. Clin. Nutr.* **2004**, *58*, 1550–1552. [CrossRef]
22. Goszcz, K.; Deakin, S.J.; Duthie, G.G.; Stewart, D.; Megson, I.L. Bioavailable concentrations of delphinidin and its metabolite, gallic acid, induce antioxidant protection associated with increased intracellular glutathione in cultured endothelial cells. *Oxidative Med. Cell. Longev.* **2017**, *2017*, 9260701. [CrossRef]
23. Nabel, E.G.; Braunwald, E.A. Tale of coronary artery disease and myocardial infarction. *N. Engl. J. Med.* **2012**, *366*, 54–63. [CrossRef] [PubMed]
24. Gustafsson, I.; Torp-Pedersen, C.; Køber, L.; Gustafsson, F.; Hildebrandt, P.; Trace Study Group. Effect of the angiotensin-converting enzyme inhibitor trandolapril on mortality and morbidity in diabetic patients with left ventricular dysfunction after acute myocardial infarction. *J. Am. Coll. Cardiol.* **1999**, *34*, 83–89. [CrossRef] [PubMed]
25. Greenberg, B.; Quinones, M.A.; Koilpillai, C.; Limacher, M.; Shindler, D.; Benedict, C.; Shelton, B. Effects of long-term enalapril therapy on cardiac structure and function in patients with left ventricular dysfunction: Results of the SOLVD echocardiography substudy. *Circulation* **1995**, *91*, 2573–2581. [CrossRef] [PubMed]
26. Quiñones, M.A.; Greenberg, B.H.; Kopelen, H.A.; Koilpillai, C.; Limacher, M.C.; Shindler, D.M.; Shelton, B.J.; Weiner, D.H.; SOLVD Investigators**. Echocardiographic predictors of clinical outcome in patients with left ventricular dysfunction enrolled in the SOLVD registry and trials: Significance of left ventricular hypertrophy. *J. Am. Coll. Cardiol.* **2000**, *35*, 1237–1244. [CrossRef]
27. Anand, I.S.; Florea, V.G. Structural Remodeling in the Development of Chronic Systolic Heart Failure: Implication for Treatment. In *Congestive Heart Failure and Cardiac Transplantation*; Springer: Cham, Switzerland, 2017; pp. 247–265.
28. Pfeffer, M.A.; Braunwald, E.; Moyé, L.A.; Basta, L.; Brown, E.J., Jr.; Cuddy, T.E.; Davis, B.R.; Geltman, E.M.; Goldman, S.; Flaker, G.C.; et al. Effect of captopril on mortality and morbidity in patients with left ventricular dysfunction after myocardial infarction: Results of the Survival and Ventricular Enlargement Trial. *N. Engl. J. Med.* **1992**, *327*, 669–677. [CrossRef]
29. Lopez-Sendon, J.; Swedberg, K.; McMurray, J.; Tamargo, J.; Maggioni, A.P.; Dargie, H.; Tendera, M.; Waagstein, F.; Kjekshus, J.; Lechat, P.; et al. Expert consensus document on angiotensin converting enzyme inhibitors in cardiovascular disease: The Task Force on ACE-inhibitors of the European Society of Cardiology. *Eur. Heart J.* **2004**, *25*, 1454–1470.
30. Fedak, P.W.; Verma, S.; Weisel, R.D.; Li, R.K. Cardiac remodeling and failure: From molecules to man (Part I). *Cardiovasc. Pathol.* **2005**, *14*, 1–11. [CrossRef]
31. Azizi, M.; Ménard, J.; Bissery, A.; Guyenne, T.T.; Bura-Rivière, A.; Vaidyanathan, S.; Camisasca, R.P. Pharmacologic demonstration of the synergistic effects of a combination of the renin inhibitor aliskiren and the AT1 receptor antagonist valsartan on the angiotensin II–renin feedback interruption. *J. Am. Soc. Nephrol.* **2004**, *15*, 3126–3133. [CrossRef]
32. King, M.K.; Coker, M.L.; Goldberg, A.; McElmurray, J.H.; Gunasinghe, H.R., 3rd; Mukherjee, R.; Zile, M.R.; O'Neill, T.P.; Spinale, F.G. Selective matrix metalloproteinase inhibition with developing heart failure: Effects on left ventricular function and structure. *Circ. Res.* **2003**, *92*, 177–185. [CrossRef]
33. Ikonomidis, J.S.; Hendrick, J.W.; Parkhurst, A.M.; Herron, A.R.; Escobar, P.G.; Dowdy, K.B.; Stroud, R.E.; Hapke, E.; Zile, M.R.; Spinale, F.G. Accelerated LV remodeling after myocardial infarction in TIMP-1-deficient mice: Effects of exogenous MMP inhibition. *Am. J. Physiol. Heart Circ. Physiol.* **2005**, *288*, H149–H158. [CrossRef]
34. Matsumura, S.; Iwanaga, S.; Mochizuki, S.; Okamoto, H.; Ogawa, S.; Okada, Y. Targeted deletion or pharmacological inhibition of MMP-2 prevents cardiac rupture after myocardial infarction in mice. *J. Clin. Investig.* **2005**, *115*, 599–609. [CrossRef] [PubMed]
35. Hu, J.; Van den Steen, P.E.; Sang, Q.X.A.; Opdenakker, G. Matrix metalloproteinase inhibitors as therapy for inflammatory and vascular diseases. *Nat. Rev. Drug Discov.* **2007**, *6*, 480–498. [CrossRef] [PubMed]
36. Vandenbroucke, R.E.; Libert, C. Is there new hope for therapeutic matrix metalloproteinase inhibition? *Nat. Rev. Drug Discov.* **2014**, *13*, 904–927. [CrossRef]
37. Fields, G.B. The rebirth of matrix metalloproteinase inhibitors: Moving beyond the dogma. *Cells* **2019**, *8*, 984. [CrossRef] [PubMed]
38. Mozaffarian, D. Dietary and policy priorities for cardiovascular disease, diabetes, and obesity: A comprehensive review. *Circulation* **2016**, *133*, 187–225. [CrossRef]
39. Chiuve, S.E.; Fung, T.T.; Rimm, E.B.; Hu, F.B.; McCullough, M.L.; Wang, M.; Stampfer, M.J.; Willett, W.C. Alternative dietary indices both strongly predict risk of chronic disease. *J. Nutr.* **2012**, *142*, 1009–1018. [CrossRef]
40. van Abeelen, A.F.; Elias, S.G.; Bossuyt, P.M.; Grobbee, D.E.; van der Schouw, Y.T.; Roseboom, T.J.; Uiterwaal, C.S. Cardiovascular consequences of famine in the young. *Eur. Heart J.* **2012**, *33*, 538–545. [CrossRef]
41. Ferguson, D.P.; Monroe, T.O.; Heredia, C.P.; Fleischmann, R.; Rodney, G.G.; Taffet, G.E.; Fiorotto, M.L. Postnatal undernutrition alters adult female mouse cardiac structure and function leading to limited exercise capacity. *J. Physiol.* **2019**, *597*, 1855–1872. [CrossRef]
42. Bensley, J.G.; Stacy, V.K.; De Matteo, R.; Harding, R.; Black, M.J. Cardiac remodelling as a result of pre-term birth: Implications for future cardiovascular disease. *Eur. Heart J.* **2010**, *31*, 2058–2066. [CrossRef]
43. Anatskaya, O.V.; Sidorenko, N.V.; Beyer, T.V.; Vinogradov, A.E. Neonatal cardiomyocyte ploidy reveals critical windows of heart development. *Int. J. Cardiol.* **2010**, *141*, 81–91. [CrossRef]

4. Mozaffarian, D.; Ludwig, D.S. Dietary guidelines in the 21st century—A time for food. *JAMA* **2010**, *304*, 681–682. [CrossRef] [PubMed]
5. LaCroix, A.Z.; Rillamas-Sun, E.; Buchner, D.; Evenson, K.R.; Di, C.; Lee, I.M.; Marshall, S.; LaMonte, M.J.; Hunt, J.; Tinker, L.F.; et al. The objective physical activity and cardiovascular disease health in older women (OPACH) study. *BMC Public Health* **2017**, *17*, 192. [CrossRef]
6. Esposito, K.; Ciotola, M.; Giugliano, D. Mediterranean diet, endothelial function and vascular inflammatory markers. *Public Health Nutr.* **2006**, *9*, 1073–1076. [CrossRef] [PubMed]
7. Casas, R.; Sacanella, E.; Urpi-Sarda, M.; Chiva-Blanch, G.; Ros, E.; Martinez-Gonzalez, M.A.; Estruch, R. The effects of the mediterranean diet on biomarkers of vascular wall inflammation and plaque vulnerability in subjects with high risk for cardiovascular disease. A randomized trial. *PLoS ONE* **2014**, *9*, e100084. [CrossRef] [PubMed]
8. Casas, R.; Urpi-Sardà, M.; Sacanella, E.; Arranz, S.; Corella, D.; Castañer, O.; Lamuela-Raventós, R.M.; Salas-Salvadó, J.; Lapetra, J.; Portillo, M.P.; et al. Anti-inflammatory effects of the Mediterranean diet in the early and late stages of atheroma plaque development. *Mediat. Inflamm.* **2017**, *2017*, 3674390. [CrossRef] [PubMed]
9. Dauchet, L.; Amouyel, P.; Dallongeville, J. Fruits, vegetables and coronary heart disease. *Nat. Rev. Cardiol.* **2009**, *6*, 599–608. [CrossRef] [PubMed]
10. Dauchet, L.; Amouyel, P.; Hercberg, S.; Dallongeville, J. Fruit and vegetable consumption and risk of coronary heart disease: A meta-analysis of cohort studies. *J. Nutr.* **2006**, *136*, 2588–2593. [CrossRef]
11. Corley, J.; Kyle, J.A.; Starr, J.M.; McNeill, G.; Deary, I.J. Dietary factors and biomarkers of systemic inflammation in older people: The Lothian Birth Cohort 1936. *Br. J. Nutr.* **2015**, *114*, 1088–1098. [CrossRef]
12. Hosseini, B.; Berthon, B.S.; Saedisomeolia, A.; Starkey, M.R.; Collison, A.; Wark, P.A.; Wood, L.G. Effects of fruit and vegetable consumption on inflammatory biomarkers and immune cell populations: A systematic literature review and meta-analysis. *Am. J. Clin. Nutr.* **2018**, *108*, 136–155. [CrossRef]
13. Arouca, A.; Michels, N.; Moreno, L.A.; González-Gil, E.M.; Marcos, A.; Gómez, S.; Díaz, L.E.; Widhalm, K.; Molnár, D.; Manios, Y.; et al. Associations between a Mediterranean diet pattern and inflammatory biomarkers in European adolescents. *Eur. J. Nutr.* **2018**, *57*, 1747–1760. [CrossRef]
14. Wongwarawipat, T.; Papageorgiou, N.; Bertsias, D.; Siasos, G.; Tousoulis, D. Olive oil-related anti-inflammatory effects on atherosclerosis: Potential clinical implications. *Endocr. Metab. Immune Disord.-Drug Targets* **2018**, *18*, 51–62. [CrossRef] [PubMed]
15. Schwingshackl, L.; Christoph, M.; Hoffmann, G. Effects of olive oil on markers of inflammation and endothelial function—A systematic review and meta-analysis. *Nutrients* **2015**, *7*, 7651–7675. [CrossRef]
16. Mente, A.; de Koning, L.; Shannon, H.S.; Anand, S.S. A systematic review of the evidence supporting a causal link between dietary factors and coronary heart disease. *Arch. Intern. Med.* **2009**, *169*, 659–669. [CrossRef] [PubMed]
17. Aune, D.; Keum, N.; Giovannucci, E.; Fadnes, L.T.; Boffetta, P.; Greenwood, D.C.; Tonstad, S.; Vatten, L.J.; Riboli, E.; Norat, T. Nut consumption and risk of cardiovascular disease, total cancer, all-cause and cause-specific mortality: A systematic review and dose-response meta-analysis of prospective studies. *BMC Med.* **2016**, *14*, 207. [CrossRef] [PubMed]
18. Guasch-Ferré, M.; Bulló, M.; Martínez-González, M.Á.; Ros, E.; Corella, D.; Estruch, R.; Fitó, M.; Arós, F.; Wärnberg, J.; Fiol, M.; et al. Frequency of nut consumption and mortality risk in the PREDIMED nutrition intervention trial. *BMC Med.* **2013**, *11*, 164. [CrossRef]
19. Olabiyi, A.A.; Carvalho, F.B.; Bottari, N.B.; Lopes, T.F.; da Costa, P.; Stefanelo, N.; Morsch, V.M.; Akindahunsi, A.A.; Oboh, G.; Schetinger, M.R. Dietary supplementation of tiger nut alters biochemical parameters relevant to erectile function in L-NAME treated rats. *Food Res. Int.* **2018**, *109*, 358–367. [CrossRef]
20. Estruch, R.; Martínez-González, M.A.; Corella, D.; Salas-Salvadó, J.; Ruiz-Gutiérrez, V.; Covas, M.I.; Fitó, M.; Gómez-Gracia, E.; López-Sabater, M.C.; Vinyoles, E.; et al. Effects of a Mediterranean-style diet on cardiovascular risk factors: A randomized trial. *Ann. Intern. Med.* **2006**, *145*, 1–11. [CrossRef]
21. Del Gobbo, L.C.; Falk, M.C.; Feldman, R.; Lewis, K.; Mozaffarian, D. Effects of tree nuts on blood lipids, apolipoproteins, and blood pressure: Systematic review, meta-analysis, and dose-response of 61 controlled intervention trials. *Am. J. Clin. Nutr.* **2015**, *102*, 1347–1356. [CrossRef] [PubMed]
22. Martini, D.; Godos, J.; Marventano, S.; Tieri, M.; Ghelfi, F.; Titta, L.; Lafranconi, A.; Trigueiro, H.; Gambera, A.; Alonzo, E.; et al. Nut and legume consumption and human health: An umbrella review of observational studies. *Int. J. Food Sci. Nutr.* **2021**, *72*, 871–878. [CrossRef] [PubMed]
23. Zhou, D.; Yu, H.; He, F.; Reilly, K.H.; Zhang, J.; Li, S.; Zhang, T.; Wang, B.; Ding, Y.; Xi, B. Nut consumption in relation to cardiovascular disease risk and type 2 diabetes: A systematic review and meta-analysis of prospective studies. *Am. J. Clin. Nutr.* **2014**, *100*, 270–277. [CrossRef] [PubMed]
24. Aramwit, P.; Kanokpanont, S.; De-Eknamkul, W.; Srichana, T. Monitoring of inflammatory mediators induced by silk sericin. *J. Biosci. Bioeng.* **2009**, *107*, 556–561. [CrossRef] [PubMed]
25. Chen, L.; Teng, H.; Jia, Z.; Battino, M.; Miron, A.; Yu, Z.; Cao, H. and Xiao, J. Intracellular signaling pathways of inflammation modulated by dietary flavonoids: The most recent evidence. *Crit. Rev. Food Sci. Nutr.* **2018**, *58*, 2908–2924. [CrossRef] [PubMed]
26. Jönsson, T.; Granfeldt, Y.; Ahrén, B.; Branell, U.C.; Pålsson, G.; Hansson, A.; Söderström, M.; Lindeberg, S. Beneficial effects of a Paleolithic diet on cardiovascular risk factors in type 2 diabetes: A randomized cross-over pilot study. *Cardiovasc. Diabetol.* **2009**, *8*, 35. [CrossRef]

67. Jew, S.; AbuMweis, S.S.; Jones, P.J. Evolution of the human diet: Linking our ancestral diet to modern functional foods as a means of chronic disease prevention. *J. Med. Food* **2009**, *12*, 925–934. [CrossRef]
68. Cordain, L. The nutritional characteristics of a contemporary diet based upon Paleolithic food groups. *J. Am. Nutraceutical. Assoc* **2002**, *5*, 15–24.
69. Österdahl, M.; Kocturk, T.; Koochek, A.; Wändell, P. Effects of a short-term intervention with a paleolithic diet in healthy volunteers. *Eur. J. Clin. Nutr.* **2008**, *62*, 682–685. [CrossRef]
70. Ghaedi, E.; Mohammadi, M.; Mohammadi, H.; Ramezani-Jolfaie, N.; Malekzadeh, J.; Hosseinzadeh, M.; Salehi-Abargouei, A. Effects of a Paleolithic Diet on Cardiovascular Disease Risk Factors: A Systematic Review and Meta-Analysis of Randomized Controlled Trials. *Adv. Nutr.* **2019**, *10*, 634–646, Erratum in *Adv. Nutr.* **2020**, *11*, 1054. [CrossRef]
71. Manheimer, E.W.; van Zuuren, E.J.; Fedorowicz, Z.; Pijl, H. Paleolithic nutrition for metabolic syndrome: Systematic review and meta-analysis. *Am. J. Clin. Nutr.* **2015**, *102*, 922–932. [CrossRef]
72. Owen, O.E.; Morgan, A.P.; Kemp, H.G.; Sullivan, J.M.; Herrera, M.G.; Cahill, G.F. Brain metabolism during fasting. *J. Clin. Investig* **1967**, *46*, 1589–1595. [CrossRef]
73. Santos, F.L.; Esteves, S.S.; da Costa Pereira, A.; Yancy, W.S.; Nunes, J.P., Jr. Systematic review and meta-analysis of clinical trials of the effects of low carbohydrate diets on cardiovascular risk factors: Low carbohydrate diets and cardiovascular risk factors. *Obes Rev.* **2012**, *13*, 1048–1066. [CrossRef] [PubMed]
74. Bueno, N.B.; de Melo, I.S.; de Oliveira, S.L.; da Rocha Ataide, T. Very-low-carbohydrate ketogenic diet v. low-fat diet for long-term weight loss: A meta-analysis of randomised controlled trials. *Br. J. Nutr.* **2013**, *110*, 1178–1187. [CrossRef] [PubMed]
75. Naude, C.E.; Schoonees, A.; Senekal, M.; Young, T.; Garner, P.; Volmink, J. Low carbohydrate versus isoenergetic balanced diets for reducing weight and cardiovascular risk: A systematic review and meta-analysis. *PLoS ONE* **2014**, *9*, e100652. [CrossRef]
76. Kosinski, C.; Jornayvaz, F.R. Effects of Ketogenic Diets on Cardiovascular Risk Factors: Evidence from Animal and Human Studies. *Nutrients* **2017**, *9*, 517. [CrossRef] [PubMed]
77. O'Neill, B.; Raggi, P. The ketogenic diet: Pros and cons. *Atherosclerosis* **2020**, *292*, 119–126. [CrossRef]
78. Xu, S.; Tao, H.; Cao, W.; Cao, L.; Lin, Y.; Zhao, S.M.; Xu, W.; Cao, J.; Zhao, J.Y. Ketogenic diets inhibit mitochondrial biogenesis and induce cardiac fibrosis. *Signal Transduct. Target Ther.* **2021**, *6*, 54. [CrossRef]
79. Gao, J.W.; Hao, Q.Y.; Zhang, H.F.; Li, X.Z.; Yuan, Z.M.; Guo, Y.; Wang, J.F.; Zhang, S.L.; Liu, P.M. Low-carbohydrate diet score and coronary artery calcium progression: Results from the CARDIA Study. *Arterioscler. Thromb. Vasc. Biol.* **2020**, *41*, 491–500. Available online: https://www.ahajournals.org/doi/10.1161/ATVBAHA.120.314838 (accessed on 29 October 2020). [CrossRef]
80. Garcia-Rios, A.; Ordovas, J.M.; Lopez-Miranda, J.; Perez-Martinez, P. New diet trials and cardiovascular risk. *Curr. Opin. Cardiol* **2018**, *33*, 423–428. [CrossRef]
81. Juraschek, S.P.; Miller III, E.R.; Chang, A.R.; Anderson, C.A.; Hall, J.E.; Appel, L.J. Effects of sodium reduction on energy metabolism, weight, thirst, and urine volume: Results from the DASH (dietary approaches to stop hypertension)-sodium trial. *Hypertension* **2020**, *75*, 723–729. [CrossRef] [PubMed]
82. Kerley, C.P. Dietary patterns and components to prevent and treat heart failure: A comprehensive review of human studies. *Nutr. Res. Rev.* **2019**, *32*, 1–27. [CrossRef]
83. Kerley, C.P. A review of plant-based diets to prevent and treat heart failure. *Card. Fail. Rev.* **2018**, *4*, 54. [CrossRef] [PubMed]
84. Oboh, G.; Olabiyi, A.A.; Akinyemi, A.J. Inhibitory effect of aqueous extract of different parts of unripe pawpaw (*Carica papaya*) fruit on Fe^{2+}-induced oxidative stress in rat pancreas in vitro. *Pharm. Biol.* **2013**, *51*, 1165–1174. [CrossRef]
85. Newman, D.J.; Cragg, G.M. Natural products as sources of new drugs from 1981 to 2014. *J. Nat. Prod.* **2016**, *79*, 629–661. [CrossRef]
86. Ray, S.; Saini, M.K. Cure and prevention of cardiovascular diseases: Herbs for heart. *Clin. Phytoscience* **2021**, *7*, 5741198. [CrossRef]
87. Patwardhan, B.; Mashelkar, R.A. Traditional medicine-inspired approaches to drug discovery: Can Ayurveda show the way forward? *Drug Discov. Today* **2009**, *14*, 804–811. [CrossRef] [PubMed]
88. Olabiyi, A.A.; Afolabi, B.A.; Reichert, K.P.; Palma, T.V.; Morsch, V.M.; Oboh, G.; Schetinger, M.R.C. Assessment of sexual behavior and neuromodulation of *Cyperus esculentus* L. and Tetracarpidium conophorum Müll. Arg dietary supplementation regulating the purinergic system in the cerebral cortex of L-NAME-challenged rats. *J. Food Biochem.* **2021**, *45*, e13862. [CrossRef] [PubMed]
89. Badole, S.L.; Bodhankar, S.L.; Patel, N.M.; Bhardwaj, S. Acute and chronic diuretic effect of ethanolic extract of leaves of *Cocculus hirsutus* (L.) Diles in normal rats. *J. Pharm. Pharmacol.* **2009**, *61*, 387–393. [CrossRef]
90. Davison, E.K.; Brimble, M.A. Natural product derived privileged scaffolds in drug discovery. *Curr. Opin. Chem. Biol.* **2019**, *52*, 1–8. [CrossRef]
91. Olabiyi, A.A.; Ajayi, K. Diet, herbs and erectile function: A good friendship! *Andrologia* **2022**, *54*, e14424. [CrossRef]
92. Shaito, A.; Thuan, D.T.B.; Phu, H.T.; Nguyen, T.H.D.; Hasan, H.; Halabi, S.; Abdelhady, S.; Nasrallah, G.K.; Eid, A.H.; Pintus, G. Herbal medicine for cardiovascular diseases: Efficacy, mechanisms, and safety. *Front. Pharmacol.* **2020**, *11*, 422. [CrossRef]
93. Silva, H.; Martins, F.G. Cardiovascular Activity of Ginkgo biloba—An Insight from Healthy Subjects. *Biology* **2022**, *12*, 15. [CrossRef] [PubMed]
94. Upadhyay, S.; Dixit, M. Role of polyphenols and other phytochemicals on molecular signaling. *Oxidative Med. Cell. Longev.* **2015**, *2015*, 504253. [CrossRef]
95. Murino Rafacho, B.P.; Portugal dos Santos, P.; Goncalves, A.D.F.; Fernandes, A.A.H.; Okoshi, K.; Chiuso-Minicucci, F.; Azevedo, P.S.; Mamede Zornoff, L.A.; Minicucci, M.F.; Wang, X.D.; et al. Rosemary supplementation (*Rosmarinus oficinallis* L.) attenuates cardiac remodeling after myocardial infarction in rats. *PLoS ONE* **2017**, *12*, e0177521. [CrossRef]

96. Butnariu, M.; Quispe, C.; Herrera-Bravo, J.; Sharifi-Rad, J.; Singh, L.; Aborehab, N.M.; Bouyahya, A.; Venditti, A.; Sen, S.; Acharya, K.; et al. The pharmacological activities of Crocus sativus L.: A review based on the mechanisms and therapeutic opportunities of its phytoconstituents. *Oxidative Med. Cell. Longev.* **2022**, *2022*, 8214821. [CrossRef] [PubMed]
97. Khazdair, M.R.; Boskabady, M.H.; Hosseini, M.; Rezaee, R.; Tsatsakis, A.M. The effects of Crocus sativus (saffron) and its constituents on nervous system: A review. *Avicenna J. Phytomedicine* **2015**, *5*, 376.
98. Mzabri, I.; Addi, M.; Berrichi, A. Traditional and modern uses of saffron (Crocus sativus). *Cosmetics* **2019**, *6*, 63. [CrossRef]
99. Sargolzaei, J.; Shabestari, M.M. The effects of Crocus Sativus, L. and its main constituents against cardiovascular diseases. *Der Pharm. Lett.* **2016**, *8*, 38–41.
100. Al-Yahya, M.A.; Mothana, R.A.; Al-Said, M.S.; El-Tahir, K.E.; Al-Sohaibani, M.; Rafatullah, S. Citrus medica "Otroj": Attenuates oxidative stress and cardiac dysrhythmia in isoproterenol-induced cardiomyopathy in rats. *Nutrients* **2013**, *5*, 4269–4283. [CrossRef]
101. Tassell, M.C.; Kingston, R.; Gilroy, D.; Lehane, M.; Furey, A. Hawthorn (Crataegus spp.) in the treatment of cardiovascular disease. *Pharmacogn. Rev.* **2010**, *4*, 32.
102. Altinterim, B. Cardiovascular effects of Hawthorn (Crataegus monogyna). *KSÜ Doğa Bilim. Derg.* **2012**, *15*, 16–18.
103. Verma, S.K.; Jain, V.; Katewa, S.S. Blood pressure lowering, fibrinolysis enhancing and antioxidant activities of cardamom (Elettaria cardamomum). *Indian J. Biochem. Biophys.* **2009**, *46*, 503–506.
104. Nagashree, S.; Archana, K.K.; Srinivas, P.; Srinivasan, K.; Sowbhagya, H.B. Anti-hypercholesterolemic influence of the spice cardamom (Elettaria cardamomum) in experimental rats. *J. Sci. Food Agric.* **2017**, *97*, 3204–3210. [CrossRef]
105. Arbeláez, L.F.G.; Pardo, A.C.; Fantinelli, J.C.; Schinella, G.R.; Mosca, S.M.; Ríos, J.L. Cardioprotection and natural polyphenols: An update of clinical and experimental studies. *Food Funct.* **2018**, *9*, 6129–6145. [CrossRef]
106. Lee, C.H.; Kim, J.H. A review on the medicinal potentials of ginseng and ginsenosides on cardiovascular diseases. *J. Ginseng Res.* **2014**, *38*, 161–166. [CrossRef] [PubMed]
107. Chan, S.W.; Tomlinson, B.; Chan, P.; Lam, C.W.K. The beneficial effects of Ganoderma lucidum on cardiovascular and metabolic disease risk. *Pharm. Biol.* **2021**, *59*, 1161–1171. [CrossRef]
108. Aviram, M.; Dornfeld, L. Pomegranate juice consumption inhibits serum angiotensin converting enzyme activity and reduces systolic blood pressure. *Atherosclerosis* **2001**, *158*, 195–198. [CrossRef]
109. Asgary, S.; Haghjooyjavanmard, S.; Setorki, M.; Rafieian, M.; Haghighi, S.; Eidi, A.; Rohani, A.H. The postprandial effect of apple juice intake on some of the biochemical risk factors of atherosclerosis in male rabbit. *J. Med. Plants Res.* **2009**, *3*, 785–790.
110. Asgary, S.; Sahebkar, A.; Afshani, M.R.; Keshvari, M.; Haghjooyjavanmard, S.; Rafieian-Kopaei, M. Clinical evaluation of blood pressure lowering, endothelial function improving, hypolipidemic and anti-inflammatory effects of pomegranate juice in hypertensive subjects. *Phytother. Res.* **2014**, *28*, 193–199. [CrossRef]
111. Setorki, M.; Nazari, B.; Asgary, S.; Eidi, A.; Rohani, A.H. Acute effects of apple cider vinegar intake on some biochemical risk factors of atherosclerosis in rabbits fed with a high cholesterol diet. *Qom Univ. Med. Sci. J.* **2010**, *3*, 10.
112. Setorki, M.; Asgary, S.; Eidi, A.; Rohani, A.H.; Esmaeil, N. Effects of apple juice on risk factors of lipid profile, inflammation and coagulation, endothelial markers and atherosclerotic lesions in high cholesterolemic rabbits. *Lipids Health Dis.* **2009**, *8*, 39. [CrossRef] [PubMed]
113. Omoni, A.O.; Aluko, R.E. The anti-carcinogenic and anti-atherogenic effects of lycopene: A review. *Trends Food Sci. Technol.* **2005**, *16*, 344–350. [CrossRef]
114. Naz, A.; Butt, M.S.; Sultan, M.T.; Qayyum, M.M.N.; Niaz, R.S. Watermelon lycopene and allied health claims. *EXCLI J.* **2014**, *13*, 650. [PubMed]
115. Chiva-Blanch, G.; Visioli, F. Polyphenols and health: Moving beyond antioxidants. *J. Berry Res.* **2012**, *2*, 63–71. [CrossRef]
116. Niki, E. Antioxidant capacity: Which capacity and how to assess it? *J. Berry Res.* **2011**, *1*, 169–176. [CrossRef]
117. Cassidy, A.; Mukamal, K.J.; Liu, L.; Franz, M.; Eliassen, A.H.; Rimm, E.B. High anthocyanin intake is associated with a reduced risk of myocardial infarction in young and middle-aged women. *Circulation* **2013**, *127*, 188–196. [CrossRef]
118. Jang, M.; Cai, L.; Udeani, G.O.; Slowing, K.V.; Thomas, C.F.; Beecher, C.W.; Fong, H.H.; Farnsworth, N.R.; Kinghorn, A.D.; Mehta, R.G.; et al. Cancer chemopreventive activity of resveratrol, a natural product derived from grapes. *Science* **1997**, *275*, 218–220. [CrossRef] [PubMed]
119. Seymour, E.M.; Singer, A.A.; Bennink, M.R.; Parikh, R.V.; Kirakosyan, A.; Kaufman, P.B.; Bolling, S.F. Chronic intake of a phytochemical-enriched diet reduces cardiac fibrosis and diastolic dysfunction caused by prolonged salt-sensitive hypertension. *J. Gerontol. Ser. A Biol. Sci. Med. Sci.* **2008**, *63*, 1034–1042. [CrossRef] [PubMed]
120. Varshney, R.; Budoff, M.J. Garlic and heart disease. *J. Nutr.* **2016**, *146*, 416S–421S. [CrossRef]
121. Ko, F.N.; Yu, S.M.; Kang, Y.F.; Teng, C.M. Characterization of the thromboxane (TP-) receptor subtype involved in proliferation in cultured vascular smooth muscle cells of rat. *Br. J. Pharmacol.* **1995**, *116*, 1801–1808. [CrossRef]
122. Pandey, K.B.; Rizvi, S.I. Plant polyphenols as dietary antioxidants in human health and disease. *Oxidative Med. Cell. Longev.* **2009**, *2*, 270–278. [CrossRef]
123. Quideau, S.; Deffieux, D.; Douat-Casassus, C.; Pouységu, L. Plant polyphenols: Chemical properties, biological activities, and synthesis. *Angew. Chem. Int. Ed.* **2011**, *50*, 586–621. [CrossRef] [PubMed]
124. Tsao, R. Chemistry and biochemistry of dietary polyphenols. *Nutrients* **2010**, *2*, 1231–1246. [CrossRef]

125. Kumar, N.; Goel, N. Phenolic acids: Natural versatile molecules with promising therapeutic applications. *Biotechnol. Rep.* 2019, 24, e00370. [CrossRef]
126. Vitrac, X.; Monti, J.P.; Vercauteren, J.; Deffieux, G.; Mérillon, J.M. Direct liquid chromatographic analysis of resveratrol derivatives and flavanonols in wines with absorbance and fluorescence detection. *Anal. Chim. Acta* 2002, 458, 103–110. [CrossRef]
127. Prasad, R.; Kawaguchi, S.; Ng, D.T. Biosynthetic mode can determine the mechanism of protein quality control. *Biochem. Biophys. Res. Commun.* 2012, 425, 689–695. [CrossRef] [PubMed]
128. Korkina, L.; Kostyuk, V.; De Luca, C.; Pastore, S. Plant phenylpropanoids as emerging anti-inflammatory agents. *Mini Rev. Med. Chem.* 2011, 11, 823–835. [CrossRef] [PubMed]
129. Saleem, M.; Kim, H.J.; Ali, M.S.; Lee, Y.S. An update on bioactive plant lignans. *Nat. Prod. Rep.* 2005, 22, 696–716. [CrossRef]
130. Ly, C.; Yockell-Lelievre, J.; Ferraro, Z.M.; Arnason, J.T.; Ferrier, J.; Gruslin, A. The effects of dietary polyphenols on reproductive health and early development. *Hum. Reprod. Update* 2015, 21, 228–248. [CrossRef]
131. Smeds, A.I.; Eklund, P.C.; Willför, S.M. Content, composition, and stereochemical characterisation of lignans in berries and seeds. *Food Chem.* 2012, 134, 1991–1998. [CrossRef]
132. Khan, N.; Mukhtar, H. Tea polyphenols for health promotion. *Life Sci.* 2007, 81, 519–533. [CrossRef]
133. Hollman, P.C.H.; Arts, I.C.W. Flavonols, flavones and flavanols–nature, occurrence and dietary burden. *J. Sci. Food Agric.* 2000, 80, 1081–1093. [CrossRef]
134. Cassidy, A.; Hanley, B.; Lamuela-Raventos, R.M. Isoflavones, lignans and stilbenes–origins, metabolism and potential importance to human health. *J. Sci. Food Agric.* 2000, 80, 1044–1062. [CrossRef]
135. Brglez Mojzer, E.; Knez Hrnčič, M.; Škerget, M.; Knez, Ž.; Bren, U. Polyphenols: Extraction Methods, Antioxidative Action, Bioavailability and Anticarcinogenic Effects. *Molecules* 2016, 21, 901. [CrossRef] [PubMed]
136. Mateos-Martín, M.L.; Fuguet, E.; Quero, C.; Pérez-Jiménez, J.; Torres, J.L. New identification of proanthocyanidins in cinnamon (*Cinnamomum zeylanicum* L.) using MALDI-TOF/TOF mass spectrometry. *Anal. Bioanal. Chem.* 2012, 402, 1327–1336. [CrossRef]
137. Han, X.; Shen, T.; Lou, H. Dietary polyphenols and their biological significance. *Int. J. Mol. Sci.* 2007, 8, 950–988. [CrossRef]
138. Raj, P.; Louis, X.L.; Thandapilly, S.J.; Movahed, A.; Zieroth, S.; Netticadan, T. Potential of resveratrol in the treatment of heart failure. *Life Sci.* 2014, 95, 63–71. [CrossRef]
139. Niu, L.; He, X.H.; Wang, Q.W.; Fu, M.Y.; Xu, F.; Xue, Y.; Wang, Z.Z.; An, X.J. Polyphenols in regulation of redox signaling and inflammation during cardiovascular diseases. *Cell Biochem. Biophys.* 2015, 72, 485–494. [CrossRef]
140. Li, M.; Jiang, Y.; Jing, W.; Sun, B.; Miao, C.; Ren, L. Quercetin provides greater cardioprotective effect than its glycoside derivative rutin on isoproterenol-induced cardiac fibrosis in the rat. *Can. J. Physiol. Pharmacol.* 2013, 91, 951–959. [CrossRef]
141. Panchal, S.K.; Poudyal, H.; Brown, L. Quercetin ameliorates cardiovascular, hepatic, and metabolic changes in diet-induced metabolic syndrome in rats. *J. Nutr.* 2012, 142, 1026–1032. [CrossRef]
142. Mak, J.C. Potential role of green tea catechins in various disease therapies: Progress and promise. *Clin. Exp. Pharmacol. Physiol.* 2012, 39, 265–273. [CrossRef]
143. Sheng, R.; Gu, Z.L.; Xie, M.L.; Zhou, W.X.; Guo, C.Y. EGCG inhibits cardiomyocyte apoptosis in pressure overload-induced cardiac hypertrophy and protects cardiomyocytes from oxidative stress in rats 1. *Acta Pharmacol. Sin.* 2007, 28, 191–201. [CrossRef] [PubMed]
144. Sheng, R.; Gu, Z.L.; Xie, M.L.; Zhou, W.X.; Guo, C.Y. EGCG inhibits proliferation of cardiac fibroblasts in rats with cardiac hypertrophy. *Planta Med.* 2009, 75, 113–120. [CrossRef] [PubMed]
145. Han, Y.S.; Lan, L.; Chu, J.; Kang, W.Q.; Ge, Z.M. Epigallocatechin gallate attenuated the activation of rat cardiac fibroblasts induced by angiotensin II via regulating β-arrestin1. *Cell. Physiol. Biochem.* 2013, 31, 338–346. [CrossRef]
146. Cai, Y.; Yu, S.S.; Chen, T.T.; Gao, S.; Geng, B.; Yu, Y.; Ye, J.T.; Liu, P.Q. EGCG inhibits CTGF expression via blocking NF-κB activation in cardiac fibroblast. *Phytomedicine* 2013, 20, 106–113. [CrossRef]
147. Cai, Y.; He, S.Q.; Hong, H.Q.; Cai, Y.P.; Zhao, L.; Zhang, M. High doses of (−)-epigallocatechin-3-gallate from green tea induces cardiac fibrosis in mice. *Biotechnol. Lett.* 2015, 37, 2371–2377. [CrossRef] [PubMed]
148. Heymans, S.; González, A.; Pizard, A.; Papageorgiou, A.P.; López-Andrés, N.; Jaisser, F.; Thum, T.; Zannad, F.; Díez, J. Searching for new mechanisms of myocardial fibrosis with diagnostic and/or therapeutic potential. *Eur. J. Heart Fail.* 2015, 17, 764–771. [CrossRef]
149. Wang, T.; Pan, D.; Zhang, Y.; Li, D.; Zhang, Y.; Xu, T.; Luo, Y.; Ma, Y. Luteolin antagonizes angiotensin II-dependent proliferation and collagen synthesis of cultured rat cardiac fibroblasts. *Curr. Pharm. Biotechnol.* 2015, 16, 430–439. [CrossRef]
150. Nakayama, A.; Morita, H.; Nakao, T.; Yamaguchi, T.; Sumida, T.; Ikeda, Y.; Kumagai, H.; Motozawa, Y.; Takahashi, T.; Imaizumi, A.; et al. A food-derived flavonoid luteolin protects against angiotensin II-induced cardiac remodeling. *PLoS ONE* 2015, 10, e0137106. [CrossRef]
151. Sun, C.D.; Zhang, B.; Zhang, J.K.; Xu, C.J.; Wu, Y.L.; Li, X.; Chen, K.S. Cyanidin-3-glucoside-rich extract from Chinese bayberry fruit protects pancreatic β cells and ameliorates hyperglycemia in streptozotocin-induced diabetic mice. *J. Med. Food* 2012, 15, 288–298. [CrossRef]
152. Skemiene, K.; Liobikas, J.; Borutaite, V. Anthocyanins as substrates for mitochondrial complex I–protective effect against heart ischemic injury. *FEBS J.* 2015, 282, 963–971. [CrossRef]
153. Škėmienė, K.; Jablonskienė, G.; Liobikas, J.; Borutaitė, V. Protecting the heart against ischemia/reperfusion-induced necrosis and apoptosis: The effect of anthocyanins. *Medicina* 2013, 49, 15. [CrossRef]

54. Chen, Y.F.; Shibu, M.A.; Fan, M.J.; Chen, M.C.; Viswanadha, V.P.; Lin, Y.L.; Lai, C.H.; Lin, K.H.; Ho, T.J.; Kuo, W.W.; et al. Purple rice anthocyanin extract protects cardiac function in STZ-induced diabetes rat hearts by inhibiting cardiac hypertrophy and fibrosis. *J. Nutr. Biochem.* **2016**, *31*, 98–105. [CrossRef] [PubMed]
55. Sunagawa, Y.; Morimoto, T.; Wada, H.; Takaya, T.; Katanasaka, Y.; Kawamura, T.; Yanagi, S.; Marui, A.; Sakata, R.; Shimatsu, A.; et al. A natural p300-specific histone acetyltransferase inhibitor, curcumin, in addition to angiotensin-converting enzyme inhibitor, exerts beneficial effects on left ventricular systolic function after myocardial infarction in rats. *Circ. J.* **2011**, *75*, 2151–2159. [CrossRef]
56. Sunagawa, Y.; Sono, S.; Katanasaka, Y.; Funamoto, M.; Hirano, S.; Miyazaki, Y.; Hojo, Y.; Suzuki, H.; Morimoto, E.; Marui, A.; et al. Optimal dose-setting study of curcumin for improvement of left ventricular systolic function after myocardial infarction in rats. *J. Pharmacol. Sci.* **2014**, *126*, 329–336. [CrossRef] [PubMed]
57. Wang, N.P.; Wang, Z.F.; Tootle, S.; Philip, T.; Zhao, Z.Q. Curcumin promotes cardiac repair and ameliorates cardiac dysfunction following myocardial infarction. *Br. J. Pharmacol.* **2012**, *167*, 1550–1562. [CrossRef]
58. Xiao, J.; Sheng, X.; Zhang, X.; Guo, M.; Ji, X. Curcumin protects against myocardial infarction-induced cardiac fibrosis via SIRT1 activation in vivo and in vitro. *Drug Des. Dev. Ther.* **2016**, *10*, 1267. [CrossRef]
59. Zeng, C.; Zhong, P.; Zhao, Y.; Kanchana, K.; Zhang, Y.; Khan, Z.A.; Chakrabarti, S.; Wu, L.; Wang, J.; Liang, G. Curcumin protects hearts from FFA-induced injury by activating Nrf2 and inactivating NF-κB both in vitro and in vivo. *J. Mol. Cell. Cardiol.* **2015**, *79*, 1–12. [CrossRef]
60. Sung, M.M.; Dyck, J.R. Therapeutic potential of resveratrol in heart failure. *Ann. N. Y. Acad. Sci.* **2015**, *1348*, 32–45. [CrossRef]
61. Song, H.; Wang, Q.; He, A.; Li, S.; Guan, X.; Hu, Y.; Feng, S. Antioxidant activity, storage stability and in vitro release of epigallocatechin-3-gallate (EGCG) encapsulated in hordein nanoparticles. *Food Chem.* **2022**, *388*, 132903. [CrossRef]
62. Qiu, C.; McClements, D.J.; Jin, Z.; Qin, Y.; Hu, Y.; Xu, X.; Wang, J. Resveratrol-loaded core-shell nanostructured delivery systems: Cyclodextrin-based metal-organic nanocapsules prepared by ionic gelation. *Food Chem.* **2020**, *317*, 126328. [CrossRef]
63. Ding, H.W.; Huang, A.L.; Zhang, Y.L.; Li, B.; Huang, C.; Ma, T.T.; Meng, X.M.; Li, J. Design, synthesis and biological evaluation of hesperetin derivatives as potent anti-inflammatory agent. *Fitoterapia* **2017**, *121*, 212–222. [CrossRef]
64. Lee, S.H.; Lee, Y.J. Synergistic anticancer activity of resveratrol in combination with docetaxel in prostate carcinoma cells. *Nutr. Res. Pract.* **2021**, *15*, 12–25. [CrossRef]
65. Quiñones, M.; Guerrero, L.; Suarez, M.; Pons, Z.; Aleixandre, A.; Arola, L.; Muguerza, B. Low-molecular procyanidin rich grape seed extract exerts antihypertensive effect in males spontaneously hypertensive rats. *Food Res. Int.* **2013**, *51*, 587–595. [CrossRef]
66. Rains, T.M.; Agarwal, S.; Maki, K.C. Antiobesity effects of green tea catechins: A mechanistic review. *J. Nutr. Biochem.* **2011**, *22*, 1–7. [CrossRef] [PubMed]
67. Koziolek, M.; Alcaro, S.; Augustijns, P.; Basit, A.W.; Grimm, M.; Hens, B.; Hoad, C.L.; Jedamzik, P.; Madla, C.M.; Maliepaard, M.; et al. The mechanisms of pharmacokinetic food-drug interactions—A perspective from the UNGAP group. *Eur. J. Pharm. Sci. Off. J. Eur. Fed. Pharm. Sci.* **2019**, *134*, 31–59. [CrossRef]
68. O'Shea, J.P.; Holm, R.; O'Driscoll, C.M.; Griffin, B.T. Food for thought: Formulating away the food effect–a PEARRL review. *J. Pharm. Pharmacol.* **2019**, *71*, 510–535. [CrossRef] [PubMed]
69. Miller, V.; Mente, A.; Dehghan, M.; Rangarajan, S.; Zhang, X.; Swaminathan, S.; Dagenais, G.; Gupta, R.; Mohan, V.; Lear, S.; et al. Fruit, vegetable, and legume intake, and cardiovascular disease and deaths in 18 countries (PURE): A prospective cohort study. *Lancet* **2017**, *390*, 2037–2049. [CrossRef]

Disclaimer/Publisher's Note: The statements, opinions and data contained in all publications are solely those of the individual author(s) and contributor(s) and not of MDPI and/or the editor(s). MDPI and/or the editor(s) disclaim responsibility for any injury to people or property resulting from any ideas, methods, instructions or products referred to in the content.

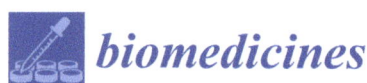

Review

Evidence and Uncertainties on Lipoprotein(a) as a Marker of Cardiovascular Health Risk in Children and Adolescents

Simonetta Genovesi [1,2,*], Marco Giussani [2], Giulia Lieti [1], Antonina Orlando [2], Ilenia Patti [1] and Gianfranco Parati [1,2]

[1] School of Medicine and Surgery, Milano-Bicocca University, 20126 Milan, Italy; g.lieti@campus.unimib.it (G.L.); a.patti8@campus.unimib.it (I.P.); dir.sci@auxologico.it (G.P.)
[2] Istituto Auxologico Italiano, Istituto Ricovero Cura Carattere Scientifico (IRCCS), 20135 Milan, Italy; dottormarcogiussani@gmail.com (M.G.); a.orlando@auxologico.it (A.O.)
* Correspondence: simonetta.genovesi@unimib.it; Tel.: +39-335243910

Abstract: Lipoprotein(a) (Lp(a)) is made up of apoprotein(a) (apo(a)) and an LDL-like particle. The *LPA* gene encodes apo(a) and thus determines the characteristics and amount of apo(a) and Lp(a). The proportion of Lp(a) in each individual is genetically determined and is only minimally modifiable by the environment or diet. Lp(a) has important pro-atherosclerotic and pro-inflammatory effects. It has been hypothesized that Lp(a) also has pro-coagulant and antifibrinolytic actions. For these reasons high Lp(a) values are an important independent risk factor for cardiovascular disease and calcific aortic valve stenosis. Numerous studies have been performed in adults about the pathophysiology and epidemiology of Lp(a) and research is under way for the development of drugs capable of reducing Lp(a) plasma values. Much less information is available regarding Lp(a) in children and adolescents. The present article reviews the evidence on this topic. The review addresses the issues of Lp(a) changes during growth, the correlation between Lp(a) values in children and those in their parents, and between Lp(a) levels in children, and the presence of cardiovascular disease in the family. Gaining information on these points is particularly important for deciding whether Lp(a) assay may be useful for defining the cardiovascular risk in children, in order to plan a prevention program early.

Keywords: lipoprotein(a); children; adolescents; cardiovascular risk

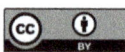

1. Introduction

Lipoprotein(a) (Lp(a)) was first described by K. Berg in 1963 [1]. For several years, interest in this lipoprotein was modest, until the sequencing of the *LPA* gene encoding apolipoprotein(a) (apo(a)), a key constituent of Lp(a) [2], and the subsequent recognition of Lp(a) as an independent risk factor for cardiovascular disease by epidemiological and Mendelian randomization studies [3,4]. Later, high Lp(a) values were also associated with calcific aortic valve stenosis [5] and increased risk of ischemic stroke [6,7].

2. Structure and Features of Lp(a)

Lp(a) consists of a very low-density lipoprotein (LDL)-like particle with apoprotein B100 being bound via a single disulfide link to a single apoprotein(a) (apo(a)) (Figure 1).

Apo(a) is a glycoprotein that has structural similarities with plasminogen. Plasminogen is made from a protein chain with a terminal part with protease activity joined to five aggregates of about 90 amino acids that have been named kringles because of their shape resembling that of a typical Northern European cake. In plasminogen, the kringles are present in single copy and are named with Roman numerals from KI to KV. Unlike plasminogen, apo(a) has an inactive protease domain and does not contain KI, KII, or KIII kringles, but consists of only one KV subtype and ten KIV subtypes, which are present in single copy except for the KIV$_2$ subtype that can repeat from one to forty times [8] (Figure 2). Polypeptide structures similar to kringle domains are found in several enzymes (thrombin, tissue plasminogen activator, hepatocyte growth factor) as well as in plasminogen and Lp(a). The KVs of plasminogen and apo(a) have strong structural homology, as do the KIVs of plasminogen and Lp(a). However, KV and KIV are quite different from each other, both structurally and as amino acid composition. In contrast, the various subtypes 1 to 10 of KIV have important structural homologies and differ in their composition by only a few amino acids. These small differences may, however, account for different activities such as, for example, the ability to create disulfide bonds between KIV9 and apoB100. The specific function of KIV2 is not known, nor is the physiological function of Lp(a). The characteristic of KIV2 is its ability to be replicated a highly variable number of times in the structure of apo(a) [9].

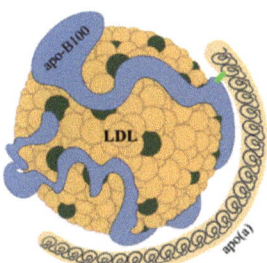

Figure 1. Structure of lipoprotein(a). Lipoprotein(a) consists of a very low-density lipoprotein (LDL)-like particle, with apoprotein B100 (apo-B100) being bound via a single disulfide link to a single apoprotein a (apo(a)).

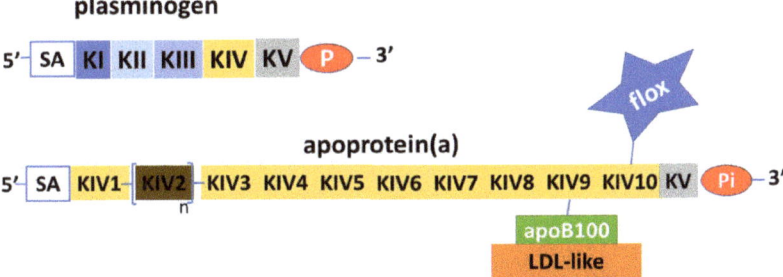

Figure 2. Schematic depiction of plasminogen and apoprotein (a). Apoprotein(a) is a glycoprotein with remarkable similarities to plasminogen, in both the protease part (P) and the inactive part (Pi), and in the kringle protein structure (K). The apoprotein(a) does not have KI to KIII, while it has KIV to KV; KV and subtypes 1 and 3 to 10 are expressed in single copy, while subtype 2 is pre-sent in variable copy numbers. Apoprotein(a) can vary greatly in length and molecular weight. Sialic acid (SA) with other N-glucans and O-glucans has structural functions and protects apoprotein(a) from proteases. Apoprotein(a) transports a considerable amount of oxidized phospholipids (flox), which, added to the LDL-like ones connected to apoprotein(a) via apoprotein B100 (ApoB100), make lipoprotein(a) the major carrier of oxidized phospholipids.

Thus, the length of apo(a) is highly variable and its molecular weight has a range from 275 to 800 kDa. Apo(a) contains a fair amount of oligosaccharides, in particular, sialic acid and other N-glycans and O-glycans, which have structural and protective functions against the activity of proteolytic enzymes [10,11]. Another relevant aspect in the structure of apo(a) is the presence of oxidized phospholipids, mainly attached to the KIV_{10} subtype. Considering also the proportion contained in the LDL-like component, Lp(a) is the major carrier of oxidized phospholipids [12], so individuals with high Lp(a) values are at greater risk of coronary heart disease and stroke. Apo(a) is produced exclusively by the endoplasmic reticulum of the liver, where it also undergoes post-translational modifications with the creation of a disulfide bond in each kringle that assumes the characteristic shape. The formation process is completed in the Golgi apparatus where the lipoprotein undergoes glycosylation [13]. The question of whether the assembly of Lp(a) with apo(a) and apoprotein B-100 takes place in the hepatocyte, on the surface or even outside, is not settled yet. Some studies suggest that an initial non-covalent bond between apo(a) and apoprotein B100 could be formed inside the hepatocyte [10], while the final disulfide bond that completes the formation of Lp(a) would be created outside the hepatocyte, in the Disse spaces of the hepatic sinusoids [14,15]. A small proportion of apo(a) remains unaggregated and is eliminated with urine; no particular function has been attributed to it [16]. The amount of circulating Lp(a) depends on how much apo(a) is produced by the liver, which, in turn, depends on the activity of the *LPA* gene, which, being made up of two codominant alleles, encodes two isoforms of apo(a) that may differ in length. In each individual, therefore, there are two different Lp(a)s which may have different molecular weights. The variability in Lp(a) levels in the general population is extremely high, and its plasma concentration can range from 0.1 to 300 mg/dL. Hepatic production of Lp(a) is 80–90% genetically determined; therefore, it is little affected by environmental factors and tends to be stable in adults [17]. Therefore, in this age group, a single Lp(a) assay may be sufficient to know the related risk profile of the individual. However, this point is a matter of debate, as it is reported that Lp(a) levels would change over time [18]; moreover, this occurs in the presence of certain diseases. First, it should be noted that Lp(a) behaves as an acute phase protein, so it tends to increase in inflammatory states [19] and this should be taken into account when scheduling the measurement. In addition, nephropathies are also associated with significant increases in Lp(a) levels, which can be explained by different mechanisms depending on the type of kidney disease. Already in the early stages of renal failure, an increase in Lp(a) can be shown, with increases proportional to the decrease in glomerular filtrate. However, in the nephrotic syndrome, Lp(a) can increase up to fourfold due to an increment of its synthesis by the liver [20]. Chronic kidney disease patients have a significantly increased risk of cardiovascular disease, related to the level of Lp(a) [21]. The amount of circulating Lp(a) is inversely proportional to the length of the apo(a), thus to the number of KIV_2 kringles. Therefore, individuals with longer apo(a) isoforms of Lp(a), thus with higher molecular weight, produce less Lp(a) than those with shorter, lower molecular weight isoforms. The lower amount of Lp(a) produced by individuals in which the higher molecular weight isoforms predominate could be due to the longer time required for its production [22] or to the greater molecular weight isoforms that have not assumed the correct conformation being translocated outside the endoplasmic reticulum, ubiquitinated and degraded [23]. In addition to length, other genetic factors may influence the increased or decreased production of Lp(a). In particular, several single nucleotide polymorphisms of the *LPA* gene are known to be associated with increased or decreased apo(a) and Lp(a) production [24,25]. Regarding cardiovascular risk, it is currently believed that it would be related to the amount of circulating Lp(a) and not to its qualitative characteristics. Thus, subjects with higher plasma concentrations of this lipoprotein, who are those with lower molecular weight isoforms of Lp(a), are most at risk [3]. Lp(a) is metabolized mainly by the liver and to a lesser extent by the kidney. Several receptors are called upon for Lp(a) uptake, such as the BI scavenger receptor, plasminogen receptors, and LDL receptors, but these aspects are not yet fully elucidated [26]. The variability of Lp(a) gives reason for the difficulties there are in developing precise laboratory methods for its assay. In particular, when polyclonal antibodies, also directed toward the repeated part of apo(a) (KIV_2), are used, larger isoforms tend to be overestimated, while smaller ones may be underestimated [27]. These difficulties can be overcome by performing analyses with calibrators containing Lp(a) of different lengths or with monoclonal antibodies directed only toward the single-copy portion of apo(a). Lp(a) assays are often expressed in mg/dL, as if directly measuring the entire lipoprotein, and thus, not only its protein part but also its cholesterol content, cholesterol esters, phospholipids, triglycerides, and carbohydrates. This is not quite correct because the assays reflect the quantitative molar ratio between apo(a) and the antibodies that interact with it. Therefore, it would be more correct to express Lp(a) values in nmol/L [27]. Again because of the variability of Lp(a), there can be no precise conversion factor between mg/dL and nmol/L. However, from a practical point of view, a conversion factor between 2 and 2.5 is still accepted [28].

3. Lp(a) and Cardiovascular Risk

Lp(a) is associated with an increased risk of cardiovascular events because of some of its structural and functional characteristics that promote atherosclerotic plaque formation and growth. In addition, it has been suggested that Lp(a) promotes coagulation processes following plaque rupture. This, however, is currently only a hypothesis and needs validation. Lp(a) contains a proportion of cholesterol that corresponds to about 30–40% of its weight [29]. This amount of cholesterol is less than that found in LDL and is negligible when circulating Lp(a) is in low concentration. However, in individuals who have high Lp(a) values, its contribution to the amount of atherogenic cholesterol can be significant, mainly due to the ease with which Lp(a) crosses the endothelium and accumulates in the inner layer of the artery wall, where it is able to activate smooth muscle cell proliferation and migration and foam cell formation [13]. Interestingly, high levels of Lp(a) promote the earlier stages of atherosclerosis and not just the more advanced phases. Imaging studies have shown that Lp(a) promotes the development of arterial wall inflammation [30] and that in the presence of coronary artery disease, high Lp(a) levels are associated with an increase in the amount of calcium and necrotic core volume from the atherosclerotic plaque [31,32]. The processes promoting inflammation and calcium deposition seem mainly related to the presence of oxidized phospholipids [33,34], which would be responsible for the secretion of chemotactic substances and proinflammatory cytokines, upregulation of adhesion molecules, and trans-endothelial migration of monocytes [30,35]. Finally, the presence in apo(a) of a protease-like domain similar to that of plasminogen, but inactive, suggests that Lp(a) might also have a role in promoting coagulation processes and reducing fibrinolysis. The latter effect of Lp(a) is still under debate [36]. However, it seems that Lp(a) has no role in venous thromboembolism events [37]. In summary, Lp(a) would have pro-atherosclerotic, pro-inflammatory, and possibly pro-coagulant and antifibrinolytic effects. Regarding calcific aortic valve stenosis, numerous studies have shown micro- and macro-calcifications of the aortic valve in adults aged 45 to 55 years with elevated Lp(a) values [5,38,39]. It is estimated that individuals with higher Lp(a) percentiles are three times more likely to develop calcific aortic valve stenosis than those with lower Lp(a) percentiles [38]. Furthermore, high plasma Lp(a) levels correlate with more rapid progression of valve stenosis [12]. The etiopathogenetic mechanisms explaining the association between Lp(a) and calcific aortic valve stenosis have yet to be elucidated; however, oxidized phospholipids would again be called into play, which, in addition to activating inflammatory processes, would stimulate the activation of genes that regulate osteoblastic processes in the cells of the valve interstitium [12,35].

Some considerations should be added regarding the relationship between hypolipidemic drug therapy and the levels of Lp(a). Statins have been reported to be associated with a tendency to increase Lp(a) levels, whereas ezetimibe would have no effect [40,41].

In contrast, apheresis [42] and drugs such as niacin [43] and PCSK9 inhibitors [44] are able to reduce plasma Lp(a) concentrations. However, while it has been shown that the decrease in Lp(a) levels induced by apheresis is approximately 75% and is associated, in subjects with extremely high Lp(a) levels, with a significant reduction in cardiovascular risk [42], the same clinical outcome is not achieved with the administration of niacin or PCSK9 inhibitors [45,46], which induce reductions in Lp(a) values of 20–30% [43,44]. On the basis of the current data, a significant reduction in cardiovascular risk by lowering Lp(a) awaits further studies. Of note, niacin and PCSK9 inhibitors do not currently have a pediatric indication.

4. Lp(a) in Adults

The plasma concentration of Lp(a) is widely variable, and in all populations, there are individuals with very-high Lp(a) values. However, important differences can be found in the distribution of Lp(a) in different ethnic groups. In fact, average Lp(a) values increase from Chinese, to South Asians, to Whites to Blacks, with average concentrations of 16, 19, 31, and 75 nmol/L, respectively [47]. Hispanics have values intermediate between South Asians and Caucasian Whites [48]. In general then, Black individuals are those with higher Lp(a) values; in fact, the mean value of the plasma Lp(a) concentration among Blacks is in the fifth quintile of the White population distribution [49]. These differences among the different ethnic groups would be largely explained by the greater presence of isoforms with lower KIV_2 kringle number in the Black, Caucasian, and Hispanic populations, respectively although mutations in the LPA gene and other yet unknown factors would play a non secondary role [50,51]. A recent large study confirms the inverse relationship between the distribution of Lp(a) values and its isoforms and the different distribution among different ethnic groups [52]. The study shows that Chinese and South Asian populations have the lowest average Lp(a) values and largest isoforms, while Africans and Arabs have the highest concentrations and smallest isoforms. Europeans, Latin Americans, and Southeast Asians rank in between for both parameters. The same study shows a correlation between the presence of Lp(a) values greater than 50 mg/dL with the risk of myocardial infarction with an odds ratio of 1.48 (95% CI: 1.32–1.67) in the entire population. The risk increased from Africans, to Arabs, Chinese, Europeans, Latin Americans to Southeast Asians who had the highest odds ratio [52]. This study suggests that ethnicity should also be taken into account when assessing the cardiovascular risk associated with Lp(a) levels, as similar Lp(a) values might be associated with different patterns of cardiovascular risk in different ethnicities. Lp(a) values could also differ according to gender. However, the reports on this issue are conflicting: some authors report that males have higher values than females [53] while for other authors, the opposite would be true [47]. In males, Lp(a) values would remain consistent throughout adult life [54], whereas in females, there would be an increase after menopause [55–58]. In adults, the correlation between Lp(a) levels and cardiovascular risk has a linear and continuous pattern. In general, individuals with Lp(a) values less than 30 mg/dL can be considered at low risk and those with values greater than 50 mg/dL at high risk. Concentrations between 30 and 50 mg/dL are considered borderline [27]. It should be emphasized, however, that in the assessment of an individual's cardiovascular risk, Lp(a) values are only one aspect, albeit an important one, that must be considered in the totality of the other known risk factors. The most recent European guidelines suggest that Lp(a) should be measured at least once in a lifetime in adults and that this information should be included in the overall estimate of the risk of developing atherosclerotic-based disease [27].

5. Lp(a) in Children and Adolescents

The number of Lp(a) studies performed in pediatric populations is much smaller than those performed in adults. This is because pediatric research on cardiovascular risk factors is often ancillary to that in adulthood, but also because cardiovascular events are exceptional in very young people. However, four studies have been published that relate to increased Lp(a) values to the occurrence of arterial ischemic stroke in infants and children [59–62]. In addition, a meta-analysis reported an OR of 6.27 (95% CI, 4.52 to 8.69) for ischemic stroke in children with elevated Lp(a) compared to children with normal values [63]. However, arterial ischemic stroke is a very rare condition in childhood, so this finding refers to a restricted aspect of the relationship between elevated Lp(a) levels and cardiovascular disease in youth. Studies that relate to Lp(a) measurement in children and adolescents are in small numbers and involve two time periods. The oldest studies date back to the 1990s, and publications have resumed in more recent times when interest around Lp(a) has grown, partly because of the possibility of specific therapy that could reduce its values.

Thus, the main questions are (i) how does Lp(a) vary during childhood and (ii) is there a correlation between Lp(a) values in children, those of their parents, and the presence of markers of atherosclerosis in adolescents and/or cardiovascular disease in the family?

In the available studies, the Lp(a) assay is expressed with different units: in milligrams/liter, in milligrams/deciliter, or in nanomoles/liter. In reporting the results of the different studies, we have kept the data as expressed in the original articles.

5.1. Changes in Lp(a) Values in Childhood

As for this topic, the questions are (i) how do Lp(a) levels vary during childhood; (ii) when do they reach adult values; (iii) will a child with high Lp(a) be an adult with high Lp(a) values?

A first study carried out in 1983 showed that Lp(a) values in neonates are very low compared to those in adults [64]. A subsequent study confirmed that the Lp(a) values at birth are very low and increase significantly by the seventh day of life and are still increasing even at 180 days after birth [65]. A later study reported Lp(a) values in 232 infants including 123 of white ethnicity and 109 of black ethnicity. The birth value of Lp(a) was 4 mg/dL with no differences by ethnicity and gender. The same study showed that Lp(a) values increased gradually from birth, reaching adult values already by the second year of life [66]. Schumacher and Wood assayed Lp(a) in 123 term infants showing a mean concentration of 13.9 mg/L in the umbilical cord blood and 10.2 mg/L in the capillary blood [67]. Subsequently, the same group published a study conducted on 625 infants and 221 children in the first year of life. The median value of Lp(a) in children less than 1 year old was 37.0 mg/L regardless of gender (males 37.1, females 37.0 mg/L) [68]. Wilcken et al. calculated the 50th and 95th percentile values of Lp(a) on a sample of more than 1000 children in the third–fifth days of life, which were found to be 30 and 130 mg/L, respectively. Repeat assays at month 8 in a subgroup of the same sample showed that the values were doubled [69]. A Turkish study conducted in 430 children with dosing at 7, 13, 24, and 36 months showed mean Lp(a) values of 84, 156, 134, and 136 mg/L, respectively. The authors also found a strong correlation between the Lp(a) concentrations of the four measurements in the individual child [70]. Two recent studies have made important contributions regarding the evolution of Lp(a) values from infancy and adolescence. In the first, the authors assayed Lp(a) in the umbilical cord, at birth at 2 months and at 15 months obtaining values of 2.2, 2.4, 4.1, and 14.6 mg/dL, respectively, showing a strong correlation between umbilical cord blood and venous blood values at birth and a moderate correlation between values at 2 and 15 months [71]. In the second, a group of Dutch researchers published data collected on a sample of nearly 3000 children and adolescents referred to an outpatient clinic dedicated to the treatment of dyslipidemia. The population had high mean LDL cholesterol values (184 mg/dL), and in about two-thirds of the cases, a diagnosis of familial hypercholesterolemia had been made and confirmed on genetic analysis. Lp(a) assays, performed by two different analytical methods, showed mean values of 117 and 103 mg/L. Lp(a) values increased with age in both the group of untreated individuals and those taking hypolipidemic drugs. In individuals in whom multiple assays had been performed at different times, at least a 20% increase in Lp(a) levels was observed. Individuals who showed high values when they were children maintained high values as adults. Finally, the researchers showed that in all of the study population, Lp(a) values increased into adulthood, and individuals treated with statins tended to have a greater increase. Subjects taking the statin/ezetimibe combination reached a plateau at age 15 years [72]. These data would confirm what has already been observed in adults in whom statin treatment would induce an increase in Lp(a) values not shown in those taking ezetimibe [40,41]. Finally, a recent study conducted in 416 Korean children with a mean age of 11.1 years, in which the mean values were 21.5 nmol/L, should be noted. The prevalence of individuals with Lp(a) values > 100 nmol/L (equal to about 50 mg/dL) was 11.3%. No age- or gender-related differences were evident [73].

5.2. Correlation between Pediatric Lp(a) Values and Clinical Data

In his study, Wilcken et al. [69] showed a correlation between Lp(a) values in children in the third–fifth day of life and those of their parents, and this correlation was even clearer in measurements performed at eight months. The study by de Boer [72] confirmed a correlation between Lp(a) values from eight years of age to adulthood, with an increase in values of about 20 percent. Qayum et al. assayed Lp(a) in 257 14-year-old adolescents referred to an outpatient cardiovascular prevention clinic based on the presence of dyslipidemia or early cardiovascular events in the family. The sample was divided into two groups based on the presence of Lp(a) values greater or less than 30 mg/dL, showing that African–American ethnicity was more represented in the group with high Lp(a) values, while there were no differences related to gender. In addition, the prevalence of early cardiovascular events in the family was higher in the group with high Lp(a) values, HDL cholesterol values were higher, and triglyceride values were lower. In contrast, there were no differences in carotid intima-media thickness or pulse wave velocity, two surrogate indices of atherosclerosis [74]. A recent study confirmed the absence of significant differences in early vascular aging in a group of young people with elevated Lp(a) compared with a control group [75]. Recently, the Italian LIPIGEN network demonstrated in a group of 653 Caucasian children and adolescents aged 2 to 17 years with clinical and/or genetic diagnosis of familial hypercholesterolemia that individuals with the highest Lp(a) values were also those with a higher prevalence of early cardiovascular events in first- or second-degree gentiles [76]. Finally, a very new publication [77] considered two studies in which the relationship between Lp(a) values in young people aged 9 to 24 years and 8 to 17 years and the incidence of cardiovascular events at the mean age of 47 years was assessed. After adjustment for several other cardiovascular risk factors, Lp(a) values > 30 mg/dL carried about twice the risk of early cardiovascular events. The concurrent presence of elevated LDL cholesterol values doubled this risk. When the data were analyzed continuously, the risk of events increased by 30 percent for every 1 standard deviation increase in Lp(a) value. In children, the clinical diagnosis of FH is based almost exclusively on LDL cholesterol values, since the other clinical signs contributing to the diagnostic scores, which are present in adults, are never found in children. Because when we assay LDL cholesterol, we cannot distinguish the amount of cholesterol carried by LDL (which increases in the presence of FH) from that related to Lp(a), the presence of high Lp(a) values could lead to misdiagnosis of heterozygous FH. De Boer's group tested this hypothesis by analyzing a sample of subjects less than 18 years of age referred for family history of FH and/or early cardiovascular disease and/or hypercholesterolemia in the family [78]. The authors noted that children with a diagnosis of FH confirmed by genetic analysis had lower Lp(a) values than those with a phenotype suggestive of FH for elevated LDL cholesterol values but with a negative genetic diagnosis. The latter group was also the one with a higher prevalence of familiarity for early cardiovascular events. These data suggest that high Lp(a) values may be a greater risk factor than carrying a genetic mutation causing heterozygous FH [79]. On the sidelines, we can mention that recently, the analysis of data from the LIPIGEN network in adults confirmed that very high Lp(a) levels can explain at least part of the clinical diagnoses of FH in subjects with very high-LDL cholesterol values and negative analysis for causative genes of this disease [80].

In conclusion, Lp(a) values at birth are very low, but they increase rapidly in the first few months of life. It is believed that definitive values are reached around the age of two years, but some data cast doubt on this assumption. There is evidence, however, of the existence of a correlation between Lp(a) values in childhood and in adulthood. There also seems to be a correlation between child and parental Lp(a) values. Finally, high Lp(a) values in children and adolescents correlate with a higher frequency of cardiovascular events in the family and an important increased risk of early cardiovascular events.

6. Role of Lp(a) in Defining Pediatric Cardiovascular Risk and Preventive Activity

Cardiovascular disease is the leading cause of death in Europe and the World [81,82] and is also a major cause of disability and health spending [83]. In low-income countries, it is not economically and organizationally feasible to provide adequate care for patients with cardiovascular disease [84,85], while in developed countries, where effective and innovative but expensive treatments are available [86], the economic burden of these diseases can become critical for welfare systems [83]. Even with these considerations in mind, primary prevention should be the key choice of a correct and forward-looking health policy. Cardiovascular disease manifests clinically in adulthood, but the underlying atherosclerotic processes are already evident even in the first decade of life [87,88]. Paradoxically, atherosclerosis could be considered a pediatric disease. Prevention of cardiovascular disease should therefore be started very early. It is well known that unhealthy lifestyles and diet, as well as exposure to environmental pollution, promote the development of atherosclerosis [89,90]. Therefore, all children and adolescents should be offered proper nutrition, adequate physical activity, and the opportunity to live in a healthy environment. However, these generalized interventions on the pediatric population should be complemented by a personalized one to early identify those children who already carry risk factors (hypertension, dyslipidemia, alterations in glucose metabolism, hyperuricemia) with the aim of stratifying the risk profile of each individual, as is already the practice for adults. Recently, it has been proposed to include Lp(a) in the algorithms for calculating the cardiovascular risk of the adult population [91]. Although less precisely than in adults, it may also be possible in children and adolescents to define an estimate of future cardiovascular risk, and this may be useful in planning individualized interventions. The questions to be answered are whether pediatric Lp(a) assay is useful, is cost-effective, should be offered to all children as screening and at what age or whether it should be reserved for particularly high-risk individuals. Currently, there is no agreement among Scientific Societies regarding the indication to perform Lp(a) assay to all individuals, despite the evidence for the correlation between Lp(a) and cardiovascular risk. The European Society of Cardiology and the European Atherosclerosis Society suggest dosing everyone at least once in a lifetime [91], while United States Scientific Societies recommend measuring Lp(a) only in at-risk individuals [92–94]. On this basis, the position expressed in 2015 by McNeal not to perform Lp(a) assay routinely in young people and to reserve it only for particular cases, suggesting healthy lifestyles for all children and adolescents [95], is consequential. More recently, Khon and colleagues have instead suggested the possibility of generalized screening in pediatric age, albeit with a number of concerns [96]. Concerns relate to the absence of a specific treatment that can reduce Lp(a) levels, the risk of creating worry in families or inducing excessive dietary restrictions in younger children, the uncertainty of what the risk thresholds of Lp(a) values are in children of different ethnicities, and, finally, the lack of evidence on what course of action to take once children with elevated Lp(a) values become adults. An argument against performing generalized pediatric screening is that since the American Academy of Pediatrics' indication to perform a lipid profile assay to all 10-year-old children is poorly followed, it would be unnecessary to add an indication to also assay Lp(a) [97]. However, the evidence that would suggest the clinical utility of performing Lp(a) dosing before the age of 20 is plentiful [96] and, certainly, it seems reasonable to perform the assay when the LDL cholesterol value is high, in suspicion of heterozygous FH [98–100]. So, there is an open discussion on this issue. In this debate, one point to be clarified is what is meant by the term screening. Should Lp(a) dosing be performed in all children, or should the assay be performed only in children at cardiovascular risk, as a component of the risk profile, in addition to family history, anthropometric parameters, blood pressure measurement, and metabolic profile assay (lipid profile, glucose profile, and serum uric acid)?

In conclusion, in our opinion, including the Lp(a) assay within the panel of pediatric cardiovascular metabolic risk factors could be of clinical utility for several reasons. Although it is not entirely clear whether, after the age of two years, the LPA gene is fully expressed or Lp(a) values continue to rise into adulthood, and children with high Lp(a) values will continue to maintain high values as adults. Lp(a) promotes all steps of atherosclerosis but it is particularly active in promoting the early stages of atherosclerosis because of its ability to enter the subendothelial layers of arteries. Thus, children with high Lp(a) will develop earlier atherosclerotic lesions and, other risk factors being equal, more rapidly progress through the steps leading to atherosclerotic plaque formation. The clinical manifestations of atherosclerosis belong almost exclusively to adulthood, yet atherosclerotic changes in the vessels progress in each individual with a speed proportional to the presence of his/her risk factors throughout life. Thus, true primary prevention is effective only if it is started from an early age. Knowing each individual's risk early, including by assessing Lp(a) levels, can help implement earlier and more effective prevention. There are currently no effective treatments available to reduce Lp(a), and when there are, young people will not be the first to be offered them. However, the presence of elevated Lp(a) recommends increased attention in controlling other modifiable risk factors and a stronger indication to lead a healthy life beginning in childhood and adolescence. Finally, the finding of elevated Lp(a) values in a child could be a stimulus for the family, in the presence of other risk factors such as excess weight and/or hypertension, to greater adherence to dietary-behavioral or pharmacological treatments that are proposed and could suggest the need for testing in parents.

A final point to clarify is whether to measure Lp(a) in all children and at which age. The value of Lp(a) is genetically determined and is randomly distributed in the population. If the value in the parents is not known, there are no other parameters to decide which children to measure. Considering that Lp(a) dosing has a low cost, it would be appropriate to measure it once in a lifetime in all children, after two years of age. As mentioned above, it would be appropriate to combine the Lp(a) assay with a comprehensive analysis of the individual's risk factors. An elevated Lp(a) value increases overall cardiovascular risk, becoming more significant in children with familial dyslipidemia, hypertension, obesity, or glucose metabolism disorders. Since the American Academy of Pediatrics recommends that all children between the ages of 9 and 11 be evaluated for lipid status [97], it may be advisable to add the Lp(a) assay at this time. If high Lp(a) values are found in one or both parents, measuring in the offspring is mandatory. The measurement, in our opinion, can be performed after the age of two, at whatever age an improvement in lifestyle and diet is deemed appropriate and effective.

7. Conclusions and Research Perspectives

Lp(a) has very low values at birth because its gene activity is not yet fully expressed, and its levels increase during childhood, but it is unclear when values proper to adults are stably reached and whether or not growth continues into adolescence. Thus, in children and adolescents, a single Lp(a) assay may not be sufficient as is suggested for adulthood. However, it seems clear that a child with high Lp(a) will almost certainly become an adult with high values of this lipoprotein, so a child with high Lp(a) values should be considered an individual with increased future cardiovascular risk. The gender and ethnicity differences known in adults have not been clearly demonstrated in pediatric age. Based on these considerations, studies in unselected pediatric populations would be needed to understand whether different Lp(a) threshold values should be defined according to age, gender, and ethnicity. Finally, the cardiovascular risk in individuals with high Lp(a) values has been defined as equal or even greater to that of heterozygous carriers of familial hypercholesterolemia [79], for whom hypolipidemic drug treatment is planned from a pediatric age [98,99]. Therefore, when drugs, currently in trials [46,101], that can reduce Lp(a) values become available, it will be appropriate to evaluate, even in pediatric age, in which individuals these medications might be useful.

Author Contributions: Conceptualization M.G. and S.G.; writing—original draft preparation, M.G. and S.G.; writing—review and editing, S.G., M.G., G.L., A.O. and I.P.; supervision G.P.; funding acquisition G.P. All authors have read and agreed to the published version of the manuscript.

Funding: This work was supported by Italian Ministry of Health-Ricerca Corrente.

Institutional Review Board Statement: Not applicable.

Informed Consent Statement: Not applicable.

Data Availability Statement: Not applicable.

Conflicts of Interest: The authors declare no conflict of interest. The funders had no role in the design of the study; in the collection, analyses, or interpretation of data; in the writing of the manuscript; or in the decision to publish the results.

References

1. Berg, K. A new serum type system in man—The lp system. *Acta Pathol. Microbiol. Scand.* **1963**, *59*, 369–382. [CrossRef] [PubMed]
2. McLean, J.W.; Tomlinson, J.E.; Kuang, W.J.; Eaton, D.L.; Chen, E.Y.; Fless, G.M.; Scanu, A.M.; Lawn, R.M. CDNA Sequence of Human Apolipoprotein(a) Is Homologous to Plasminogen. *Nature* **1987**, *330*, 132–137. [CrossRef] [PubMed]
3. Erqou, S.; Thompson, A.; Di Angelantonio, E.; Saleheen, D.; Kaptoge, S.; Marcovina, S.; Danesh, J. Apolipoprotein(a) Isoforms and the Risk of Vascular Disease: Systematic Review of 40 Studies Involving 58,000 Participants. *J. Am. Coll. Cardiol.* **2010**, *55*, 2160–2167. [CrossRef] [PubMed]
4. Kamstrup, P.R.; Tybjaerg-Hansen, A.; Steffensen, R.; Nordestgaard, B.G. Genetically Elevated Lipoprotein(a) and Increased Risk of Myocardial Infarction. *JAMA* **2009**, *301*, 2331–2339. [CrossRef] [PubMed]
5. Thanassoulis, G.; Campbell, C.Y.; Owens, D.S.; Smith, J.G.; Smith, A.V.; Peloso, G.M.; Kerr, K.F.; Pechlivanis, S.; Budoff, M.J.; Harris, T.B.; et al. Genetic Associations with Valvular Calcification and Aortic Stenosis. *N. Engl. J. Med.* **2013**, *368*, 503–512. [CrossRef]
6. Langsted, A.; Nordestgaard, B.G.; Kamstrup, P.R. Elevated Lipoprotein(a) and Risk of Ischemic Stroke. *J. Am. Coll. Cardiol.* **2019**, *74*, 54–66. [CrossRef]
7. Koschinsky, M.L.; Kronenberg, F. The Long Journey of Lipoprotein(a) from Cardiovascular Curiosity to Therapeutic Target. *Atherosclerosis* **2022**, *349*, 1–6. [CrossRef]
8. van der Hoek, Y.Y.; Wittekoek, M.E.; Beisiegel, U.; Kastelein, J.J.; Koschinsky, M.L. The Apolipoprotein(a) Kringle IV Repeats Which Differ from the Major Repeat Kringle Are Present in Variably-Sized Isoforms. *Hum. Mol. Genet.* **1993**, *2*, 361–366. [CrossRef]
9. Santonastaso, A.; Maggi, M.; De Jonge, H.; Scotti, C. High Resolution Structure of Human Apolipoprotein (a) Kringle IV Type 2: Beyond the Lysine Binding Site. *J. Lipid Res.* **2020**, *61*, 1687–1696. [CrossRef]
10. Garner, B.; Merry, A.H.; Royle, L.; Harvey, D.J.; Rudd, P.M.; Thillet, J. Structural Elucidation of the N- and O-Glycans of Human Apolipoprotein(a): Role of o-Glycans in Conferring Protease Resistance. *J. Biol. Chem.* **2001**, *276*, 22200–22208. [CrossRef]
11. Kostner, G.M. Lp(a) Biochemistry, Composition, and Structure. In *Lipoprotein(a)*; Kostner, K., Kostner, G.M., Toth, P.P., Eds.; Contemporary Cardiology; Springer International Publishing: Cham, Switzerland, 2023; pp. 39–54. ISBN 978-3-031-24575-6.
12. Zheng, K.H.; Tsimikas, S.; Pawade, T.; Kroon, J.; Jenkins, W.S.A.; Doris, M.K.; White, A.C.; Timmers, N.K.L.M.; Hjortnaes, J.; Rogers, M.A.; et al. Lipoprotein(a) and Oxidized Phospholipids Promote Valve Calcification in Patients with Aortic Stenosis. *J. Am. Coll. Cardiol.* **2019**, *73*, 2150–2162. [CrossRef] [PubMed]
13. Chemello, K.; Chan, D.C.; Lambert, G.; Watts, G.F. Recent Advances in Demystifying the Metabolism of Lipoprotein(a). *Atherosclerosis* **2022**, *349*, 82–91. [CrossRef]
14. Koschinsky, M.L.; Marcovina, S.M. Structure-Function Relationships in Apolipoprotein(a): Insights into Lipoprotein(a) Assembly and Pathogenicity. *Curr. Opin. Lipidol.* **2004**, *15*, 167–174. [CrossRef] [PubMed]
15. Becker, L.; Nesheim, M.E.; Koschinsky, M.L. Catalysis of Covalent Lp(a) Assembly: Evidence for an Extracellular Enzyme Activity That Enhances Disulfide Bond Formation. *Biochemistry* **2006**, *45*, 9919–9928. [CrossRef]
16. Mooser, V.; Marcovina, S.M.; White, A.L.; Hobbs, H.H. Kringle-Containing Fragments of Apolipoprotein(a) Circulate in Human Plasma and Are Excreted into the Urine. *J. Clin. Investig.* **1996**, *98*, 2414–2424. [CrossRef]
17. Borrelli, M.J.; Youssef, A.; Boffa, M.B.; Koschinsky, M.L. New Frontiers in Lp(a)-Targeted Therapies. *Trends Pharmacol. Sci.* **2019**, *40*, 212–225. [CrossRef] [PubMed]
18. Pagnan, A.; Kostner, G.; Braggion, M.; Ziron, L. Relationship between "sinking Pre-Beta-Lipoprotein" (Lp(a) Lipoprotein) and Age in a Family Kindred. *Gerontology* **1982**, *28*, 381–385. [CrossRef]
19. Reyes-Soffer, G.; Westerterp, M. Beyond Lipoprotein(a) Plasma Measurements: Lipoprotein(a) and Inflammation. *Pharmacol. Res.* **2021**, *169*, 105689. [CrossRef]
20. Kronenberg, F. Causes and Consequences of Lipoprotein(a) Abnormalities in Kidney Disease. *Clin. Exp. Nephrol.* **2014**, *18*, 234–237. [CrossRef]

21. Barbagelata, L.; Masson, W.; Corral, P.; Lavalle-Cobo, A.; Nogueira, J.P.; Rosa Diez, G. Relationship between Lipoprotein(a) Levels, Cardiovascular Outcomes and Death in Patients with Chronic Kidney Disease: A Systematic Review of Prospective Studies. *J. Nephrol.* **2023**. [CrossRef]
22. Chan, D.C.; Watts, G.F.; Coll, B.; Wasserman, S.M.; Marcovina, S.M.; Barrett, P.H.R. Lipoprotein(a) Particle Production as a Determinant of Plasma Lipoprotein(a) Concentration Across Varying Apolipoprotein(a) Isoform Sizes and Background Cholesterol-Lowering Therapy. *J. Am. Heart Assoc.* **2019**, *8*, e011781. [CrossRef] [PubMed]
23. Boffa, M.B.; Koschinsky, M.L. Understanding the Ins and Outs of Lipoprotein (a) Metabolism. *Curr. Opin. Lipidol.* **2022**, *33*, 185–192. [CrossRef] [PubMed]
24. Coassin, S.; Kronenberg, F. Lipoprotein(a) beyond the Kringle IV Repeat Polymorphism: The Complexity of Genetic Variation in the *LPA* Gene. *Atherosclerosis* **2022**, *349*, 17–35. [CrossRef]
25. Noureen, A.; Fresser, F.; Utermann, G.; Schmidt, K. Sequence Variation within the KIV-2 Copy Number Polymorphism of the Human *LPA* Gene in African, Asian, and European Populations. *PLoS ONE* **2015**, *10*, e0121582. [CrossRef] [PubMed]
26. McCormick, S.P.A.; Schneider, W.J. Lipoprotein(a) Catabolism: A Case of Multiple Receptors. *Pathology* **2019**, *51*, 155–164. [CrossRef]
27. Cegla, J.; France, M.; Marcovina, S.M.; Neely, R.D.G. Lp(a): When and How to Measure It. *Ann. Clin. Biochem.* **2021**, *58*, 16–21. [CrossRef] [PubMed]
28. Kronenberg, F. Lipoprotein(a) Measurement Issues: Are We Making a Mountain out of a Molehill? *Atherosclerosis* **2022**, *349*, 123–135. [CrossRef]
29. Kinpara, K.; Okada, H.; Yoneyama, A.; Okubo, M.; Murase, T. Lipoprotein(a)-Cholesterol: A Significant Component of Serum Cholesterol. *Clin. Chim. Acta* **2011**, *412*, 1783–1787. [CrossRef]
30. van der Valk, F.M.; Bekkering, S.; Kroon, J.; Yeang, C.; Van den Bossche, J.; van Buul, J.D.; Ravandi, A.; Nederveen, A.J.; Verberne, H.J.; Scipione, C.; et al. Oxidized Phospholipids on Lipoprotein(a) Elicit Arterial Wall Inflammation and an Inflammatory Monocyte Response in Humans. *Circulation* **2016**, *134*, 611–624. [CrossRef]
31. Garg, P.K.; Guan, W.; Karger, A.B.; Steffen, B.T.; Budoff, M.; Tsai, M.Y. Lipoprotein (a) and Risk for Calcification of the Coronary Arteries, Mitral Valve, and Thoracic Aorta: The Multi-Ethnic Study of Atherosclerosis. *J. Cardiovasc. Comput. Tomogr.* **2021**, *15*, 154–160. [CrossRef]
32. Kaiser, Y.; Daghem, M.; Tzolos, E.; Meah, M.N.; Doris, M.K.; Moss, A.J.; Kwiecinski, J.; Kroon, J.; Nurmohamed, N.S.; van der Harst, P.; et al. Association of Lipoprotein(a) With Atherosclerotic Plaque Progression. *J. Am. Coll. Cardiol.* **2022**, *79*, 223–233. [CrossRef] [PubMed]
33. Leibundgut, G.; Scipione, C.; Yin, H.; Schneider, M.; Boffa, M.B.; Green, S.; Yang, X.; Dennis, E.; Witztum, J.L.; Koschinsky, M.L.; et al. Determinants of Binding of Oxidized Phospholipids on Apolipoprotein (a) and Lipoprotein (a). *J. Lipid Res.* **2013**, *54*, 2815–2830. [CrossRef] [PubMed]
34. Koschinsky, M.L.; Boffa, M.B. Oxidized Phospholipid Modification of Lipoprotein(a): Epidemiology, Biochemistry and Pathophysiology. *Atherosclerosis* **2022**, *349*, 92–100. [CrossRef] [PubMed]
35. Dzobo, K.E.; Kraaijenhof, J.M.; Stroes, E.S.G.; Nurmohamed, N.S.; Kroon, J. Lipoprotein(a): An Underestimated Inflammatory Mastermind. *Atherosclerosis* **2022**, *349*, 101–109. [CrossRef]
36. Boffa, M.B.; Koschinsky, M.L. Lipoprotein (a): Truly a Direct Prothrombotic Factor in Cardiovascular Disease? *J. Lipid Res.* **2016**, *57*, 745–757. [CrossRef]
37. Nordestgaard, B.G.; Langsted, A. Lipoprotein (a) as a Cause of Cardiovascular Disease: Insights from Epidemiology, Genetics, and Biology. *J. Lipid Res.* **2016**, *57*, 1953–1975. [CrossRef]
38. Kaiser, Y.; Singh, S.S.; Zheng, K.H.; Verbeek, R.; Kavousi, M.; Pinto, S.-J.; Vernooij, M.W.; Sijbrands, E.J.G.; Boekholdt, S.M.; de Rijke, Y.B.; et al. Lipoprotein(a) Is Robustly Associated with Aortic Valve Calcium. *Heart* **2021**, *107*, 1422–1428. [CrossRef]
39. Kaltoft, M.; Sigvardsen, P.E.; Afzal, S.; Langsted, A.; Fuchs, A.; Kühl, J.T.; Køber, L.; Kamstrup, P.R.; Kofoed, K.F.; Nordestgaard, B.G. Elevated Lipoprotein(a) in Mitral and Aortic Valve Calcification and Disease: The Copenhagen General Population Study. *Atherosclerosis* **2022**, *349*, 166–174. [CrossRef]
40. Tsimikas, S.; Gordts, P.L.S.M.; Nora, C.; Yeang, C.; Witztum, J.L. Statin Therapy Increases Lipoprotein(a) Levels. *Eur. Heart J.* **2020**, *41*, 2275–2284. [CrossRef]
41. Awad, K.; Mikhailidis, D.P.; Katsiki, N.; Muntner, P.; Banach, M. Lipid and Blood Pressure Meta-Analysis Collaboration (LBPMC) Group Effect of Ezetimibe Monotherapy on Plasma Lipoprotein(a) Concentrations in Patients with Primary Hypercholesterolemia: A Systematic Review and Meta-Analysis of Randomized Controlled Trials. *Drugs* **2018**, *78*, 453–462. [CrossRef]
42. Jaeger, B.R.; Richter, Y.; Nagel, D.; Heigl, F.; Vogt, A.; Roeseler, E.; Parhofer, K.; Ramlow, W.; Koch, M.; Utermann, G.; et al. Longitudinal cohort study on the effectiveness of lipid apheresis treatment to reduce high lipoprotein(a) levels and prevent major adverse coronary events. *Nat. Clin. Pract. Cardiovasc. Med.* **2009**, *6*, 229–239. [CrossRef] [PubMed]
43. AIM-HIGH Investigators; Boden, W.E.; Probstfield, J.L.; Anderson, T.; Chaitman, B.R.; Desvignes-Nickens, P.; Koprowicz, K.; McBride, R.; Teo, K.; Weintraub, W. Niacin in Patients with Low HDL Cholesterol Levels Receiving Intensive Statin Therapy. *N. Engl. J. Med.* **2011**, *365*, 2255–2267. [CrossRef] [PubMed]
44. O'Donoghue, M.L.; Fazio, S.; Giugliano, R.P.; Stroes, E.S.G.; Kanevsky, E.; Gouni-Berthold, I.; Im, K.; Lira Pineda, A.; Wasserman, S.M.; Češka, R.; et al. Lipoprotein(a), PCSK9 Inhibition, and Cardiovascular Risk. *Circulation* **2019**, *139*, 1483–1492. [CrossRef] [PubMed]

5. Tsushima, T.; Tsushima, Y.; Sullivan, C.; Hatipoglu, B. Lipoprotein(a) and Atherosclerotic Cardiovascular Disease, the Impact of Available Lipid-Lowering Medications on Lipoprotein(a): An Update on New Therapies. *Endocr. Pract.* **2022**, S1530-891X(22)00901-6. [CrossRef] [PubMed]
6. Ibrahim, S.; Stroes, E.S.G. Therapy of Elevated Lipoprotein(a). In *Lipoprotein(a)*; Kostner, K., Kostner, G.M., Toth, P.P., Eds.; Contemporary Cardiology; Springer International Publishing: Cham, Switzerland, 2023; pp. 347–357. ISBN 978-3-031-24575-6.
7. Mehta, A.; Jain, V.; Saeed, A.; Saseen, J.J.; Gulati, M.; Ballantyne, C.M.; Virani, S.S. Lipoprotein(a) and Ethnicities. *Atherosclerosis* **2022**, *349*, 42–52. [CrossRef]
8. Patel, A.P.; Wang, M.; Pirruccello, J.P.; Ellinor, P.T.; Ng, K.; Kathiresan, S.; Khera, A.V. Lp(a) (Lipoprotein[a]) Concentrations and Incident Atherosclerotic Cardiovascular Disease: New Insights from a Large National Biobank. *Arterioscler. Thromb. Vasc. Biol.* **2021**, *41*, 465–474. [CrossRef]
9. Virani, S.S.; Brautbar, A.; Davis, B.C.; Nambi, V.; Hoogeveen, R.C.; Sharrett, A.R.; Coresh, J.; Mosley, T.H.; Morrisett, J.D.; Catellier, D.J.; et al. Associations between Lipoprotein(a) Levels and Cardiovascular Outcomes in Black and White Subjects: The Atherosclerosis Risk in Communities (ARIC) Study. *Circulation* **2012**, *125*, 241–249. [CrossRef]
10. Tsimikas, S.; Clopton, P.; Brilakis, E.S.; Marcovina, S.M.; Khera, A.; Miller, E.R.; de Lemos, J.A.; Witztum, J.L. Relationship of Oxidized Phospholipids on Apolipoprotein B-100 Particles to Race/Ethnicity, Apolipoprotein(a) Isoform Size, and Cardiovascular Risk Factors: Results from the Dallas Heart Study. *Circulation* **2009**, *119*, 1711–1719. [CrossRef]
11. Deo, R.C.; Wilson, J.G.; Xing, C.; Lawson, K.; Kao, W.H.L.; Reich, D.; Tandon, A.; Akylbekova, E.; Patterson, N.; Mosley, T.H.; et al. Single-Nucleotide Polymorphisms in *LPA* Explain Most of the Ancestry-Specific Variation in Lp(a) Levels in African Americans. *PLoS ONE* **2011**, *6*, e14581. [CrossRef]
12. Paré, G.; Çaku, A.; McQueen, M.; Anand, S.S.; Enas, E.; Clarke, R.; Boffa, M.B.; Koschinsky, M.; Wang, X.; Yusuf, S.; et al. Lipoprotein(a) Levels and the Risk of Myocardial Infarction Among 7 Ethnic Groups. *Circulation* **2019**, *139*, 1472–1482. [CrossRef]
13. Varvel, S.; McConnell, J.P.; Tsimikas, S. Prevalence of Elevated Lp(a) Mass Levels and Patient Thresholds in 532 359 Patients in the United States. *Arterioscler. Thromb. Vasc. Biol.* **2016**, *36*, 2239–2245. [CrossRef] [PubMed]
14. Trinder, M.; Paruchuri, K.; Haidermota, S.; Bernardo, R.; Zekavat, S.M.; Gilliland, T.; Januzzi, J.; Natarajan, P. Repeat Measures of Lipoprotein(a) Molar Concentration and Cardiovascular Risk. *J. Am. Coll. Cardiol.* **2022**, *79*, 617–628. [CrossRef] [PubMed]
15. Jenner, J.L.; Ordovas, J.M.; Lamon-Fava, S.; Schaefer, M.M.; Wilson, P.W.; Castelli, W.P.; Schaefer, E.J. Effects of Age, Sex, and Menopausal Status on Plasma Lipoprotein(a) Levels. The Framingham Offspring Study. *Circulation* **1993**, *87*, 1135–1141. [CrossRef] [PubMed]
16. Derby, C.A.; Crawford, S.L.; Pasternak, R.C.; Sowers, M.; Sternfeld, B.; Matthews, K.A. Lipid Changes during the Menopause Transition in Relation to Age and Weight: The Study of Women's Health Across the Nation. *Am. J. Epidemiol.* **2009**, *169*, 1352–1361. [CrossRef] [PubMed]
17. Anagnostis, P.; Antza, C.; Trakatelli, C.; Lambrinoudaki, I.; Goulis, D.G.; Kotsis, V. The Effect of Menopause on Lipoprotein (a) Concentrations: A Systematic Review and Meta-Analysis. *Maturitas* **2023**, *167*, 39–45. [CrossRef]
18. Simony, S.B.; Mortensen, M.B.; Langsted, A.; Afzal, S.; Kamstrup, P.R.; Nordestgaard, B.G. Sex Differences of Lipoprotein(a) Levels and Associated Risk of Morbidity and Mortality by Age: The Copenhagen General Population Study. *Atherosclerosis* **2022**, *355*, 76–82. [CrossRef]
19. Nowak-Göttl, U.; Sträter, R.; Heinecke, A.; Junker, R.; Koch, H.G.; Schuierer, G.; von Eckardstein, A. Lipoprotein (a) and Genetic Polymorphisms of Clotting Factor V, Prothrombin, and Methylenetetrahydrofolate Reductase Are Risk Factors of Spontaneous Ischemic Stroke in Childhood. *Blood* **1999**, *94*, 3678–3682. [CrossRef]
20. Nowak-Göttl, U.; Debus, O.; Findeisen, M.; Kassenböhmer, R.; Koch, H.G.; Pollmann, H.; Postler, C.; Weber, P.; Vielhaber, H. Lipoprotein (a): Its Role in Childhood Thromboembolism. *Pediatrics* **1997**, *99*, E11. [CrossRef]
21. Nowak-Göttl, U.; Sträter, R.; Dübbers, A.; Oleszuk-Raschke, K.; Vielhaber, H. Ischaemic Stroke in Infancy and Childhood: Role of the Arg506 to Gln Mutation in the Factor V Gene. *Blood Coagul. Fibrinolysis* **1996**, *7*, 684–688. [CrossRef]
22. Peynet, J.; Beaudeux, J.-L.; Woimant, F.; Flourié, F.; Giraudeaux, V.; Vicaut, E.; Launay, J.-M. Apolipoprotein(a) Size Polymorphism in Young Adults with Ischemic Stroke. *Atherosclerosis* **1999**, *142*, 233–239. [CrossRef]
23. Chan, A.; Iorio, A.; Kenet, G. Impact of Thrombophilia on Risk of Arterial Ischemic Stroke or Cerebral Sinovenous Thrombosis in Neonates and Children: A Systematic Review and Meta-Analysis of Observational Studies. *Circulation* **2010**, *121*, 1838–1847.
24. Strobl, W.; Widhalm, K.; Kostner, G.; Pollak, A. Serum Apolipoproteins and Lipoprotein (a) during the First Week of Life. *Acta Paediatr. Scand.* **1983**, *72*, 505–509. [CrossRef] [PubMed]
25. Van Biervliet, J.P.; Labeur, C.; Michiels, G.; Usher, D.C.; Rosseneu, M. Lipoprotein(a) Profiles and Evolution in Newborns. *Atherosclerosis* **1991**, *86*, 173–181. [CrossRef] [PubMed]
26. Rifai, N.; Heiss, G.; Doetsch, K. Lipoprotein(a) at Birth, in Blacks and Whites. *Atherosclerosis* **1992**, *92*, 123–129. [CrossRef]
27. Schumacher, M.; Kessler, A.; Meier, A.; Weigert, S.; Wood, W.G. Lipoprotein(a) Concentrations in Cord and Capillary Blood from Newborns and in Serum from in-Patient Children, Adolescents and Adults. *Eur. J. Clin. Chem. Clin. Biochem.* **1994**, *32*, 341–347. [CrossRef]
28. Wood, W.G.; Schumacher, M.; Weigert, S. (Apo)Lipoprotein(a) Concentrations at Birth and in the First Days and Months of Life—Studies on the Distribution of Serum Levels and the Predictive Value of Measurements Made at This Time. *Eur. J. Clin. Chem. Clin. Biochem.* **1995**, *33*, 139–145. [CrossRef]

69. Wilcken, D.E.; Wang, X.L.; Dudman, N.P. The Relationship between Infant and Parent Lp(a) Levels. *Chem. Phys. Lipids* **1994**, *67–68*, 299–304. [CrossRef]
70. Routi, T.; Rönnemaa, T.; Viikari, J.S.; Leino, A.; Välimäki, I.A.; Simell, O.G. Tracking of Serum Lipoprotein (a) Concentration and Its Contribution to Serum Cholesterol Values in Children from 7 to 36 Months of Age in the STRIP Baby Study. Special Turku Coronary Risk Factor Intervention Project for Babies. *Ann. Med.* **1997**, *29*, 541–547. [CrossRef]
71. Strandkjær, N.; Hansen, M.K.; Nielsen, S.T.; Frikke-Schmidt, R.; Tybjærg-Hansen, A.; Nordestgaard, B.G.; Tabor, A.; Bundgaard, H.; Iversen, K.; Kamstrup, P.R. Lipoprotein(a) Levels at Birth and in Early Childhood: The COMPARE Study. *J. Clin. Endocrinol Metab.* **2022**, *107*, 324–335. [CrossRef]
72. de Boer, L.M.; Hof, M.H.; Wiegman, A.; Stroobants, A.K.; Kastelein, J.J.P.; Hutten, B.A. Lipoprotein(a) Levels from Childhood to Adulthood: Data in Nearly 3000 Children Who Visited a Pediatric Lipid Clinic. *Atherosclerosis* **2022**, *349*, 227–232. [CrossRef]
73. Choi, R.; Lee, S.G.; Lee, E.H. Lipoprotein(a) in the Korean Pediatric Population Visiting Local Clinics and Hospitals. *Nutrients* **2022**, *14*, 2820. [CrossRef] [PubMed]
74. Qayum, O.; Alshami, N.; Ibezim, C.F.; Reid, K.J.; Noel-MacDonnell, J.R.; Raghuveer, G. Lipoprotein (a): Examination of Cardiovascular Risk in a Pediatric Referral Population. *Pediatr. Cardiol.* **2018**, *39*, 1540–1546. [CrossRef] [PubMed]
75. Papadopoulou-Legbelou, K.; Triantafyllou, A.; Vampertzi, O.; Koletsos, N.; Douma, S.; Papadopoulou-Alataki, E. Similar Myocardial Perfusion and Vascular Stiffness in Children and Adolescents with High Lipoprotein (a) Levels, in Comparison with Healthy Controls. *Pulse* **2021**, *9*, 64–71. [CrossRef] [PubMed]
76. Pederiva, C.; Capra, M.E.; Biasucci, G.; Banderali, G.; Fabrizi, E.; Gazzotti, M.; Casula, M.; Catapano, A.L.; Lipigen Paediatric Group; Members of the Lipigen Steering Committee; et al. Lipoprotein(a) and Family History for Cardiovascular Disease in Paediatric Patients: A New Frontier in Cardiovascular Risk Stratification. Data from the LIPIGEN Paediatric Group. *Atherosclerosis* **2022**, *349*, 233–239. [CrossRef]
77. Raitakari, O.; Kartiosuo, N.; Pahkala, K.; Hutri-Kähönen, N.; Bazzano, L.A.; Chen, W.; Urbina, E.M.; Jacobs, D.R.; Sinaiko, A.; Steinberger, J.; et al. Lipoprotein(a) in Youth and Prediction of Major Cardiovascular Outcomes in Adulthood. *Circulation* **2023**, *147*, 23–31. [CrossRef]
78. de Boer, L.M.; Hutten, B.A.; Zwinderman, A.H.; Wiegman, A. Lipoprotein(a) Levels in Children with Suspected Familial Hypercholesterolaemia: A Cross-Sectional Study. *Eur. Heart J.* **2023**, *44*, 1421–1428. [CrossRef]
79. Averna, M.R.; Cefalù, A.B. Lp(a): A Genetic Cause of Clinical FH in Children. *Eur. Heart J.* **2023**, *44*, 1429–1431. [CrossRef]
80. Olmastroni, E.; Gazzotti, M.; Averna, M.; Arca, M.; Tarugi, P.; Calandra, S.; Bertolini, S.; Catapano, A.L.; Casula, M.; LIPIGEN Study Group. Lipoprotein(a) Genotype Influences the Clinical Diagnosis of Familial Hypercholesterolemia. *J. Am. Heart Assoc.* **2023**, *12*, e029223. [CrossRef]
81. WHO Mortality Database—WHO. Available online: https://www.who.int/data/data-collection-tools/who-mortality-database (accessed on 28 February 2023).
82. Global Health Estimates. Available online: https://www.who.int/data/global-health-estimates (accessed on 28 February 2023).
83. Birger, M.; Kaldjian, A.S.; Roth, G.A.; Moran, A.E.; Dieleman, J.L.; Bellows, B.K. Spending on Cardiovascular Disease and Cardiovascular Risk Factors in the United States: 1996 to 2016. *Circulation* **2021**, *144*, 271–282. [CrossRef]
84. Moran, A.E.; Forouzanfar, M.H.; Roth, G.A.; Mensah, G.A.; Ezzati, M.; Murray, C.J.L.; Naghavi, M. Temporal Trends in Ischemic Heart Disease Mortality in 21 World Regions, 1980 to 2010: The Global Burden of Disease 2010 Study. *Circulation* **2014**, *129*, 1483–1492. [CrossRef]
85. Roth, G.A.; Mensah, G.A.; Johnson, C.O.; Addolorato, G.; Ammirati, E.; Baddour, L.M.; Barengo, N.C.; Beaton, A.Z.; Benjamin, E.J.; Benziger, C.P.; et al. Global Burden of Cardiovascular Diseases and Risk Factors, 1990–2019. *J. Am. Coll. Cardiol.* **2020**, *76*, 2982–3021. [CrossRef] [PubMed]
86. Takura, T.; Yokoi, H.; Tanaka, N.; Matsumoto, N.; Yoshida, E.; Nakata, T.; J-CONCIOUS Investigators. Health Economics-Based Verification of Functional Myocardial Ischemia Evaluation of Stable Coronary Artery Disease in Japan: A Long-Term Longitudinal Study Using Propensity Score Matching. *J. Nucl. Cardiol.* **2022**, *29*, 1356–1369. [CrossRef] [PubMed]
87. Berenson, G.S.; Srinivasan, S.R.; Bao, W.; Newman, W.P.; Tracy, R.E.; Wattigney, W.A. Association between Multiple Cardiovascular Risk Factors and Atherosclerosis in Children and Young Adults. The Bogalusa Heart Study. *N. Engl. J. Med.* **1998**, *338*, 1650–1656. [CrossRef] [PubMed]
88. Milei, J.; Ottaviani, G.; Lavezzi, A.M.; Grana, D.R.; Stella, I.; Matturri, L. Perinatal and Infant Early Atherosclerotic Coronary Lesions. *Can. J. Cardiol.* **2008**, *24*, 137–141. [CrossRef]
89. Lechner, K.; von Schacky, C.; McKenzie, A.L.; Worm, N.; Nixdorff, U.; Lechner, B.; Kränkel, N.; Halle, M.; Krauss, R.M.; Scherr, J.; Lifestyle Factors and High-Risk Atherosclerosis: Pathways and Mechanisms beyond Traditional Risk Factors. *Eur. J. Prev. Cardiol.* **2020**, *27*, 394–406. [CrossRef]
90. Adar, S.D.; Sheppard, L.; Vedal, S.; Polak, J.F.; Sampson, P.D.; Diez Roux, A.V.; Budoff, M.; Jacobs, D.R.; Barr, R.G.; Watson, K.; et al. Fine Particulate Air Pollution and the Progression of Carotid Intima-Medial Thickness: A Prospective Cohort Study from the Multi-Ethnic Study of Atherosclerosis and Air Pollution. *PLoS Med.* **2013**, *10*, e1001430. [CrossRef]
91. Kronenberg, F.; Mora, S.; Stroes, E.S.G.; Ference, B.A.; Arsenault, B.J.; Berglund, L.; Dweck, M.R.; Koschinsky, M.; Lambert, G.; Mach, F.; et al. Lipoprotein(a) in Atherosclerotic Cardiovascular Disease and Aortic Stenosis: A European Atherosclerosis Society Consensus Statement. *Eur. Heart J.* **2022**, *43*, 3925–3946. [CrossRef]

92. Wilson, D.P.; Jacobson, T.A.; Jones, P.H.; Koschinsky, M.L.; McNeal, C.J.; Nordestgaard, B.G.; Orringer, C.E. Use of Lipoprotein(a) in Clinical Practice: A Biomarker Whose Time Has Come. A Scientific Statement from the National Lipid Association. *J. Clin. Lipidol.* **2019**, *13*, 374–392. [CrossRef]
93. Arnett, D.K.; Blumenthal, R.S.; Albert, M.A.; Buroker, A.B.; Goldberger, Z.D.; Hahn, E.J.; Himmelfarb, C.D.; Khera, A.; Lloyd-Jones, D.; McEvoy, J.W.; et al. 2019 ACC/AHA Guideline on the Primary Prevention of Cardiovascular Disease: A Report of the American College of Cardiology/American Heart Association Task Force on Clinical Practice Guidelines. *Circulation* **2019**, *140*, e596–e646. [CrossRef]
94. Jellinger, P.S.; Handelsman, Y.; Rosenblit, P.D.; Bloomgarden, Z.T.; Fonseca, V.A.; Garber, A.J.; Grunberger, G.; Guerin, C.K.; Bell, D.S.H.; Mechanick, J.I.; et al. American association of clinical endocrinologists and american college of endocrinology guidelines for management of dyslipidemia and prevention of cardiovascular disease. *Endocr. Pract.* **2017**, *23*, 1–87. [CrossRef]
95. McNeal, C.J. Lipoprotein(a): Its Relevance to the Pediatric Population. *J. Clin. Lipidol.* **2015**, *9*, S57–S66. [CrossRef] [PubMed]
96. Kohn, B.; Ashraf, A.P.; Wilson, D.P. Should Lipoprotein(a) Be Measured in Youth? *J. Pediatr.* **2021**, *228*, 285–289. [CrossRef] [PubMed]
97. Simon, G.R.; Baker, C.; Barden, G.A.; Brown, O.W.; Hardin, A.; Lessin, H.R.; Meade, K.; Moore, S.; Rodgers, C.T.; Committee on Practice and Ambulatory Medicine; et al. 2014 Recommendations for Pediatric Preventive Health Care. *Pediatrics* **2014**, *133*, 568–570. [CrossRef]
98. Daniels, S.R.; Gidding, S.S.; de Ferranti, S.D. Pediatric Aspects of Familial Hypercholesterolemias: Recommendations from the National Lipid Association Expert Panel on Familial Hypercholesterolemia. *J. Clin. Lipidol.* **2011**, *5*, S30–S37. [CrossRef] [PubMed]
99. Descamps, O.S.; Tenoutasse, S.; Stephenne, X.; Gies, I.; Beauloye, V.; Lebrethon, M.-C.; De Beaufort, C.; De Waele, K.; Scheen, A.; Rietzschel, E.; et al. Management of Familial Hypercholesterolemia in Children and Young Adults: Consensus Paper Developed by a Panel of Lipidologists, Cardiologists, Paediatricians, Nutritionists, Gastroenterologists, General Practitioners and a Patient Organization. *Atherosclerosis* **2011**, *218*, 272–280. [CrossRef]
100. Watts, G.F.; Gidding, S.; Wierzbicki, A.S.; Toth, P.P.; Alonso, R.; Brown, W.V.; Bruckert, E.; Defesche, J.; Lin, K.K.; Livingston, M.; et al. Integrated Guidance on the Care of Familial Hypercholesterolaemia from the International FH Foundation. *Int. J. Cardiol.* **2014**, *171*, 309–325. [CrossRef]
101. Koutsogianni, A.; Liamis, G.; Liberopoulos, E.; Adamidis, P.S.; Florentin, M. Effects of Lipid-Modifying and Other Drugs on Lipoprotein(a) Levels—Potent Clinical Implications. *Pharmaceuticals* **2023**, *16*, 750. [CrossRef]

Disclaimer/Publisher's Note: The statements, opinions and data contained in all publications are solely those of the individual author(s) and contributor(s) and not of MDPI and/or the editor(s). MDPI and/or the editor(s) disclaim responsibility for any injury to people or property resulting from any ideas, methods, instructions or products referred to in the content.

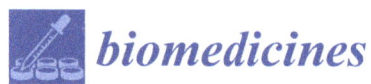

Review

Biomarkers of Atrial Fibrillation Recurrence in Patients with Paroxysmal or Persistent Atrial Fibrillation Following External Direct Current Electrical Cardioversion

Ozan Demirel [1], Alexander E. Berezin [1,2,*], Moritz Mirna [1], Elke Boxhammer [1], Sarah X. Gharibeh [1], Uta C. Hoppe [1] and Michael Lichtenauer [1]

[1] Department of Internal Medicine II, Division of Cardiology, Paracelsus Medical University Salzburg, 5020 Salzburg, Austria; o.demirel@salk.at (O.D.); m.mirna@salk.at (M.M.); e.boxhammer@salk.at (E.B.); s.gharibeh@salk.at (S.X.G.); u.hoppe@salk.at (U.C.H.); m.lichtenauer@salk.at (M.L.)
[2] Internal Medicine Department, Zaporozhye State Medical University, 69035 Zaporozhye, Ukraine
* Correspondence: aeberezin@gmail.com

Abstract: Atrial fibrillation (AF) is associated with atrial remodeling, cardiac dysfunction, and poor clinical outcomes. External direct current electrical cardioversion is a well-developed urgent treatment strategy for patients presenting with recent-onset AF. However, there is a lack of accurate predictive serum biomarkers to identify the risks of AF relapse after electrical cardioversion. We reviewed the currently available data and interpreted the findings of several studies revealing biomarkers for crucial elements in the pathogenesis of AF and affecting cardiac remodeling, fibrosis, inflammation, endothelial dysfunction, oxidative stress, adipose tissue dysfunction, myopathy, and mitochondrial dysfunction. Although there is ample strong evidence that elevated levels of numerous biomarkers (such as natriuretic peptides, C-reactive protein, galectin-3, soluble suppressor tumorigenicity-2, fibroblast growth factor-23, turn-over collagen biomarkers, growth differential factor-15) are associated with AF occurrence, the data obtained in clinical studies seem to be controversial in terms of their predictive ability for post-cardioversion outcomes. Novel circulating biomarkers are needed to elucidate the modality of this approach compared with conventional predictive tools. Conclusions: Biomarker-based strategies for predicting events after AF treatment require extensive investigation in the future, especially in the presence of different gender and variable comorbidity profiles. Perhaps, a multiple biomarker approach exerts more utilization for patients with different forms of AF than single biomarker use.

Keywords: atrial fibrillation; electrical cardioversion; post-procedural complications; biomarkers

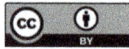

1. Introduction

Atrial fibrillation (AF) is the most common form of sustained cardiac arrhythmia in the world [1]. The prevalence of AF advances with increasing age. After the age of 80, atrial fibrillation affects 10–17% of the population [2]. The morbidity is increased and mortality rises up to 3.5-fold in men and women [3]. Along with it, AF frequently occurs in patients at higher risk of cardiovascular diseases (CVD) as well as among individuals with known CVD [4]. Unfortunately, AF and CVD exacerbate each other and mutually intervene in prognosis. Indeed, patients with any form of AF demonstrated poorer clinical outcomes if there is concomitant heart failure (HF), coronary artery disease (CAD), type 2 diabetes mellitus (T2DM), obesity, obstructive sleep apnea, chronic kidney disease (CKD), or peripheral artery disease [5–7]. Further, the prognosis of patients with AF is poorer than the prognosis of patients with various CVD and comorbid conditions (i.e., HF, CKD) without AF [8]. Multi-morbidity among patients with AF seems to play a pivotal role in natural evolution of primary and secondary AF through direct and indirect impact on the structural and/or electrophysiological abnormalities that occur in AF [9,10]. AF influences electrical remodeling, i.e., shortening of refractoriness due to the high atrial rate itself, resulting in adverse cardiac remodeling [11]. Yet, the persistence of AF itself modulates the risk of cerebrovascular and cardiovascular events [12,13].

The management of AF includes either rhythm restoration or rate control along with comorbidity management, prevention of stroke, and systemic thromboembolism [14]. Synchronized electrical cardioversion can terminate AF. Combined with sedation, it is a safe procedure and highly effective, restoring sinus rhythm in more than 90% [15–17]. It is important to detect AF recurrence after successful electrical cardioversion. In this case, early cardioversion could prolong the subsequent duration of sinus rhythm and slow disease progression compared to delayed sinus rhythm restoration [18].

Although the current clinical protocol of initial AF management seems to be very useful in practice [1], it poses challenges in predicting incidental AF and early detection of AF-related complications [19,20]. There are many factors associated with AF recurrence, such as duration of AF, higher age, sex, HF, LA volume index, chronic obstructive pulmonary disease, hypertension, obstructive sleep apnea, hyperthyroidism, smoking, and obesity [21,22]. However, the role of biomarkers reflecting the different stages of AF pathogenesis has not been completely understood. The purpose of the study is to summarize the current evidence on the value of various biomarkers in predicting the likelihood of AF recurrence after electrical cardioversion.

2. Promoting Factors and Electrophysiological/Anatomical Substrates of AF

Vulnerable substrates for the occurrence, support, and recurrence of AF are electrophysiological and adverse cardiac remodeling, along with structural remodeling, mechanical dysfunction, and trigger activity, which are mediated by genetic ion channel alterations, concomitant cardiovascular (CV) diseases (acute and chronic coronary syndromes, multifocal atherosclerosis, primary and secondary cardiomyopathy, etc.), CV risk factors (hypertension, smoking, obesity, diabetes mellitus, resistance to insulin, and dyslipidemia), and comorbidities (chronic obstructive pulmonary disease, bronchial asthma, chronic kidney disease) (Figure 1). In addition, concomitant hemodynamic factors as a result of numerous diseases (heart failure, atrial cardiomyopathy, pulmonary hypertension, inherited and acquired heart diseases, myocarditis) and conditions (chemotherapy, cardiac toxicity) play a crucial role in secondary structural remodeling of the heart [23–25]. These factors contribute to AF occurrence by maintaining afterdepolarization-induced triggered ectopic activity, focal enhanced automaticity, altered function of ion channels, micro-reentrant circus rotor, less dynamic head–tail interactions during re-entry in cardiac tissue, altered ion accumulation on the dynamics of re-entry and electrical heterogeneity [26]. Indeed, head–tail interactions have previously been known to have a causative impact on the dynamics of the reentrant action potential, which plays a pivotal role in inducing AF [26]. To note, intracellular ions, mainly Ca^{2+} and Na^+, accumulated during reentrant arrhythmia through the rapid repetitive cellular excitation may lead to spontaneous termination of re-entry or break-up of the re-entry loop into multiple pathways resulting in AF. Along with it, the initiation and persistence of AF are controlled by both parasympathetic and sympathetic stimulation, as well as hormonal influences, which also seem to play a role in AF recurrence [27]. However, the continuous interaction between electrophysiological, structural, and anatomical remodeling leads to intercellular uncoupling and a pro-fibrotic response, which is crucial for trigger activity, the presence of AF, and the transformation of cardiac dysfunction into HF [28].

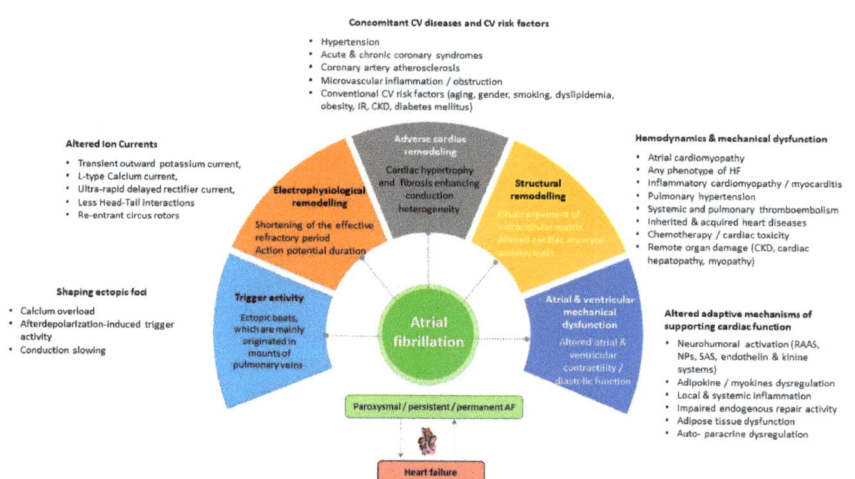

Figure 1. Promoting factors and plausible pathogenetic mechanisms of AF. Abbreviations: AF, atrial fibrillation; CV, cardiovascular; CKD, chronic kidney disease; SAS, sympathoadrenal system; IR, insulin resistance; HF, heart failure; RAAS, renin-angiotensin-aldosterone system.

2.1. Electrophysiological Remodeling

Electrophysiological remodeling affects variable changes in specific ionic currents, such as a reduction in transient outward potassium current, L-type calcium current, and ultra-rapid delayed rectifier current, as well as shortening of the effective refractory period and prolongation of the action potential, which are also associated with the increase in the stimulation rate [29,30]. The overload of intracellular calcium in cardiac myocytes and its spontaneous release from the sarcoplasmic reticulum seems to be a major factor in the occurrence of delayed afterdepolarizations and triggered ectopic activity in the myocardium [30]. Although sympathetic activation and direct stimulation by angiotensin-II are classic mechanisms of enhancing propensity for AF, there are numerous other mechanisms that intervene in altered afterdepolarizations. They mainly include a reduced inward rectifier, as well as increased activity of the Na/Ca exchanger and residual beta-adrenergic responsiveness [31,32]. Yet, alterations in the regulation and accumulation of intracellular calcium can be a result of properly persistent AF and alternative arrhythmogenic mechanisms (intramural decremented conduction, transmural heterogeneity of repolarization, prolongation of QT-interval, and block of the premature impulse), which are activated due to progress of pre-exciting CV diseases including HF and coronary artery syndromes [33]. To note, asynchronous down-regulation of voltage-dependent potassium currents and L-type calcium currents between layers of myocardium through the calcium/calmodulin-dependent kinase II signal pathway activated by hemodynamic factors (fluid overload, hypertension), ischemia/hypoxia, hormonal dysfunction (hyperthyroidism), perivascular edema due to microvascular inflammation, impaired mitochondrial metabolism and oxidative stress due to metabolic diseases/conditions (diabetes mellitus, obesity, myopathy, insulin resistance) and cardiac hypertrophy may support electrophysiological remodeling [34–39]. Although the role of hemodynamic factors and ischemia in shaping AF risk is well established [34,35], the impact of metabolic influences on electrophysiological remodeling is not always obvious. For instance, among patients with thyroid dysfunction, free thyroxine levels but not thyroid-stimulating hormone concentrations are associated with an increased risk of incident AF regardless of preexisting CV disease [37]. On the other hand, a hypothyroid state may directly induce myocardial fibrosis via stimulating autophagy and inhibiting TGF-β1/Smad2 signal transduction pathway [38]. Obesity and T2DM link glycemic fluctuations to electrophysiological remodeling that leads to the onset and maintenance of AF through mitochondrial dysfunction, oxidative stress, and inflammation [39].

Chan YH et al. (2019) [40] reported that insulin resistance (IR) was associated with significantly increased sarcoplasmic reticulum calcium content and diastolic calcium sparks in the atrial myocardium. Moreover, IR increased collagen accumulation and superoxide production in the atrial myocardium through increased synthesis of transforming growth factor beta 1 (TGF-β1) and abnormal upregulation of calcium-homeostasis-related proteins, such as oxidized CaMKIIδ, phosphorylated-phospholamban, phosphorylated-RyR-2, and sodium–calcium exchanger [40].

Yet, subcellular mechanisms underlying electrophysiological remodeling seem to relate to the alteration of connexin 43 expression, which is a principal ventricular gap junction protein [40,41]. However, significant changes in connexin 43 phosphorylation were found to be more closely associated with timing AF persistence and the presence of HF [42]. In particular, these changes can even explain an association of such powerful components of electrophysiological features as increased transmural dispersion in refractoriness and conduction with increased inducibility of AF and low efficacy of electrical cardioversion [43,44]. Moreover, this may be a novel paradigm of electrophysiological remodeling based on the timing of conduction abnormalities in connection to dynamic changes in connexin 43 isoforms, cardiac dysfunction, and comorbidities [43,44]. Indeed, there is strong evidence of the fact that apelin-13-an aliphatic multifunctional peptide, mainly originated from the myocardium, skeletal muscles, and liver-increased connexin 43 through autophagy inhibition and inducing AKT and mTOR phosphorylation and thereby decreases susceptibility to cardiac arrhythmias including AF and cardiomyocyte death [45,46]. Yang M et al. (2022) [47] recently reported that the apelin/AMPK/mTOR signaling pathway, which regulates angiotensin II-mediated autophagy and apoptosis of cardiac myocytes, is under close control of miRNA-122-5p. The overexpression of miRNA-122-5p leads to exacerbation of cardiac and vascular hypertrophy, cardiac fibrosis, and dysfunction. Thus, the overexpression of miRNA-122-5p may be an underlying mechanism of binding myocardial fibroblasts and activation of AF. On the other hand, angiotensin-II acts as a promoter of expression of pro-apoptotic molecules, such as P62 and Bax, and as a mediator of mTOR phosphorylation, which downregulates LC3II, beclin-1, and contributes to the imbalance of autophagy and apoptosis in the myocardium. These changes were associated with increased myocardial accumulation of collagen I and collagen III, overexpression of TGF-beta-1 and connective tissue growth factor (CTGF), as well as downregulation of myocardial expression of apelin, angiotensin-converting enzyme-2 (ACE2), and growth differential factor-15 (GDF-15) [47–49]. These facts confirm a close interplay between the Apelin-APJ axis and ACE2-GDF-15-porimin signaling in angiotensin-II-mediated myocardial hypertrophy and fibrosis, which are crucial substrates for AF occurrence and prolongation. Therefore, they modulate the relationship between electrophysiological and anatomical cardiac remodeling.

2.2. Adverse Cardiac Remodeling

Adverse cardiac remodeling in AF patients includes AF-related atrial remodeling and cardiac remodeling due to concomitant CV diseases [50]. Both variants may be associated with sinus node dysfunction, variability in conduction gaps due to parasympathetic/sympathetic stimulation and epigenetic regulation of intercellular communication, cardiac cell-to-cell heterogeneity, and extracellular matrix alteration [50–53]. Therefore, the overlap between both variants of remodeling is mediated by concomitant hemodynamic changes such as valvular regurgitation [54]. AF-related alteration of atrial structure starts with the differentiation of cardiac fibroblasts into myofibroblasts, which is regulated by numerous triggers, including angiotensin-II, noradrenaline, thyroid hormones, inflammatory cytokines, chemokines, matrix metalloproteinases, galectine-3, soluble suppression of tumorigenesis-2 (sST2), TGF-beta-1 and microRNAs (Figure 2).

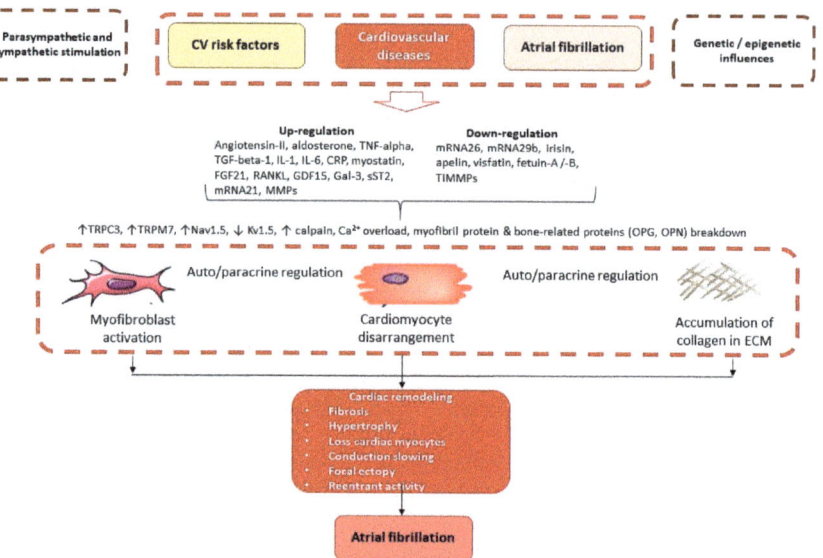

Figure 2. Molecular mechanisms of AF. Abbreviations: CV, cardiovascular; CRP, C-reactive protein; ECM, extracellular matrix; FGF21, fibroblast growth factor-21; GDF15, growth differential factor-15; Gal-3, galectine-3; TGF-beta-1 transforming growth factor beta-1, TNFα tumor necrosis factor alpha; TRPC3 transient receptor potential channel-3; TRPM7, transient receptor potential cation channel, subfamily M, member 7; Nav1.5, voltage-gated sodium channel, Kv1.5, voltage-gated potassium channel; MMPs. Matrix metalloproteinases; sST2, soluble suppression of tumorigenesis-2; RANKL, tumor necrosis factor ligand superfamily member 11; OPG, osteoprotegerin.

These triggers contribute to the altered expression of several ion channel proteins, such as transient receptor potential channel-3 (TRPM3) and member 7 TRPC3, which regulate intracellular calcium flow, and mediate dysfunction of the ion channels on the surfaces of target cells [54]. Angiotensin-II, aldosterone, endothelin, and catecholamines, as well as several inflammatory cytokines (TNF-alpha, interleukin-2) acting as signaling molecules contribute to fibroblast proliferation via Ca^{2+} entry via transient receptor potential channels (voltage-gated sodium [Nav1.5] and potassium channels [Kv1.5]) [55]. In addition, myofibril protein breakdown is stimulated by overexpressed calpain, which is activated by intracellular Ca^{2+} loading [56]. As a result, activated myofibroblasts not only produce several types of collagens shaping collagen deposition and cardiac fibrosis but also directly interact with cardiomyocytes promoting AF [57]. Moreover, myofibroblasts and fibrotic areas interfere with atrial tissue conduction and lead to intercellular uncoupling. Indeed, interactions between myofibroblast and cardiomyocyte alter conduction and elicit focal activity in the atria [58]. Finally, cell uncoupling, along with cardiac myocyte disarmament and extensive fibrosis, lead to gap junctions and non-uniformity of anisotropy modulating AF. In addition, pre-exceeding CV diseases, such as myocardial infarction, cardiomyopathies, myocarditis, and cardiac hypertrophy, through the strength of local mechanical forces, loss of cardiac myocytes and extensive fibrosis intervene in anisotropy modality of cardiac electrical conductivity and shaping arrhythmogenic substrate [59].

Although collagen accumulation in the myocardium is regulated by autocrine/paracrin and neurohumoral mechanisms, the atria are more prone to extracellular matrix remodeling and collagen deposition than the ventricles. Possibly, it depends on the distinguished presence of matrix metalloproteinases, their inhibitors, and pro-inflammatory molecules involved in the subsequent regulation of collagen synthesis and degradation. The accumulation of collagen, other matrix proteins (elastin, fibronectin 1, fibrillin 1), and proteoglycans in abundance lead to severe heterogeneous areas in the atria with variable alteration of electrophysiological properties [59]. This eventually leads to changes in myocardial cell architecture, such as elongation and disturbed alignment of demarcated fibers. This subsequently causes anisotropic changes in the entire myocardium, mediating a discrepancy between transverse and longitudinal electrical conduction leading to AF.

3. Electrical Cardioversion of AF: Safety and Outcomes

It seems that standard external direct current electrical cardioversion is a well-developed urgent treatment strategy for patients presenting recent-onset AF [1,60]. Numerous retrospective one-center studies and multicenter trials yielded 86–88% efficacy of the approach in restoring sinus rhythm along with 6–10% relapse of AF in a short-term perspective (7–28 days) [61–63]. Overall, electrical cardioversion in AF patients who required emergency department transportation was associated with infrequent hospital admission and few mild-to-moderate complications [61]. However, the duration of AF in the majority of studies was less than 48 h in 99% of the patients. Burton JH et al. (2004) [61] observed in a retrospective multicenter study that electrical cardioversion had an 86% success rate, and only 10% of the patients returned to the emergency department within 7 days. Fried AM et al. (2021) [16] reported that the efficacy of this procedure, defined as restoration of sinus rhythm, reached 88% in routine clinical practice, whereas major complications (post-cardioversion stroke, thromboembolic events, jaw thrust maneuver for hypoxia, and overnight observation for hypotension) and predefined minor adverse events (frequently related to general anesthesia, skin burns) were detected in 0.3% and 14%, respectively. In addition, electrical cardioversion was about 2.5 times more effective than conventional pharmacological treatment in restoring sinus rhythm [62,63]. Although there are numerous potential complications of electrical cardioversion (i.e., ventricular fibrillation, thromboembolism due to inadequate anticoagulant therapy, nonsustained ventricular tachycardia, various forms of atrial arrhythmias, bradycardia, transient left bundle branch block, myocardial necrosis, asymptomatic myocardial dysfunction, acute HF, transient hypotension, pulmonary edema, and stroke), they occur less frequently than recurrent AF. Further, 6.4% of patients revisited the emergency department within 30 days, and 4.8% returned with AF or atrial flutter. It is noteworthy that the return visit rate for patients with relapsed AF varies between 3% and 17% [64].

Overall, 30-day all-cause mortality among AF patients undergoing direct-current electrical cardioversion was 0.8% [65]. Data received from the FIRE (Atrial Fibrillation/flutter Italian Registry) registry showed that predictors of unsuccessful electrical cardioversion were onset of AF > 48 h, concomitant HF, increasing age, syncope, transient ischemic attack (TIA)/stroke as well as previous admission to a non-cardiology department [66]. The investigators also found several predictors of in-hospital mortality in this patient population, including age, HF, diabetes mellitus, previous admission to a non-cardiology department, and TIA/stroke [66]. Thus, patients at low risk for thromboembolic complications, including stroke and heart failure, seem to benefit more from electric cardioversion than other individuals with recent-onset AF [67].

Another reason for physicians to use this approach may be cost savings and a short period of emergency department admission [67,68]. Houghton AR et al. (2000) [69] and Boriani G. et al. (2007) [70] did not identify concise hemodynamic predictors of successful external electrical cardioversion or relapses after electrical cardioversion among patients with persistent AF or atrial flutter. However, only two predictors (duration of arrhythmia ≥1 year and previous cardioversion) were found to be powerful for this matter [69,70], whereas, in previous investigations, relapse of AF was associated with reduced left ventricular ejection fraction [71]. Along with it, standard external biphasic direct current electrical cardioversion has better efficacy than monophasic electrical cardioversion (360-J) for restoration of sinus rhythm in AF patients, although dual external monophasic 360-J cardioversion may increase the success rate as a rescue technique after failing standard external direct current cardioversion [72,73]. In this concept, the prediction of plausible cardiovascular events, including relapsed AF, with a biomarker strategy seems promising in patients with recent-onset AF.

4. Predictors for AF Recurrence Following Electrical Cardioversion

Biomarkers reflecting the complex pathophysiological mechanisms underlying AF seem to be an effective tool to predict rhythm status after cardioversion as well as other AF-related complications, which can intervene in mortality, hospital admission, cardiovascular (CV), and non-CV outcomes (Table A1).

4.1. Natriuretic Peptides

Natriuretic peptides (brain natriuretic peptide [BNP], N-terminal pro-B-type natriuretic peptide (NT-proBNP), mid-regional pro-A type natriuretic peptide (MR-proANP)) serve as circulating cardiac biomarkers of biomechanical stress, adverse cardiac remodeling, and fluid overload with established diagnostic and predictive values for acute and chronic HF involving any phenotypes [74,75]. Along with it, elevated levels of NPs were strongly associated with all-cause and CV mortality and urgent hospitalization among patients with AF, T2DM, CKD, hypertension, and cardiac hypertrophy [76,77]. Moreover, NT-proBNP and BNP were found to be predictors for AF [78–80]. However, it has been suggested that restoration of sinus rhythm through effective electric cardioversion may associate with a reduction in NP concentrations and thereby predict the recurrence of new episodes of arrhythmia. Xu X et al. (2017) [81] observed in a meta-analysis that low levels of BNP and NT-proBNP were associated with the maintenance of sinus rhythm and that the baseline concentrations of both biomarkers may be a predictor of AF recurrence after successful electrical cardioversion. Ari H. et al. (2008) [82] reported that a significant decrease in BNP levels 30 min after electric cardioversion corresponded to six-month maintenance of sinus rhythm in follow-up.

In the GAPP-AF (The gene expression patterns for the prediction of atrial fibrillation) study, Meyre PB (2022) [83] investigated 21 conventional and new circulating biomarkers reflecting inflammation, myocardial injury, cardiac biomechanical stress, and renal dysfunction before and 30 days after electrical cardioversion and evaluated plausible associations of changes in circulating biomarker levels with rhythm status at 30-day follow-up. The patients included in the study had no acute HF, severe valvular disease, or life-limiting active or chronic serious concomitant diseases. The authors found that low levels of NT-proBNP were independently associated with sinus rhythm restoration after electric cardioversion On the other hand, initial levels of BNP and NT-proBNP in patients with persistent AF without established CVD did not predict long-term sinus rhythm maintenance, although conversion to sinus rhythm related to a significant decrease in circulating BNP but not NT-proBNP level [84]. In contrast, NT-proBNP levels were found to be a predictor of AF recurrence 30 days after successful electric cardioversion among patients with persistent AF and CV risk factors, including hypertension and dyslipidemia [85]. In another study, pre-procedural NT-proBNP levels, but not post-procedural levels of the peptide, independently predicted the relapse of AF after successful electrical cardioversion [86]. These controversial issues perhaps may relate to the presence of concomitant HF. Indeed, in the CAPRAF (Candesartan in the Prevention of Relapsing Atrial Fibrillation) trial, plasma NT-proBNP concentrations measured before electrical cardioversion did not predict cardioversion success nor the relapse of AF in patients without HF [87]. Mabuchi N et al. (2000) [88] noticed that low atrial natriuretic peptide (ANP) and high BNP levels before electric cardioversion were independent predictors of recurrent AF in mild chronic HF patients. Moreover, the authors established that ANP to BNP ratio <0.44 was a significant risk factor for AF recurrence [88]. The BNP level of 700 fmol/mL or higher on day 7 after cardioversion was most predictive for AF recurrence (sensitivity, 78%; specificity, 71%), whereas ANP did not predict the relapse of AF [89]. Buccelletti F. et al. (2011) [90] measured the levels of NT-proBNP in 200 patients admitted to the emergency department due to new-onset AF (<2 weeks) regardless of HF presence. The authors found that NT-proBNP levels of either ≤450 pg/mL or >1800 pg/mL seem to show positive and negative predictive values for cardioversion in rate-control and rhythm-control strategies, respectively. In the range of 450 to 1800 pg/mL, NT-proBNP did not exhibit serious clinical utility [90]. However, it remained unclear whether continuous monitoring of the dynamic changes of NPs after sinus rhythm restoration predicts recurrent AF [91]. Overall, the restoration of sinus rhythm after electric cardioversion in AF patients is associated with a decrease in circulating levels of NPs and low levels of NT-proBNP predicts a sustainable maintains of sinus rhythm in follow-up.

4.2. Biomarkers of Fibrosis

Cardiac fibrosis was found to be closely associated with AF. Circulating biomarkers of fibrosis have already been proposed as a promising tool in its evaluation, but which biomarkers are most appropriate for AF remains unclear [92]. There are a large number of circulating biomarkers, which characterize the accumulation of extracellular matrix components and fibrosis, such as soluble suppressor tumorigenicity-2 (sST2), galectin-3 (Gal-3), procollagen type III N terminal peptide (PIIINP), type I collagen carboxyl telopeptide (ICTP), and fibroblast growth factor 23 (FGF-23) [93].

4.2.1. Galectin-3

Gal-3 is a multifunctional galactose-binding protein that belongs to the transforming growth factor beta superfamily and a biomarker of fibrosis, involved in atrial remodeling, cardiac fibrosis, and AF [94]. Previous studies revealed that patients with AF had higher Gal-3 values than non-AF patients, regardless of their comorbidity profile [95,96]. Moreover, elevated Gal-3 levels were independently associated with paroxysmal non-valvular AF [97].

There is ample evidence of a close relation between elevated Gal-3 levels, atrial remodeling (i.e., parameters of left atrial dimension, volume, compliance, and contractility) and AF recurrence following successful electrical cardioversion [98–100]. Gürses KM et al. (2019) [98] reported that pre-cardioversion Gal-3 levels in persistent AF corresponded to a higher left atrial volume index and were associated with early AF recurrence following successful sinus rhythm restoration. In contrast, Cichoń M et al. (2021) [101] did not find any link between circulating Gal-3 levels and the risk of recurrent AF in obese and non-obese patients with persistent AF. The same results were obtained in another study involving 75 non-HF patients with paroxysmal or persistent AF referred for electrical cardioversion [102]. Although the authors of the study established a correlation between the Gal-3 levels and oxidative stress and inflammation in AF patients, only circulating myeloperoxidase, but not Gal-3, was associated with the maintenance of sinus rhythm in a multivariate model, possibly due to the small number of patients and relatively early stage of AF [102]. Whether these changes may be explained in connection with single nuclear polymorphisms of the Gal-3 gene has not been fully elucidated [103]. Thus, the predictive ability of Gal-3 for sinus rhythm restoration following successful electrical cardioversion requires thorough investigations in face-to-face comparison with other biomarkers before implementation in clinical practice.

4.2.2. sST2

Soluble suppression of Tumorigenicity 2 protein (sST2) is part of the interleukin 1 receptor/Toll-like superfamily, which is related to cardiac inflammation, fibrosis, and also remodeling. Current clinical guidelines for HF consider sST2 as an alternative biomarker of all-cause and CV mortality as well as HF-related complications, including hospital admission, especially in HF with preserved ejection fraction (HFpEF) [74,75]. Although sST2 is involved in cardiac fibrosis, local and systemic inflammation, and atrial and ventricular remodeling, its role in predicting clinical outcomes of electrical cardioversion of AF remains uncertain [104,105]. In patients with HF and acute myocardial infarction, elevated sST2 levels were a powerful risk factor for new-onset AF [106,107]. Moreover, in AF patients without concomitant cardiovascular disease, sST2 concentrations were positively associated with LV myocardial strain and T1 mapping indices [108]. Previous studies have demonstrated significant predictability of AF recurrence after cryoballoon and radiofrequency ablation using sST2 [109–111].

It appears that limited evidence exists regarding a discriminatory effect of sST2 measured before and after electrical cardioversion on AF recurrence. Wałek P. et al. (2020) [112] found that sST2, but not Gal-3, predicted sinus rhythm maintenance after successful electrical cardioversion of AF in patients without HF. Perhaps, sST2 may be considered as part of a multimarker panel for the prediction of AF recurrence along with NPs and Gal-3. Overall, sST2 seems to be a promising predictive biomarker for AF recurrence after electrical cardioversion, cryoballoon, and radiofrequency ablation.

4.2.3. Other Biomarkers of Fibrosis

Begg GA (2017) [113] investigated an association of biomarkers related to fibrosis and collagen metabolism with procedural risk and AF recurrence rates among 79 patients undergoing external direct current cardioversion in comparison with 40 age-and-disease-matched volunteers. The authors found that Gal-3, PIIINP, and ICTP were not predictive for AF recurrence after electrical cardioversion, whereas FGF-23 had a weak predictive ability for relapsing AF [113]. In contrast, Kawamura M. et al. (2012) [114] found no discriminatory levels of interleukin-6, high-sensitivity C-reactive protein, BNP, renin, and aldosterone for the 24-month recurrence rate of AF, whereas baseline serum levels of PIIINP > 0.72 U/mL predicted AF relapse. Thus, there is a serious discrepancy between biomarker levels corresponding to the presence of atrial fibrosis confirmed by cardiac magnetic resonance imaging and their discriminatory properties for recurrent AF [115–117].

Furthermore, elevated serum levels of FGF-23 strongly correlated with the total number of major cardiovascular events and left atrial dimension in paroxysmal AF patients as well as with new-onset AF in sinus rhythm patients presenting CV risk factors, but not with the maintenance of sinus rhythm during follow-up [117–119]. Meta-analysis of 15 clinical studies, enrolling 36,017 participants, revealed that elevated serum FGF-23 levels, but not GDF15 levels, were associated with the risk of AF [120]. A meta-analysis of 15 clinical trials involving 36,017 participants found that elevated serum FGF-23 levels, but not GDF15 levels, were associated with AF risk [120]. However, it remains unclear whether these results also apply to patients undergoing electrical cardioversion.

4.3. Biomarkers of Inflammation

4.3.1. GDF15

GDF15 is a member of the TGF-beta superfamily whose expression is increased in response to biomechanical myocardial stress, inflammation, or ischemia/hypoxia [121]. GDF15 is involved in the regulation of energy homeostasis, thermogenesis, and eating behavior [122]. Yet, GDF15 also exerts anti-inflammatory and anti-proliferative properties, although the underlying molecular mechanisms are still unclear [123]. Elevated GDF15 levels were found in patients with any phenotypes of chronic HF, stroke, AF, and T2DM [124–128]. In the general population, GDF-15 did not show a positive association with the prevalence of AF and the risk of AF occurrence [129]. The suitability of GDF15 for predicting bleeding and/or atrial thrombosis during anticoagulant therapy remains questionable [130]. Clinical evidence for the discriminative value of GDF15 for AF relapse or sinus rhythm maintenance is extremely limited. There is one small study that prospectively included 82 patients with persistent AF [101]. Although log10 serum GDF-15 levels correlated positively with the CHA2DS2-VASc score, there was no close association between GDF-15 levels and sinus rhythm maintenance in patients after successful electric cardioversion [101]. Thus, a discriminative potency of GDF15 for the prediction of clinical efficacy of electrical cardioversion among patients with nonvalvular/valvular AF is not completely understood and requires scrutiny in large clinical studies.

4.3.2. hs-CRP

High-sensitivity C-reactive protein (hs-CRP) is a classic biomarker of inflammation and is a component of the inflammatory profile observed in AF patients. Elevated hs-CRP levels were found in patients with all forms of nonvalvular/valvular AF, regardless of etiology and concomitant comorbidities [131,132]. hs-CRP predicted new-onset AF both in the general population as well as in patients with established cardiovascular or metabolic diseases, such as HF, acute myocardial infarction, T2DM, and metabolic syndrome [133–135]. Among patients with AF complicated by systemic thromboembolism, the levels of hs-CRP correlated positively with the CHA2DS2-VASc score [136].

Loricchio ML et al. (2007) [137] investigated plausible predictors for a 1-year risk of AF recurrence after electrical cardioversion. In a Cox regression analysis, the authors found that age, gender, hypertension, T2DM, LVEF, left atrial diameter, use of various antiarrhythmic and antihypertensive (including angiotensin-converting enzyme inhibitors or angiotensin II antagonists) drugs, and statins were not associated with relapsing AF. On the contrary, a low quartile of hs-CRP levels was found to be a strong predictor for this outcome [137]. Lombardi F. et al. (2008) [138] did not find any changes in hs-CRP levels after cardioversion in patients with persistent AF and preserved LVEF, regardless of the post-procedural underlying rhythm. However, NT-proBNP levels decreased significantly in patients who maintained sinus rhythm but not in those who had AF. Yet, baseline hs-CRP levels, but not echocardiographic features of atrial dysfunction and initial NT-proBNP levels, predicted recurrences of AF after cardioversion in patients without pre-existing left ventricular dysfunction [138]. Barassi A et al. (2012) [139] and Korantzopoulos P et al. (2008) [140] confirmed that in patients with persistent AF and preserved LVEF, elevated hs-CRP levels independently predicted subacute AF recurrence rate, whereas NT-proBNP concentrations were not associated with arrhythmic outcome but corresponded to the alterations of cardiac hemodynamics secondary to the presence of AF.

Overall, there is ample strong evidence that elevated preprocedural hs-CRP levels may provide independent predictive information for both successful electrical cardioversion of AF and maintenance of sinus rhythm after conversion [141,142]. The meta-analysis by Liu et al. [143], which included six prospective observational studies (n = 366 patients), showed that peripheral blood CRP levels were higher in patients with failed electric cardioversion than in those with successful restoration of sinus rhythm. In another meta-analysis by Yo CH et al. (2014) [144], a cut-off value of 1.9 mg/L hs-CRP predicted long-term AF recurrence (77% sensitivity, 65% specificity), and more than 3 mg/L predicted short-term AF relapse (73% sensitivity, 71% specificity). Thus, the measurement of CRP levels before the procedure may provide additional prognostic information about the success of sinus rhythm maintenance.

In addition, there are data illustrating that hs-CRP levels measured shortly after electrical cardioversion may be a powerful biomarker for assessing the risk of relapsing AF in the long-term. In particular, Celebi OO et al. (2011) [145] reported that hs-CRP levels measured before and 2 days after electrical cardioversion predicted the 1-year risk of AF relapse. Whether postprocedural hs-CRP provides more information to predict the event than preprocedural hs-CRP is still unclear. However, elevated levels of hs-CRP predicted new-onset AF in the general population and among patients with known cardiovascular diseases, while their role as a marker of sustainable sinus rhythm control places under question.

4.4. Myokines and Adipocytokines

Several interdependent canonic signaling pathways, such as the renin-angiotensin-aldosterone system; TGF-beta pathway, inflammatory chemokines, and cytokines lead to cardiac fibrosis through modulation of oxidative stress and inflammation. However, the direct mechanical stretch may act as a modulator of extracellular matrix remodeling by attenuating the expression of matrix metalloproteinases and their inhibitors. Recently, another signaling pathway has been identified that induces atrial fibrosis via the secretion of adipokines from epicardial, perivascular, and adipose tissue white adipocytes. In addition, recent studies have shown that myokines derived from cardiac and skeletal muscle myocytes may act as adaptive regulators of extracellular matrix remodeling and can attenuate fibrosis [146,147]. Depending on their origin, adipokines and myokines may modulate myofibroblast capabilities, regulate myocyte energy homeostasis and protect against inflammation and fibrosis [148,149]. However, some pro-fibrotic adipokines and myokines can switch a generation of reactive oxygen species to pro-inflammatory and pro-fibrotic stimuli, stimulate myofibroblast differentiation through JAK/STAT3 and JNK/c-Jun signaling, interfere with myocyte electrophysiology, and promote fibrosis in the myocardium [150–152]. Numerous previous studies have shown that resistin, apelin, and adiponectin are adipokines associated with several known risk factors for AF and risk of AF [153–156]. A recent meta-analysis of 34 studies (total number of patients = 31,479) showed that some adipokines, mainly adiponectin, apelin, and resistin, were associated with the risk of AF in the pooled univariate data, whereas the associations were not apparent after multivariate adjustment [157]. However, there is limited evidence of the relation between adipokine and myokine signatures and the risk of AF-related outcomes after electric cardioversion.

4.4.1. Apelin

Apelin is a multifunctional regulatory peptide with potential cytoprotective properties. It is a ligand of the angiotensin II protein J receptor (APJ) receptor and belongs to the G protein-coupled receptor family [158]. Apelin mRNA is widely expressed in tissues such as the cardiovascular, central nervous, adipose, skeletal muscles, and gastrointestinal systems. The Apelin/APJ axis mediates signal transduction for regulating energy homeostasis including glucose and lipid metabolism, mitochondrial function, angiogenesis, cellular proliferation, and differentiation [159]. Furthermore, apelin inhibits apoptosis, decreases myocardial infarction size, and prevents myocardial ischemia/reperfusion injury via the PI3K/Akt and ERK1/2 caspase signaling. It is also engaged in the autophagy pathway, attenuation of inflammatory reactions, and prevention of atherosclerotic plaque formation [160]. Several controversial issues remain regarding whether the apelin/APJ system is essential for regulating atrial and ventricular remodeling by alleviating myocardial hypertrophy induced by angiotensin II, oxidative stress, and TGF-beta1 [161–163]. Nevertheless, it has been shown that atrial wall stretching can activate the myocardial APJ axis [164]. Moreover, APJ was found to be essential for stretch-induced contractility and may also induce ectopic electrical activity by Ca^{2+} sensitization of myofilaments. It is believed that apelin counteracts APJ's stretch-triggered hypertrophy signaling by suppressing Ca^{2+} transients [164]. Along with it, there are a variety of vascular effects of apelin that include regulation of systolic and diastolic blood pressure through vasorelaxation and an increase in regional blood flow [165,166].

Previous studies have shown that circulating levels of apelin were sufficiently lower in patients with established cardiovascular diseases (coronary artery disease, myocardial infarction, acute coronary syndrome, HF), T2DM, and obesity than in healthy volunteers [167,168]. A meta-analysis of 30 studies revealed a negative association of apelin serum levels with cardiovascular diseases [169]. However, peripheral blood apelin concentrations were not only significantly decreased in AF patients compared with healthy controls but also independently predicted recurrent AF in patients with persistent AF. This included cases occurring after pulmonary vein isolation in subjects without structural heart disease [170–172]. It has been suggested that low apelin levels may interfere with AF susceptibility through elevated atrial NADPH-dependent oxidative stress and the TGF-β/Smad2/α-SMA pathway associated with mitochondrial dysfunction and myocardial fibrosis [173,174]. In addition, the apelin/APJ axis might be involved in atrial thrombus formation among AF patients, possibly as a result of concomitant downstream plasminogen activator inhibitor-1 (PAI-1) [175].

The predictive role of apelin for AF occurrence after electric cardioversion remains uncertain. In a small comparative study, Kallergis EM et al. (2010) [176] showed that baseline apelin levels did not independently predict AF recurrence, whereas NT-proBNP did. Interestingly, maintenance of sinus rhythm after electrical cardioversion resulted in an increase in serum apelin levels and a decrease in serum NT-pro-BNP levels. However, more studies are needed to clarify apelin's discriminative potency for AF recurrence in AF patients after electrical cardioversion, with comparisons of apelin's predictive value to other conventional and promising biomarkers.

4.4.2. Irisin

Irisin was previously described as a hormone-like myokine, which is mainly secreted by skeletal muscle and myocardium and is a derivative of the membrane protein fibronectin type III domain-containing 5 (FNDC5) [177]. Exercise increases serum levels of irisin, which exert cytoprotective effects on remote organs and tissues, including the heart, kidney, vasculature, bones, and brain [177,178]. Irisin interacts with $\alpha V/\beta 5$ integrin on the surface of target cells and induces a wide range of biological effects, including stimulation of glucose and lipid metabolism, increase in insulin resistance, browning of visceral adipose tissue, thermogenesis, angiogenesis, survival of osteoblasts, and production of bone-related proteins such as sclerostin [179–182].

Serum irisin levels were significantly decreased in obese and T2DM patients compared with nondiabetic controls, as well as in patients with known cardiovascular disease (cardiac hypertrophy, stable coronary artery disease, chronic HF, multifocal atherosclerosis) compared with healthy volunteers [183,184]. On the contrary, acute HF, acute coronary syndrome, and acute myocardial infarction were associated with an increase in irisin levels, which is considered an adaptive factor that reduces endothelial damage by inhibiting inflammatory reactions and suppressing oxidative stress [185–187]. A low irisin level was described as an independent predictor of clinical outcomes in HF patients [188,189]. Although patients with HFpEF and AF had significantly lower irisin levels than those without AF [190], the role of irisin in predicting AF-related events, including relapse after electric cardioversion, has not yet been investigated.

4.4.3. Bone-Related Proteins

There is growing strong evidence that inflammatory responses are involved in the development of AF and its complications. Bone-related proteins are matricellular peptides that mediate diverse biological functions and are involved in many pathological conditions in cardiovascular disease, including fibrosis, microvascular inflammation, calcification, extracellular remodeling, and atherosclerotic plaque formation [191]. Bone-related proteins, such as osteoprotegerin (OPG) and TNF-related apoptosis-inducing ligand (TRAIL), mediate a link between cardiovascular comorbidities and diseases, such as diabetes mellitus, CKD, atherosclerosis, HF, vascular calcification, and the occurrence of AF [192]. Indeed, cardiovascular comorbidities were associated with higher OPG levels and lower TRAIL levels immediately after the first hours of AF paroxysm [125,193]. Furthermore, osteopontine (OPN) levels were related to an increased risk of systemic thromboembolism and ischemic stroke in patients with AF [194]. OPG and OPN were found to be predictors of HF outcomes independent of AF presence and have been included in a multiple-scoring system to predict survival in chronic HF [195]. In a small clinical study involving 100 non-CVD patients with and without AF recurrence, low levels of bone morphogenetic protein 10 exhibited predictive value for sinus rhythm maintenance with a striking similarity to NT-proBNP [83]. However, it remains unclear whether these biomarkers have prognostic abilities for the maintenance of sinus rhythm in AF patients after electrical cardioversion.

4.5. Biomarkers of Oxidative Stress and Endothelial Dysfunction

4.5.1. Cell-Free Circulating DNA

Cell-free circulating DNA (cfcDNA) circulates in two main pools: circular and single-stranded molecules belonging to mitochondrial-derived and nuclear-derived subpopulations, reflecting patterns of DNA methylation and a variety of neutrophil extracellular traps (NETosis) [196,197]. The cfcDNA are determined in subdetectable concentrations under certain physiological conditions, such as physical exercise, whereas increased circulating levels of these fragments are strongly associated with cardiovascular, autoimmune, rheumatic diseases, infections, and malignancy [198–202]. The main causes of cfcDNA production are mitochondrial dysfunction and inflammation, which are powerful drivers of numerous diseases and conditions, including AF [203].

Wiersma M. et al. (2020) [204] reported that levels of cell-free circulating mitochondrial DNA (cfc-mtDNA) were significantly increased in patients with paroxysmal AF undergoing AF treatment, especially in men and in patients with AF recurrence after electrical cardioversion or pulmonary vein isolation. In contrast, cfc-mtDNA levels gradually decreased in patients with persistent AF and long-standing persistent AF. Nevertheless, the authors suggested that cfc-mtDNA levels might be associated with the stage of AF and the risk of AF recurrence after treatment, especially in men. Gender differences in descriptive values of cfc-mtDNA for AF recurrence remain poorly understood but could be related to different comorbidities in both subpopulations. However, another study found no significant changes in mtDNA copy number in the peripheral blood of AF patients of different sex and age [205]. Perhaps, cfcDNA may be included in the multiple biomarker models with the aim of improving their predictive potency in AF patients with low levels of NT-proBNP or in AF patients with malignancy who are treated with chemotherapy.

4.5.2. mRNA

MicroRNAs (miRNAs) participate in atrial remodeling and cardiac fibrosis, contributing to the development of AF [206]. Garcia-Elias A et al. (2021) [207] established that circulating levels of miR-199a-5p and miR-22-5p, which regulate fibrogenic response in the myocardium, were higher in HFrEF patients with AF than in those without AF [207]. MiR-21, which corresponds to atrial fibrosis, is associated with the risk of persistent AF in patients with left atrial enlargement [208]. Interestingly, increased circulating levels of miR-1-3p, which is a myosine gene regulator involved in hypertrophy, myocardial infarction, and cardiac arrhythmogenesis, predicted a high risk of subclinical AF [209]. MiR423, which downregulates fibrosis-related genes such as collagen I, collagen III, fibronectin, and TGF-beta, may be a pivotal factor in stratifying patients at risk of AF occurrence and persistence [210]. Moreover, differences in miRNA expression in the atrial myocardium of men and women may mediate a sex-specific association between circulating miRNAs in plasma and AF at the population level [206]. In addition, there is evidence that epigenetic regulation of NETosis may participate in the development of AF susceptibility. As a matter of fact, miR-146a and miR21 may provide prognostic information in patients with AF [211,212] due to its direct effects on NETosis. In a study by da Silva AMG (2018) [213], miR-21, miR-133b, and miR-499, which are directly involved in the downregulation of apoptosis and fibrosis, were found to be directly involved in AF. However, it remains to be determined whether a signature of mi-Rs can be used to predict poor response to AF treatment, including electrical cardioversion. At the same time, Zhou Q et al. (2018) [213] reported that among 123 miRs affecting cardiac fibrosis, hypertrophy, and inflammation by relation with the SMAD7 and FASLG genes, only miR-21 demonstrated a positive correlation with left atrial low-voltage areas in patients with persistent AF and was associated with post-ablation outcome. Overall, the signature of miRs appears to be a more promising tool for higher AF risk than for outcomes after treatment, although this conjecture needs to be further investigated in the future.

4.5.3. Asymmetric Dimethylarginine

Asymmetric dimethylarginine (ADMA) is a well-known biomarker of endothelial dysfunction that indirectly reflects vascular NO production and exhibits certain predictive information for mortality and morbidity of cardiovascular diseases, including AF [214,215]. In the population-based Gutenberg Health Study (n = 5000), ADMA levels were correlated with left ventricular hypertrophy and AF prevalence [216]. An ARISTOTLE (Apixaban for Reduction in Stroke and Other Thromboembolic Events in Atrial Fibrillation) substudy showed that elevated ADMA levels exhibited a weak association with thromboembolic events in AF patients treated with anticoagulants (warfarin or apixaban) for a median of 1.9 years [217]. The investigators found that tertile groups of ADMA levels were sufficiently associated with death, stroke, and systemic embolism and that incorporating ADMA into CHA2DS2-VASc or HAS-BLED predictive models significantly improved C-indices for those clinical outcomes [217].

There is strong evidence that acute and persistent episodes of AF seem to show elevated ADMA levels accompanied by increased biomarkers of ischemic myocardial injury like cardiac troponins [218]. In the animal AF model, ADMA concentrations in peripheral blood returned to normal within 24 h after successful electrical cardioversion [218]. Along with it, increased circulating levels of ADMA in AF may be reduced by a Mediterranean diet and statin treatment [219,220]. Thus, being closely associated with thrombus formation and CHADS2/CHA2DS2-VASc score, ADMA is a biomarker for predicting pro-thrombotic risk in AF [221,222].

There are controversial data for ADMA's predictive ability regarding AF recurrence after electrical cardioversion. Xia W et al. (208) [223] reported that elevated ADMA levels were strongly associated with an increased risk of AF relapse within 1 month after electrical cardioversion. On the contrary, Tveit A et al. (2010) [224] found that the levels of ADMA and the L-arginine/ADMA ratio did not exert predictive ability for sinus rhythm maintenance after electrical cardioversion, while the L-arginine/ADMA ratio remained elevated in patients with sinus rhythm for 6 months compared with patients with AF recurrence. The discriminative potency of ADMA may be strongly related to comorbidities. Indeed, serum ADMA levels were not associated with incident AF in the general population after adjusting for other cardiovascular risk factors [224]. Overall, the utility of ADMA refines clinical risk stratification in AF regardless of the treatment strategy.

5. Conclusions

Previous clinical studies demonstrated limited ability to predict the efficacy of electrical cardioversion with conventional biomarkers, which described adverse cardiac remodeling, biomechanical stress, fibrosis, inflammation, endothelial dysfunction, oxidative stress, and mitochondrial dysfunction. Epigenetic biomarkers such as miRs and biomarkers of oxidative stress and inflammation such as cfcDNA appear to show highly variable results in predicting post-procedural events. A biomarker-based strategy for predicting events after AF treatment requires extensive future investigation, especially in different gender and variable comorbidity profiles. Therefore, a multiple biomarker approach may be more useful than using a single biomarker for patients with different forms of AF. Large clinical trials are needed to make direct face-to-face comparisons with different biomarkers and their combinations.

Author Contributions: Conceptualization, O.D. and M.L.; methodology, A.E.B.; software, O.D.; formal analysis, O.D.; investigation, O.D.; resources, O.D.; data curation, A.E.B.; writing—original draft preparation, O.D., M.L. and A.E.B.; writing—review and editing, O.D., U.C.H., M.M., E.B., S.X.G., M.L. and A.E.B.; supervision, A.E.B.; project administration, O.D.; advice for analysis and interpretation of the data: U.C.H., M.M., E.B. and S.X.G. All authors have participated in drafting the manuscript. All authors have read and agreed to the published version of the manuscript.

Funding: This research received no external funding.

Institutional Review Board Statement: Not applicable.

Informed Consent Statement: Not applicable.

Data Availability Statement: Not applicable.

Conflicts of Interest: The authors declare no conflict of interest.

Appendix A

Table A1. Predictive values of different biomarkers in prediction of AF-related complications after electrical cardioversion.

Biomarkers	Population	Observation Period	Significance/Outcomes	References
Biomechanical stress				
BNP	58 patients with persistent AF and preserved LVEF	6 months	Baseline BNP level and the magnitude of its decrease after successful cardioversion predicted AF recurrence	[82]
NT-proBNP and BMP10	100 non-CVD patients with and without AF recurrence	30-day follow-up	Low NT-proBNP levels and BMP10 levels after electric cardioversion predicted sinus rhythm restoration	[83]
BNP and NT-proBNP	43 patients with persistent AF	18 months	Pre- and post-procedural levels of BNP and NT-proBNP did not predict new episodes of AF	[84]
NT-proBNP	199 patients with persistent AF	30 days	The levels of NT-proBNP > 500 ng/L predicted recurrence of AF in 30 days after successful electrical cardioversion	[85]
NT-pro-BNP	40 patients with persistent AF	1 month	Elevated baseline NT-pro-BNP predicted AF recurrence after electric cardioversion	[86]
NT-pro-BNP	171 patients with persistent AF without HF	1 month	Pre-cardioversion and post-cardioversion NT-pro-BNP levels did not predict a relapse of AF in patients without HF	[87]
ANP and BNP	71 HF patients with persistent AF	1 month	Low ANP and high BNP levels before electric cardioversion independently predicted recurrent AF	[88]
ANP and BNP	60 patients with persistent AF	12 months	The BNP level ≥700 fmol/mL on day 7 after cardioversion predicted AF recurrence. ANP level was not predictive of AF recurrence	[89]
NT-proBNP	200 patients with newly onset AF with and without HF	1 month	NT-proBNP levels of either ≤450 pg/mL or >1800 pg/mL had positive and negative predictive values for cardioversion in rate-control and rhythm-control strategies	[90]
Cardiac fibrosis				
Gal-3	90 patients with persistent AF	3 months	Serum Gal-3 level independently predicted early AF recurrence following successful direct-current electrical cardioversion.	[98]
Gal-3	82 patients with persistent AF	1 month	Baseline serum levels of Gal-3 were not associated with a risk of recurrent AF	[101]
Gal-3	75 non-HF patients with paroxysmal or persistent AF	1 year	Pre-procedural Gal-3 levels did not predict recurrent AF	[102]

Table A1. *Cont.*

Biomarkers	Population	Observation Period	Significance/Outcomes	References
sST2	80 patients with persistent AF without HF	12 months	Serum levels of sST2 predict sinus rhythm maintenance after cardioversion of AF in patients without HF	[112]
FGF-23	79 patients with persistent AF	12 months	FGF-23, but not Gal-3, PIIINP, and ICTP, had weak predictive ability for relapsing AF	[113]
PIIINP	88 patients with maintenance of sinus rhythm and 54 patients with AF recurrence	24 months	Baseline PIIINP levels >0.72 U/mL independently predicted AF recurrence after electric cardioversion	[114]
		Inflammation		
GDF15	82 patients with persistent AF	1 month	GDF-15 levels correlated positively with the CHA2DS2-VASc score, but not associated with a risk of recurrent AF after electric cardioversion	[101]
hs-CRP	102 patients with non-valvular persistent AF	1 year	Low levels of hs-CRP were associated with long-term maintenance of sinus rhythm after electrical cardioversion for AF	[137]
hs-CRP	53 patients with persistent AF and a mean LVEF of 58.7 ± 6%	3 weeks	No changes in hs-CRP levels and decrease in NT-proBNP levels after effective cardioversion. Pre-procedural levels of hs-CRP predicted recurrence rate of AF	[138]
hs-CRP	57 patients with a mean LVEF of 58.7 ± 6%	3 weeks	Pre-procedural levels of hs-CRP, but not NT-proBNP, predicted recurrence rate of AF	[139]
hs-CRP	60 patients who received amiodarone for sinus rhythm maintenance	3 years	Pre-procedural levels of CRP >0.43 mg/dL were an independent predictor of AF recurrence	[140]
hs-CRP	106 patients with a history of symptomatic AF lasting ≥ 1 day	36 days	Pre-procedural hs-CRP levels ≥0.06 mg/dL predicted both AF recurrence and maintenance of sinus rhythm	[141]
hs-CRP	56 patients with persistent AF	180 days	Pre-procedural hs-CRP <0.8 mg/L was significantly associated with lower AF recurrence rates and maintenance of sinus rhythm	[142]
hs-CRP	216 patients with persistent AF	12 months	The baseline and 2-day levels of hs-CRP levels contributed a risk of AF recurrence	[145]
Apelin and NT-proBNP	40 patients with persistent AF and 15 controls in sinus rhythm	1 month	Pre-procedural apelin levels were lower and NT-pro-BNP levels were higher in patients with AF compared to controls. Cardioversion led to an increase in apelin levels and a decrease in NT-proBNP levels. Apelin did not predict AF recurrence, but NT-proBNP did	[176]

Table A1. Cont.

Biomarkers	Population	Observation Period	Significance/Outcomes	References
Biomarkers of oxidative stress and mitochondrial dysfunction				
cfc-mtDNA	59 non-AF patients undergoing cardiac surgery, 100 patients with paroxysmal AF, 116 patients with persistent AF, 20 longstanding-persistent AF individuals and 84 control individuals	-	Elevated cfc-mtDNA levels were found in patients with paroxysmal AF undergoing electrical cardioversion or pulmonary vein isolation, as well as in patients with AF relapse after AF treatment. In patients with persistent AF and longstanding persistent AF, the levels of cfc-mtDNA gradually decreased	[204]
miR-199a-5p and miR-22-5p	49 HFrEF with AF and 49 HFrEF with sinus rhythm	-	Elevated levels of circulating miR-199a-5p and miR-22-5p were associated with AF in HFrEF patients	[207]
miR-21	60 persistent AF patients and 60 matched sinus rhythm volunteers	-	Circulating miR-21 positively correlates with the quantification of left atrial fibrosis and is associated with the risk of persistent AF in patients with left atrial enlargement	[208]
miR-1-3p	64 consecutive patients with cryptogenic stroke, 9 patients with AF and 9 individuals with sinus rhythm	6 and 12 months	Elevated plasma levels of miR-1-3p predicted AF	[209]
miR-21, miR-133a, miR-133b, miR-150, miR-328, and miR-499	5 acute new-onset AF patients, 16 well-controlled AF and 15 control	-	miR-21, miR-133b, and miR-499, which downregulate apoptosis and fibrosis, were found to be directly related to AF	[213]
Biomarkers of endothelial dysfunction				
ADMA	64 patients with persistent AF	1 month	High levels of ADMA were strongly associated with an increased risk of AF relapse after electrical cardioversion	[222]
ADMA	98 patients with persistent AF	6 months	Changes in ADMA did not predict rhythm outcome after electrical cardioversion	[223]

Abbreviations: ADMA, asymmetric dimethylarginine; ANP, atrial natriuretic peptide; CVD, cardiovascular disease; BNP, brain natriuretic peptide; BMP10, bone morphogenetic protein 10; HF, heart failure; hs-CRP, high-sensitivity C-reactive protein; LVEF, left ventricular ejection fraction; NT-proBNP, N-terminal pro-B-type natriuretic peptide; sST2, soluble suppressor tumorigenisity-2; Gal-3, galectin-3; PIIINP, procollagen type III N terminal peptide; ICTP, type I collagen carboxyl telopeptide; FGF-23, fibroblast growth factor 23, cfc-mtDNA, cell-free circulating mitochondrial DNA.

References

1. Hindricks, G.; Potpara, T.; Dagres, N.; Arbelo, E.; Bax, J.J.; Blomström-Lundqvist, C.; Boriani, G.; Castella, M.; Dan, G.-A.; Dilaveris, P.E.; et al. 2020 ESC Guidelines for the Diagnosis and Management of Atrial Fibrillation Developed in Collaboration with the European Association for Cardio-Thoracic Surgery (EACTS): The Task Force for the Diagnosis and Management of Atrial Fibrillation of the European Society of Cardiology (ESC) Developed with the Special Contribution of the European Heart Rhythm Association (EHRA) of the ESC. *Eur. Heart J.* **2021**, *42*, 373–498. [CrossRef] [PubMed]
2. Zoni-Berisso, M.; Lercari, F.; Carazza, T.; Domenicucci, S. Epidemiology of Atrial Fibrillation: European Perspective. *Clin. Epidemiol.* **2014**, *6*, 213–220. [CrossRef]
3. Magnussen, C.; Niiranen, T.J.; Ojeda, F.M.; Gianfagna, F.; Blankenberg, S.; Njølstad, I.; Vartiainen, E.; Sans, S.; Pasterkamp, G.; Hughes, M.; et al. Sex Differences and Similarities in Atrial Fibrillation Epidemiology, Risk Factors, and Mortality in Community Cohorts: Results from the BiomarCaRE Consortium (Biomarker for Cardiovascular Risk Assessment in Europe). *Circulation* **2017**, *136*, 1588–1597. [CrossRef] [PubMed]
4. Wachter, R. Vorhofflimmern als Komorbidität bei Herzinsuffizienz. *Internist* **2018**, *59*, 415–419. [CrossRef]

6. Alonso, A.; Almuwaqqat, Z.; Chamberlain, A. Mortality in Atrial Fibrillation: Is It Changing? *Trends Cardiovasc. Med.* **2021**, *31*, 469–473. [CrossRef] [PubMed]
7. Walczak-Galezewska, M.; Markowska, M.; Braszak, A.; Bryl, W.; Bogdanski, P. Atrial Fibrillation and Obesity: Should Doctors Focus on This Comorbidity? *Minerva Med.* **2019**, *110*, 175–176. [CrossRef] [PubMed]
8. Hong, K.L.; Glover, B.M. The Impact of Lifestyle Intervention on Atrial Fibrillation. *Curr. Opin. Cardiol.* **2018**, *33*, 14–19. [CrossRef] [PubMed]
9. Shaikh, F.; Pasch, L.B.; Newton, P.J.; Bajorek, B.V.; Ferguson, C. Addressing Multimorbidity and Polypharmacy in Individuals with Atrial Fibrillation. *Curr. Cardiol. Rep.* **2018**, *20*, 32. [CrossRef] [PubMed]
10. Heijman, J.; Linz, D.; Schotten, U. Dynamics of Atrial Fibrillation Mechanisms and Comorbidities. *Annu. Rev. Physiol.* **2021**, *83*, 83–106. [CrossRef] [PubMed]
11. Schoonderwoerd, B.A.; Van Gelder, I.C.; Van Veldhuisen, D.J.; Van den Berg, M.P.; Crijns, H.J.G.M. Electrical and Structural Remodeling: Role in the Genesis and Maintenance of Atrial Fibrillation. *Prog. Cardiovasc. Dis.* **2005**, *48*, 153–168. [CrossRef] [PubMed]
12. Cha, T.-J.; Ehrlich, J.R.; Zhang, L.; Shi, Y.-F.; Tardif, J.-C.; Leung, T.K.; Nattel, S. Dissociation between Ionic Remodeling and Ability to Sustain Atrial Fibrillation during Recovery from Experimental Congestive Heart Failure. *Circulation* **2004**, *109*, 412–418. [CrossRef] [PubMed]
13. Vanbeselaere, V.; Truyers, C.; Elli, S.; Buntinx, F.; De Witte, H.; Degryse, J.; Henrard, S.; Vaes, B. Association between Atrial Fibrillation, Anticoagulation, Risk of Cerebrovascular Events and Multimorbidity in General Practice: A Registry-Based Study. *BMC Cardiovasc. Disord.* **2016**, *16*, 61. [CrossRef]
14. Bernard, M.L. Atrial Fibrillation and Multimorbidity. *Mayo Clin. Proc.* **2019**, *94*, 2381–2382. [CrossRef] [PubMed]
15. Kwok, C.S.; Lip, G.Y.H. The Patient Pathway Review for Atrial Fibrillation. *Crit. Pathw. Cardiol.* **2022**, *21*, 96–102. [CrossRef] [PubMed]
16. Furniss, S.S.; Sneyd, J.R. Safe Sedation in Modern Cardiological Practice. *Heart* **2015**, *101*, 1526–1530. [CrossRef] [PubMed]
17. Fried, A.M.; Strout, T.D.; Perron, A.D. Electrical Cardioversion for Atrial Fibrillation in the Emergency Department: A Large Single-Center Experience. *Am. J. Emerg. Med.* **2021**, *42*, 115–120. [CrossRef]
18. Brandes, A.; Crijns, H.J.G.M.; Rienstra, M.; Kirchhof, P.; Grove, E.L.; Pedersen, K.B.; Van Gelder, I.C. Cardioversion of Atrial Fibrillation and Atrial Flutter Revisited: Current Evidence and Practical Guidance for a Common Procedure. *EP Eur.* **2020**, *22*, 1149–1161. [CrossRef]
19. Voskoboinik, A.; Kalman, E.; Plunkett, G.; Knott, J.; Moskovitch, J.; Sanders, P.; Kistler, P.M.; Kalman, J.M. A Comparison of Early versus Delayed Elective Electrical Cardioversion for Recurrent Episodes of Persistent Atrial Fibrillation: A Multi-Center Study. *Int. J. Cardiol.* **2019**, *284*, 33–37. [CrossRef]
20. Yoon, M.; Yang, P.-S.; Jang, E.; Yu, H.T.; Kim, T.-H.; Uhm, J.-S.; Kim, J.-Y.; Sung, J.-H.; Pak, H.-N.; Lee, M.-H.; et al. Improved Population-Based Clinical Outcomes of Patients with Atrial Fibrillation by Compliance with the Simple ABC (Atrial Fibrillation Better Care) Pathway for Integrated Care Management: A Nationwide Cohort Study. *Thromb. Haemost.* **2019**, *119*, 1695–1703. [CrossRef]
21. Cheung, C.C.; Nattel, S.; Macle, L.; Andrade, J.G. Management of Atrial Fibrillation in 2021: An Updated Comparison of the Current CCS/CHRS, ESC, and AHA/ACC/HRS Guidelines. *Can. J. Cardiol.* **2021**, *37*, 1607–1618. [CrossRef] [PubMed]
22. Toufan, M.; Kazemi, B.; Molazadeh, N. The Significance of the Left Atrial Volume Index in Prediction of Atrial Fibrillation Recurrence after Electrical Cardioversion. *J. Cardiovasc. Thorac. Res.* **2017**, *9*, 54–59. [CrossRef] [PubMed]
23. Ecker, V.; Knoery, C.; Rushworth, G.; Rudd, I.; Ortner, A.; Begley, D.; Leslie, S.J. A Review of Factors Associated with Maintenance of Sinus Rhythm after Elective Electrical Cardioversion for Atrial Fibrillation. *Clin. Cardiol.* **2018**, *41*, 862–870. [CrossRef]
24. Conte, M.; Petraglia, L.; Cabaro, S.; Valerio, V.; Poggio, P.; Pilato, E.; Attena, E.; Russo, V.; Ferro, A.; Formisano, P.; et al. Epicardial Adipose Tissue and Cardiac Arrhythmias: Focus on Atrial Fibrillation. *Front. Cardiovasc. Med.* **2022**, *9*, 932262. [CrossRef]
25. Abe, I.; Teshima, Y.; Kondo, H.; Kaku, H.; Kira, S.; Ikebe, Y.; Saito, S.; Fukui, A.; Shinohara, T.; Yufu, K.; et al. Association of fibrotic remodeling and cytokines/chemokines content in epicardial adipose tissue with atrial myocardial fibrosis in patients with atrial fibrillation. *Heart Rhythm* **2018**, *15*, 1717–1727. [CrossRef] [PubMed]
26. Michniewicz, E.; Mlodawska, E.; Lopatowska, P.; Tomaszuk-Kazberuk, A.; Malyszko, J. Patients with atrial fibrillation and coronary artery disease—Double trouble. *Adv. Med. Sci.* **2018**, *63*, 30–35. [CrossRef] [PubMed]
27. Huang, T.; Nairn, D.; Chen, J.; Mueller-Edenborn, B.; Pilia, N.; Mayer, L.; Eichenlaub, M.; Moreno-Weidmann, Z.; Allgeier, J.; Trenk, D.; et al. Structural and electrophysiological determinants of atrial cardiomyopathy identify remodeling discrepancies between paroxysmal and persistent atrial fibrillation. *Front. Cardiovasc. Med.* **2023**, *9*, 1101152. [CrossRef]
28. Sánchez-Quintana, D.; López-Mínguez, J.R.; Pizarro, G.; Murillo, M.; Cabrera, J.A. Triggers and anatomical substrates in the genesis and perpetuation of atrial fibrillation. *Curr. Cardiol. Rev.* **2012**, *8*, 310–326. [CrossRef] [PubMed]
29. Gomez, J.F.; Cardona, K.; Martinez, L.; Saiz, J.; Trenor, B. Electrophysiological and structural remodeling in heart failure modulate arrhythmogenesis. 2D simulation study. *PLoS ONE* **2014**, *9*, e103273. [CrossRef]
30. Wang, Y.; Hill, J.A. Electrophysiological remodeling in heart failure. *J. Mol. Cell. Cardiol.* **2010**, *48*, 619–632. [CrossRef]
31. Janse, M.J. Electrophysiological changes in heart failure and their relationship to arrhythmogenesis. *Cardiovasc. Res.* **2004**, *61*, 208–217. [CrossRef]

31. Coronel, R.; Wilders, R.; Verkerk, A.O.; Wiegerinck, R.F.; Benoist, D.; Bernus, O. Electrophysiological changes in heart failure and their implications for arrhythmogenesis. *Biochim. Biophys. Acta* **2013**, *1832*, 2432–2441. [CrossRef]
32. Aistrup, G.L.; Balke, C.W.; Wasserstrom, J.A. Arrhythmia triggers in heart failure: The smoking gun of [Ca^{2+}]i dysregulation. *Heart Rhythm* **2011**, *8*, 1804–1808. [CrossRef]
33. Akar, F.G.; Rosenbaum, D.S. Transmural electrophysiological heterogeneities underlying arrhythmogenesis in heart failure. *Circ. Res.* **2003**, *93*, 638–645. [CrossRef] [PubMed]
34. Shi, C.; Wang, X.; Dong, F.; Wang, Y.; Hui, J.; Lin, Z.; Yang, J.; Xu, Y. Temporal alterations and cellular mechanisms of transmural repolarization during progression of mouse cardiac hypertrophy and failure. *Acta Physiol.* **2013**, *208*, 95–110. [CrossRef]
35. Yang, X.; Chen, Y.; Li, Y.; Ren, X.; Xing, Y.; Shang, H. Effects of Wenxin Keli on Cardiac Hypertrophy and Arrhythmia via Regulation of the Calcium/Calmodulin Dependent Kinase II Signaling Pathway. *Biomed. Res. Int.* **2017**, *2017*, 1569235. [CrossRef]
36. Kuba, K.; Sato, T.; Imai, Y.; Yamaguchi, T. Apelin and Elabela/Toddler; double ligands for APJ/Apelin receptor in heart development, physiology, and pathology. *Peptides* **2019**, *111*, 62–70. [CrossRef] [PubMed]
37. Baumgartner, C.; da Costa, B.R.; Collet, T.H.; Feller, M.; Floriani, C.; Bauer, D.C.; Cappola, A.R.; Heckbert, S.R.; Ceresini, G.; Gussekloo, J.; et al. Thyroid Function within the Normal Range, Subclinical Hypothyroidism, and the Risk of Atrial Fibrillation. *Circulation* **2017**, *136*, 2100–2116. [CrossRef] [PubMed]
38. Song, X.; Nie, L.; Long, J.; Zhao, J.; Liu, X.; Wang, L.; Liu, D.; Wang, S.; Liu, S.; Yang, J. Hydrogen sulfide alleviates hypothyroidism induced myocardial fibrosis in rats through stimulating autophagy and inhibiting TGF-β1/Smad2 pathway. *Korean J. Physiol. Pharmacol.* **2023**, *27*, 1–8. [CrossRef]
39. Karam, B.S.; Chavez-Moreno, A.; Koh, W.; Akar, J.G.; Akar, F.G. Oxidative stress and inflammation as central mediators of atrial fibrillation in obesity and diabetes. *Cardiovasc. Diabetol.* **2017**, *16*, 120. [CrossRef]
40. Chan, Y.H.; Chang, G.J.; Lai, Y.J.; Chen, W.J.; Chang, S.H.; Hung, L.M.; Kuo, C.T.; Yeh, Y.H. Atrial fibrillation and its arrhythmogenesis associated with insulin resistance. *Cardiovasc. Diabetol.* **2019**, *18*, 125. [CrossRef]
41. Glukhov, A.V.; Fedorov, V.V.; Kalish, P.W.; Ravikumar, V.K.; Lou, Q.; Janks, D.; Schuessler, R.B.; Moazami, N.; Efimov, I.R. Conduction remodeling in human end-stage nonischemic left ventricular cardiomyopathy. *Circulation* **2012**, *125*, 1835–1847. [CrossRef]
42. Wiegerinck, R.F.; van Veen, T.A.; Belterman, C.N.; Schumacher, C.A.; Noorman, M.; de Bakker, J.M.; Coronel, R. Transmural dispersion of refractoriness and conduction velocity is associated with heterogeneously reduced connexin-43 in a rabbit model of heart failure. *Heart Rhythm* **2008**, *5*, 1178–1185. [CrossRef]
43. Akar, F.G.; Nass, R.D.; Hahn, S.; Cingolani, E.; Shah, M.; Hesketh, G.G.; DiSilvestre, D.; Tunin, R.S.; Kass, D.A.; Tomaselli, G.F. Dynamic changes in conduction velocity and gap junction properties during development of pacing-induced heart failure. *Am. J. Physiol. Heart Circ. Physiol.* **2007**, *293*, H1223–H1230. [CrossRef]
44. Yan, J.; Killingsworth, C.; Walcott, G.; Zhu, Y.; Litovsky, S.; Huang, J.; Ai, X.; Pogwizd, S.M. Molecular remodeling of Cx43, but not structural remodeling, promotes arrhythmias in an arrhythmogenic canine model of nonischemic heart failure. *J. Mol. Cell. Cardiol.* **2021**, *158*, 72–81. [CrossRef]
45. Poelzing, S.; Rosenbaum, D.S. Altered connexin43 expression produces arrhythmia substrate in heart failure. *Am. J. Physiol. Heart Circ. Physiol.* **2004**, *287*, H1762–H1770. [CrossRef] [PubMed]
46. Vitale, E.; Rosso, R.; Lo Iacono, M.; Cristallini, C.; Giachino, C.; Rastaldo, R. Apelin-13 Increases Functional Connexin-43 through Autophagy Inhibition via AKT/mTOR Pathway in the Non-Myocytic Cell Population of the Heart. *Int. J. Mol. Sci.* **2022**, *23*, 13073. [CrossRef] [PubMed]
47. Chen, Y.; Qiao, X.; Zhang, L.; Li, X.; Liu, Q. Apelin-13 regulates angiotensin ii-induced Cx43 downregulation and autophagy via the AMPK/mTOR signaling pathway in HL-1 cells. *Physiol. Res.* **2020**, *69*, 813–822. [CrossRef] [PubMed]
48. Yang, M.; Song, J.J.; Yang, X.C.; Zhong, G.Z.; Zhong, J.C. MiRNA-122-5p inhibitor abolishes angiotensin II-mediated loss of autophagy and promotion of apoptosis in rat cardiofibroblasts by modulation of the apelin-AMPK-mTOR signaling. *In Vitro Cell. Dev. Biol. Anim.* **2022**, *58*, 136–148. [CrossRef]
49. Song, J.; Zhang, Z.; Dong, Z.; Liu, X.; Liu, Y.; Li, X.; Xu, Y.; Guo, Y.; Wang, N.; Zhang, M.; et al. MicroRNA-122-5p Aggravates Angiotensin II-Mediated Myocardial Fibrosis and Dysfunction in Hypertensive Rats by Regulating the Elabela/Apelin-APJ and ACE2-GDF15-Porimin Signaling. *J. Cardiovasc. Transl. Res.* **2022**, *15*, 535–547. [CrossRef]
50. Beyer, C.; Tokarska, L.; Stühlinger, M.; Feuchtner, G.; Hintringer, F.; Honold, S.; Fiedler, L.; Schönbauer, M.S.; Schönbauer, R.; Plank, F. Structural Cardiac Remodeling in Atrial Fibrillation. *JACC Cardiovasc. Imaging* **2021**, *14*, 2199–2208. [CrossRef] [PubMed]
51. Jackson, L.R., 2nd; Rathakrishnan, B.; Campbell, K.; Thomas, K.L.; Piccini, J.P.; Bahnson, T.; Stiber, J.A.; Daubert, J.P. Sinus Node Dysfunction and Atrial Fibrillation: A Reversible Phenomenon? *Pacing Clin. Electrophysiol.* **2017**, *40*, 442–450. [CrossRef] [PubMed]
52. Elliott, J.; Mainardi, L.; Rodriguez Matas, J.F. Cellular heterogeneity and repolarisation across the atria: An in silico study. *Med. Biol. Eng. Comput.* **2022**, *60*, 3153–3168. [CrossRef]
53. Da Costa, A.; Mourot, S.; Roméyer-Bouchard, C.; Thévenin, J.; Samuel, B.; Kihel, A.; Isaaz, K. Anatomic and electrophysiological differences between chronic and paroxysmal forms of common atrial flutter and comparison with controls. *Pacing Clin. Electrophysiol.* **2004**, *27*, 1202–1211. [CrossRef]

4. Soulat-Dufour, L.; Lang, S.; Addetia, K.; Ederhy, S.; Adavane-Scheuble, S.; Chauvet-Droit, M.; Jean, M.L.; Nhan, P.; Ben Said, R.; Kamami, I.; et al. Restoring Sinus Rhythm Reverses Cardiac Remodeling and Reduces Valvular Regurgitation in Patients with Atrial Fibrillation. *J. Am. Coll. Cardiol.* **2022**, *79*, 951–961. [CrossRef] [PubMed]
5. Jacquemet, V.; Henriquez, C.S. Modelling cardiac fibroblasts: Interactions with myocytes and their impact on impulse propagation. *Europace* **2007**, *9* (Suppl. S6), vi29–vi37. [CrossRef]
6. Duffy, H.S. Fibroblasts, myofibroblasts, and fibrosis: Fact, fiction, and the future. *J. Cardiovasc. Pharmacol.* **2011**, *57*, 373–375. [CrossRef]
7. Rohr, S. Cardiac fibroblasts in cell culture systems: Myofibroblasts all along? *J. Cardiovasc. Pharmacol.* **2011**, *57*, 389–399. [CrossRef]
8. Dhein, S.; Salameh, A. Remodeling of Cardiac Gap Junctional Cell-Cell Coupling. *Cells* **2021**, *10*, 2422. [CrossRef]
9. Ravens, U.; Peyronnet, R. Electrical Remodelling in Cardiac Disease. *Cells* **2023**, *12*, 230. [CrossRef] [PubMed]
10. Wolfes, J.; Ellermann, C.; Frommeyer, G.; Eckardt, L. Evidence-based treatment of atrial fibrillation around the globe: Comparison of the latest ESC, AHA/ACC/HRS, and CCS guidelines on the management of atrial fibrillation. *Rev. Cardiovasc. Med.* **2022**, *23*, 56. [CrossRef] [PubMed]
11. Burton, J.H.; Vinson, D.R.; Drummond, K.; Strout, T.D.; Thode, H.C.; McInturff, J.J. Electrical cardioversion of emergency department patients with atrial fibrillation. *Ann. Emerg. Med.* **2004**, *44*, 20–30. [CrossRef]
12. Michael, J.A.; Stiell, I.G.; Agarwal, S.; Mandavia, D.P. Cardioversion of paroxysmal atrial fibrillation in the emergency department. *Ann. Emerg. Med.* **1999**, *33*, 379–387. [CrossRef] [PubMed]
13. Dankner, R.; Shahar, A.; Novikov, I.; Agmon, U.; Ziv, A.; Hod, H. Treatment of stable atrial fibrillation in the emergency department: A population-based comparison of electrical direct-current versus pharmacological cardioversion or conservative management. *Cardiology* **2009**, *112*, 270–278. [CrossRef]
14. Von Besser, K.; Mills, A.M. Is discharge to home after emergency department cardioversion safe for the treatment of recent-onset atrial fibrillation? *Ann. Emerg. Med.* **2011**, *58*, 517–520. [CrossRef]
15. Xavier Scheuermeyer, F.; Grafstein, E.; Stenstrom, R.; Innes, G.; Poureslami, I.; Sighary, M. Thirty-day outcomes of emergency department patients undergoing electrical cardioversion for atrial fibrillation or flutter. *Acad. Emerg. Med.* **2010**, *17*, 408–415. [CrossRef] [PubMed]
16. Santini, M.; De Ferrari, G.M.; Pandozi, C.; Alboni, P.; Capucci, A.; Disertori, M.; Gaita, F.; Lombardi, F.; Maggioni, A.P.; Mugelli, A.; et al. Atrial fibrillation requiring urgent medical care. Approach and outcome in the various departments of admission. Data from the atrial Fibrillation/flutter Italian REgistry (FIRE). *Ital. Heart J.* **2004**, *5*, 205–213. [PubMed]
17. Cohn, B.G.; Keim, S.M.; Yealy, D.M. Is emergency department cardioversion of recent-onset atrial fibrillation safe and effective? *J. Emerg. Med.* **2013**, *45*, 117–127. [CrossRef]
18. Cristoni, L.; Tampieri, A.; Mucci, F.; Iannone, P.; Venturi, A.; Cavazza, M.; Lenzi, T. Cardioversion of acute atrial fibrillation in the short observation unit: Comparison of a protocol focused on electrical cardioversion with simple antiarrhythmic treatment. *Emerg. Med. J.* **2011**, *28*, 932–937. [CrossRef]
19. Houghton, A.R.; Sharman, A.; Pohl, J.E. Determinants of successful direct current cardioversion for atrial fibrillation and flutter: The importance of rapid referral. *Br. J. Gen. Pract.* **2000**, *50*, 710–711.
20. Boriani, G.; Diemberger, I.; Biffi, M.; Domenichini, G.; Martignani, C.; Valzania, C.; Branzi, A. Electrical cardioversion for persistent atrial fibrillation or atrial flutter in clinical practice: Predictors of long-term outcome. *Int. J. Clin. Pract.* **2007**, *61*, 748–756. [CrossRef] [PubMed]
21. Larsen, M.T.; Lyngborg, K.; Pedersen, F.; Corell, P. Predictive factors of maintenance of sinus rhythm after direct current (DC) cardioversion of atrial fibrillation/atrial flutter. *Ugeskr. Laeger* **2005**, *167*, 3408–3412. [PubMed]
22. Mittal, S.; Ayati, S.; Stein, K.M.; Schwartzman, D.; Cavlovich, D.; Tchou, P.J.; Markowitz, S.M.; Slotwiner, D.J.; Scheiner, M.A.; Lerman, B.B. Transthoracic cardioversion of atrial fibrillation: Comparison of rectilinear biphasic versus damped sine wave monophasic shocks. *Circulation* **2000**, *101*, 1282–1287. [CrossRef] [PubMed]
23. Inácio, J.F.; da Rosa Mdos, S.; Shah, J.; Rosário, J.; Vissoci, J.R.; Manica, A.L.; Rodrigues, C.G. Monophasic and biphasic shock for transthoracic conversion of atrial fibrillation: Systematic review and network meta-analysis. *Resuscitation* **2016**, *100*, 66–75. [CrossRef]
24. McDonagh, T.A.; Metra, M.; Adamo, M.; Gardner, R.S.; Baumbach, A.; Böhm, M.; Burri, H.; Butler, J.; Čelutkienė, J.; Chioncel, O.; et al. 2021 ESC Guidelines for the diagnosis and treatment of acute and chronic heart failure. *Eur. Heart J.* **2021**, *42*, 3599–3726. [CrossRef]
25. Heidenreich, P.A.; Bozkurt, B.; Aguilar, D.; Allen, L.A.; Byun, J.J.; Colvin, M.M.; Deswal, A.; Drazner, M.H.; Dunlay, S.M.; Evers, L.R.; et al. 2022 AHA/ACC/HFSA Guideline for the Management of Heart Failure: A Report of the American College of Cardiology/American Heart Association Joint Committee on Clinical Practice Guidelines. *Circulation* **2022**, *145*, e895–e1032. [CrossRef]
26. Cui, K.; Huang, W.; Fan, J.; Lei, H. Midregional pro-atrial natriuretic peptide is a superior biomarker to N-terminal pro-B-type natriuretic peptide in the diagnosis of heart failure patients with preserved ejection fraction. *Medicine* **2018**, *97*, e12277. [CrossRef]
27. Okutucu, S.; Gorenek, B. Current Recommendations on Atrial Fibrillation: A Comparison of the Recent European and Canadian Guidelines. *Cardiology* **2022**, *147*, 81–89. [CrossRef] [PubMed]

78. Schnabel, R.B.; Larson, M.G.; Yamamoto, J.F.; Sullivan, L.M.; Pencina, M.J.; Meigs, J.B.; Tofler, G.H.; Selhub, J.; Jacques, P.F.; Wolf, P.A.; et al. Relations of biomarkers of distinct pathophysiological pathways and atrial fibrillation incidence in the community. *Circulation* **2010**, *121*, 200–207. [CrossRef] [PubMed]
79. Fan, J.; Cao, H.; Su, L.; Ling, Z.; Liu, Z.; Lan, X.; Xu, Y.; Chen, W.; Yin, Y. NT-proBNP, but not ANP and C-reactive protein, is predictive of paroxysmal atrial fibrillation in patients undergoing pulmonary vein isolation. *J. Interv. Card. Electrophysiol.* **2012**, *33*, 93–100. [CrossRef] [PubMed]
80. Beck-da-Silva, L.; de Bold, A.; Fraser, M.; Williams, K.; Haddad, H. Brain natriuretic peptide predicts successful cardioversion in patients with atrial fibrillation and maintenance of sinus rhythm. *Can. J. Cardiol.* **2004**, *20*, 1245–1248.
81. Xu, X.; Tang, Y. Relationship between Brain Natriuretic Peptide and Recurrence of Atrial Fibrillation after Successful Electrical Cardioversion: An Updated Meta-Analysis. *Braz. J. Cardiovasc. Surg.* **2017**, *32*, 530–535. [CrossRef] [PubMed]
82. Ari, H.; Binici, S.; Ari, S.; Akkaya, M.; Koca, V.; Bozat, T.; Gürdoğan, M. The predictive value of plasma brain natriuretic peptide for the recurrence of atrial fibrillation six months after external cardioversion. *Turk. Kardiyol. Dern. Ars.* **2008**, *36*, 456–460.
83. Meyre, P.B.; Aeschbacher, S.; Blum, S.; Voellmin, G.; Kastner, P.M.; Hennings, E.; Kaufmann, B.A.; Kühne, M.; Osswald, S.; Conen, D. Biomarkers associated with rhythm status after cardioversion in patients with atrial fibrillation. *Sci. Rep.* **2022**, *12*, 1680. [CrossRef] [PubMed]
84. Wozakowska-Kapłon, B.; Bartkowiak, R.; Grabowska, U.; Janiszewska, G. B-type natriuretic peptide level after sinus rhythm restoration in patients with persistent atrial fibrillation—clinical significance. *Kardiol. Pol.* **2010**, *68*, 781–786.
85. Andersson, J.; Rosenqvist, M.; Tornvall, P.; Boman, K. NT-proBNP predicts maintenance of sinus rhythm after electrical cardioversion. *Thromb. Res.* **2015**, *135*, 289–291. [CrossRef]
86. Kallergis, E.M.; Manios, E.G.; Kanoupakis, E.M.; Mavrakis, H.E.; Goudis, C.A.; Maliaraki, N.E.; Saloustros, I.G.; Milathianaki, M.E.; Chlouverakis, G.I.; Vardas, P.E. Effect of sinus rhythm restoration after electrical cardioversion on apelin and brain natriuretic Peptide prohormone levels in patients with persistent atrial fibrillation. *Am. J. Cardiol.* **2010**, *105*, 90–94. [CrossRef] [PubMed]
87. Tveit, A.; Seljeflot, I.; Grundvold, I.; Abdelnoor, M.; Arnesen, H.; Smith, P. Candesartan, NT-proBNP and recurrence of atrial fibrillation after electrical cardioversion. *Int. J. Cardiol.* **2009**, *131*, 234–239. [CrossRef]
88. Mabuchi, N.; Tsutamoto, T.; Maeda, K.; Kinoshita, M. Plasma cardiac natriuretic peptides as biochemical markers of recurrence of atrial fibrillation in patients with mild congestive heart failure. *Jpn. Circ. J.* **2000**, *64*, 765–771. [CrossRef]
89. Lewicka, E.; Dudzińska-Gehrmann, J.; Dąbrowska-Kugacka, A.; Zagożdżon, P.; Stepnowska, E.; Liżewska, A.; Kozłowski, D.; Raczak, G. Plasma biomarkers as predictors of recurrence of atrial fibrillation. *Pol. Arch. Med. Wewn.* **2015**, *125*, 424–433. [CrossRef]
90. Buccelletti, F.; Gilardi, E.; Marsiliani, D.; Carroccia, A.; Silveri, N.G.; Franceschi, F. Predictive value of NT-proBNP for cardioversion in a new onset atrial fibrillation. *Eur. J. Emerg. Med.* **2011**, *18*, 157–161. [CrossRef]
91. Koniari, I.; Artopoulou, E.; Velissaris, D.; Ainslie, M.; Mplani, V.; Karavasili, G.; Kounis, N.; Tsigkas, G. Biomarkers in the clinical management of patients with atrial fibrillation and heart failure. *J. Geriatr. Cardiol.* **2021**, *18*, 908–951. [CrossRef]
92. Scalise, R.F.M.; De Sarro, R.; Caracciolo, A.; Lauro, R.; Squadrito, F.; Carerj, S.; Bitto, A.; Micari, A.; Bella, G.D.; Costa, F.; et al. Fibrosis after Myocardial Infarction: An Overview on Cellular Processes, Molecular Pathways, Clinical Evaluation and Prognostic Value. *Med. Sci.* **2021**, *9*, 16. [CrossRef] [PubMed]
93. Kawamura, M.; Ito, H.; Onuki, T.; Miyoshi, F.; Watanabe, N.; Asano, T.; Tanno, K.; Kobayashi, Y. Candesartan decreases type III procollagen-N-peptide levels and inflammatory marker levels and maintains sinus rhythm in patients with atrial fibrillation. *J. Cardiovasc. Pharmacol.* **2010**, *55*, 511–517. [CrossRef]
94. Clementy, N.; Piver, E.; Bisson, A.; Andre, C.; Bernard, A.; Pierre, B.; Fauchier, L.; Babuty, D. Galectin-3 in Atrial Fibrillation: Mechanisms and Therapeutic Implications. *Int. J. Mol. Sci.* **2018**, *19*, 976. [CrossRef] [PubMed]
95. Ho, J.E.; Yin, X.; Levy, D.; Vasan, R.S.; Magnani, J.W.; Ellinor, P.T.; McManus, D.D.; Lubitz, S.A.; Larson, M.G.; Benjamin, E.J. Galectin 3 and incident atrial fibrillation in the community. *Am. Heart J.* **2014**, *167*, 729–734.e1. [CrossRef]
96. Takemoto, Y.; Ramirez, R.J.; Yokokawa, M.; Kaur, K.; Ponce-Balbuena, D.; Sinno, M.C.; Willis, B.C.; Ghanbari, H.; Ennis, S.R.; Guerrero-Serna, G.; et al. Galectin-3 Regulates Atrial Fibrillation Remodeling and Predicts Catheter Ablation Outcomes. *JACC Basic Transl. Sci.* **2016**, *1*, 143–154. [CrossRef]
97. Yalcin, M.U.; Gurses, K.M.; Kocyigit, D.; Canpinar, H.; Canpolat, U.; Evranos, B.; Yorgun, H.; Sahiner, M.L.; Kaya, E.B.; Hazirolan, T.; et al. The Association of Serum Galectin-3 Levels with Atrial Electrical and Structural Remodeling. *J. Cardiovasc. Electrophysiol.* **2015**, *26*, 635–640. [CrossRef]
98. Gürses, K.M.; Yalçın, M.U.; Koçyiğit, D.; Canpınar, H.; Ateş, A.H.; Canpolat, U.; Yorgun, H.; Güç, D.; Aytemir, K. Serum galectin-3 level predicts early recurrence following successful direct-current cardioversion in persistent atrial fibrillation patients. *Turk. Kardiyol. Dern. Ars.* **2019**, *47*, 564–571. [CrossRef] [PubMed]
99. Wałek, P.; Grabowska, U.; Cieśla, E.; Sielski, J.; Roskal-Wałek, J.; Wożakowska-Kapłon, B. Analysis of the Correlation of Galectin-3 Concentration with the Measurements of Echocardiographic Parameters Assessing Left Atrial Remodeling and Function in Patients with Persistent Atrial Fibrillation. *Biomolecules* **2021**, *11*, 1108. [CrossRef]
100. Gong, M.; Cheung, A.; Wang, Q.S.; Li, G.; Goudis, C.A.; Bazoukis, G.; Lip, G.Y.H.; Baranchuk, A.; Korantzopoulos, P.; Letsas, K.P.; et al. Galectin-3 and risk of atrial fibrillation: A systematic review and meta-analysis. *J. Clin. Lab. Anal.* **2020**, *34*, e23104. [CrossRef]

1. Cichoń, M.; Mizia-Szubryt, M.; Olszanecka-Glinianowicz, M.; Bożentowicz-Wikarek, M.; Owczarek, A.J.; Michalik, R.; Mizia-Stec, K. Biomarkers of left atrial overload in obese and nonobese patients with atrial fibrillation qualified for electrical cardioversion. *Kardiol. Pol.* **2021**, *79*, 269–276. [CrossRef]
2. Pauklin, P.; Zilmer, M.; Eha, J.; Tootsi, K.; Kals, M.; Kampus, P. Markers of Inflammation, Oxidative Stress, and Fibrosis in Patients with Atrial Fibrillation. *Oxid. Med. Cell. Longev.* **2022**, *2022*, 4556671. [CrossRef] [PubMed]
3. Saez-Maleta, R.; Merino-Merino, A.; Gundin-Menendez, S.; Salgado-Aranda, R.; Al Kassam-Martinez, D.; Pascual-Tejerina, V.; Martin-Gonzalez, J.; Garcia-Fernandez, J.; Perez-Rivera, J.A. sST2 and Galectin-3 genotyping in patients with persistent atrial fibrillation. *Mol. Biol. Rep.* **2021**, *48*, 1601–1606. [CrossRef] [PubMed]
4. Liu, J.H.; Han, Q.F.; Mo, D.G. The progress of the soluble suppression of tumorigenicity 2 (sST2) in atrial fibrillation. *J. Interv. Card. Electrophysiol.* **2022**, *65*, 591–592. [CrossRef] [PubMed]
5. Fan, J.; Li, Y.; Yan, Q.; Wu, W.; Xu, P.; Liu, L.; Luan, C.; Zhang, J.; Zheng, Q.; Xue, J. Higher serum sST2 is associated with increased left atrial low-voltage areas and atrial fibrillation recurrence in patients undergoing radiofrequency ablation. *J. Interv. Card. Electrophysiol.* **2022**, *64*, 733–742. [CrossRef] [PubMed]
6. Chen, L.; Chen, W.; Shao, Y.; Zhang, M.; Li, Z.; Wang, Z.; Lu, Y. Association of Soluble Suppression of Tumorigenicity 2 with New-Onset Atrial Fibrillation in Acute Myocardial Infarction. *Cardiology* **2022**, *147*, 381–388. [CrossRef]
7. Tseng, C.C.S.; Huibers, M.M.H.; van Kuik, J.; de Weger, R.A.; Vink, A.; de Jonge, N. The interleukin-33/ST2 pathway is expressed in the failing human heart and associated with pro-fibrotic remodeling of the myocardium. *J. Cardiovasc. Transl. Res.* **2018**, *11*, 15–21. [CrossRef]
8. Zhao, L.; Li, S.; Zhang, C.; Tian, J.; Lu, A.; Bai, R.; An, J.; Greiser, A.; Huang, J.; Ma, X. Cardiovascular magnetic resonance-determined left ventricular myocardium impairment is associated with C-reactive protein and ST2 in patients with paroxysmal atrial fibrillation. *J. Cardiovasc. Magn. Reson.* **2021**, *23*, 30. [CrossRef] [PubMed]
9. Sun, W.P.; Du, X.; Chen, J.J. Biomarkers for Predicting the Occurrence and Progression of Atrial Fibrillation: Soluble Suppression of Tumorigenicity 2 Protein and Tissue Inhibitor of Matrix Metalloproteinase-1. *Int. J. Clin. Pract.* **2022**, *2022*, 6926510. [CrossRef] [PubMed]
10. Okar, S.; Kaypakli, O.; Şahin, D.Y.; Koç, M. Fibrosis Marker Soluble ST2 Predicts Atrial Fibrillation Recurrence after Cryoballoon Catheter Ablation of Nonvalvular Paroxysmal Atrial Fibrillation. *Korean Circ. J.* **2018**, *48*, 920–929. [CrossRef]
11. Liu, H.; Wang, K.; Lin, Y.; Liang, X.; Zhao, S.; Li, M.; Chen, M. Role of sST2 in predicting recurrence of atrial fibrillation after radiofrequency catheter ablation. *Pacing Clin. Electrophysiol.* **2020**, *43*, 1235–1241. [CrossRef]
12. Wałek, P.; Gorczyca, I.; Grabowska, U.; Spałek, M.; Wożakowska-Kapłon, B. The prognostic value of soluble suppression of tumourigenicity 2 and galectin-3 for sinus rhythm maintenance after cardioversion due to persistent atrial fibrillation in patients with normal left ventricular systolic function. *Europace* **2020**, *22*, 1470–1479. [CrossRef]
13. Begg, G.A.; Lip, G.Y.; Plein, S.; Tayebjee, M.H. Circulating biomarkers of fibrosis and cardioversion of atrial fibrillation: A prospective, controlled cohort study. *Clin. Biochem.* **2017**, *50*, 11–15. [CrossRef] [PubMed]
14. Kawamura, M.; Munetsugu, Y.; Kawasaki, S.; Onishi, K.; Onuma, Y.; Kikuchi, M.; Tanno, K.; Kobayashi, Y. Type III procollagen-N-peptide as a predictor of persistent atrial fibrillation recurrence after cardioversion. *Europace* **2012**, *14*, 1719–1725. [CrossRef] [PubMed]
15. Çöteli, C.; Hazırolan, T.; Aytemir, K.; Erdemir, A.G.; Bakır, E.N.; Canpolat, U.; Yorgun, H.; Ateş, A.H.; Kaya, E.B.; Dikmen, Z.G.; et al. Evaluation of atrial fibrosis in atrial fibrillation patients with three different methods. *Turk. J. Med. Sci.* **2022**, *52*, 175–187. [CrossRef]
16. Dong, Q.; Li, S.; Wang, W.; Han, L.; Xia, Z.; Wu, Y.; Tang, Y.; Li, J.; Cheng, X. FGF23 regulates atrial fibrosis in atrial fibrillation by mediating the STAT3 and SMAD3 pathways. *J. Cell. Physiol.* **2019**, *234*, 19502–19510. [CrossRef] [PubMed]
17. Chen, J.M.; Zhong, Y.T.; Tu, C.; Lan, J. Significance of serum fibroblast growth factor-23 and miR-208b in pathogenesis of atrial fibrillation and their relationship with prognosis. *World J. Clin. Cases* **2020**, *8*, 3458–3464. [CrossRef]
18. Mizia-Stec, K.; Wieczorek, J.; Polak, M.; Wybraniec, M.T.; Woźniak-Skowerska, I.; Hoffmann, A.; Nowak, S.; Wikarek, M.; Wnuk-Wojnar, A.; Chudek, J.; et al. Lower soluble Klotho and higher fibroblast growth factor 23 serum levels are associated with episodes of atrial fibrillation. *Cytokine* **2018**, *111*, 106–111. [CrossRef]
19. Chua, W.; Purmah, Y.; Cardoso, V.R.; Gkoutos, G.V.; Tull, S.P.; Neculau, G.; Thomas, M.R.; Kotecha, D.; Lip, G.Y.H.; Kirchhof, P.; et al. Data-driven discovery and validation of circulating blood-based biomarkers associated with prevalent atrial fibrillation. *Eur. Heart J.* **2019**, *40*, 1268–1276. [CrossRef]
20. Tan, Z.; Song, T.; Huang, S.; Liu, M.; Ma, J.; Zhang, J.; Yu, P.; Liu, X. Relationship between serum growth differentiation factor 15, fibroblast growth factor-23 and risk of atrial fibrillation: A systematic review and meta-analysis. *Front. Cardiovasc. Med.* **2022**, *9*, 899667. [CrossRef]
21. Wang, D.; Day, E.A.; Townsend, L.K.; Djordjevic, D.; Jørgensen, S.B.; Steinberg, G.R. GDF15: Emerging biology and therapeutic applications for obesity and cardiometabolic disease. *Nat. Rev. Endocrinol.* **2021**, *17*, 592–607. [CrossRef]
22. Breit, S.N.; Brown, D.A.; Tsai, V.W. The GDF15-GFRAL Pathway in Health and Metabolic Disease: Friend or Foe? *Annu. Rev. Physiol.* **2021**, *83*, 127–151. [CrossRef]
23. Perrone, M.A.; Aimo, A.; Bernardini, S.; Clerico, A. Inflammageing and Cardiovascular System: Focus on Cardiokines and Cardiac-Specific Biomarkers. *Int. J. Mol. Sci.* **2023**, *24*, 844. [CrossRef]

124. Aulin, J.; Hijazi, Z.; Lindbäck, J.; Alexander, J.H.; Gersh, B.J.; Granger, C.B.; Hanna, M.; Horowitz, J.; Lopes, R.D.; McMurray, J.J.V.; et al. Biomarkers and heart failure events in patients with atrial fibrillation in the ARISTOTLE trial evaluated by a multi-state model. *Am. Heart J.* **2022**, *251*, 13–24. [CrossRef] [PubMed]
125. Hijazi, Z.; Wallentin, L.; Lindbäck, J.; Alexander, J.H.; Connolly, S.J.; Eikelboom, J.W.; Ezekowitz, M.D.; Granger, C.B.; Lopes, R.D.; Pol, T.; et al. Screening of Multiple Biomarkers Associated with Ischemic Stroke in Atrial Fibrillation. *J. Am. Heart Assoc.* **2020**, *9*, e018984. [CrossRef]
126. Charafeddine, K.; Zakka, P.; Bou Dargham, B.; Abdulhai, F.; Zakka, K.; Zouein, F.A.; Refaat, M. Potential Biomarkers in Atrial Fibrillation: Insight into Their Clinical Significance. *J. Cardiovasc. Pharmacol.* **2021**, *78*, 184–191. [CrossRef] [PubMed]
127. Shao, Q.; Liu, H.; Ng, C.Y.; Xu, G.; Liu, E.; Li, G.; Liu, T. Circulating serum levels of growth differentiation factor-15 and neuregulin-1 in patients with paroxysmal non-valvular atrial fibrillation. *Int. J. Cardiol.* **2014**, *172*, e311–e313. [CrossRef]
128. Eddy, A.C.; Trask, A.J. Growth differentiation factor-15 and its role in diabetes and cardiovascular disease. *Cytokine Growth Factor Rev.* **2021**, *57*, 11–18. [CrossRef] [PubMed]
129. Lyngbakken, M.N.; Rønningen, P.S.; Solberg, M.G.; Berge, T.; Brynildsen, J.; Aagaard, E.N.; Kvisvik, B.; Røsjø, H.; Steine, K.; Tveit, A.; et al. Prediction of incident atrial fibrillation with cardiac biomarkers and left atrial volumes. *Heart* **2023**, *109*, 356–363. [CrossRef] [PubMed]
130. Matusik, P.T.; Małecka, B.; Lelakowski, J.; Undas, A. Association of NT-proBNP and GDF-15 with markers of a prothrombotic state in patients with atrial fibrillation off anticoagulation. *Clin. Res. Cardiol.* **2020**, *109*, 426–434. [CrossRef]
131. Ding, B.; Liu, P.; Zhang, F.; Hui, J.; He, L. Predicting Values of Neutrophil-to-Lymphocyte Ratio (NLR), High-Sensitivity C-Reactive Protein (hs-CRP), and Left Atrial Diameter (LAD) in Patients with Nonvalvular Atrial Fibrillation Recurrence After Radiofrequency Ablation. *Med. Sci. Monit.* **2022**, *28*, e934569. [CrossRef]
132. Li, X.; Peng, S.; Wu, X.; Guan, B.; Tse, G.; Chen, S.; Zhou, G.; Wei, Y.; Gong, C.; Lu, X.; et al. C-reactive protein and atrial fibrillation. Insights from epidemiological and Mendelian randomization studies. *Nutr. Metab. Cardiovasc. Dis.* **2022**, *32*, 1519–1527. [CrossRef]
133. Fu, Y.; Pan, Y.; Gao, Y.; Yang, X.; Chen, M. Predictive value of CHA2DS2-VASc score combined with hs-CRP for new-onset atrial fibrillation in elderly patients with acute myocardial infarction. *BMC Cardiovasc. Disord.* **2021**, *21*, 175. [CrossRef]
134. Sinning, C.; Kempf, T.; Schwarzl, M.; Lanfermann, S.; Ojeda, F.; Schnabel, R.B.; Zengin, E.; Wild, P.S.; Lackner, K.J.; Munzel, T.; et al. Biomarkers for characterization of heart failure–Distinction of heart failure with preserved and reduced ejection fraction. *Int. J. Cardiol.* **2017**, *227*, 272–277. [CrossRef] [PubMed]
135. Georgakopoulos, C.; Vlachopoulos, C.; Lazaros, G.; Tousoulis, D. Biomarkers of Atrial Fibrillation in Metabolic Syndrome. *Curr. Med. Chem.* **2019**, *26*, 898–908. [CrossRef]
136. Sun, J.; Xu, J.; Yang, Q. Expression and predictive value of NLRP3 in patients with atrial fibrillation and stroke. *Am. J. Transl. Res.* **2022**, *14*, 3104–3112. [PubMed]
137. Loricchio, M.L.; Cianfrocca, C.; Pasceri, V.; Bianconi, L.; Auriti, A.; Calo, L.; Lamberti, F.; Castro, A.; Pandozi, C.; Palamara, A.; et al. Relation of C-reactive protein to long-term risk of recurrence of atrial fibrillation after electrical cardioversion. *Am. J. Cardiol.* **2007**, *99*, 1421–1424. [CrossRef]
138. Lombardi, F.; Tundo, F.; Belletti, S.; Mantero, A.; Melzi D'eril, G.V. C-reactive protein but not atrial dysfunction predicts recurrences of atrial fibrillation after cardioversion in patients with preserved left ventricular function. *J. Cardiovasc. Med.* **2008**, *9*, 581–588. [CrossRef] [PubMed]
139. Barassi, A.; Pezzilli, R.; Morselli-Labate, A.M.; Lombardi, F.; Belletti, S.; Dogliotti, G.; Corsi, M.M.; Merlini, G.; Melzi d'Eril, G.V. Serum amyloid a and C-reactive protein independently predict the recurrences of atrial fibrillation after cardioversion in patients with preserved left ventricular function. *Can. J. Cardiol.* **2012**, *28*, 537–541. [CrossRef]
140. Korantzopoulos, P.; Kalantzi, K.; Siogas, K.; Goudevenos, J.A. Long-term prognostic value of baseline C-reactive protein in predicting recurrence of atrial fibrillation after electrical cardioversion. *Pacing Clin. Electrophysiol.* **2008**, *31*, 1272–1276. [CrossRef] [PubMed]
141. Watanabe, E.; Arakawa, T.; Uchiyama, T.; Kodama, I.; Hishida, H. High-sensitivity C-reactive protein is predictive of successful cardioversion for atrial fibrillation and maintenance of sinus rhythm after conversion. *Int. J. Cardiol.* **2006**, *108*, 346–353. [CrossRef]
142. Henningsen, K.M.; Therkelsen, S.K.; Bruunsgaard, H.; Krabbe, K.S.; Pedersen, B.K.; Svendsen, J.H. Prognostic impact of hs-CRP and IL-6 in patients with persistent atrial fibrillation treated with electrical cardioversion. *Scand. J. Clin. Lab. Investig.* **2009**, *69*, 425–432. [CrossRef]
143. Liu, T.; Li, L.; Korantzopoulos, P.; Goudevenos, J.A.; Li, G. Meta-analysis of association between C-reactive protein and immediate success of electrical cardioversion in persistent atrial fibrillation. *Am. J. Cardiol.* **2008**, *101*, 1749–1752. [CrossRef] [PubMed]
144. Yo, C.H.; Lee, S.H.; Chang, S.S.; Lee, M.C.; Lee, C.C. Value of high-sensitivity C-reactive protein assays in predicting atrial fibrillation recurrence: A systematic review and meta-analysis. *BMJ Open* **2014**, *4*, e004418. [CrossRef]
145. Celebi, O.O.; Celebi, S.; Canbay, A.; Ergun, G.; Aydogdu, S.; Diker, E. The effect of sinus rhythm restoration on high-sensitivity C-reactive protein levels and their association with long-term atrial fibrillation recurrence after electrical cardioversion. *Cardiology* **2011**, *118*, 168–174. [CrossRef]
146. Krishnan, A.; Chilton, E.; Raman, J.; Saxena, P.; McFarlane, C.; Trollope, A.F.; Kinobe, R.; Chilton, L. Are Interactions between Epicardial Adipose Tissue, Cardiac Fibroblasts and Cardiac Myocytes Instrumental in Atrial Fibrosis and Atrial Fibrillation? *Cells* **2021**, *10*, 2501. [CrossRef] [PubMed]

47. Berezin, A.E.; Berezin, A.A.; Lichtenauer, M. Myokines and Heart Failure: Challenging Role in Adverse Cardiac Remodeling, Myopathy, and Clinical Outcomes. *Dis. Markers* **2021**, *2021*, 6644631. [CrossRef] [PubMed]
48. Suffee, N.; Moore-Morris, T.; Jagla, B.; Mougenot, N.; Dilanian, G.; Berthet, M.; Proukhnitzky, J.; Le Prince, P.; Tregouet, D.A.; Pucéat, M.; et al. Reactivation of the Epicardium at the Origin of Myocardial Fibro-Fatty Infiltration During the Atrial Cardiomyopathy. *Circ. Res.* **2020**, *126*, 1330–1342. [CrossRef] [PubMed]
49. Fujita, K.; Maeda, N.; Sonoda, M.; Ohashi, K.; Hibuse, T.; Nishizawa, H.; Nishida, M.; Hiuge, A.; Kurata, A.; Kihara, S.; et al. Adiponectin protects against angiotensin II-induced cardiac fibrosis through activation of PPAR-alpha. *Arterioscler. Thromb. Vasc. Biol.* **2008**, *28*, 863–870. [CrossRef]
50. Kim, Y.; Lim, J.H.; Kim, E.N.; Hong, Y.A.; Park, H.J.; Chung, S.; Choi, B.S.; Kim, Y.S.; Park, J.Y.; Kim, H.W.; et al. Adiponectin receptor agonist ameliorates cardiac lipotoxicity via enhancing ceramide metabolism in type 2 diabetic mice. *Cell Death Dis.* **2022**, *13*, 282. [CrossRef] [PubMed]
51. Singh, R.; Kaundal, R.K.; Zhao, B.; Bouchareb, R.; Lebeche, D. Resistin induces cardiac fibroblast-myofibroblast differentiation through JAK/STAT3 and JNK/c-Jun signaling. *Pharmacol. Res.* **2021**, *167*, 105414. [CrossRef] [PubMed]
52. Martínez-Martínez, E.; Jurado-López, R.; Valero-Muñoz, M.; Bartolomé, M.V.; Ballesteros, S.; Luaces, M.; Briones, A.M.; López-Andrés, N.; Miana, M.; Cachofeiro, V. Leptin induces cardiac fibrosis through galectin-3, mTOR and oxidative stress: Potential role in obesity. *J. Hypertens.* **2014**, *32*, 1104–1114; discussion 1114. [CrossRef]
53. Rienstra, M.; Sun, J.X.; Lubitz, S.A.; Frankel, D.S.; Vasan, R.S.; Levy, D.; Magnani, J.W.; Sullivan, L.M.; Meigs, J.B.; Ellinor, P.T.; et al. Plasma resistin, adiponectin, and risk of incident atrial fibrillation: The Framingham Offspring Study. *Am. Heart J.* **2012**, *163*, 119–124.e1. [CrossRef]
54. Peller, M.; Kapłon-Cieślicka, A.; Rosiak, M.; Tymińska, A.; Ozierański, K.; Eyileten, C.; Kondracka, A.; Mirowska-Guzel, D.; Opolski, G.; Postuła, M.; et al. Are adipokines associated with atrial fibrillation in type 2 diabetes? *Endokrynol. Pol.* **2020**, *71*, 34–41. [CrossRef] [PubMed]
55. Velliou, M.; Sanidas, E.; Papadopoulos, D.; Iliopoulos, D.; Mantzourani, M.; Toutouzas, K.; Barbetseas, J. Adipokines and atrial fibrillation: The important role of apelin. *Hell. J. Cardiol.* **2021**, *62*, 89–91. [CrossRef] [PubMed]
56. Agbaedeng, T.A.; Zacharia, A.L.; Iroga, P.E.; Rathnasekara, V.M.; Munawar, D.A.; Bursill, C.; Noubiap, J.J. Associations between adipokines and atrial fibrillation: A systematic review and meta-analysis. *Nutr. Metab. Cardiovasc. Dis.* **2022**, *32*, 853–862. [CrossRef] [PubMed]
57. Antushevich, H.; Wójcik, M. Review: Apelin in disease. *Clin. Chim. Acta* **2018**, *483*, 241–248. [CrossRef] [PubMed]
58. Ilaghi, M.; Soltanizadeh, A.; Amiri, S.; Kohlmeier, K.A.; Shabani, M. The apelin/APJ signaling system and cytoprotection: Role of its cross-talk with kappa opioid receptor. *Eur. J. Pharmacol.* **2022**, *936*, 175353. [CrossRef] [PubMed]
59. Liu, J.; Liu, M.; Chen, L. Novel pathogenesis: Regulation of apoptosis by Apelin/APJ system. *Acta Biochim. Biophys. Sin.* **2017**, *49*, 471–478. [CrossRef] [PubMed]
60. Lu, L.; Wu, D.; Li, L.; Chen, L. Apelin/APJ system: A bifunctional target for cardiac hypertrophy. *Int. J. Cardiol.* **2017**, *230*, 164–170. [CrossRef]
61. Rikitake, Y. The apelin/APJ system in the regulation of vascular tone: Friend or foe? *J. Biochem.* **2021**, *169*, 383–386. [CrossRef] [PubMed]
62. Li, C.; Cheng, H.; Adhikari, B.K.; Wang, S.; Yang, N.; Liu, W.; Sun, J.; Wang, Y. The Role of Apelin-APJ System in Diabetes and Obesity. *Front. Endocrinol.* **2022**, *13*, 820002. [CrossRef]
63. Parikh, V.N.; Liu, J.; Shang, C.; Woods, C.; Chang, A.C.; Zhao, M.; Charo, D.N.; Grunwald, Z.; Huang, Y.; Seo, K.; et al. Apelin and APJ orchestrate complex tissue-specific control of cardiomyocyte hypertrophy and contractility in the hypertrophy-heart failure transition. *Am. J. Physiol. Heart Circ. Physiol.* **2018**, *315*, H348–H356. [CrossRef] [PubMed]
64. Mughal, A.; O'Rourke, S.T. Vascular effects of apelin: Mechanisms and therapeutic potential. *Pharmacol. Ther.* **2018**, *190*, 139–147. [CrossRef] [PubMed]
65. Charles, C.J. Putative role for apelin in pressure/volume homeostasis and cardiovascular disease. *Cardiovasc. Hematol. Agents Med. Chem.* **2007**, *5*, 1–10. [CrossRef]
66. Askin, L.; Askin, H.S.; Tanrıverdi, O.; Ozyildiz, A.G.; Duman, H. Serum apelin levels and cardiovascular diseases. *North Clin. Istanb.* **2022**, *9*, 290–294. [CrossRef] [PubMed]
67. Riazian, M.; Khorrami, E.; Alipoor, E.; Moradmand, S.; Yaseri, M.; Hosseinzadeh-Attar, M.J. Assessment of Apelin Serum Levels in Persistent Atrial Fibrillation and Coronary Artery Disease. *Am. J. Med. Sci.* **2016**, *352*, 354–359. [CrossRef] [PubMed]
68. Akbari, H.; Hosseini-Bensenjan, M.; Salahi, S.; Moazzen, F.; Aria, H.; Manafi, A.; Hosseini, S.; Niknam, M.; Asadikaram, G. Apelin and its ratio to lipid factors are associated with cardiovascular diseases: A systematic review and meta-analysis. *PLoS ONE* **2022**, *17*, e0271899. [CrossRef]
69. Bohm, A.; Urban, L.; Tothova, L.; Bezak, B.; Uher, T.; Musil, P.; Kyselovic, J.; Lipton, J.; Olejnik, P.; Hatala, R. Concentration of apelin inversely correlates with atrial fibrillation burden. *Bratisl. Lek. Listy* **2021**, *122*, 165–171. [CrossRef]
70. Wang, Y.Z.; Fan, J.; Zhong, B.; Xu, Q. Apelin: A novel prognostic predictor for atrial fibrillation recurrence after pulmonary vein isolation. *Medicine* **2018**, *97*, e12580. [CrossRef]
71. Falcone, C.; Buzzi, M.P.; D'Angelo, A.; Schirinzi, S.; Falcone, R.; Rordorf, R.; Capettini, A.C.; Landolina, M.; Storti, C.; Pelissero, G. Apelin plasma levels predict arrhythmia recurrence in patients with persistent atrial fibrillation. *Int. J. Immunopathol. Pharmacol.* **2010**, *23*, 917–925. [CrossRef]

172. Kim, Y.M.; Lakin, R.; Zhang, H.; Liu, J.; Sachedina, A.; Singh, M.; Wilson, E.; Perez, M.; Verma, S.; Quertermous, T.; et al. Apelin increases atrial conduction velocity, refractoriness, and prevents inducibility of atrial fibrillation. *JCI Insight* **2020**, *5*, e126525. [CrossRef] [PubMed]
173. Lv, W.; Zhang, L.; Cheng, X.; Wang, H.; Qin, W.; Zhou, X.; Tang, B. Apelin Inhibits Angiotensin II-Induced Atrial Fibrosis and Atrial Fibrillation via TGF-β1/Smad2/α-SMA Pathway. *Front. Physiol.* **2020**, *11*, 583570. [CrossRef]
174. Cheng, H.; Chen, Y.; Li, X.; Chen, F.; Zhao, J.; Hu, J.; Shan, A.; Qiao, S.; Wei, Z.; He, G.; et al. Involvement of Apelin/APJ Axis in Thrombogenesis in Valve Heart Disease Patients with Atrial Fibrillation. *Int. Heart J.* **2019**, *60*, 145–150. [CrossRef] [PubMed]
175. Baba, M.; Yoshida, K.; Ieda, M. Clinical Applications of Natriuretic Peptides in Heart Failure and Atrial Fibrillation. *Int. J. Mol. Sci.* **2019**, *20*, 2824. [CrossRef] [PubMed]
176. Colaianni, G.; Cinti, S.; Colucci, S.; Grano, M. Irisin and musculoskeletal health. *Ann. New York Acad. Sci.* **2017**, *1402*, 5–9. [CrossRef] [PubMed]
177. Kim, H.; Wrann, C.D.; Jedrychowski, M.; Vidoni, S.; Kitase, Y.; Nagano, K.; Zhou, C.; Chou, J.; Parkman, V.A.; Novick, S.J.; et al. Irisin Mediates Effects on Bone and Fat via αV Integrin Receptors. *Cell* **2018**, *175*, 1756–1768.e17. [CrossRef]
178. Gamas, L.; Matafome, P.; Seiça, R. Irisin and Myonectin Regulation in the Insulin Resistant Muscle: Implications to Adipose Tissue: Muscle Crosstalk. *J. Diabetes Res.* **2015**, *2015*, 359159. [CrossRef]
179. Moreno-Navarrete, J.M.; Ortega, F.; Serrano, M.; Guerra, E.; Pardo, G.; Tinahones, F.; Ricart, W.; Fernández-Real, J.M. Irisin is expressed and produced by human muscle and adipose tissue in association with obesity and insulin resistance. *J. Clin. Endocrinol. Metab.* **2013**, *98*, E769–E778. [CrossRef] [PubMed]
180. Yang, Z.; Chen, X.; Chen, Y.; Zhao, Q. Decreased irisin secretion contributes to muscle insulin resistance in high-fat diet mice. *Int. J. Clin. Exp. Pathol.* **2015**, *8*, 6490–6497. [PubMed]
181. Polyzos, S.A.; Anastasilakis, A.D.; Efstathiadou, Z.A.; Makras, P.; Perakakis, N.; Kountouras, J.; Mantzoros, C.S. Irisin in metabolic diseases. *Endocrine* **2018**, *59*, 260–274. [CrossRef]
182. Shoukry, A.; Shalaby, S.M.; El-Arabi Bdeer, S.; Mahmoud, A.A.; Mousa, M.M.; Khalifa, A. Circulating serum irisin levels in obesity and type 2 diabetes mellitus. *IUBMB Life* **2016**, *68*, 544–556. [CrossRef] [PubMed]
183. Ho, M.Y.; Wang, C.Y. Role of Irisin in Myocardial Infarction, Heart Failure, and Cardiac Hypertrophy. *Cells* **2021**, *10*, 2103. [CrossRef]
184. Luna-Ceron, E.; González-Gil, A.M.; Elizondo-Montemayor, L. Current Insights on the Role of Irisin in Endothelial Dysfunction. *Curr. Vasc. Pharmacol.* **2022**, *20*, 205–220. [CrossRef]
185. Hsieh, I.C.; Ho, M.Y.; Wen, M.S.; Chen, C.C.; Hsieh, M.J.; Lin, C.P.; Yeh, J.K.; Tsai, M.L.; Yang, C.H.; Wu, V.C.; et al. Serum irisin levels are associated with adverse cardiovascular outcomes in patients with acute myocardial infarction. *Int. J. Cardiol.* **2018**, *261*, 12–17. [CrossRef]
186. Abd El-Motaleb, N.A.; Galal, H.M.; El Maghraby, K.M.; Gadallah, A.I. Serum irisin level in myocardial infarction patients with or without heart failure. *Can. J. Physiol. Pharmacol.* **2019**, *97*, 932–938. [CrossRef] [PubMed]
187. Berezin, A.A.; Lichtenauer, M.; Boxhammer, E.; Fushtey, I.M.; Berezin, A.E. Serum Levels of Irisin Predict Cumulative Clinical Outcomes in Heart Failure Patients with Type 2 Diabetes Mellitus. *Front. Physiol.* **2022**, *13*, 922775. [CrossRef] [PubMed]
188. Berezin, A.A.; Lichtenauer, M.; Boxhammer, E.; Stöhr, E.; Berezin, A.E. Discriminative Value of Serum Irisin in Prediction of Heart Failure with Different Phenotypes among Patients with Type 2 Diabetes Mellitus. *Cells* **2022**, *11*, 2794. [CrossRef] [PubMed]
189. Bosanac, J.; Straus, L.; Novaković, M.; Košuta, D.; Božič Mijovski, M.; Tasič, J.; Jug, B. HFpEF and Atrial Fibrillation: The Enigmatic Interplay of Dysmetabolism, Biomarkers, and Vascular Endothelial Dysfunction. *Dis. Markers* **2022**, *2022*, 9539676. [CrossRef]
190. Shirakawa, K.; Sano, M. Osteopontin in Cardiovascular Diseases. *Biomolecules* **2021**, *11*, 1047. [CrossRef]
191. Berezin, A.E.; Kremzer, A.A. Circulating osteopontin as a marker of early coronary vascular calcification in type two diabetes mellitus patients with known asymptomatic coronary artery disease. *Atherosclerosis* **2013**, *229*, 475–481. [CrossRef]
192. Rewiuk, K.; Grodzicki, T. Osteoprotegerin and TRAIL in Acute Onset of Atrial Fibrillation. *Biomed. Res. Int.* **2015**, *2015*, 259843. [CrossRef] [PubMed]
193. Lin, M.; Bao, Y.; Du, Z.; Zhou, Y.; Zhang, N.; Lin, C.; Xie, Y.; Zhang, R.; Li, Q.; Quan, J.; et al. Plasma protein profiling analysis in patients with atrial fibrillation before and after three different ablation techniques. *Front. Cardiovasc. Med.* **2023**, *9*, 1077992. [CrossRef] [PubMed]
194. Berezin, A.E.; Kremzer, A.A.; Martovitskaya, Y.V.; Samura, T.A.; Berezina, T.A.; Zulli, A.; Klimas, J.; Kruzliak, P. The utility of biomarker risk prediction score in patients with chronic heart failure. *Int. J. Clin. Exp. Med.* **2015**, *8*, 18255–18264. [CrossRef]
195. Lo, Y.M.D.; Han, D.S.C.; Jiang, P.; Chiu, R.W.K. Epigenetics, fragmentomics, and topology of cell-free DNA in liquid biopsies. *Science* **2021**, *372*, eaaw3616. [CrossRef]
196. Luo, H.; Wei, W.; Ye, Z.; Zheng, J.; Xu, R.H. Liquid Biopsy of Methylation Biomarkers in Cell-Free DNA. *Trends Mol. Med.* **2021**, *27*, 482–500. [CrossRef] [PubMed]
197. Grosse, G.M.; Blume, N.; Abu-Fares, O.; Götz, F.; Ernst, J.; Leotescu, A.; Gabriel, M.M.; van Gemmeren, T.; Worthmann, H.; Lichtinghagen, R.; et al. Endogenous Deoxyribonuclease Activity and Cell-Free Deoxyribonucleic Acid in Acute Ischemic Stroke: A Cohort Study. *Stroke* **2022**, *53*, 1235–1244. [CrossRef]

98. Berezina, T.A.; Kopytsya, M.P.; Petyunina, O.V.; Berezin, A.A.; Obradovic, Z.; Schmidbauer, L.; Lichtenauer, M.; Berezin, A.E. Lower Circulating Cell-Free Mitochondrial DNA Is Associated with Heart Failure in Type 2 Diabetes Mellitus Patients. *Cardiogenetics* **2023**, *13*, 15–30. [CrossRef]
99. Li, X.; Hu, R.; Luo, T.; Peng, C.; Gong, L.; Hu, J.; Yang, S.; Li, Q. Serum cell-free DNA and progression of diabetic kidney disease: A prospective study. *BMJ Open Diabetes Res. Care* **2020**, *8*, e001078. [CrossRef]
100. Gianni, C.; Palleschi, M.; Merloni, F.; Di Menna, G.; Sirico, M.; Sarti, S.; Virga, A.; Ulivi, P.; Cecconetto, L.; Mariotti, M.; et al. Cell-Free DNA Fragmentomics: A Promising Biomarker for Diagnosis, Prognosis and Prediction of Response in Breast Cancer. *Int. J. Mol. Sci.* **2022**, *23*, 14197. [CrossRef] [PubMed]
101. Hashimoto, T.; Ueki, S.; Kamide, Y.; Miyabe, Y.; Fukuchi, M.; Yokoyama, Y.; Furukawa, T.; Azuma, N.; Oka, N.; Takeuchi, H.; et al. Increased Circulating Cell-Free DNA in Eosinophilic Granulomatosis with Polyangiitis: Implications for Eosinophil Extracellular Traps and Immunothrombosis. *Front. Immunol.* **2022**, *12*, 801897. [CrossRef]
102. Yamazoe, M.; Sasano, T.; Ihara, K.; Takahashi, K.; Nakamura, W.; Takahashi, N.; Komuro, H.; Hamada, S.; Furukawa, T. Sparsely methylated mitochondrial cell free DNA released from cardiomyocytes contributes to systemic inflammatory response accompanied by atrial fibrillation. *Sci. Rep.* **2021**, *11*, 5837. [CrossRef]
103. Wiersma, M.; van Marion, D.M.S.; Bouman, E.J.; Li, J.; Zhang, D.; Ramos, K.S.; Lanters, E.A.H.; de Groot, N.M.S.; Brundel, B.J.J.M. Cell-Free Circulating Mitochondrial DNA: A Potential Blood-Based Marker for Atrial Fibrillation. *Cells* **2020**, *9*, 1159. [CrossRef]
104. Soltész, B.; Urbancsek, R.; Pös, O.; Hajas, O.; Forgács, I.N.; Szilágyi, E.; Nagy-Baló, E.; Szemes, T.; Csanádi, Z.; Nagy, B. Quantification of peripheral whole blood, cell-free plasma and exosome encapsulated mitochondrial DNA copy numbers in patients with atrial fibrillation. *J. Biotechnol.* **2019**, *299*, 66–71. [CrossRef] [PubMed]
105. Geurts, S.; Mens, M.M.J.; Bos, M.M.; Ikram, M.A.; Ghanbari, M.; Kavousi, M. Circulatory MicroRNAs in Plasma and Atrial Fibrillation in the General Population: The Rotterdam Study. *Genes* **2021**, *13*, 11. [CrossRef] [PubMed]
106. Garcia-Elias, A.; Tajes, M.; Yáñez-Bisbe, L.; Enjuanes, C.; Comín-Colet, J.; Serra, S.A.; Fernández-Fernández, J.M.; Aguilar-Agon, K.W.; Reilly, S.; Martí-Almor, J.; et al. Atrial Fibrillation in Heart Failure Is Associated with High Levels of Circulating microRNA-199a-5p and 22-5p and a Defective Regulation of Intracellular Calcium and Cell-to-Cell Communication. *Int. J. Mol. Sci.* **2021**, *22*, 10377. [CrossRef]
107. Chen, H.; Zhang, F.; Zhang, Y.L.; Yang, X.C. Relationship between circulating miRNA-21, atrial fibrosis, and atrial fibrillation in patients with atrial enlargement. *Ann. Palliat. Med.* **2021**, *10*, 12742–12749. [CrossRef] [PubMed]
108. Benito, B.; García-Elías, A.; Ois, Á.; Tajes, M.; Vallès, E.; Ble, M.; Yáñez Bisbe, L.; Giralt-Steinhauer, E.; Rodríguez-Campello, A.; Cladellas Capdevila, M.; et al. Plasma levels of miRNA-1-3p are associated with subclinical atrial fibrillation in patients with cryptogenic stroke. *Rev. Esp. Cardiol. (Engl. Ed.)* **2022**, *75*, 717–726, (In English and Spanish). [CrossRef]
109. Park, H.; Park, H.; Park, J. Circulating microRNA-423 attenuates the phosphorylation of calcium handling proteins in atrial fibrillation. *Mol. Med. Rep.* **2022**, *25*, 186. [CrossRef]
110. Arroyo, A.B.; de Los Reyes-García, A.M.; Rivera-Caravaca, J.M.; Valledor, P.; García-Barberá, N.; Roldán, V.; Vicente, V.; Martínez, C.; González-Conejero, R. MiR-146a Regulates Neutrophil Extracellular Trap Formation That Predicts Adverse Cardiovascular Events in Patients with Atrial Fibrillation. *Arterioscler. Thromb. Vasc. Biol.* **2018**, *38*, 892–902. [CrossRef] [PubMed]
111. Da Silva, A.M.G.; de Araújo, J.N.G.; de Oliveira, K.M.; Novaes, A.E.M.; Lopes, M.B.; de Sousa, J.C.V.; Filho, A.A.A.; Luchessi, A.D.; de Rezende, A.A.; Hirata, M.H.; et al. Circulating miRNAs in acute new-onset atrial fibrillation and their target mRNA network. *J. Cardiovasc. Electrophysiol.* **2018**, *29*, 1159–1166. [CrossRef]
112. Zhou, Q.; Maleck, C.; von Ungern-Sternberg, S.N.I.; Neupane, B.; Heinzmann, D.; Marquardt, J.; Duckheim, M.; Scheckenbach, C.; Stimpfle, F.; Gawaz, M.; et al. Circulating MicroRNA-21 Correlates with Left Atrial Low-Voltage Areas and Is Associated with Procedure Outcome in Patients Undergoing Atrial Fibrillation Ablation. *Circ. Arrhythm. Electrophysiol.* **2018**, *11*, e006242. [CrossRef]
113. Rochette, L.; Lorin, J.; Zeller, M.; Guilland, J.C.; Lorgis, L.; Cottin, Y.; Vergely, C. Nitric oxide synthase inhibition and oxidative stress in cardiovascular diseases: Possible therapeutic targets? *Pharmacol. Ther.* **2013**, *140*, 239–257. [CrossRef] [PubMed]
114. Büttner, P.; Bahls, M.; Böger, R.H.; Hindricks, G.; Thiele, H.; Schwedhelm, E.; Kornej, J. Arginine derivatives in atrial fibrillation progression phenotypes. *J. Mol. Med.* **2020**, *98*, 999–1008. [CrossRef] [PubMed]
115. Ramuschkat, M.; Appelbaum, S.; Atzler, D.; Zeller, T.; Bauer, C.; Ojeda, F.M.; Sinning, C.R.; Hoffmann, B.; Lackner, K.J.; Böger, R.H.; et al. ADMA, subclinical changes and atrial fibrillation in the general population. *Int. J. Cardiol.* **2016**, *203*, 640–646. [CrossRef]
116. Horowitz, J.D.; De Caterina, R.; Heresztyn, T.; Alexander, J.H.; Andersson, U.; Lopes, R.D.; Steg, P.G.; Hylek, E.M.; Mohan, P.; Hanna, M.; et al. Asymmetric and Symmetric Dimethylarginine Predict Outcomes in Patients with Atrial Fibrillation: An ARISTOTLE Substudy. *J. Am. Coll. Cardiol.* **2018**, *72*, 721–733. [CrossRef]
117. Goette, A.; Hammwöhner, M.; Bukowska, A.; Scalera, F.; Martens-Lobenhoffer, J.; Dobrev, D.; Ravens, U.; Weinert, S.; Medunjanin, S.; Lendeckel, U.; et al. The impact of rapid atrial pacing on ADMA and endothelial NOS. *Int. J. Cardiol.* **2012**, *154*, 141–146. [CrossRef]
118. Goni, L.; Razquin, C.; Toledo, E.; Guasch-Ferré, M.; Clish, C.B.; Babio, N.; Wittenbecher, C.; Atzeni, A.; Li, J.; Liang, L.; et al. Arginine catabolism metabolites and atrial fibrillation or heart failure risk: 2 case-control studies within the Prevención con Dieta Mediterránea (PREDIMED) trial. *Am. J. Clin. Nutr.* **2022**, *116*, 653–662. [CrossRef] [PubMed]

219. Li, J.; Xia, W.; Feng, W.; Qu, X. Effects of rosuvastatin on serum asymmetric dimethylarginine levels and atrial structural remodeling in atrial fibrillation dogs. *Pacing Clin. Electrophysiol.* **2012**, *35*, 456–464. [CrossRef]
220. Lao, M.C.; Liu, L.J.; Luo, C.F.; Lu, G.H.; Zhai, Y.S.; Chen, X.L.; Gao, X.R. Effect of asymmetrical dimethylarginine for predicting pro-thrombotic risk in atrial fibrillation. *Zhonghua Yi Xue Za Zhi* **2016**, *96*, 2059–2063. (In Chinese) [CrossRef] [PubMed]
221. Chao, T.F.; Lu, T.M.; Lin, Y.J.; Tsao, H.M.; Chang, S.L.; Lo, L.W.; Hu, Y.F.; Tuan, T.C.; Hsieh, M.H.; Chen, S.A. Plasma asymmetric dimethylarginine and adverse events in patients with atrial fibrillation referred for coronary angiogram. *PLoS ONE* **2013**, *8*, e71675. [CrossRef] [PubMed]
222. Xia, W.; Qu, X.; Yu, Y.; Zhang, X.; Feng, W.; Song, Y. Asymmetric dimethylarginine concentration and early recurrence of atrial fibrillation after electrical cardioversion. *Pacing Clin. Electrophysiol.* **2008**, *31*, 1036–1040. [CrossRef] [PubMed]
223. Tveit, A.; Arnesen, H.; Smith, P.; Bratseth, V.; Seljeflot, I. L-arginine, asymmetric dimethylarginine and rhythm outcome after electrical cardioversion for atrial fibrillation. *Cardiology* **2010**, *117*, 176–180. [CrossRef] [PubMed]
224. Schnabel, R.B.; Maas, R.; Wang, N.; Yin, X.; Larson, M.G.; Levy, D.; Ellinor, P.T.; Lubitz, S.A.; McManus, D.D.; Magnani, J.W. et al. Asymmetric dimethylarginine, related arginine derivatives, and incident atrial fibrillation. *Am. Heart J.* **2016**, *176*, 100–106. [CrossRef] [PubMed]

Disclaimer/Publisher's Note: The statements, opinions and data contained in all publications are solely those of the individual author(s) and contributor(s) and not of MDPI and/or the editor(s). MDPI and/or the editor(s) disclaim responsibility for any injury to people or property resulting from any ideas, methods, instructions or products referred to in the content.

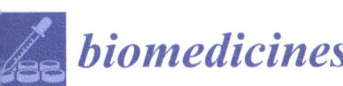

Review

Thyroid Hormone and Heart Failure: Charting Known Pathways for Cardiac Repair/Regeneration

Polyxeni Mantzouratou [1], Eleftheria Malaxianaki [1], Domenico Cerullo [2], Angelo Michele Lavecchia [2], Constantinos Pantos [1], Christodoulos Xinaris [2] and Iordanis Mourouzis [1,*]

1 Department of Pharmacology, University of Athens, 11527 Athens, Greece
2 Centro Anna Maria Astori, Istituto di Ricerche Farmacologiche Mario Negri IRCCS, 24126 Bergamo, Italy
* Correspondence: imour@med.uoa.gr

Abstract: Heart failure affects more than 64 million people worldwide, having a serious impact on their survival and quality of life. Exploring its pathophysiology and molecular bases is an urgent need in order to develop new therapeutic approaches. Thyroid hormone signaling, evolutionarily conserved, controls fundamental biological processes and has a crucial role in development and metabolism. Its active form is L-triiodothyronine, which not only regulates important gene expression by binding to its nuclear receptors, but also has nongenomic actions, controlling crucial intracellular signalings. Stressful stimuli, such as acute myocardial infarction, lead to changes in thyroid hormone signaling, and especially in the relation of the thyroid hormone and its nuclear receptor, which are associated with the reactivation of fetal development programmes, with structural remodeling and phenotypical changes in the cardiomyocytes. The recapitulation of fetal-like features of the signaling may be partially an incomplete effort of the myocardium to recapitulate its developmental program and enable cardiomyocytes to proliferate and finally to regenerate. In this review, we will discuss the experimental and clinical evidence about the role of the thyroid hormone in the recovery of the myocardium in the setting of heart failure with reduced and preserved ejection fraction and its future therapeutic implications.

Keywords: thyroid hormone; thyroid receptors; low T3 syndrome; heart failure; coronary disease; cardiac remodeling

1. Introduction

Heart failure (HF) is a clinical syndrome with specific symptoms and signs (e.g., breathlessness, peripheral edema) due to structural or functional cardiac abnormalities that result in elevated intracardial pressure and/or impaired cardiac output [1]. Although the prognosis of patients has considerably improved over the last few decades, HF still affects more than 64 million people worldwide, having a serious impact on their survival and quality of life [2]. Hospitalizations because of HF represent 1–2% of all admissions in Western countries, and HF is the most common cause of hospitalization of individuals >65 years. Around 30–40% of HF patients have a history of hospital admission, and 50% are readmitted within 1 year of their initial diagnosis. Mortality is high, with the 1-year risk being between 15–30% and the 5-year risk up to 75% in several populations [2]. The current health care costs per year for every HF patient are up to EUR 25,000 in the Western world, while the increasing prevalence of HF is expected to lead to prohibitive costs, even for developed countries [2]. Therefore, there is an urgent need to better understand the pathophysiology and molecular basis of HF in order to develop new therapeutic approaches.

Thyroid hormone (TH) signaling, evolutionarily conserved, controls fundamental biological processes and has a crucial role in development and metabolism [3]. The active form of TH is L-triiodothyronine (T3), which regulates important gene expression by

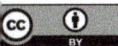

binding to its nuclear receptors, TH receptors (TRs; TRalpha1-2 and TRbeta1-2) [4]. In the heart, ventricular cardiomyocytes mostly express TRalpha1, while both TRalpha1 and TRbeta1 are expressed in the peripheral ventricular conduction system [5]. TRs are transcription factors that reside in the nucleus but also rapidly shuttle between the cytoplasm and nucleus. Genomic actions of TRs include interactions with TH response elements in specific genes [6]. Nongenomic actions of TH regulate important intracellular signaling pathways and are mediated via cytosolic TRs or via the membrane integrin receptor $\alpha v\beta 3$ [6].

One of the best-characterized TRs in mammals is TRalpha1, which is present and well described in the heart [7]. Interestingly, during fetal life, due to low levels of T3, TRalpha1, highly expressed, is in an unliganded state, acting as an aporeceptor, repressing the expression of the adult gene program and allowing the proliferation of cardiomyocytes and an increase in cardiac mass. After birth, a burst of T3 results in the liganded state of TRalpha1, which, acting as a holoreceptor, triggers the expression of adult genes promoting heart maturation and development [8]. It is of great interest that TRalpha1 seems to act like a "molecular switch" during heart development, since its status as an apo- or a holoreceptor controls the proliferation and differentiation of the cardiomyocytes, and thereby this role can be of great clinical relevance [9]. Indeed, in a recent study, a dominant negative TRalpha1—which is unable to bind T3 and become a holoreceptor—in a mouse heart, prevented myocardial cells from complete differentiation and permitted their proliferation—and thus the regeneration—of the myocardium after acute myocardial infarction (AMI) [10]. Importantly, in adult life after stressful stimuli and during disease states, such as in HF, the fetal profile of the TRalpha1-T3 axis recurs. This recapitulation of fetal-like features of the signaling may be an incomplete effort of the myocardium to recapitulate its developmental program and enable cardiomyocytes to proliferate and finally to regenerate [8]. In organs with very limited regenerative potential, such as the heart, the fetal profile of the TRalpha1-T3 axis during stress results in cell hypertrophy without progressing to reductive mitosis. This hypertrophy can temporally compensate the dysfunction, but when accompanied by adoption of a low energy profile, it becomes maladaptive and leads to failure [11]. Therefore, after stress, a drop in T3 serum levels takes place—a phenomenon known as "low T3 syndrome"—whilst the unliganded TRalpha1 moves to the nucleus to induce dedifferentiation and reactivation of fetal genes, as well as growth in cardiomyocytes. The main regulators of T3 concentration at the tissue level are enzymes called deiodinases, which mediate the activation or inactivation of TH. Types 1, 2, and 3 iodothyronine deiodinases have unique catalytic properties and tissue distributions [12–14]. Deiodinase type 3 (D3) has a high affinity in inactivating T3, playing a critical role in T3 availability in the systematic level as well as locally in the injured tissue [13]. Interestingly, D3 is highly expressed in the heart after myocardial injury [15]. In addition, the shuttling of TRalpha1 to the nucleus is shown to be controlled by the activation of the adrenergic system [16], which is thought to be involved in fetal gene reactivation and cardiac remodeling. Milestones of the fetal-like shift in the myocardium are an increase in the beta myosin heavy chain (the predominantly fetal type of myosin, which is slower and less energy-consuming than the adult alpha type of myosin), the decreased ratio of sarcoplasmic reticulum-calcium ATPase (SERCA) to phospholamban (PLN), and the "energy shift" of the stressed myocardium to the use of glucose as an energy substrate instead of fatty acids (like in fetal life) [17,18]. Although this transcriptional shift in the short term allows the cardiomyocytes to recover to a less energy-demanding state by having a lower maximum shortening velocity [19], in the long term it becomes detrimental, leading to further deterioration of the organ's structure and function [20] (Figure 1).

Exogenous administration of T3 in the setting of acute or chronic heart injury turns TRalpha1 to its holoreceptor form, promoting the expression of the adult transcriptional program and ameliorating cardiac structure and function [9]. In accordance, a series of epidemiological studies reveal an association of low T3 levels after stress with adverse clinical outcomes in cardiological patients such as the ones with HF, while exogenous T3 treatment has promising results [7].

In this review, we will discuss the experimental and clinical evidence about the role of TH in the recovery of the myocardium in HF with reduced and preserved ejection fraction (HFrEF, HFpEF) and its future therapeutic implications.

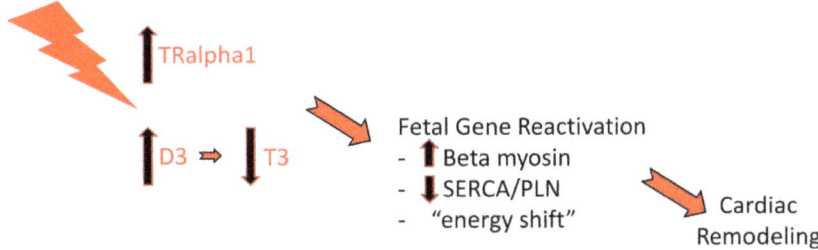

Figure 1. After stress, TRalpha1 increases in the nucleus while T3 is inactivated by D3. As a consequence, TRalpha1 acts as an aporeceptor, leading to fetal gene reactivation and cardiac remodeling.

2. TH and HFrEF

Cardiac dysfunction results from myocardial injury and/or changes in the viable nonischemic myocardium, a process known as cardiac remodeling. This response is characterized by altered cardiac chamber geometry, a shift in cardiomyocyte protein expression to a fetal pattern, energy deficit, and the induction of fibrosis [21,22]. Despite the advances in current treatments, cardiac remodeling occurs in nearly 30–40% of patients with AMI treated with reperfusion, and results in progressive dilatation and HF, making coronary artery disease the most common cause of HfrEF [23].

2.1. Preclinical Studies

Significant changes in TH signaling take place during cardiac remodeling after acute myocardial injury. In a model of AMI in rats, T3 levels drop within a week, and TH-related genes, such as myosin isoforms and SERCA, normalize after TH administration [18]. A distinct pattern of TRalpha1 alteration is also present after acute injury and in the course of HF. During the compensatory stage of HF, TRalpha1 expression increases and declines thereafter with the progression to the noncompensatory left ventricular dysfunction [24]. Interestingly, the pharmacological inactivation of TRalpha1 in the postischemic myocardium in mice results in a decreased ratio of SERCA to PLN and in activated proapoptotic p38 mitogen-activated protein kinase (MAPK). Therefore, there is a further dramatic deterioration of postischemic heart function [25], and this makes the emerging role of TH signaling in the response to stress after myocardial injury clear. In more detail, mice with AMI, which are treated with the selective TRalpha1 inhibitor debutyl-dronedarone, exhibit a significantly depressed left ventricular (LV) function with lower ejection fraction (EF) and higher wall tension index compared to the control group. These changes are accompanied by a marked activation of the proapoptotic p38 MAPK, known for its negative inotropic effect. On the other hand, when TH is administered to the same model of acute myocardial injury and HFrEF, in a replacement dose, there is a significant improvement of LV function and geometry, a decrease in the expression of the fetal type of myosin (beta myosin), and an enhancement of the prosurvival signaling Akt [26]. Likewise, in a rat model of ischemic heart disease, TH treatment results in improved LV geometry as well as function, inhibits the expansion of the scar over time [27], and reduces apoptosis by activating Akt again [28]. Early and constant replacement of T3 levels in the same model also prevents the progression towards HF, likely due to increased capillary formation and mitochondrial protection [29]. Even with the presence of comorbidities, such as diabetes, TH administration improves wall stress, increases cardiac mass, and ameliorates cardiac remodeling [30]. Moreover, TH pretreatment in ex vivo rat models of ischemia show a protective effect against ischemia–

reperfusion injury by suppressing the activation of the proapoptotic p38 kinase cascade [31], while T3 treatment at reperfusion significantly helps the recovery of function and reduces apoptosis and tissue necrosis [32].

2.2. Epidemiological Studies

On the basis of the aforementioned experimental evidence, TH signaling appears to be essential for the response of the myocardium to stress in the setting of acute myocardial injury. In fact, in numerous epidemiological studies, researchers have noticed the association of TH levels with clinical outcomes in the clinical conditions of acute myocardial ischemia and HF. In patients with AMI followed by percutaneous coronary intervention (PCI), the levels of T3 six months after the incidence appear to be an independent predictor of recovery of cardiac function [33]. In the same setting, patients younger than 75 years old with low free T3 levels have higher mortality [34], while patients with elective or primary PCI and subclinical hypothyroidism have worse outcomes of repeat revascularization and cardiac death following PCI [35]. Interestingly, patients with ST segment elevation myocardial infarction, treated with PCI who developed cardiogenic shock, have lower free T3 (FT3) and higher free T4 (FT4) upon admission compared to those without cardiogenic shock. During 2.5 years of follow-up, those with low FT3 (<2.85 pg/mL) and high FT4 ($\geq$0.88 ng/dL) have the highest all-cause mortality (18.2%), while those with high FT3 and low FT4 have the lowest (3.8%) [36]. The prognostic value of the ratio FT3 to FT4 is also examined in patients with myocardial infarction with nonobstructive coronary arteries. Patients with lower ratio have a higher incidence of major adverse cardiovascular events (MACE) (10.0%, 13.9%, 18.2%; $p = 0.005$) over the median follow-up over 41.7 months. The risk of MACE also increases when FT3/FT4 is decreased after multivariate adjustment, and a low level of FT3/FT4 ratio is strongly connected to a poor prognosis [37]. The association between low T3 levels and mortality was once again highlighted by a ThyAMI-1 study in which patients with AMI and low T3 syndrome had significantly higher all-cause mortality [38]. In patients with chronic HF, Pingitore et al. also showed that low T3 levels are an independent predictor of mortality [39]. Significantly worse one-year all-cause mortality was also identified in patients with decompensated acute HF [40]. In those patients, levels of T3 are proposed to be used for their risk stratification [41]. In hospitalized patients with chronic HF, low T3 is associated with higher cardiac and all-cause mortality [42], while exercise capacity, as an indicator of functional status, is reduced in patients with HF and low T3 levels [43]. Kannan et al. showed that in patients with pre-existing HF, subclinical hypothyroidism with thyroid stimulating hormone (TSH) $\geq$7 mIU/L and low T3 levels is associated with poor prognosis [44]. Interestingly, in patients with idiopathic dilated cardiomyopathy, low FT3 level is also associated with myocardial fibrosis and perfusion/metabolism abnormalities as evaluated by cardiac magnetic resonance imaging (CMR), single-photon emission computed tomography (SPECT), and positron emission tomography (PET) [45].

2.3. Clinical Trials

Based on the above clinical findings and on the aforementioned experimental evidence, TH treatment has been used in several trials in patients with HF or ischemic heart disease. A study of acute intravenous administration of T3 in a small number of patients with advanced HF established the basis for further investigation into the safety and potential benefits of TH treatment. An intravenous bolus dose of T3 was administered to 23 patients with advanced HFrEF without adverse events. T3 administration increased cardiac output along with a reduction in systemic vascular resistance in patients receiving the largest dose [46]. In another study, short-term synthetic L-T3 replacement therapy in patients with HF had positive results [47]. A total of 20 patients with ischemic or nonischemic HF and low T3 syndrome, clinically stable, were enrolled. The study group (10 patients) underwent 3-d synthetic L-T3 infusion in order to restore normal T3 levels as rapidly as possible without adverse effects. The control group (10 patients) underwent placebo infusion. The main finding of the study was the positive effect in the cardiac function and neuroendocrine profile of the patients. Thus, the study group had an improved stroke volume of the LV and a significantly reduced noradrenalin, aldosterone, and N-terminal-pro-B-type natriuretic peptide (NTproBNP) [47]. On the contrary, in a small randomized, double-blind, crossover, placebo-controlled interventional study, oral T3 given twice daily for three months in patients with low T3 levels, chronic HF, and modestly reduced LVEF did not improve cardiac function and neurohormonal profile [48]. Although this could be partly explained by the small sample size and the oral type of treatment for a relatively short time of period, another randomized double-blind, placebo-controlled trial had different results. In more detail, fifty adult patients with clinically stable HF and low T3 levels received oral liothyronine or placebo for 6 weeks. Liothyronine had an important impact in patients' functional status by significantly improving the 6 min walk test, their neurohormonal profile, and cardiac LVEF [49]. Although the above studies examine the effect of T3 in patients with HF and low T3 syndrome, an ongoing multicenter, open-label, randomized, parallel group trial (ThyroHeart-CHF), aims to evaluate the efficacy and safety of levothyroxine replacement on the exercise capability in chronic systolic HF patients with subclinical hypothyroidism without examining T3 levels [50]. In more detail, eligible patients have to be 18 years or older, with systolic HF (New York heart association (NYHA) class II–III), LVEF $\leq$ 40%, and subclinical hypothyroidism. They will be randomly 1:1 assigned in order to receive thyroxine replacement therapy along with standard chronic HF treatment or only standard HF therapy. The initial levothyroxine dose will be 12.5 µg once a day and will be titrated until TSH normalization (T3 or T4 values are not examined). The primary endpoints include the difference in 6 min walk test results between 24 weeks and baseline. Secondary endpoints are the differences in neurohormonal and serum lipid profiles, changes in the NYHA classification, cardiovascular death, rehospitalization, differences in heart structure and function as assessed by echocardiogram and CMR imaging measures, and Minnesota living with heart failure questionnaire results between 24 weeks and baseline.

In the last few years, several phase II studies have been conducted for the first time to investigate the potential of TH treatment after AMI to prevent the development of cardiac remodeling and HF. Pingitore et al. investigated whether TH replacement therapy is safe in patients after AMI with low T3 syndrome and whether it has an impact on the infarct size and LV volumes and function. In this study, 37 patients with AMI were randomly treated or untreated with T3 for 6 months in addition to the standard therapy. At discharge and at 6 months, the LV volumes, LVEF, wall motion score index (WMSI), and infarct extent were measured by CMR. At follow-up, there was a significant reduction in WMSI for patients in both groups, while the difference value (discharge/follow-up) was significantly higher in the T3-treated group. In addition, stroke volume increased significantly at follow-up after T3 treatment, which appeared to be safe and able to improve regional dysfunction in patients with AMI. However, no effect of TH replacement therapy was found in infarct extent, LV volumes, and EF [51].

In another double-blind, randomized clinical trial, 95 patients with AMI were randomized to receive either levothyroxine (starting at 25 µg) or a placebo for 52 weeks, and cardiac function was assessed by CMR imaging at baseline and at the end of the study. Treatment with levothyroxine was shown to be safe but did not significantly improve EF, LV volumes, or infarct size after 52 weeks [52]. The dose and timing of administration may play a significant role in these trials. Upon ischemic stress, there is an impaired conversion of T4 to T3, while T3 inactivation is increased due to alterations in deiodinase activity. Furthermore, changes at the level of TH receptors take place and modify the response of the myocardium to THs [7]. More recently, a pilot, randomized, double-blind, placebo-controlled trial (ThyRepair study) investigated potential effects of acute, high-dose LT3 treatment in patients with ST-elevation anterior AMI. LT3 treatment started after primary PCI with an intravenous bolus injection of LT3 followed by a constant infusion for 48 h. Data were analyzed from 37 patients who had CMR at hospital discharge and 6 months follow-up. Acute LT3 treatment resulted in significant lower LV end-diastolic volume index and LV systolic volume index at hospital discharge, while CMR infarct volume was lower in the LT3-treated group at 6 months. These findings may be of high clinical relevance. Early LV dilatation, as assessed by CMR, was shown to carry 57% long-term mortality vs 27% and 26% of late and absence of dilatation, respectively [53]. Moreover, after adjustment for LVEF and age, early dilatation was the exclusive independent predictor of long-term mortality [53]. The primary endpoint of the present study, LVEF%, was found increased in the LT3-treated group of compared to the placebo, although without statistical significance. It seems that at this stage, LV with higher dilatation, which was found in untreated patients, could contribute to higher LVEF% via Starling's law effect [53]. However, LVEF% difference between groups, evident at 6 months of follow-up, was at a magnitude of 5 units, and this is of clinical relevance since an LVEF% change of higher than 5 units is a powerful predictor of both HF hospitalizations and survival [54], although a bigger sample size was necessary to designate a significant change in LVEF% at this stage. Furthermore, it is also interesting that ECG QRS duration at 6 months follow-up was significantly lower in the LT3-treated group, indicating a potential positive effect of T3 on electrical remodeling of the heart. In fact, the prolonged duration of QRS after AMI shows adverse electrical remodeling and correlates with increased mortality [55]. Despite a tendency for increased incidence of atrial fibrillation during the first 48 h, serious, life-threatening events related to LT3 treatment were not observed [56].

Interestingly, TH therapy has been also used for the hemodynamic support of heart donors in cardiac transplantation, having a protective role against ischemic injury. This effect was evident in a series of 66,629 organ donors, where T3 or T4 treatment was connected to the attainment of a significantly higher number of cardiac grafts. Astonishingly, this effect was also associated with increased graft survival after transplantation and was also independent of other factors [57,58].

We could consider several variables in any attempt to explain inconsistencies between the above trials, such as the time and dosing of administration, intrinsic methodological differences in the analysis tools, and clinical endpoints and the nature and severity of injury/disease. Based on the above, the exogenous administration of TH seems to be both safe and beneficial for patients with HF and ischemic heart disease. However, large-scale trials are needed in order to validate these results (Table 1).

Table 1. Clinical studies with TH administration in HF and AMI settings.

Clinical Study	Patients (N)	Setting	Treatment	Outcome	Safety
Hamilton et al. [46]	23	Advanced HF and low T3	0.15–2.7 ìg/kg (iv) T3 for 6–12 h	Increased CO and reduction in SVR	No AEs
Pingitore et al. [47]	20	HF and low T3	35.6 ìg LT3 (iv) in the first 24 h and 15 ìg/day until 72 h	Increased SV and lower HR; decrease in NT-proBNP, noradrenaline, and aldosterone	No AEs
Holmager et al. [48]	13	Stable systolic HF and low T3	20 μg oral T3 per day for 3 months	No changes in cardiac function and neurohormonal profile	No AEs
Amin et al. [49]	50	Chronic stable HF and low T3	T3 replacement dose by oral liothyronine for 6 weeks	Increased 6 min walk test, decreased hsCRP, decrease in NTproBNP	No AEs
Zhang et al. [50]	124 (estimated)	Chronic HF and low T3	Oral levothyroxine with a starting dose of 12.5 μg	Ongoing	Ongoing
Pingitore et al. [51]	37	AMI and low T3	Oral liothyronine (T3) (maximum dosage 15 mcg/m^2/die for 6 months	Significant reduction in WMSI difference value (discharge/follow-up), increased stroke volume at follow-up	No AEs

Table 1. Cont.

Clinical Study	Patients (N)	Setting	Treatment	Outcome	Safety
Jabbar et al. [52]	95	AMI and subclinical hypothyroidism	Oral levothyroxine (25 µg titrated to serum thyrotropin levels between 0.4 and 2.5 mU/L	No significant differences	No AEs
Pantos et al. [56]	52	Anterior STEMI undergoing PCI	(i.v.) bolus injection of 0.8 µg/kg of LT3 followed by a constant infusion of 0.113 µg/kg/h i.v. for 48 h	Significantly lower LV end-diastolic volume index and LV end-systolic volume index at discharge, CMR IV tended to be lower in the LT3-treated group at 6 months	Tendency for an increased incidence of AF during the first 48 h

2.4. TH and HFpEF

Although the prevalence of HFpEF is rapidly growing, due to the aging population and an increase in pathological conditions such as hypertension and diabetes [59], its therapy remains challenging [60]. Pathophysiologicaly, diastolic impairment with abnormal relaxation and increased passive stiffness predominate [61]. Myocardial stiffening can be attributed to the giant cytoskeletal protein titin as well as to the extracellular matrix, and HFpEF patients have both increased collagen content and titin-dependent stiffness. Changes in calcium homeostasis, including increased diastolic calcium levels [62], are also quite important contributors to abnormal relaxation in HFpEF, while impaired bioenergetics have also been proposed as a key mechanism [63]. Interestingly, TH biological actions can pleiotropically affect the underlining pathophysiology of HFpEF. It is known that THs not only stimulate cell growth and neoangiogenesis, but also decrease cardiac fibrosis by enhancing metalloproteinase activity [64]. It is also of great importance that THs enhance the expression of genes encoding SERCA and negatively regulate the transcription of PLN. The increase in SERCA and the inhibition of PLN not only increase the calcium available in systole, but also improve its reuptake into the sarcoplasmic reticulum during relaxation of the heart [65]. In terms of bioenergetics, importantly, THs stimulate cardiac mitochondrial biogenesis and improve oxidative phosphorylation, and this can have a great impact not only in systolic but also in diastolic cardiac function [66].

Indeed, abnormal and especially low TH levels are associated with diastolic cardiac impairment [67]. Patients with subclinical hypothyroidism that were evaluated by Doppler echocardiography showed significant prolongation of the isovolumic relaxation time, reduced E/A ratio, and an increased A wave [68]. In the subgroup of patients that were re-evaluated after TH profile normalization, diastolic abnormalities were reversed [68]. In patients with overt HFpEF, subclinical hypothyroidism and low T3 syndrome are quite common. The inflammatory process in HFpEF, along with the intracellular hypoxia, may contribute to the increased D3 gene expression, which results in the degradation of T3 into inactive metabolites and in local hypothyroidism [15,69]. In an interesting study, among 89 patients with HFpEF, 22% exhibited low T3 levels, which were associated with markers of severity, such as B-type natriuretic peptides as well as echocardiographic parameters of diastolic impairment [70]. Data from animal models of HFpEF suggest an improvement in diastolic function after TH treatment. Longstanding hypertension, in animal models, results in low T3 in serum and heart tissue along with increased collagen and a fetal phenotype shift in myosins. Treatment with low doses of T3 in the long term not only normalizes serum and cardiac tissue T3 levels, but also restores α/β myosin protein levels, collagen, and systolic wall stress, tending to improve diastolic function [71]. In a rat model of type II diabetes, T3 treatment prevents tissue fibrosis, cardiomyocyte dedifferentiation and cytoarchitectural alterations, reverses the diabetes-induced reactivation of fetal genes and pathological growth, and improves myocardium ultrastructure (unpublished data).

There are no clinical trials that have investigated the effects of TH treatment in patients with HFpEF. Interestingly, a phase II randomized trial aims to determine the feasibility, safety, and preliminary efficacy of oral LT3 therapy in patients with HfpEF, and is expected to be completed in 2023. The design includes a treatment during an approximate period of 8 weeks, with every week titration of study drug for 4 weeks, a maintenance dose of 4 weeks, then a 2-week washout, and finally crossing over to the other arm (drug/placebo) LT3 is titrated based on serum T3 levels. The minimum LT3 dose is set to 2.5 mcg three times daily and the maximum LT3 dose to 12.5 mcg three times daily. Endpoints of efficacy include the peak maximal rate of oxygen consumption during exercise (VO2 Max), quality of life, and NT-proBNP levels [72].

Effective treatments for HFpEF are lacking. Thus, understanding the potential therapeutic role of TH in this syndrome could prove the missing link in the quest for novel treatments for diastolic dysfunction.

3. The Challenge of Clinical Translation

Exogenous administration of TH in experimental models of HF has showed, as already mentioned, great therapeutic potential. Nevertheless, translating this new therapeutic strategy into clinical practice has proven a great challenge. The coronary drug project was the first randomized, placebo-controlled trial that investigated the effect of a TH analog, dextrothyroxine (DT4), in patients after AMI. In this old study, in an era when reperfusion with PCI or thrombolysis did not exist, DT4 was given at high doses for several months, and resulted in small but significant increases in arrhythmia and mortality, which caused the discontinuation of this treatment arm [73]. In another, more recent study, patients with chronic HF were treated with excessive doses of another TH analog, diiodothyropropionic acid (DITPA), for 6 months. DITPA improved some hemodynamic parameters, such as cardiac index and vascular resistance, but was poorly tolerated, mainly due to fatigue [74]. Several preclinical studies published during the last few years have increased our knowledge about the favorable or detrimental actions of TH treatment in cardiovascular diseases. In the injured or failing heart, the conversion of T4 to T3 is impaired and deactivation of T3 is enhanced due to increased D3 activity. Furthermore, changes occur in the expression and/or shuttling of TRs, resulting in an altered response of the myocardium to THs compared to the normal myocardium [7]. Thus, high doses of TH are needed in order to increase T3 levels locally in the diseased heart. However, in dose-dependent preclinical studies, long-term administration of high doses of T4 and T3 have shown adverse effects in cardiac remodeling and increased mortality [26]. The dose, timing, and duration of administration are probably critical points in translating the beneficial effects of TH. As reported above, three recent phase II randomized, double-blind, placebo-controlled trials were performed in patients with AMI, and three different therapeutic approaches were tested: low-dose (replacement) LT4 treatment for 52 weeks [52]; low-dose (replacement) LT3 treatment for 6 months [51]; and high-dose (7–10 times the replacement dose), acute LT3 treatment for 48 h [56]. The safety of the treatment was observed in each case. LT4 did not show any beneficial effect, while some secondary beneficial effects were seen after LT3 treatment for 6 months. On the other hand, acute, high-dose LT3 showed great therapeutic potential, improving LV dilatation and reducing infarct volume. However, some concerns were raised due to a trend towards a higher incidence of early reversible atrial fibrillation in LT3-treated patients. Furthermore, there was a modest increase in heart rate, and nervousness was observed in some patients during the period of administration [56].

A different or complementary therapeutic approach could include the development of drugs that enhance local tissue T3 levels indirectly by potentiating the conversion of T4 to T3 or by inhibiting D3 activity [75]. In fact, a beneficial role of vitamin D supplementation has been shown in the conversion of LT4 to LT3 via D2 in experimental studies. In addition, in a recent clinical study in AMI patients, a relationship between hypovitaminosis D and LT3 levels has been found, indicating that vitamin D supplementation could potentially act to restore local T3 levels [76].

The development and synthesis of novel TH analogs could also prove valuable in order to selectively target specific TRs [77]. In this regard, TH analogs lacking iodine molecules would be resistant to deiodinase activity and could specifically activate TR receptors of interest in low doses.

Specific delivery and targeting of injured tissues could also be achieved through novel nanotechnology approaches. Recently, Karakus et al. formulated and characterized chemically modified polymeric nanoparticles (NPs) incorporating T3 in the surface in order to target membrane integrin receptor $\alpha v \beta 3$ in such a manner that only the nongenomic effects are activated [78]. Modified T3 was conjugated to polylactide-co-glycolide (PLGA), which is a biodegradable and hydrophobic FDA-approved drug delivery carrier, in order to enhance T3 delivery and restrict its nuclear translocation [79,80]. Interestingly, PLGA-T3 NPs showed an enhanced cardioprotective effect, improved mitochondrial function, energy status, and preserved cytoskeletal integrity under hypoxic conditions. This nanotargeted delivery of T3 can prolong the circulation half-life of T3 and allows for the encapsulation of different bioactive molecules such as phosphocreatine, which could further improve the energy status of cardiomyocytes. In the field of HFpEF, nanomedicine-based approaches could be of utmost importance for the specific delivery of TH in the heart and the avoidance or minimization of TH-associated adverse effects. One recent attempt (funded by the EuroNanoMed III) incorporates computational, chemistry, and cellular biology approaches to develop a nanoparticle-based drug delivery system that will target and deliver T3 in diabetes-injured cells in order to restore cardiac and renal function. Both polymeric and lipid nanoparticles are functionalized with specific molecules in the surface that permit targeting and uptake from stressed cells. After uptake, T3 is released in the cell and acts on TRs. The main advantages of these smart nanocarriers are that adverse effects such as tachycardia, arrhythmias (mainly atrial fibrillation), kidney hyperfiltration, nervousness, and disruption of the thyroid axis could be avoided [81].

4. Conclusions

HF greatly affects patients' quality of life and survival, and novel therapeutic approaches for its treatment are quite necessary. TH signaling, on the other hand, has a crucial role in the pathophysiology of HF and ischemic heart disease, while past and ongoing studies are promising, regarding TH's therapeutic results. Novel or complementary therapeutic approaches with the use of cutting-edge technologies could become an important tool to highlight and enhance TH therapeutic potential, at the same time avoiding probable adverse effects.

Funding: Part of this research has been funded from the EuroNanoMed3 project entitled "Regenerating the diabetic heart and kidney by using stress-specific thyroid hormone nanocarriers" (T11EPA4-00079).

Institutional Review Board Statement: Not applicable.

Informed Consent Statement: Not applicable.

Data Availability Statement: Not applicable.

Conflicts of Interest: C.P. and I.M. are the inventors and hold royalties in relation to the patent PCT/EP2019/087056. Other authors have no disclosures to report.

References

1. McDonagh, T.A.; Metra, M.; Adamo, M.; Gardner, R.S.; Baumbach, A.; Böhm, M.; Burri, H.; Butler, J.; Čelutkienė, J.; Chioncel, O.; et al. 2021 ESC Guidelines for the diagnosis and treatment of acute and chronic heart failure. *Eur. Heart J.* **2021**, *42*, 3599–3726. [CrossRef] [PubMed]
2. Savarese, G.; Becher, P.M.; Lund, L.H.; Seferovic, P.; Rosano, G.M.C.; Coats, A. Global burden of heart failure: A comprehensive and updated review of epidemiology. *Cardiovasc. Res.* **2022**, *118*, 3272–3287. [CrossRef] [PubMed]
3. Mantzouratou, P.; Lavecchia, A.M.; Xinaris, C. Thyroid Hormone Signalling in Human Evolution and Disease: A Novel Hypothesis. *J. Clin. Med.* **2021**, *11*, 43. [CrossRef] [PubMed]
4. Brent, G.A. Mechanisms of thyroid hormone action. *J. Clin. Investig.* **2012**, *122*, 3035–3043. [CrossRef] [PubMed]

5. Stoykov, I.; Zandieh-Doulabi, B.; Moorman, A.F.M.; Christoffels, V.; Wiersinga, W.M.; Bakker, O. Expression pattern and ontogenesis of thyroid hormone receptor isoforms in the mouse heart. *J. Endocrinol.* **2006**, *189*, 231–245. [CrossRef]
6. Anyetei-Anum, C.S.; Roggero, V.R.; Allison, L.A. Thyroid hormone receptor localization in target tissues. *J. Endocrinol.* **2018**, *237*, R19–R34. [CrossRef]
7. Pantos, C.; Mourouzis, I. Thyroid hormone receptor α1 as a novel therapeutic target for tissue repair. *Ann. Transl. Med.* **2018**, *6*, 254. [CrossRef]
8. Mourouzis, I.; Lavecchia, A.M.; Xinaris, C. Thyroid Hormone Signalling: From the Dawn of Life to the Bedside. *J. Mol. Evol.* **2020**, *88*, 88–103. [CrossRef]
9. Pantos, C.; Mourouzis, I. The emerging role of TRα1 in cardiac repair: Potential therapeutic implications. *Oxid. Med. Cell Longev.* **2014**, *2014*, 481482. [CrossRef]
10. Hirose, K.; Payumo, A.Y.; Cutie, S.; Hoang, A.; Zhang, H.; Guyot, R.; Lunn, D.; Bigley, R.B.; Yu, H.; Wang, J.; et al. Evidence for hormonal control of heart regenerative capacity during endothermy acquisition. *Science* **2019**, *364*, 184–188. [CrossRef]
11. Lavecchia, A.M.; Pelekanos, K.; Mavelli, F.; Xinaris, C. Cell Hypertrophy: A 'Biophysical Roadblock' to Reversing Kidney Injury. *Front. Cell Dev. Biol.* **2022**, *10*, 854998. [CrossRef]
12. Luongo, C.; Dentice, M.; Salvatore, D. Deiodinases and their intricate role in thyroid hormone homeostasis. *Nat. Rev. Endocrinol.* **2019**, *15*, 479–488. [CrossRef]
13. Dentice, M.; Marsili, A.; Zavacki, A.; Larsen, P.R.; Salvatore, D. The deiodinases and the control of intracellular thyroid hormone signaling during cellular differentiation. *Biochim. Biophys. Acta* **2013**, *1830*, 3937–3945. [CrossRef]
14. Barca-Mayo, O.; Liao, X.H.; Alonso, M.; Di Cosmo, C.; Hernandez, A.; Refetoff, S.; Weisse, R.E. Thyroid hormone receptor α and regulation of type 3 deiodinase. *Mol. Endocrinol.* **2011**, *25*, 575–583. [CrossRef]
15. Simonides, W.S.; Mulcahey, M.A.; Redout, E.M.; Muller, A.; Zuidwijk, M.J.; Visser, T.J.; Wassen, F.W.J.S.; Crescenzi, A.; da-Silva, W.S.; Harney, J.; et al. Hypoxia-inducible factor induces local thyroid hormone inactivation during hypoxic-ischemic disease in rats. *J. Clin. Investig.* **2008**, *118*, 975–983. [CrossRef]
16. Pantos, C.; Xinaris, C.; Mourouzis, I.; Perimenis, P.; Politi, E.; Spanou, D.; Cokkinos, D.V. Thyroid hormone receptor alpha 1: A switch to cardiac cell 'metamorphosis'? *J. Physiol. Pharmacol.* **2008**, *59*, 253–269.
17. Pantos, C.; Mourouzis, I.; Xinaris, C.; Papadopoulou-Daifoti, Z.; Cokkinos, D. Thyroid hormone and 'cardiac metamorphosis': Potential therapeutic implications. *Pharmacol. Ther.* **2008**, *118*, 277–294. [CrossRef]
18. Ojamaa, K.; Kenessey, A.; Shenoy, R.; Klein, I. Thyroid hormone metabolism and cardiac gene expression after acute myocardial infarction in the rat. *Am. J. Physiol. Endocrinol. Metab.* **2000**, *279*, E1319–E1324. [CrossRef]
19. Alpert, N.R.; Brosseau, C.; Federico, A.; Krenz, M.; Robbins, J.; Warshaw, D.M. Molecular mechanics of mouse cardiac myosin isoforms. *Am. J. Physiol. Heart Circ. Physiol.* **2002**, *283*, H1446–H1454. [CrossRef]
20. Pantos, C.; Mourouzis, I.; Cokkinos, D.V. New insights into the role of thyroid hormone in cardiac remodeling: Time to reconsider? *Heart Fail. Rev.* **2011**, *16*, 79–96. [CrossRef]
21. Rajabi, M.; Kassiotis, C.; Razeghi, P.; Taegtmeyer, H. Return to the fetal gene program protects the stressed heart: A strong hypothesis. *Heart Fail. Rev.* **2007**, *12*, 331–343. [CrossRef]
22. Swynghedauw, B. Molecular mechanisms of myocardial remodeling. *Physiol. Rev.* **1999**, *79*, 215–262. [CrossRef] [PubMed]
23. Bolognese, L.; Neskovic, A.N.; Parodi, G.; Cerisano, G.; Buonamici, P.; Santoro, G.M.; Antoniucci, D. Left ventricular remodeling after primary coronary angioplasty: Patterns of left ventricular dilation and long-term prognostic implications. *Circulation* **2002**, *106*, 2351–2357. [CrossRef] [PubMed]
24. Pantos, C.; Mourouzis, I.; Galanopoulos, G.; Gavra, M.; Perimenis, P.; Spanou, D.; Cokkinos, D.V. Thyroid hormone receptor alpha1 downregulation in postischemic heart failure progression: The potential role of tissue hypothyroidism. *Horm. Metab. Res. Horm. Stoffwechs. Horm. Metab.* **2010**, *42*, 718–724. [CrossRef] [PubMed]
25. Mourouzis, I.; Kostakou, E.; Galanopoulos, G.; Mantzouratou, P.; Pantos, C. Inhibition of thyroid hormone receptor α1 impairs post-ischemic cardiac performance after myocardial infarction in mice. *Mol. Cell Biochem.* **2013**, *379*, 97–105. [CrossRef]
26. Mourouzis, I.; Mantzouratou, P.; Galanopoulos, G.; Kostakou, E.; Roukounakis, N.; Kokkinos, A.D.; Cokkinos, D.V.; Pantos, C. Dose-dependent effects of thyroid hormone on post-ischemic cardiac performance: Potential involvement of Akt and ERK signalings. *Mol. Cell Biochem.* **2012**, *363*, 235–243. [CrossRef]
27. Iliopoulou, I.; Mourouzis, I.; Lambrou, G.I.; Iliopoulou, D.; Koutsouris, D.D.; Pantos, C. Time-dependent and independent effects of thyroid hormone administration following myocardial infarction in rats. *Mol. Med. Rep.* **2018**, *18*, 864–876. [CrossRef]
28. Chen, Y.F.; Kobayashi, S.; Chen, J.; Redetzke, R.A.; Said, S.; Liang, Q.; Gerdes, A.M. Short term triiodo-L-thyronine treatment inhibits cardiac myocyte apoptosis in border area after myocardial infarction in rats. *J. Mol. Cell Cardiol.* **2008**, *44*, 180–187. [CrossRef]
29. Forini, F.; Lionetti, V.; Ardehali, H.; Pucci, A.; Cecchetti, F.; Ghanefar, M.; Nicolini, G.; Ichikawa, Y.; Nannipieri, M.; Recchia, F.A.; et al. Early long-term L-T3 replacement rescues mitochondria and prevents ischemic cardiac remodelling in rats. *J. Cell Mol. Med.* **2011**, *15*, 514–524. [CrossRef]
30. Mourouzis, I.; Giagourta, I.; Galanopoulos, G.; Mantzouratou, P.; Kostakou, E.; Kokkinos, A.D.; Tentolouris, N.; Pantos, C. Thyroid hormone improves the mechanical performance of the post-infarcted diabetic myocardium: A response associated with up-regulation of Akt/mTOR and AMPK activation. *Metabolism* **2013**, *62*, 1387–1393.

1. Pantos, C.; Malliopoulou, V.; Paizis, I.; Moraitis, P.; Mourouzis, I.; Tzeis, S.; Karamanoli, E.; Cokkinos, D.D.; Carageorgiou, H.; Varonos, D.; et al. Thyroid hormone and cardioprotection: Study of p38 MAPK and JNKs during ischaemia and at reperfusion in isolated rat heart. *Mol. Cell Biochem.* **2003**, *242*, 173–180. [CrossRef]
2. Pantos, C.; Mourouzis, I.; Saranteas, T.; Clavé, G.; Ligeret, H.; Noack-Fraissignes, P.; Renard, P.-Y.; Massonneau, M.; Perimenis, P.; Spanou, D.; et al. Thyroid hormone improves postischaemic recovery of function while limiting apoptosis: A new therapeutic approach to support hemodynamics in the setting of ischaemia-reperfusion? *Basic Res. Cardiol.* **2009**, *104*, 69–77. [CrossRef]
3. Lymvaios, I.; Mourouzis, I.; Cokkinos, D.V.; Dimopoulos, M.A.; Toumanidis, S.T.; Pantos, C. Thyroid hormone and recovery of cardiac function in patients with acute myocardial infarction: A strong association? *Eur. J. Endocrinol.* **2011**, *165*, 107–114. [CrossRef]
4. Lazzeri, C.; Sori, A.; Picariello, C.; Chiostri, M.; Gensini, G.F.; Valente, S. Nonthyroidal illness syndrome in ST-elevation myocardial infarction treated with mechanical revascularization. *Int. J. Cardiol.* **2012**, *158*, 103–104. [CrossRef]
5. Lee, Y.; Lim, Y.H.; Shin, J.H.; Park, J.; Shin, J. Impact of subclinical hypothyroidism on clinical outcomes following percutaneous coronary intervention. *Int. J. Cardiol.* **2018**, *253*, 155–160. [CrossRef]
6. Xue, Y.; Zhu, Y.; Shen, J.; Zhou, W.; Xiang, J.; Xiang, Z.; Wang, L.; Luo, S. The Association of Thyroid Hormones With Cardiogenic Shock and Prognosis in Patients with ST Segment Elevation Myocardial Infarction (STEMI) Treated with Primary PCI. *Am. J. Med. Sci.* **2022**, *363*, 251–258. [CrossRef]
7. Gao, S.; Ma, W.; Huang, S.; Lin, X.; Yu, M. Predictive Value of Free Triiodothyronine to Free Thyroxine Ratio in Euthyroid Patients With Myocardial Infarction With Nonobstructive Coronary Arteries. *Front. Endocrinol.* **2021**, *12*, 708216. [CrossRef]
8. Jabbar, A.; Ingoe, L.; Thomas, H.; Carey, P.; Junejo, S.; Addison, C.; Vernazza, J.; Austin, D.; Greenwood, J.P.; Zaman, A. Prevalence, predictors and outcomes of thyroid dysfunction in patients with acute myocardial infarction: The ThyrAMI-1 study. *J. Endocrinol. Investig.* **2021**, *44*, 1209–1218. [CrossRef] [PubMed]
9. Pingitore, A.; Landi, P.; Taddei, M.C.; Ripoli, A.; L'Abbate, A.; Iervasi, G. Triiodothyronine levels for risk stratification of patients with chronic heart failure. *Am. J. Med.* **2005**, *118*, 132–136. [CrossRef] [PubMed]
10. Xinke, Z.; Rongcheng, Z.; Hugang, J.; Kai, L.; Chengxu, M.; Ming, B.; Tao, A.; Younan, Y.; Xinqiang, W.; Ming, W.; et al. Combined Use of Low T3 Syndrome and NT-proBNP as Predictors for Death in Patients with Acute Decompensated Heart Failure. *BMC Endocr. Disord.* **2021**, *21*, 140.
11. Rothberger, G.D.; Gadhvi, S.; Michelakis, N.; Kumar, A.; Calixte, R.; Shapiro, L.E. Usefulness of Serum Triiodothyronine (T3) to Predict Outcomes in Patients Hospitalized with Acute Heart Failure. *Am. J. Cardiol.* **2017**, *119*, 599–603. [CrossRef] [PubMed]
12. Sato, Y.; Yoshihisa, A.; Kimishima, Y.; Kiko, T.; Kanno, Y.; Yokokawa, T.; Abe, S.; Misaka, T.; Sato, T.; Oikawa, M.; et al. Low T3 Syndrome Is Associated with High Mortality in Hospitalized Patients With Heart Failure. *J. Card. Fail.* **2019**, *25*, 195–203. [CrossRef]
13. Fontana, M.; Passino, C.; Poletti, R.; Zyw, L.; Prontera, C.; Scarlattini, M.; Clerico, A.; Emdin, M.; Iervasi, G. Low triiodothyronine and exercise capacity in heart failure. *Int. J. Cardiol.* **2012**, *154*, 153–157. [CrossRef]
14. Kannan, L.; Shaw, P.A.; Morley, M.P.; Brandimarto, J.; Fang, J.C.; Sweitzer, N.K.; Cappola, T.P.; Cappola, A.R. Thyroid Dysfunction in Heart Failure and Cardiovascular Outcomes. *Circ. Heart Fail.* **2018**, *11*, e005266. [CrossRef]
15. Wang, W.; Guan, H.; Fang, W.; Zhang, K.; Gerdes, A.M.; Iervasi, G.; Tang, Y.D. Free Triiodothyronine Level Correlates with Myocardial Injury and Prognosis in Idiopathic Dilated Cardiomyopathy: Evidence from Cardiac MRI and SPECT/PET Imaging. *Sci. Rep.* **2016**, *6*, 39811. [CrossRef]
16. Hamilton, M.A.; Stevenson, L.W.; Fonarow, G.C.; Steimle, A.; Goldhaber, J.I.; Child, J.S.; Chopra, I.J.; Moriguchi, J.D.; Hage, A. Safety and hemodynamic effects of intravenous triiodothyronine in advanced congestive heart failure. *Am. J. Cardiol.* **1998**, *81*, 443–447. [CrossRef]
17. Pingitore, A.; Galli, E.; Barison, A.; Iervasi, A.; Scarlattini, M.; Nucci, D.; L'abbate, A.; Mariotti, R.; Iervasi, G. Acute effects of triiodothyronine (T3) replacement therapy in patients with chronic heart failure and low-T3 syndrome: A randomized, placebo-controlled study. *J. Clin. Endocrinol. Metab.* **2008**, *93*, 1351–1358. [CrossRef]
18. Holmager, P.; Schmidt, U.; Mark, P.; Andersen, U.; Dominguez, H.; Raymond, I.; Zerahn, B.; Nygaard, B.; Kistorp, C.; Faber, J. Long-term L-Triiodothyronine (T3) treatment in stable systolic heart failure patients: A randomised, double-blind, cross-over, placebo-controlled intervention study. *Clin. Endocrinol.* **2015**, *83*, 931–937. [CrossRef]
19. Amin, A.; Chitsazan, M.; Taghavi, S.; Ardeshiri, M. Effects of triiodothyronine replacement therapy in patients with chronic stable heart failure and low-triiodothyronine syndrome: A randomized, double-blind, placebo-controlled study. *ESC Heart Fail.* **2015**, *2*, 5–11. [CrossRef]
20. Zhang, X.; Wang, W.; Zhang, K.; Tian, J.; Zheng, J.L.; Chen, J.; An, S.M.; Wang, S.Y.; Liu, Y.P.; Zhao, Y.; et al. Efficacy and safety of levothyroxine (L-T4) replacement on the exercise capability in chronic systolic heart failure patients with subclinical hypothyroidism: Study protocol for a multi-center, open label, randomized, parallel group trial (ThyroHeart-CHF). *Trials* **2019**, *20*, 143. [CrossRef]
21. Pingitore, A.; Mastorci, F.; Piaggi, P.; Aquaro, G.D.; Molinaro, S.; Ravani, M.; De Caterina, A.; Trianni, G.; Ndreu, R.; Berti, S.; et al. Usefulness of Triiodothyronine Replacement Therapy in Patients with ST Elevation Myocardial Infarction and Border-line/Reduced Triiodothyronine Levels (from the THIRST Study). *Am. J. Cardiol.* **2019**, *123*, 905–912. [CrossRef] [PubMed]

52. Jabbar, A.; Ingoe, L.; Junejo, S.; Carey, P.; Addison, C.; Thomas, H.; Parikh, J.D.; Austin, D.; Hollingsworth, K.G.; Stocken, D.D. et al. Effect of Levothyroxine on Left Ventricular Ejection Fraction in Patients With Subclinical Hypothyroidism and Acute Myocardial Infarction: A Randomized Clinical Trial. *JAMA* **2020**, *324*, 249–258. [CrossRef] [PubMed]
53. Sinn, M.R.; Lund, G.K.; Muellerleile, K.; Freiwald, E.; Saeed, M.; Avanesov, M.; Lenz, A.; Starekova, J.; von Kodolitsch, Y.; Blankenberg, S.; et al. Prognosis of early pre-discharge and late left ventricular dilatation by cardiac magnetic resonance imaging after acute myocardial infarction. *Int. J. Cardiovasc. Imaging* **2021**, *37*, 1711–1720. [CrossRef] [PubMed]
54. Breathett, K.; Allen, L.A.; Udelson, J.; Davis, G.; Bristow, M. Changes in Left Ventricular Ejection Fraction Predict Survival and Hospitalization in Heart Failure With Reduced Ejection Fraction. *Circ. Heart Fail.* **2016**, *9*, e002962. [CrossRef] [PubMed]
55. Yerra, L.; Anavekar, N.; Skali, H.; Zelenkofske, S.; Velazquez, E.; McMurray, J.; Pfeffer, M.; Solomon, S.D. Association of QRS duration and outcomes after myocardial infarction: The VALIANT trial. *Heart Rhythm* **2006**, *3*, 313–316. [CrossRef]
56. Pantos, C.I.; Trikas, A.G.; Pissimisis, E.G.; Grigoriou, K.P.; Stougiannos, P.N.; Dimopoulos, A.K.; Linardakis, S.I.; Alexopoulos, N.A.; Evdoridis, C.G.; Gavrielatos, G.D.; et al. Effects of Acute Triiodothyronine Treatment in Patients with Anterior Myocardial Infarction Undergoing Primary Angioplasty: Evidence from a Pilot Randomized Clinical Trial (ThyRepair Study). *Thyroid* **2022**, *32*, 714–724. [CrossRef]
57. Novitzky, D.; Mi, Z.; Sun, Q.; Collins, J.F.; Cooper, D.K. Thyroid hormone therapy in the management of 63,593 brain-dead organ donors: A retrospective review. *Transplantation* **2014**, *98*, 1119–1127. [CrossRef]
58. Novitzky, D.; Cooper, D.K. Thyroid hormones and the stunned myocardium. *J. Endocrinol.* **2014**, *223*, R1–R8. [CrossRef]
59. Omote, K.; Verbrugge, F.H.; Borlaug, B.A. Heart Failure with Preserved Ejection Fraction: Mechanisms and Treatment Strategies. *Annu. Rev. Med.* **2022**, *73*, 321–337. [CrossRef]
60. Gevaert, A.B.; Kataria, R.; Zannad, F.; Sauer, A.J.; Damman, K.; Sharma, K.; Shah, S.J.; Van Spall, H.G.C. Heart failure with preserved ejection fraction: Recent concepts in diagnosis, mechanisms and management. *Heart Br. Card Soc.* **2022**, *108*, 1342–1350 [CrossRef]
61. Gevaert, A.B.; Boen, J.R.A.; Segers, V.F.; Van Craenenbroeck, E.M. Heart Failure with Preserved Ejection Fraction: A Review of Cardiac and Noncardiac Pathophysiology. *Front. Physiol.* **2019**, *10*, 638. [CrossRef]
62. Runte, K.E.; Bell, S.P.; Selby, D.E.; Häußler, T.N.; Ashikaga, T.; LeWinter, M.M.; Palmer, B.M.; Meyer, M. Relaxation and the Role of Calcium in Isolated Contracting Myocardium from Patients with Hypertensive Heart Disease and Heart Failure With Preserved Ejection Fraction. *Circ. Heart Fail.* **2017**, *10*, e004311. [CrossRef]
63. Neves, J.S.; Vale, C.; von Hafe, M.; Borges-Canha, M.; Leite, A.R.; Almeida-Coelho, J.; Lourenço, A.; Falcão-Pires, I.; Carvalho, D.; Leite-Moreira, A. Thyroid hormones and modulation of diastolic function: A promising target for heart failure with preserved ejection fraction. *Ther. Adv. Endocrinol. Metab.* **2020**, *11*, 2042018820958331. [CrossRef]
64. von Hafe, M.; Neves, J.S.; Vale, C.; Borges-Canha, M.; Leite-Moreira, A. The impact of thyroid hormone dysfunction on ischemic heart disease. *Endocr. Connect.* **2019**, *8*, R76–R90. [CrossRef]
65. Dan, G.-A. Thyroid Hormones and the Heart. *Heart Fail. Rev.* **2016**, *21*, 357–359. [CrossRef]
66. Madathil, A.; Hollingsworth, K.G.; Blamire, A.M.; Razvi, S.; Newton, J.L.; Taylor, R.; Weaver, J.U. Levothyroxine Improves Abnormal Cardiac Bioenergetics in Subclinical Hypothyroidism: A Cardiac Magnetic Resonance Spectroscopic Study. *J. Clin. Endocrinol. Metab.* **2015**, *100*, E607–E610. [CrossRef]
67. Vale, C.; Neves, J.S.; von Hafe, M.; Borges-Canha, M.; Leite-Moreira, A. The Role of Thyroid Hormones in Heart Failure. *Cardiovasc. Drugs Ther.* **2019**, *33*, 179–188. [CrossRef]
68. Biondi, B.; Fazio, S.; Palmieri, E.A.; Carella, C.; Panza, N.; Cittadini, A.; Bonè, F.; Lombardi, G.; Saccà, L. Left ventricular diastolic dysfunction in patients with subclinical hypothyroidism. *J. Clin. Endocrinol. Metab.* **1999**, *84*, 2064–2067. [CrossRef]
69. Razvi, S. Novel uses of thyroid hormones in cardiovascular conditions. *Endocrine* **2019**, *66*, 115–123. [CrossRef]
70. Selvaraj, S.; Klein, I.; Danzi, S.; Akhter, N.; Bonow, R.O.; Shah, S.J. Association of serum triiodothyronine with B-type natriuretic peptide and severe left ventricular diastolic dysfunction in heart failure with preserved ejection fraction. *Am. J. Cardiol.* **2012**, *110*, 234–239. [CrossRef]
71. Weltman, N.Y.; Pol, C.J.; Zhang, Y.; Wang, Y.; Koder, A.; Raza, S.; Zucchi, R.; Saba, A.; Colligiani, D.; Gerdes, A.M. Long-term physiological T3 supplementation in hypertensive heart disease in rats. *Am. J. Physiol. Heart Circ. Physiol.* **2015**, *309*, H1059–H1065. [CrossRef] [PubMed]
72. Coppola, A. Developing Oral LT3 Therapy for Heart Failure with Preserved Ejection Fraction. clinicaltrials.gov. 2021 Dec. Report No.: NCT04111536. Available online: https://clinicaltrials.gov/ct2/show/NCT04111536 (accessed on 9 June 2022).
73. The Coronary Drug Project. Findings leading to discontinuation of the 2.5-mg day estrogen group. The coronary Drug Project Research Group. *JAMA* **1973**, *226*, 652–657. [CrossRef]
74. Goldman, S.; McCarren, M.; Morkin, E.; Ladenson, P.W.; Edson, R.; Warren, S.; Ohm, J.; Thai, H.; Churby, L.; Barnhill, J.; et al. DITPA (3,5-Diiodothyropropionic Acid), a thyroid hormone analog to treat heart failure: Phase II trial veterans affairs cooperative study. *Circulation* **2009**, *119*, 3093–3100. [CrossRef] [PubMed]
75. Trivieri, M.G.; Oudit, G.Y.; Sah, R.; Kerfant, B.G.; Sun, H.; Gramolini, A.O.; Pan, Y.; Wickenden, A.D.; Croteau, W.; Morreale de Escobar, G.; et al. Cardiac-specific elevations in thyroid hormone enhance contractility and prevent pressure overload-induced cardiac dysfunction. *Proc. Natl. Acad. Sci. USA* **2006**, *103*, 6043–6048. [CrossRef]
76. Pingitore, A.; Mastorci, F.; Berti, S.; Sabatino, L.; Palmieri, C.; Iervasi, G.; Vassalle, C. Hypovitaminosis D and Low T3 Syndrome: A Link for Therapeutic Challenges in Patients with Acute Myocardial Infarction. *J. Clin. Med.* **2021**, *10*, 5267. [CrossRef]

7. Pantos, C.; Mourouzis, I. Translating thyroid hormone effects into clinical practice: The relevance of thyroid hormone receptor α1 in cardiac repair. *Heart Fail. Rev.* **2015**, *20*, 273–282. [CrossRef]
8. Karakus, O.O.; Darwish, N.H.E.; Sudha, T.; Salaheldin, T.A.; Fujioka, K.; Dickinson, P.C.T.; Weil, B.; Mousa, S.A. Development of Triiodothyronine Polymeric Nanoparticles for Targeted Delivery in the Cardioprotection against Ischemic Insult. *Biomedicines* **2021**, *9*, 1713. [CrossRef]
9. Makadia, H.K.; Siegel, S.J. Poly Lactic-co-Glycolic Acid (PLGA) as Biodegradable Controlled Drug Delivery Carrier. *Polymers* **2011**, *3*, 1377–1397. [CrossRef]
10. Rezvantalab, S.; Drude, N.I.; Moraveji, M.K.; Güvener, N.; Koons, E.K.; Shi, Y.; Lammers, T.; Kiessling, F. PLGA-Based Nanoparticles in Cancer Treatment. *Front. Pharmacol.* **2018**, *9*, 1260. [CrossRef]
11. Regenerating the Diabetic Heart and Kidney by Using Stress-Specific Thyroid Hormone Nanocarriers—ERA-LEARN. Available online: https://www.era-learn.eu/network-information/networks/euronanomed-iii/joint-transnational-call-2019/regenerating-the-diabetic-heart-and-kidney-by-using-stress-specific-thyroid-hormone-nanocarriersAuthor (accessed on 13 June 2022).

Disclaimer/Publisher's Note: The statements, opinions and data contained in all publications are solely those of the individual author(s) and contributor(s) and not of MDPI and/or the editor(s). MDPI and/or the editor(s) disclaim responsibility for any injury to people or property resulting from any ideas, methods, instructions or products referred to in the content.

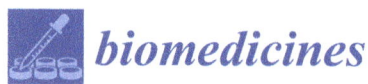

Review

The Perspectives of Platelet Proteomics in Health and Disease

Preeti Kumari Chaudhary, Sachin Upadhayaya, Sanggu Kim and Soochong Kim *

Laboratory of Veterinary Pathology and Platelet Signaling, College of Veterinary Medicine, Chungbuk National University, Cheongju 28644, Republic of Korea; chaudharypreety11@gmail.com (P.K.C.); dr.supadhayaya@gmail.com (S.U.); tkdrnfld@naver.com (S.K.)
* Correspondence: skim0026@cbu.ac.kr; Tel.: +82-43-249-1846

Abstract: Cardiovascular thromboembolic diseases and cancer continue to be a leading cause of death and disability worldwide. Therefore, it is crucial to advance their diagnoses and treatment in the context of individualized medicine. However, the disease specificity of the currently available markers is limited. Based on analyses of a subset of peptides and matching proteins in disease vs. healthy platelets, scientists have recently shown that focused platelet proteomics enables the quantification of disease-specific biomarkers in humans. In this review, we explored the potential of accurate platelet proteomic research, which is required to identify novel diagnostic and pharmaceutical targets by comprehending the proteome variety of healthy individuals and patients for personalized and precision medicine.

Keywords: platelet; proteomics; CVDs; cancer; transfusion

Citation: Chaudhary, P.K.;
Upadhayaya, S.; Kim, S.; Kim, S. The
Perspectives of Platelet Proteomics in
Health and Disease. *Biomedicines*
2024, *12*, 585. https://doi.org/
10.3390/biomedicines12030585

Academic Editor: Alfredo Caturano

Received: 3 January 2024
Revised: 8 February 2024
Accepted: 8 February 2024
Published: 6 March 2024

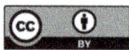

Copyright: © 2024 by the authors. Licensee MDPI, Basel, Switzerland. This article is an open access article distributed under the terms and conditions of the Creative Commons Attribution (CC BY) license (https:// creativecommons.org/licenses/by/ 4.0/).

1. Introduction

Platelets are small anucleated cell fragments that play a central role in regulating thrombosis and hemostasis in the body. They contain more than 1500 proteins, including those involved in platelet activity, and are composed of alpha granules, dense granules, lysosomal granules, and glycogen [1]. Due to platelets' high granular content of growth factors (GFs), cytokines, and other biological modulators that can respond to a variety of signals and regulate a wide variety of biological processes, including inflammation, angiogenesis, stem cell migration, and cell proliferation, scientific research and technology have recently offered a new perspective on platelets and their functions.

Recently, the objective identification and quantification of the protein profile, the so-called proteome of cells, tissues, or organs, has drawn interest from several sectors as it provides extra useful information for research problems. This tool has been utilized to comprehend disease and to find biomarkers for the prognosis and diagnosis of diseases with various etiologies. Proteomics and platelet biology are sciences that are growing quickly and have great promise. Platelets are thought to act as biosensors for both health and diseases, and their proteome may be used to recognize the telltale signs of both [1]. It is known that platelet production is affected by one's health status and that they can even take up molecules from nearby cells and release microvesicles into the bloodstream [2–4]. Therefore, the clinical management of some pathologies in which platelets play a significant role necessitates the development of alternative therapies, as is the case in patients whose thrombosis–bleeding balance is disturbed, and a proteomics approach may help in the identification of novel targets in such cases.

It may be possible to find biomarkers that might be employed in early diagnosis, illness prediction, or therapy response by understanding how the platelet protein functions physiologically and how this may be changed in the case of disease. Additionally, because platelets are naturally lacking in a nucleus, proteomics can be one of the most intriguing methods for studying them. Moreover, studying platelet proteomics could make it possible to find new targets for developing individualized treatment plans. On the other hand, platelet proteomics could offer a substantial biomarker-finding tool in other disorders, outside those primarily connected to platelets, given the varied and diversified activities of platelets throughout ontogeny or in inflammation.

2. The Principal Role of Platelet: Hemostasis and Thrombosis

Platelets are tiny (2–3 µM in diameter) cell fragments that are the second-most prevalent component of blood circulation, after red blood cells (RBCs). They originate from the cytoplasm of megakaryocytes (MK) present in the lungs and bone marrow. After they become senile, they circulate for 7–10 days in the circulatory system before being eliminated in the spleen or liver [5]. Platelets execute many tasks from primary hemostasis to inflammation depending on their activation. Platelets have various receptors on their surface and biological components kept in various granules that play a role in their activation. Upon platelet activation, the platelet secretes a milieu of physiologically active metabolites and proteins from its granules in a well-regulated manner, and these are effectively transported to their sites of action, which strengthens the coagulative response in a positive-feedback loop [6]. There are three distinct types of granules in platelets: α-granules that consist of a variety of proteins, cytokines, chemokines, and GFs; dense-granules that house small molecules, such as serotonin, adenosine diphosphate (ADP), polyphosphates, and calcium; and lysosomes that house deteriorating enzymes (Table 1) [7]. These contents are secreted through an open canalicular system (OCS), a unique surface-connected network of channels. Toll-like receptor 9 (TLR9), protein disulfide isomerase (PDI), and vesicle-associated membrane protein 8 (VAMP-8) are present in T-granules, and it has been hypothesized that these molecules are attracted to the cell surface and aid in secretion [8].

Table 1. Various proteins present in platelet granules.

Granule	Type	Contents	Role
α-granules	Adhesive proteins	P-selectin, Fibrinogen, von Willebrand factor, Fibronectin, Thrombospondin-1/2, Laminin-8, Vitronectin	• Promoting adherence of WBCs to activated platelets and endothelium. Promotion of leukocyte adherence to activated platelets and endothelium • Binding to GpIIb/IIIa receptors, factor VIII, integrin $\alpha 5\beta 1$, $\alpha v\beta 3$, $\beta 1$, $\alpha IIb\beta 3$, $\alpha v\beta 3$, $\alpha 3\beta 1$, and $\alpha 6\beta 1$, and uPAR
	Growth factors	Epidermal-growth factor, Insulin-like-growth factor, Hepatocyte-growth factor, Platelet-derived-growth factor	• Stimulating/inhibiting the proliferation of fibroblasts, epithelial cells, and smooth muscle cells. • The major mediator of growth hormone-stimulated somatic growth and growth hormone-independent anabolic responses. The primary mediator of growth hormone (GH)-stimulated somatic growth and GH-independent anabolic responses • Metabolic flux of glucose in different insulin-sensitive cell types; plays a key role in β-cell homeostasis. Metabolic flux of glucose in various types of insulin-sensitive cells; plays a key role in the homeostasis of beta cells
	Angiogenic factors	Growth factor from vascular endothelium, Platelet-derived growth factor, Fibroblast	• Enhance the proliferation, migration, survival, and invasion of endothelial cells • Enhance permeability of existing vessels, forming a lattice network for endothelial cell migration, chemotaxis, and homing of bone marrow-derived vascular precursor cells. Improvement of the permeability of existing vessels, formation of a lattice network for the migration of endothelial cells, chemotaxis, and homing of vascular progenitor cells derived from the bone marrow • Modulating the proliferation and recruitment of perivascular cells • Activation of a serine-rich protein or serine-rich phosphorylating kinase network regulating alternative splicing of vascular endothelial growth factor receptor 1 (VEGFR1) in endothelial cells.

Table 1. Cont.

Granule	Type	Contents	Role
	Chemokines	CXCL8/7/1/5/2/6/12	• Activating and recruiting neutrophils
		CCL5/3/2/7	• Helps in the recruitment of basophils, macrophages, monocytes, eosinophils, polymorph nuclear WBCs, and neutrophils
		IL1β	• Recruitment and activation of WBCs
	Clotting factors	Factor V	• Cleavage of prothrombin to thrombin
		Protein S	• Anticoagulant by inhibition of factor IXa
		Factor XI	• Hemostasis by activating factor IX
		Factor XIII	• Fibrin network stabilization
		Kininogens	• Activating factor XI
		Plasminogen	• Fibrinolysis by means of binding to the fibrin clot
	Integral membrane proteins	Integrin αIIbβ3, GPIba-IX-V, GPVI, TLT-1, P-selectin	• Activation of platelets, adjacent platelets aggregation, formation of thrombus. Plays a role in inflammatory insult-induced bleeding. Promotes the adhesion of WBCs to activated platelets and endothelium
	Immune mediators	Complement C3/C4 precursor Factor D/H, C1 inhibitor, Immunoglobulins	• Triggers inflammation, phagocytosis, cell lysis, and cell activation by cleaving to C3a and C3b by intruders • Inhibition of activation of early clotting proteins and the classical complement pathway • Antigenic binding and neutralization
	Protease inhibitors	α2-antiplasmin, PAI-1, α2-antitrypsin, α2-macroglobulin, TFPI, C1-inhibitor	• Inhibition of plasminogen binding to fibrin and fibrin cross-linking • Binding to and inhibition of tissue-type plasminogen activator and urokinase-type plasminogen activator • Anti-inflammatory properties through the destruction of major proteases • Binding of foreign peptides, acting as a humoral barrier against pathogens • Blocks the initial steps of the extrinsic coagulation pathway by inhibiting Factor Xa and Factor VIIa • Inhibits activation of early coagulation proteins and the classical complement pathway
	Proteoglycans	MMP2/9	• Degradation of collagen, elastin, fibronectin, gelatin, and laminin and remodeling of the extracellular matrix
Dense granules	Amines	Serotonin, Histamine	• Minimize blood loss by inducing constriction of injured blood vessels and enhancing platelet aggregation • Provides aggregation and immunological stimuli
	Bivalent cations	Ca^{2+}, Mg^{2+}	
	Nucleotides	ATP, ADP, GTP, GDP	
Lysosome granules	Acid proteases	Cathepsin D and E, Carboxypeptidases (A, B), Prolinecarboxypeptidase, Collagenase, Acid phosphatase, Arylsulphatase	
	Glycohydrolases	Heparinase, β-N-acetyl-glucosaminidase	

3. Activation of Platelets

Platelets become activated upon exposure to extracellular matrix proteins including collagen, von Willebrand factor (vWF), or fibronectin when there is any endothelial damage (Figure 1). Normally, endothelial cells help to keep them inactive by secreting prostaglandin I_2 (prostacyclin, PGI_2) and nitric oxide (NO), and by expressing CD39 (ectonucleotidase that cleaves ADP/ATP). Platelets react fast to damage to the vessel wall; they adhere to the affected regions and become activated to close the wound [9]. vWF, which is generated from plasma, alters the shape of platelets in high-shear circumstances and enables their binding to the exposed collagen via glycoprotein (GP) VI and αIIbβ3 integrin at the injured region [10]. In addition, the GPIb-V-IX complex is necessary to maintain platelet adherence to the vascular surface under high-shear circumstances [11]. Collagen binding by the integrin α2β1 at low-shear circumstances also plays a significant part in platelet adherence to the damaged endothelium.

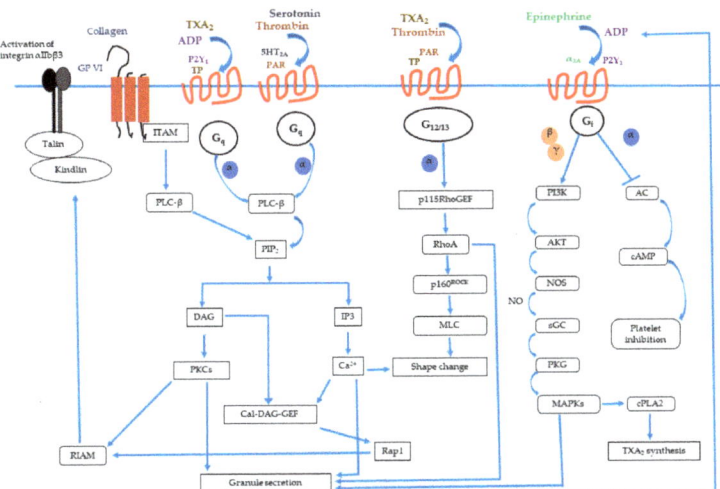

Figure 1. Overall signaling mechanism of platelet activation.

Through GPVI, a member of the immunoglobulin family that is connected to the Fc receptor (FcR), collagen starts the activation of platelets. Immune receptor tyrosine-based activation motif (ITAM), which is present in the cytoplasmic tail of FcR, is phosphorylated by Src kinases [12]. Upon activation, platelets undergo a shapeshift from discoid to a more spherical shape, develop filopodia, and completely expand into lamellipodia. Activated platelets function in a paracrine and autocrine manner to recruit more circulating platelets and further activate after adhesion. Thromboxane A_2 (TxA_2) synthesis and the ADP release from dense granules stimulate TxA_2 and $P2Y_{(1\ and\ 12)}$ receptors, respectively, by coupling to G-protein to facilitate the activation process.

The second messengers inositol 1,4,5-triphosphate (IP_3) and diacylglycerol (DAG), which are derived from the membrane phospholipid phosphatidylinositol 4,5-bisphosphate (PIP_2), are produced when the G-protein and ITAM-coupled receptors are activated. While DAG will activate several protein kinase C (PKC) isoforms, IP_3 will cause the release of Ca^{2+} from intracellular reserves [13]. Several platelet reactions, including cytoskeletal modifications, integrin activation, and degranulation, are triggered by an increase in Ca^{2+}. The guanine nucleotide exchange factor CalDAG-GEFI, in turn, activates the small GTPase Rap1 in response to an increase in Ca^{2+} [14]. Rap1 then attracts talin to the plasma membrane, further activating integrin αIIβ3 as a result. To regulate the additional cytoskeletal remodeling required for complete platelet spreading and clot retraction, active αIIβ3 will convey outside-in signaling upon binding to its ligands (such as fibrinogen, vWF, etc.) [15]. By attaching platelets to one another, this binding also helps to stabilize aggregates. Last but not least, exposed injured tissue releases tissue factor, which encourages the production of thrombin. Thrombin cleaves fibrinogen into fibrin, which will further strengthen aggregation [16]. As a result of secondary hemostasis, actin-myosin platelet retraction mediates the clot's ultimate stability. However, unbalanced clot formation (thrombosis) could result in the occlusion of the vessels in certain pathological conditions when the balance between the platelet stimulatory and inhibitory pathways is disrupted. This could result in myocardial infarction, stroke, or venous thromboembolism [17]. In conclusion, it is critical to tightly control platelet activation to guarantee a correct platelet functional response and avoid the development of unintended thrombi that might have serious pathological consequences.

4. Platelet Proteomics

A proteome is the complete set of proteins expressed within a defined sample under specific conditions that may be highly complex, as the composition depends on the phase, fate, and environment of a cell, as well being modulated by metabolic pathways and post-translational modifications (PTM). In nucleated cells, there are thought to be about 10,000 distinct proteins, among which 2000–6000 proteins have been shown to be analyzed by proteomic assays. Although platelets are anucleated cells, they retain a large portion of their cytoplasmic content from MKs and thus contain RNA, which carries messages for several platelet proteins including chemokines, FcRs, plasminogen activator inhibitor-1 (PAI-1), and PKC (Table 1). Combining proteomics with platelets will help us to analyze the total protein components of platelets under certain conditions.

Theoretically, the total expression of protein-coding genes in platelets is now predicted to be 1400 proteins based on data from the genome-wide platelet transcriptome. As far as we now understand, mitochondrial, metabolic, signaling/adaptor and transcription proteins are notably prevalent in the discovered platelet proteome [18]. A lot of progress has been achieved in the last 10 years in determining the protein makeup of platelets which are newly separated from human blood samples. The number of proteins has grown from 1300 proteins discovered by mass spectrometry and label-free analysis in 2011 to 5400 proteins, of which 3700 have estimated copy numbers [19–21]. The 500 proteins with the greatest copy numbers were analyzed, and it was found that proteins involved in signaling, small GTPases, the actin and microtubule cytoskeletons, and α-granules were the most abundant [22]. Numerous virtually intact 20 S and 26 S proteasomes were also found, supporting normal protein degradation in platelets [23]. A study also showed that 80 proteins (9%) associated with plasma proteins and signaling proteins had different abundances in small and big platelets generated from single healthy donors [24].

5. Methods of Platelet Proteomic Analysis

Platelet isolation without contamination is a challenging procedure and is performed by the centrifugation of whole blood. Indeed, various factors including the recent administration of a drug (aspirin, prednisolone), quick isolation after blood collection, age, and platelet suspension temperature may modify the protein of platelets [23,25–27]. Therefore, various methods are used to prepare the proteomics sample depending upon the purpose of the experiments [28]. The most widely used method is the lysis of platelets to extract the protein in them, and several lysis methods have been used, among which glycerol lysis appeared to be the most reproducible and efficient [29].

Protein separation can be done by two processes: Sodium dodecyl sulfate–polyacrylamide gel electrophoresis (SDS–PAGE) and two-dimensional gel electrophoresis (2-DE). In SDS-PAGE, proteins are separated according to polypeptide size using polyacrylamide gel in which low to medium-size separation occurs [30]. In the high-resolution 2-DE process of protein separation, proteins are separated by their two distinct properties: initially by their isoelectric point and then according to their relative molecular mass [31]. The composition of platelets' subcellular organelles, such as lipid rafts, membranes, secretory granules, and platelet microparticles, as well as the identification of proteins and the mapping protein phosphorylation of resting and active platelets, have all been studied using this technique. The rough relative measurement and monitoring of platelet differences under various physiological and pathological situations were made possible by further protein comparison staining or pre-labeling of the proteins from various biological samples and mixing them before separation. Mass spectrometry (MS) has increasingly become the method of choice for the analysis of complex protein samples and is currently proteomics' most important tool, as it measures the femtoliter concentration of protein [32]. For the digestion of protein to generate peptides in MS, enzymatic digestion by trypsin is known to be the best method used [33]. To minimize the complexity of the mixture, high-performance liquid chromatography (HPLC) is used in combination with electrospray ionization coupled to MS. The mass analysis and detection of peptide ions are performed by the MS. MS analysis of the peptides is divided into peptide mass fingerprinting and tandem MS (MS/MS) [34]. MS/MS allows for the sequencing of proteins and peptides, which is why it is an indispensable tool for the recognition of proteins, detection of the site of phosphorylation, structure illustration, and characterization of PTMs [35]. In MS/MS, labeling leucine is performed in protein identification [36]. The advantages and disadvantages of each method of platelet proteomics analysis are listed in Table 2.

Table 2. Advantages and disadvantages of gel-based and gel-free platelet proteomics analysis.

	Gel-Based (2D)	Gel-Free (LCMS/MS)
Advantages	1. Detection of isoforms on protein level 2. Relative quantification	1. High sensitivity 2. High throughput 3. High dynamic range 4. PTMs site location 5. Precise quantification 6. Application in clinics
Disadvantages	1. Low throughput 2. Low sensitivity 3. Low protein coverage 4. Time-consuming sample processing 5. Limited detection of hydrophobic proteins	1. Expensive analytical equipment 2. Sophisticated data analysis

To determine the quality of protein, quantitative proteomics can be performed. There are two different approaches for the quantification of protein which are label-free and isobaric labeling (tandem mass taqs or isobaric tags for relative and absolute quantification; iTRAQ). The label-free quantification approach has been the most popular and is the simpler technique, and measures the absolute concentrations of all proteins based on summarized ion counts. After protein biosynthesis, PTM is performed to control multiple biological functions of protein: protein folding, localization, and interaction with other biomolecules [37]. In the case of platelets, PMTs are studied for the phosphorylation sites, ubiquitylation, and proteolysis of proteins, as well as some special interest in platelet activation [34]. Additionally, pathway and network analysis techniques have become increasingly popular, as these aim to identify activated pathways and pathway modules from functional proteomic data [38]. Pathway analysis also helps to organize a long list of proteins in a short list of pathway knowledge maps, which makes the interpretation of molecular mechanisms easier when they are involved in protein alteration and their expression.

Validation of the proteomics analysis is a crucial step to confirm the data and can be performed by several methods including western blot, ELISA, immunoblotting, and immunoprecipitation [39].

6. Platelet Proteome in Health and Diseases

When platelets are activated, they release a variety of chemicals that can have an impact on various pathophysiological processes, such as inflammation, tissue regeneration and repair, cancer growth, and cardiovascular diseases (CVDs) (Figure 2). Earlier studies on platelet proteomics, phosphorylation, and other PTMs are done in resting and activated states where the composition and copy numbers of human and mouse platelets are thoroughly described [20,21,40]. Additionally, the "platelet release", the term for the proteomic composition of the granules released by activated platelets, is described and characterized [6]. A thorough map of human platelets and an examination of inter- and intra-donor variation also revealed that 85% of the platelet proteome is stable [21,41]. Since the fundamentals are already established, this can be used to investigate how various illnesses change platelets and, hopefully, to understand how to target those signaling pathways with drugs.

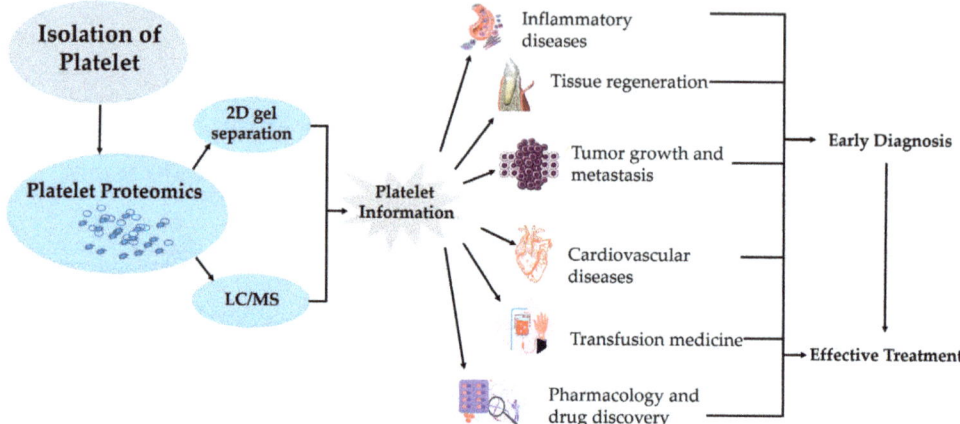

Figure 2. Schematic diagram of platelet proteomics and its application.

CVDs are the primary cause of death in developed countries, and it is well-known that platelets play a significant role in their development. Methods for the detection and prognostication of CVD progression are urgently needed, but the underlying signal transduction is still poorly understood. Acute coronary syndrome and stable coronary artery disease may now be distinguished using comparative proteomics of "platelet releasates" [42]. A study showed that 6 out of 400 proteins that were tested had distinct expression patterns in individuals with acute and chronic coronary syndromes [43]. In a small cohort of 10–30 participants that compared acute vs. chronic coronary syndromes in individuals, it was established that the differently regulated proteins have a role in the cell structure, morphology, and cell assembly processes, all of which are crucial for platelet activation [34]. In particular, signaling, glycolysis, and cytoskeletal-related platelet proteins were shown to be differentially altered in two groups of patients with acute coronary syndrome [44,45].

Likewise, in contrast to circulating platelets, gel-based proteomics found a change in 16 platelet proteins including integrin αIIb and thrombospondin-1 collected from the intracoronary culprit site in patients with ST-elevation myocardial infarction (STEMI) [46]. Furthermore, a platelet phosphoproteomic study of STEMI patients showed an elevation in critical tyrosine phosphorylation upon GPVI activation, raising the idea that GPVI might be used as an antithrombotic target in STEMI [46,47]. Platelet releasate from individuals with stable angina pectoris and whole platelets from patients with lupus anticoagulant-related thrombosis showed that only a small number of proteins are changed [48].

According to targeted mass spectrometry, the difference in integrin αIIbβ3 was found to be only 5% for platelets from control participants compared to patients with type I Glanzmann thrombasthenia, a severe bleeding disease [49]. In addition, as compared to control platelets, plasma proteins endocytosed by integrin αIIbβ3 seemed to be downregulated, including fibrinogen, factor XIII, plasminogen, and carboxypeptidase 2B. Quantitative proteomics analysis on platelets from a patient with Scott syndrome, a rare moderate bleeding condition, showed that 134 (6%) proteins were either up- or down-regulated, including the full absence of the phospholipid scramblase anoctamin-6 and low levels of the platelet-morphology-regulating calpain-1 protease [50]. Likewise, in patients with the severe bleeding condition X-linked thrombocytopenia with thalassemia, 83 changed proteins along with cyclooxygenase 1 (COX1) and a number of the cytoskeleton and proteasome proteins were discovered by quantitative proteomics [51]. Additionally, 123 platelet proteins were primarily downregulated in 5 out of 47 gray platelet syndrome patients (a milder bleeding condition) with novel variations in NBEAL2, with the majority being granule-associated and cargo proteins at unchanged mRNA expression levels [52].

Although several studies have looked at the platelets from individuals with cardiovascular conditions, complete platelet proteomic evidence is still lacking. Large-scale validation studies are necessary to determine whether platelet proteomics may be a valuable tool in cardiology treatment and clinical practice, even though prior research has shown that platelet activation varies across certain cardiovascular illnesses. With the most recent technology, it is possible to monitor the protein abundance in "platelet releasates" to assess uneven platelet reactivity and probable future thrombus development.

Some proteomic studies have looked at platelets from individuals with somatic mutations in cancer or genetically less well-defined disorders in addition to uncommon congenital defects. Quantitative proteome analysis research revealed disease regulation by a wide range of platelet proteins from 12 patients with early-stage malignancies, in contrast to healthy participants [53]. The majority of these proteins returned to normal following surgical resection. It has been suggested that the platelet proteome contains variably expressed proteins linked to early-stage cancer, and as a result, platelet proteins are identified as a novel source of potential biomarkers [53]. However, these findings were supported by proof-of-concept research conducted only on a small cohort of patients with lung or pancreatic cancer. Additional focus is required in this area as some of the proteins that are controlled by platelets may serve as biomarkers for certain malignancies.

Platelet function issues also are linked to chronic kidney disease, which can result in bleeding and thrombotic problems, leading to high morbidity and mortality [54,55]. Platelet glycoproteins GPIIb/IIIa, serotonin, and ADP release, as well as problems with the metabolism of arachidonic acid and prostaglandins, are potential contributory factors [54]. Additionally, uremic toxins have been demonstrated to affect endothelial cells, vascular smooth muscle cells, macrophages, and platelets, increasing inflammation and causing platelet activation and aggregation [56]. Due to platelets' multifactorial nature, disease stage-associated variability, and interpatient variability, unraveling the factors that contribute to platelet dysfunction through proteomics analysis for diagnostic and prognostic interests would substantially aid in the recognition of risk factors and treatment alternatives.

Significantly, the amounts of plasma proteins involved in immunological responses and inflammation were increased, which showed that these patients may also have an immune deficiency. Plasma proteins including fibrinogen and 2-macroglobulin, which are associated with enhanced endocytosis or stickiness of the patient's platelets, were shown to be raised in the platelet proteome of individuals with progressive multiple sclerosis [57]. Platelet quantitative proteomics found roughly 300 regulated proteins in dengue virus-infected individuals [58]. A total of 360 differently regulated proteins were discovered, among which four of them, PHB, UQCRH, GP1BA, and FINC, were effective in differentiating between patients and healthy controls during the platelet proteomic analysis of patients with mild and severe cognitive impairment in the search for an Alzheimer's disease biomarker [59].

Neutrophil Extracellular Traps (NETs) are formed by neutrophils during the immune response by a controlled cell death process called NETosis and are web-like structures composed of DNA and histones [60]. TLR2 and TLR4 are involved in the activation of neutrophils [61]. Histones within NETs can also activate platelets directly via TLR2 and TLR4, enhancing platelet aggregation and thrombin production [62]. Histones also stimulate the release of vWF from vascular endothelial cells, mediating further platelet adhesion and aggregation. Importantly, platelet activation can cause the dysregulation of NETosis, which can result in immune-mediated scattered microthrombi, hypercoagulability, and tissue damage through the vWF–NETs axis, leading to multiple organ failure and death [63,64]. For example, the vWF–NET axis has been noted to contribute to thrombotic complications in acute ischemic stroke and COVID-19 [65]. It has been observed that NETs cause patients with gastric cancer to have hypercoagulable platelets by upregulating the cell-surface expression of P-selectin and phosphatidylserine [66,67]. Malignant tumors may also trigger immunothrombosis by stimulating neutrophils and/or platelets, which is followed by the formation of a NET [68]. Furthermore, Guglietta et al. provided a link between NETs and platelets in an animal model of small intestinal tumors [69]. There is evidence that the interaction between platelets and NET causes autoimmune diseases like systemic lupus erythematosus by affecting coagulation [70]. It has now been demonstrated that type 1 diabetes and the platelet–neutrophil interaction are related [71]. The pancreas of non-obese diabetes mice showed a correlation between an increase in platelet–neutrophil aggregates in the circulatory system and NET markers, indicating that platelets may stimulate neutrophils for transmigration into islets, which is followed by NETosis and islet destruction. The TLR4–ERK5 platelet axis has been shown to facilitate NET formation in the lung and further promote metastasis [72]. Taken together, the TLR-mediated vWF–NET signaling pathway plays an important role in immune response and is linked to the prothrombotic state in various diseases. The detailed analysis of proteins involved in vWF–NET axis-mediated thrombosis and inflammation may be a valuable tool in identifying novel biomarkers and therapeutic targets in CVDs and other diseases associated with thrombosis.

7. Platelet Proteomics in Transfusion Medicine

A long-standing problem is how to optimally store platelets to preserve their functions after transfusion [73]. Proteomics is being actively used to describe temperature-induced platelet changes. According to transcriptome-based research, freshly separated platelets have a limited potential for protein synthesis and are continuously degrading RNA species [74]. Frequently, platelet concentrates used in transfusions may be kept in storage for a few days before the platelets begin to lose their functional characteristics, a condition known as platelet storage lesion [75]. Numerous investigations on the protein alterations of aging platelets have been conducted to determine the source of this lesion. In an early study, the majority of the 2900 identified proteins were found to have new N-termini, which showed that platelet storage included significant proteolytic processing [76]. Endocytosis- and cytoskeleton-related proteins were shown to alter with platelet age to enrich younger circulating platelets in a platelet apheresis intervention program [77]. According to two quantitative proteomic investigations, changed proteins in particular had a role in degranulation as the storage duration increased [78,79]. Due to the stimulation of glycoprotein shedding, platelets kept at 2–6 °C were shown to exhibit lower levels of glycoproteins and higher amounts of surface activation indicators, although their viability was unaffected [80]. In the wake of the transfusion of aging platelets, several organizations are looking for proteins present in the platelet that might justify harmful transfusion responses that harm the health of patients. In terms of pathogen inactivation, the exposure of concentrated platelets to riboflavin and ultraviolet light for two days led to the production of reactive oxygen species, which led to a slight increase in the number of oxidized peptides when compared to the 18% of the 9400 identified platelet peptides that were already oxidized [81,82]. Age-related upregulation of proinflammatory cytokines (CCL5, PF4) and metabolic proteins (such as glycolysis and lactate synthesis) was seen in proteomic investigations on extracellular vesicles produced by aging platelets [83].

As technology advanced, proteomic research using label-free quantification showed that prolonged storage for 13–16 days decreased the levels of proteins involved in platelet degranulation, secretion, and exocytosis while increasing the levels of 2-macroglobulin, glycogenin, and Ig chain C region [78]. Wang et al. discovered that varied storage temperatures resulted in various PSLs after comparing the proteomic signatures of platelets kept at 22 °C, 10 °C, and 80 °C. While cold storage affects SNARE interactions in vesicular transport and vasopressin-regulated water reabsorption, the storage duration mostly affects endocytosis, Fc gamma R-mediated phagocytosis, and actin rearrangement [79]. Concentrated platelets for customized transfusions may become available in the future of precision medicine.

8. Hurdles in Accurate Platelet Proteome Research

While studying platelets by proteomics may appear simple and straightforward, there are several issues, mostly with the quality control of samples used in this proteomics research. The use of high-throughput proteomics to study platelet biology raises several issues, as accepted by all industry professionals. These range from the collection of blood samples, such as the isolation method, use of anticoagulant, and sample processing, to components of mass spectrometry technology and data analysis, such as protein detection low-abundance, modifiable protein abundance, etc.

Washed platelets are often employed in platelet proteome studies today. Reliable proteome analysis depends on the platelet purity, quantity, and activation state. Although washed platelets have been isolated in most studies with a high purity (99–99.99%), the presence of proteins from plasma, RBCs, and white blood cells (WBCs) cannot be totally ruled out [18]. The platelet separation process is often built upon a series of low-speed centrifugation stages that separate whole blood into distinct blood components depending on their densities while leaving the tiny, light platelets floating in the liquid plasma [84,85]. However, because platelets in direct contact with blood plasma have a prolonged open canicular system, leftover plasma proteins are always present in the majority of listed platelet proteomes [18]. Although the ability to separate platelets from whole blood has increased throughout the years, earlier studies with platelet proteomics demonstrated a broad range of platelet purities, platelet concentrations, and protein use quantities per sample under analysis. In the first proteomics investigation on mice, protein abundance patterns were examined along several purification processes to separate real platelet proteins from impurities in plasma, WBCs, and RBCs [40]. The study showed that there can be the presence of more than 200 impurities (mostly RBC components or extremely abundant plasma proteins such as apolipoproteins, and complement factors due to the clustering of proteins at various purification stages) [40].

It was claimed that the OptiPrepTM density gradient centrifugation method could recover more than half the population of platelets with a 99.99% platelet purity and little WBC contamination, but it has not been used for proteomic investigations. Microfluidic platelet preparation or a completely automated method that offers a high yield and purity (>99%) with the reduced activation of platelets are suggested to be used in place of centrifugation methods for analyzing the platelet transcriptome [86].

For high-throughput research, additional controls should be created to guarantee full platelet lysis and digestion, low peptide loss during the preparation of samples, and automation for the analysis of a large number of samples. In the laboratories working with platelets' biological and translational applications, quality control methods of mass spectrometry-based proteomics data acquisition must be established. For example, a cloud-based quality control system or web-based apps can be applied [86–88]. Label-free analysis, which allows for infinite numbers of samples to be compared at the level of the proteome, can be done for greater throughput applications [78].

Searching known databases of fragmentation spectra is the most often utilized method for proteomic data analysis. It provides a useful summary of current bioinformatics approaches for the identification and quantification of proteins [89]. Data normalization, which involves applying adjustments in accordance with predetermined standards to eliminate inconsistent data points followed by statistical testing/screening for false discovery rates, is a crucial stage in the analysis. A changing protein abundance should not be the reason for the apparent regulation of a phosphorylation site in phosphoproteomics [90]. Special methods must be used to determine a phosphorylated peptide's site of phosphorylation and the kinase that is involved with platelet function [91].

One of the major drawbacks that has been observed in several studies is the inclusion of just a few platelet samples for comparison. Because of this, even when comparing healthy individuals to those who are sick, it has become challenging to make conclusions about inter-subject variances. Other technical drawbacks include inadequate protein abundance that is associated with inadequate peptide coverage, difficult spectral data processing, missing hydrophobic peptide sequences, and uncertain functions for several newly found proteins [92]. Therefore, the quantity of samples is another aspect that cannot be overlooked in platelet proteomic research. Strategies must be established in the future that allow for the use of only a few microliters of blood for platelets-based proteome study.

Since many studies only use a small number of samples and mass spectrometry proteome analyses are still expensive, it is difficult for institutions to conduct research with the ideal number of samples needed for careful data interpretation. Proteomics analysis is complicated and needs educated employees, which prevents the widespread use of the technology at diagnostic clinical laboratories. The equipment may not be inexpensive for clinical institutions. This raises questions about how well platelet proteomics may be applied in the therapeutic setting. It is recommended that standard protocols and areas of concern need to be created for platelet preparation, sample processing, and data analysis in order to increase the reproducibility of platelet research.

Most importantly, PTMs are another big hurdle in studying platelet biology. PTM is defined as the addition, subtraction, exchange, or rearrangement of functional groups to the side chains of amino acids and the N- and C-termini of proteins. After biosynthesis, proteins are subjected to PTMs, which are known to regulate a variety of biological processes, including protein activity, folding, localization, and interactions with other biomolecules [93]. Although more than 400 PTMs have been characterized, the full extent of their physiological functions is yet unknown. Phosphorylation, ubiquitylation, and proteolysis are the PTMs for platelets that have been extensively researched, while glycosylation, acetylation, and palmitoylation are given little consideration. The interaction of platelet PTMs during activation is also particularly intriguing.

Although there will be a lot of difficulties in making this shift, the development of proteomics as a basic tool for platelet research and moving this field from the discovery stage into the biology and preclinical application stage is important. In summary, for the field to advance, standardized criteria that enhance the repeatability of platelet preparation, proteomic sample processing, and complicated data analysis across laboratories should be implemented.

9. Is Clinical Translation between Mouse Platelet Proteome to Human Clinical Studies Possible?

Preclinical models have enabled a wide range of clinical uses, including surgery, vaccine development, illness detection, and therapy, among others. According to the thorough understanding thus far drawn from interspecies investigations, conclusions gained from animal research cannot be casually extrapolated to humans. Nevertheless, some research topics need the use of animal preclinical models, where researchers may phenocopy human illnesses, pathologies, or diseases in order to better understand the process underlying these qualities and test possible innovative therapies.

Human and mouse platelets share a substantially conserved proteome, thus providing evidence for the application of the proteomics technique in both intra- and inter-species fields [94]. This is also supported by an increasing number of preclinical or clinically applicable investigations in humans. Additionally, the similarity of the physiological, anatomical, and genetic characteristics between mice and humans justifies the use of mice as preclinical models, despite the evident differences between the two species [95]. Moreover, we have the ability to modify them genetically and physiologically. Therefore, although there are differences between the platelet formation processes in humans and mice, it is possible to study the megakaryopoiesis, thrombopoiesis, and platelet function of humans using mice as a model [95,96]. Murine preclinical models can enable us to illustrate how different proteins, including transcription factors, receptors, signaling molecules, hormones, cytokines, etc., function pathophysiologically in humans [97,98].

10. Conclusions and Future Perspectives

Myocardial infarction, ischemic stroke, and pulmonary embolism are just a few examples of cardiovascular thromboembolic diseases that continue to be the leading causes of death and disability in the world. Therefore, it is crucial to advance diagnoses and treatment in the context of individualized medicine. The disease specificity of currently available indicators is restricted, despite the fact that traditional platelet-activation markers are sensitive in detecting excessive or faulty activation states. Recent studies of platelet proteomics signatures, in contrast, demonstrate an enhanced disease specificity. Based on analyses of peptides and matching proteins in disease vs. healthy individuals, it has recently been shown that focused human platelet proteomics enables the quantification of CVD and other thrombotic disease biomarkers. In a customized and precision medicine scenario, it will become more critical to analyze the individual diversities in the proteomes of healthy people and patients.

Although the studies on the subject must be further validated by various independent investigations, the recent advances in mass spectrometer technology have made it possible to analyze numerous previously unidentified and newly discovered proteins quantitatively and to reveal the intricate phosphorylation patterns of proteins, many of whose functions are still unknown. The discovery of novel platelet proteins as possible biomarkers for diseases would be another breakthrough in the proteomic discipline. Some of the altered proteins that are indicative of an increased risk for CVDs and other platelet-associated disease states, reflecting alternations in platelet function and signaling pathways, are listed in Table 3.

Table 3. Various key platelet protein biomarkers involved in CVDs and other platelet-associated disease conditions.

Biomarker	Disease Conditions	References
Podoplanin	Tumor-induced platelet activation and tumor metastasis and invasion.	[99–104]
CD40 ligand	Acute coronary syndromes, coronary revascularization procedures, atherosclerosis, and inflammatory processes.	[105–107]
Platelet-derived growth factors (PDGFs)	Gliomas, sarcomas, leukemias, and epithelial cancers.	[108,109]
P-selectin	Coronary heart disease, hypertension, arterial fibrillation, congestive heart failure, stroke, atherosclerosis.	[110–114]
Glycoprotein IIb/IIIa	Platelet aggregation, thrombosis, hemostasis, carotid atherosclerosis, and diabetes.	[115–118]
Thrombospondin	Myocardial infarction, heart failure, coronary artery disease, coronary heart disease, abdominal aortic aneurysms.	[119–122]
Advanced glycation end products	Peripheral artery disease increases thrombotic effect in diabetes and coronary heart diseases.	[123–125]
Troponin	Myocardial infarction, heart failure, arterial fibrillation, Takotsubo cardiomyopathy, stroke, atherosclerosis.	[126–130],
Signal transducer and activator of transcription	Chronic inflammation, osteosarcoma, and prostate cancer.	[131,132]
Vascular endothelial growth factor	Breast cancer progression, invasion, and migration, angiogenesis.	[133–135]

Table 3. Cont.

Biomarker	Disease Conditions	References
β2-Glycoprotein I	Autoimmune condition antiphospholipid syndrome, thrombosis.	[136]
Oxidized LDL receptors	Atherosclerosis.	[137]
Vasodilator stimulated phosphoprotein	Metastasis in colorectal cancer.	[138]
Myeloperoxidase	Atherosclerosis, coronary artery disease, myocardial infarction, heart failure, inflammation, colon cancer, breast cancer.	[139–141]
RANTES	Acute coronary syndrome, atherosclerosis, inflammation. Development and progression of atherosclerosis, inflammation, thrombosis, diabetes, myocardial infarction, and atherothrombosis.	[142–152]
Platelet factor 4	Liposarcoma, mammary adenocarcinoma, and osteosarcoma, inflammation, atherosclerosis, myocardial infraction.	[153–156]
VWF	Atherosclerosis, hepatic carcinoma, hemostasis and thrombus formation.	[157–160]
Beta amyloid precursor protein II	Alzheimer's disease.	[161–163]
IL-1B	Atherosclerosis, inflammation, diabetes, coronary heart disease, stroke, peripheral vascular disease.	[164–167]
Autoantibody against platelet protein	Immune thrombocytopenia.	[168]
Facotor XII	Coronary heart disease, atherosclerosis, ischemic and hemorrhagic stroke, myocardial infraction.	[169–172]
ADAMTS13	Thrombotic microangiopathies, Thrombotic thrombocytopenic purpura, hepatocellular carcinoma, peripheral arterial disease, coronary heart disease, stroke, heart failure, myocardial infarction, liver cirrhosis.	[158,173]
Neutrophil extracellular traps (NETs) interacting protein	Autoimmune and inflammatory disorders, atherosclerosis, thrombosis.	[174–177]
Neutrophil elastase	Colorectal cancer, gastric cancer, pulmonary arterial hypertension.	[178–180]
Citrullinated histones	Thrombosis, inflammation, thromboembolism.	[181,182]
ERK5	Inflammation, atherosclerosis, hypertension.	[183–185]
Autotaxin	Alzheimer's disease, ischemic dilated cardiomyopathy, calcified aortic valve stenosis.	[186,187]
Cyclooxygenase	Atherosclerosis, aneurysm	[188,189]
Platelet-derived microvesicle	Development and progression of atherosclerosis, inflammation, thrombosis, diabetes, myocardial infarction, and atherothrombosis.	[145–152]

Despite wide variations in mass spectrometry and spectrum analysis techniques, the exact composition of the 'typical' human platelet proteome is still unknown. The attainable human platelet proteome will need to be defined through a coordinated multi-laboratory effort. The manner and purity of sample preparation, including the platelet concentration, activation state, and all sample processing, differ significantly between the studies done to date. In order to compare new research results more effectively, inter-laboratory standardization is expected to be required. Independent methods to confirm conclusions about protein up- or down-regulation have led to the inconsistency and non-repeatability of the research results.

The physiological roles in platelets of many proteins of putative biomarker importance remain unknown, and more complex protein function studies than general pathway studies are needed (e.g., using Gene Ontology). This objective may be accomplished with the use of a recent categorization scheme of all proteins predicted to be or present in platelets. Mass spectrometry can be substituted by less expensive, immune-based, or flow-cytometry techniques in bigger/clinical research if a biomarker is confirmed.

Low sample sizes have prevented published studies of patients from examining common intersubject factors, including blood cell characteristics, gender, age, and health history. The simultaneous comparison of several platelet samples is possible thanks to new high-throughput analytic techniques that combine label-free quantification approaches with data-independent acquisition, which is necessary for these clinically pertinent concerns.

Detailed information regarding protein distributions in healthy volunteers and patients will be provided by quantitative proteomics research. The phosphorylation patterns of platelets will also be helpful in comprehending platelet activation and finding potential new treatment approaches. Beyond the conventional depiction of linear pathways, a greater knowledge of platelet signaling will be possible thanks, in particular, to quantitative phosphoproteomic research. Over the past decade, although these unique technical approaches have and will continue to produce important discoveries, signaling has proven to be much more dynamic than expected in comparison to existing techniques. To identify previously unidentified post-translational changes, the unsupervised elucidation of platelet signaling using artificial intelligence may become increasingly significant in the future. In order to merge traditional biochemical knowledge with unexpected discoveries from big data methods, fresh data analysis strategies are needed to handle the enormous quantity of data generated by quantitative proteomics investigations.

Author Contributions: Conceptualization, S.K. (Soochong Kim) and P.K.C.; validation, S.K. (Soochong Kim); investigation, P.K.C.; writing—original draft, P.K.C., S.U. and S.K. (Sanggu Kim); writing—review and editing, S.K. (Soochong Kim); supervision, S.K. (Soochong Kim). All authors have read and agreed to the published version of the manuscript.

Funding: This research was funded by the National Research Foundation of Korea (NRF-2022R1 A2C1003638) and the Basic Research Lab Program (2022R1A4A1025557) through the NRF of Korea funded by the Ministry of Science and ICT.

Conflicts of Interest: The authors declare no conflicts of interest.

References

1. Chaudhary, P.K.; Kim, S.; Kim, S. An insight into recent advances on platelet function in health and disease. *Int. J. Mol. Sci.* **2022**, *23*, 6022. [CrossRef]
2. Villa-Fajardo, M.; Palma, M.C.Y.; Acebes-Huerta, A.; Martínez-Botía, P.; Meinders, M.; Nolte, M.A.; Cuesta, C.B.; Eble, J.A.; Del Castillo, J.G.; Martín-Sánchez, F.J. Platelet number and function alterations in preclinical models of sterile inflammation and sepsis patients: Implications in the pathophysiology and treatment of inflammation. *Transfus. Apher. Sci.* **2022**, *61*, 103413. [CrossRef] [PubMed]
3. Gianazza, E.; Brioschi, M.; Baetta, R.; Mallia, A.; Banfi, C.; Tremoli, E. Platelets in healthy and disease states: From biomarkers discovery to drug targets identification by proteomics. *Int. J. Mol. Sci.* **2020**, *21*, 4541. [CrossRef]
4. Antunes-Ferreira, M.; Koppers-Lalic, D.; Würdinger, T. Circulating platelets as liquid biopsy sources for cancer detection. *Mol. Oncol.* **2021**, *15*, 1727–1743. [CrossRef] [PubMed]
5. Humphrey, J. Origin of blood platelets. *Nature* **1955**, *176*, 38. [CrossRef] [PubMed]
6. Pagel, O.; Walter, E.; Jurk, K.; Zahedi, R.P. Taking the stock of granule cargo: Platelet releasate proteomics. *Platelets* **2017**, *28*, 119–128. [CrossRef] [PubMed]
7. Heijnen, H.; Van Der Sluijs, P. Platelet secretory behaviour: As diverse as the granules... or not? *J. Thromb.* **2015**, *13*, 2141–2151. [CrossRef] [PubMed]
8. Thon, J.N.; Peters, C.G.; Machlus, K.R.; Aslam, R.; Rowley, J.; Macleod, H.; Devine, M.T.; Fuchs, T.A.; Weyrich, A.S.; Semple, J.W. T granules in human platelets function in TLR9 organization and signaling. *J. Cell Biol.* **2012**, *198*, 561–574. [CrossRef]
9. Michelson, A.D.; Cattaneo, M.; Frelinger, A.; Newman, P. *Platelets*; Academic Press: Cambridge, MA, USA, 2019.
10. Ghoshal, K.; Bhattacharyya, M. Overview of platelet physiology: Its hemostatic and nonhemostatic role in disease pathogenesis. *Sci. World* **2014**, *20*, 14. [CrossRef]
11. Nuyttens, B.P.; Thijs, T.; Deckmyn, H.; Broos, K. Platelet adhesion to collagen. *Thromb. J.* **2011**, *127*, S26–S29. [CrossRef]

12. Schmaier, A.A.; Zou, Z.; Kazlauskas, A.; Emert-Sedlak, L.; Fong, K.P.; Neeves, K.B.; Maloney, S.F.; Diamond, S.L.; Kunapuli, S.P.; Ware, J. Molecular priming of Lyn by GPVI enables an immune receptor to adopt a hemostatic role. *Proc. Natl. Acad. Sci. USA* **2009**, *106*, 21167–21172. [CrossRef]
13. Heemskerk, J.W.; Harper, M.T.; Cosemans, J.M.; Poole, A.W. Unravelling the different functions of protein kinase C isoforms in platelets. *FEBS Lett.* **2011**, *585*, 1711–1716. [CrossRef]
14. Crittenden, J.R.; Bergmeier, W.; Zhang, Y.; Piffath, C.L.; Liang, Y.; Wagner, D.D.; Housman, D.E.; Graybiel, A.M. CalDAG-GEFI integrates signaling for platelet aggregation and thrombus formation. *Nat. Med.* **2004**, *10*, 982–986. [CrossRef]
15. Durrant, T.N.; van den Bosch, M.T.; Hers, I. Integrin αIIbβ3 outside-in signaling. *Blood Am. Soc. Hematol.* **2017**, *130*, 1607–1619. [CrossRef]
16. Sang, Y.; Roest, M.; de Laat, B.; de Groot, P.G.; Huskens, D. Interplay between platelets and coagulation. *Blood Rev.* **2021**, *46*, 100733. [CrossRef] [PubMed]
17. Koupenova, M.; Clancy, L.; Corkrey, H.A.; Freedman, J.E. Circulating platelets as mediators of immunity, inflammation, and thrombosis. *Circ. Res.* **2018**, *122*, 337–351. [CrossRef]
18. Huang, J.; Swieringa, F.; Solari, F.A.; Provenzale, I.; Grassi, L.; De Simone, I.; Baaten, C.C.; Cavill, R.; Sickmann, A.; Frontini, M. Assessment of a complete and classified platelet proteome from genome-wide transcripts of human platelets and megakaryocytes covering platelet functions. *Sci. Rep.* **2021**, *11*, 12358. [CrossRef]
19. Dowal, L.; Yang, W.; Freeman, M.R.; Steen, H.; Flaumenhaft, R. Proteomic analysis of palmitoylated platelet proteins. *Blood Am. J. Hematol.* **2011**, *118*, e62–e73. [CrossRef]
20. Lee, H.; Chae, S.; Park, J.; Bae, J.; Go, E.-B.; Kim, S.-J.; Kim, H.; Hwang, D.; Lee, S.-W.; Lee, S.-Y. Comprehensive proteome profiling of platelet identified a protein profile predictive of responses to an antiplatelet agent sarpogrelate. *Mol. Cell Proteom.* **2016**, *15*, 3461–3472. [CrossRef] [PubMed]
21. Burkhart, J.M.; Vaudel, M.; Gambaryan, S.; Radau, S.; Walter, U.; Martens, L.; Geiger, J.; Sickmann, A.; Zahedi, R.P. The first comprehensive and quantitative analysis of human platelet protein composition allows the comparative analysis of structural and functional pathways. *Blood Am. Soc. Hematol.* **2012**, *120*, e73–e82. [CrossRef] [PubMed]
22. Burkhart, J.M.; Gambaryan, S.; Watson, S.P.; Jurk, K.; Walter, U.; Sickmann, A.; Heemskerk, J.W.; Zahedi, R.P. What can proteomics tell us about platelets? *Circ. Res.* **2014**, *114*, 1204–1219. [CrossRef]
23. Thon, J.N.; Schubert, P.; Devine, D.V. Platelet storage lesion: A new understanding from a proteomic perspective. *Transfus. Med. Rev.* **2008**, *22*, 268–279. [CrossRef]
24. Handtke, S.; Steil, L.; Palankar, R.; Conrad, J.; Cauhan, S.; Kraus, L.; Ferrara, M.; Dhople, V.; Wesche, J.; Völker, U. Role of platelet size revisited—Function and protein composition of large and small platelets. *Thromb. Haemost.* **2019**, *119*, 407–420. [CrossRef]
25. Kim, S.; Chaudhary, P.K.; Kim, S. Role of Prednisolone in Platelet Activation by Inhibiting TxA(2) Generation through the Regulation of cPLA(2) Phosphorylation. *Animals* **2023**, *13*, 1299. [CrossRef]
26. Patrono, C.; Rocca, B. Aspirin, 110 years later. *J. Thromb. Haemost.* **2009**, *7*, 258–261. [CrossRef]
27. Egidi, M.G.; D'Alessandro, A.; Mandarello, G.; Zolla, L. Troubleshooting in platelet storage temperature and new perspectives through proteomics. *Blood Transfus.* **2010**, *8*, 73–81.
28. Canas, B.; Pineiro, C.; Calvo, E.; Lopez-Ferrer, D.; Gallardo, J.M. Trends in sample preparation for classical and second generation proteomics. *J. Chromatogr. A* **2007**, *1153*, 235–258. [CrossRef]
29. Barber, A.J.; Pepper, D.S.; Jamieson, G.A. A comparison of methods for platelet lysis and the isolation of platelet membranes. *Thromb. Diath. Haemorrh.* **1971**, *26*, 38–57. [CrossRef] [PubMed]
30. Zufferey, A.; Fontana, P.; Reny, J.L.; Nolli, S.; Sanchez, J.C. Platelet proteomics. *Mass. Spectrom. Rev.* **2012**, *31*, 331–351. [CrossRef] [PubMed]
31. Gorg, A.; Obermaier, C.; Boguth, G.; Harder, A.; Scheibe, B.; Wildgruber, R.; Weiss, W. The current state of two-dimensional electrophoresis with immobilized pH gradients. *Electrophoresis* **2000**, *21*, 1037–1053. [CrossRef]
32. Aebersold, R.; Goodlett, D.R. Mass spectrometry in proteomics. *Nature* **2001**, *101*, 269–295. [CrossRef]
33. Burkhart, J.M.; Schumbrutzki, C.; Wortelkamp, S.; Sickmann, A.; Zahedi, R.P. Systematic and quantitative comparison of digest efficiency and specificity reveals the impact of trypsin quality on MS-based proteomics. *J. Proteom.* **2012**, *75*, 1454–1462. [CrossRef]
34. Shevchuk, O.; Begonja, A.J.; Gambaryan, S.; Totzeck, M.; Rassaf, T.; Huber, T.B.; Greinacher, A.; Renne, T.; Sickmann, A. Proteomics: A Tool to Study Platelet Function. *Int. J. Mol. Sci.* **2021**, *22*, 4776. [CrossRef]
35. Hunt, D.F.; Yates, J.R.; Shabanowitz, J.; Winston, S.; Hauer, C.R. Protein sequencing by tandem mass spectrometry. *Proc. Natl. Acad. Sci. USA* **1986**, *83*, 6233–6237. [CrossRef] [PubMed]
36. Pratt, J.M.; Robertson, D.H.; Gaskell, S.J.; Riba-Garcia, I.; Hubbard, S.J.; Sidhu, K.; Oliver, S.G.; Butler, P.; Hayes, A.; Petty, J.; et al. Stable isotope labelling in vivo as an aid to protein identification in peptide mass fingerprinting. *Proteomics* **2002**, *2*, 157–163. [CrossRef] [PubMed]
37. Mnatsakanyan, R.; Shema, G.; Basik, M.; Batist, G.; Borchers, C.H.; Sickmann, A.; Zahedi, R.P. Detecting post-translational modification signatures as potential biomarkers in clinical mass spectrometry. *Expert. Rev. Proteom.* **2018**, *15*, 515–535. [CrossRef] [PubMed]
38. Wu, X.; Hasan, M.A.; Chen, J.Y. Pathway and network analysis in proteomics. *J. Theor. Biol.* **2014**, *362*, 44–52. [CrossRef] [PubMed]
39. Dittrich, M.; Birschmann, I.; Mietner, S.; Sickmann, A.; Walter, U.; Dandekar, T. Platelet protein interactions: Map, signaling components, and phosphorylation groundstate. *Arterioscler. Thromb. Vasc. Biol.* **2008**, *28*, 1326–1331. [CrossRef] [PubMed]

70. Zeiler, M.; Moser, M.; Mann, M. Copy number analysis of the murine platelet proteome spanning the complete abundance range. *Mol. Cell Proteom.* **2014**, *13*, 3435–3445. [CrossRef]
71. Winkler, W.; Zellner, M.; Diestinger, M.; Babeluk, R.; Marchetti, M.; Goll, A.; Zehetmayer, S.; Bauer, P.; Rappold, E.; Miller, I. Biological variation of the platelet proteome in the elderly population and its implication for biomarker research. *Mol. Cell Proteom.* **2008**, *7*, 193–203. [CrossRef]
72. Maguire, P.B.; Parsons, M.E.; Szklanna, P.B.; Zdanyte, M.; Münzer, P.; Chatterjee, M.; Wynne, K.; Rath, D.; Comer, S.P.; Hayden, M. Comparative platelet releasate proteomic profiling of acute coronary syndrome versus stable coronary artery disease. *Front. Cardiovasc. Med.* **2020**, *7*, 101. [CrossRef] [PubMed]
73. Gutmann, C.; Joshi, A.; Mayr, M. Platelet "-omics" in health and cardiovascular disease. *Atherosclerosis* **2020**, *307*, 87–96. [CrossRef]
74. Fernandez Parguina, A.; Grigorian-Shamajian, L.; Agra, R.M.; Teijeira-Fernández, E.; Rosa, I.; Alonso, J.; Viñuela-Roldán, J.E.; Seoane, A.; González-Juanatey, J.R.; Garcia, A. Proteins involved in platelet signaling are differentially regulated in acute coronary syndrome: A proteomic study. *PLoS ONE* **2010**, *5*, e13404. [CrossRef] [PubMed]
75. López-Farré, A.J.; Zamorano-Leon, J.J.; Azcona, L.; Modrego, J.; Mateos-Cáceres, P.J.; González-Armengol, J.; Villarroel, P.; Moreno-Herrero, R.; Rodríguez-Sierra, P.; Segura, A. Proteomic changes related to "bewildered" circulating platelets in the acute coronary syndrome. *Proteomics* **2011**, *11*, 3335–3348. [CrossRef] [PubMed]
76. Vélez, P.; Ocaranza-Sánchez, R.; López-Otero, D.; Grigorian-Shamagian, L.; Rosa, I.; Bravo, S.B.; González-Juanatey, J.R.; García, Á. 2D-DIGE-based proteomic analysis of intracoronary versus peripheral arterial blood platelets from acute myocardial infarction patients: Upregulation of platelet activation biomarkers at the culprit site. *Proteom. Clin. Appl.* **2016**, *10*, 851–858. [CrossRef]
77. Vélez, P.; Izquierdo, I.; Rosa, I.; García, Á. A 2D-DIGE-based proteomic analysis reveals differences in the platelet releasate composition when comparing thrombin and collagen stimulations. *Sci. Rep.* **2015**, *5*, 8198. [CrossRef]
78. Hell, L.; Lurger, K.; Mauracher, L.-M.; Grilz, E.; Reumiller, C.M.; Schmidt, G.J.; Ercan, H.; Koder, S.; Assinger, A.; Basilio, J. Altered platelet proteome in lupus anticoagulant (LA)-positive patients—Protein disulfide isomerase and NETosis as new players in LA-related thrombosis. *Exp. Mol. Med.* **2020**, *52*, 66–78. [CrossRef]
79. Loroch, S.; Trabold, K.; Gambaryan, S.; Reiß, C.; Schwierczek, K.; Fleming, I.; Sickmann, A.; Behnisch, W.; Zieger, B.; Zahedi, R.P. Alterations of the platelet proteome in type I Glanzmann thrombasthenia caused by different homozygous delG frameshift mutations in ITGA2B. *Thromb. Haemost.* **2017**, *117*, 556–569. [CrossRef]
80. van Kruchten, R.; Mattheij, N.J.; Saunders, C.; Feijge, M.A.; Swieringa, F.; Wolfs, J.L.; Collins, P.W.; Heemskerk, J.W.; Bevers, E.M. Both TMEM16F-dependent and TMEM16F-independent pathways contribute to phosphatidylserine exposure in platelet apoptosis and platelet activation. *Blood Am. Soc. Hematol.* **2013**, *121*, 1850–1857. [CrossRef]
81. Bergemalm, D.; Ramström, S.; Kardeby, C.; Hultenby, K.; Eremo, A.G.; Sihlbom, C.; Bergström, J.; Palmblad, J.; Åström, M. Platelet proteome and function in X− linked thrombocytopenia with thalassemia and in silico comparisons with gray platelet syndrome. *Haematologica* **2021**, *106*, 2947. [CrossRef]
82. Sims, M.C.; Mayer, L.; Collins, J.H.; Bariana, T.K.; Megy, K.; Lavenu-Bombled, C.; Seyres, D.; Kollipara, L.; Burden, F.S.; Greene, D. Novel manifestations of immune dysregulation and granule defects in gray platelet syndrome. *Blood Am. Soc. Hematol.* **2020**, *136*, 1956–1967. [CrossRef]
83. Sabrkhany, S.; Kuijpers, M.J.; Knol, J.C.; Damink, S.W.O.; Dingemans, A.-M.C.; Verheul, H.M.; Piersma, S.R.; Pham, T.V.; Griffioen, A.W.; Oude Egbrink, M.G. Exploration of the platelet proteome in patients with early-stage cancer. *J. Proteom.* **2018**, *177*, 65–74. [CrossRef]
84. Jalal, D.I.; Chonchol, M.; Targher, G. In Disorders of hemostasis associated with chronic kidney disease. *Semin. Thromb. Hemost.* **2010**, *2010*, 34–40. [CrossRef]
85. Lutz, J.; Menke, J.; Sollinger, D.; Schinzel, H.; Thürmel, K. Haemostasis in chronic kidney disease. *Nephrol. Dial. Transpl.* **2014**, *29*, 29–40. [CrossRef]
86. Ravid, J.D.; Chitalia, V.C. Molecular mechanisms underlying the cardiovascular toxicity of specific uremic solutes. *Cells* **2020**, *9*, 2024. [CrossRef] [PubMed]
87. Bijak, M.; Olejnik, A.; Rokita, B.; Morel, A.; Dziedzic, A.; Miller, E.; Saluk-Bijak, J. Increased level of fibrinogen chains in the proteome of blood platelets in secondary progressive multiple sclerosis patients. *J. Cell. Mol. Med.* **2019**, *23*, 3476–3482. [CrossRef] [PubMed]
88. Trugilho, M.R.d.O.; Hottz, E.D.; Brunoro, G.V.F.; Teixeira-Ferreira, A.; Carvalho, P.C.; Salazar, G.A.; Zimmerman, G.A.; Bozza, F.A.; Bozza, P.T.; Perales, J. Platelet proteome reveals novel pathways of platelet activation and platelet-mediated immunoregulation in dengue. *PLoS Pathog.* **2017**, *13*, e1006385. [CrossRef] [PubMed]
89. Yu, H.; Liu, Y.; He, B.; He, T.; Chen, C.; He, J.; Yang, X.; Wang, J.Z. Platelet biomarkers for a descending cognitive function: A proteomic approach. *Aging Cell* **2021**, *20*, e13358. [CrossRef] [PubMed]
90. Fuchs, T.A.; Abed, U.; Goosmann, C.; Hurwitz, R.; Schulze, I.; Wahn, V.; Weinrauch, Y.; Brinkmann, V.; Zychlinsky, A. Novel cell death program leads to neutrophil extracellular traps. *J. Cell Biol.* **2007**, *176*, 231–241. [CrossRef] [PubMed]
91. Labib, D.A.; Ashmawy, I.; Elmazny, A.; Helmy, H.; Ismail, R.S. Toll-like receptors 2 and 4 expression on peripheral blood lymphocytes and neutrophils of Egyptian multiple sclerosis patients. *Int. J. Neurosci.* **2022**, *132*, 323–327. [CrossRef] [PubMed]
92. Semeraro, F.; Ammollo, C.T.; Morrissey, J.H.; Dale, G.L.; Friese, P.; Esmon, N.L.; Esmon, C.T. Extracellular histones promote thrombin generation through platelet-dependent mechanisms: Involvement of platelet TLR2 and TLR4. *Blood* **2011**, *118*, 1952–1961. [CrossRef] [PubMed]

63. Fuchs, T.A.; Brill, A.; Duerschmied, D.; Schatzberg, D.; Monestier, M.; Myers, D.D., Jr.; Wrobleski, S.K.; Wakefield, T.W.; Hartwig, J.H.; Wagner, D.D. Extracellular DNA traps promote thrombosis. *Proc. Natl. Acad. Sci. USA* **2010**, *107*, 15880–15885. [CrossRef] [PubMed]
64. Engelmann, B.; Massberg, S. Thrombosis as an intravascular effector of innate immunity. *Nat. Rev. Immunol.* **2013**, *13*, 34–45. [CrossRef] [PubMed]
65. van den Berg, J.; Haslbauer, J.D.; Stalder, A.K.; Romanens, A.; Mertz, K.D.; Studt, J.D.; Siegemund, M.; Buser, A.; Holbro, A.; Tzankov, A. Von Willebrand factor and the thrombophilia of severe COVID-19: In situ evidence from autopsies. *Res. Pract. Thromb. Haemost.* **2023**, *7*, 100182. [CrossRef] [PubMed]
66. Kaltenmeier, C.; Simmons, R.L.; Tohme, S.; Yazdani, H.O. Neutrophil Extracellular Traps (NETs) in Cancer Metastasis. *Cancers* **2021**, *13*, 6131. [CrossRef] [PubMed]
67. Etulain, J.; Martinod, K.; Wong, S.L.; Cifuni, S.M.; Schattner, M.; Wagner, D.D. P-selectin promotes neutrophil extracellular trap formation in mice. *Blood* **2015**, *126*, 242–246. [CrossRef] [PubMed]
68. Demers, M.; Krause, D.S.; Schatzberg, D.; Martinod, K.; Voorhees, J.R.; Fuchs, T.A.; Scadden, D.T.; Wagner, D.D. Cancers predispose neutrophils to release extracellular DNA traps that contribute to cancer-associated thrombosis. *Proc. Natl. Acad. Sci. USA* **2012**, *109*, 13076–13081. [CrossRef]
69. Guglietta, S.; Chiavelli, A.; Zagato, E.; Krieg, C.; Gandini, S.; Ravenda, P.S.; Bazolli, B.; Lu, B.; Penna, G.; Rescigno, M. Coagulation induced by C3aR-dependent NETosis drives protumorigenic neutrophils during small intestinal tumorigenesis. *Nat. Commun.* **2016**, *7*, 11037. [CrossRef]
70. Yalavarthi, S.; Gould, T.J.; Rao, A.N.; Mazza, L.F.; Morris, A.E.; Nunez-Alvarez, C.; Hernandez-Ramirez, D.; Bockenstedt, P.L.; Liaw, P.C.; Cabral, A.R.; et al. Release of neutrophil extracellular traps by neutrophils stimulated with antiphospholipid antibodies: A newly identified mechanism of thrombosis in the antiphospholipid syndrome. *Arthritis Rheumatol.* **2015**, *67*, 2990–3003. [CrossRef]
71. Popp, S.K.; Vecchio, F.; Brown, D.J.; Fukuda, R.; Suzuki, Y.; Takeda, Y.; Wakamatsu, R.; Sarma, M.A.; Garrett, J.; Giovenzana, A.; et al. Circulating platelet-neutrophil aggregates characterize the development of type 1 diabetes in humans and NOD mice. *JCI Insight* **2022**, *7*, e153993. [CrossRef]
72. Ren, J.; He, J.; Zhang, H.; Xia, Y.; Hu, Z.; Loughran, P.; Billiar, T.; Huang, H.; Tsung, A. Platelet TLR4-ERK5 Axis Facilitates NET-Mediated Capturing of Circulating Tumor Cells and Distant Metastasis after Surgical Stress. *Cancer Res.* **2021**, *81*, 2373–2385. [CrossRef]
73. Pang, A.; Cui, Y.; Chen, Y.; Cheng, N.; Delaney, M.K.; Gu, M.; Stojanovic-Terpo, A.; Zhu, C.; Du, X. Shear-induced integrin signaling in platelet phosphatidylserine exposure, microvesicle release, and coagulation. *Blood Am. Soc. Hematol.* **2018**, *132*, 533–543. [CrossRef]
74. Zimmerman, G.A.; Weyrich, A.S. Signal-dependent protein synthesis by activated platelets: New pathways to altered phenotype and function. *Arterioscler. Thromb. Vasc. Biol.* **2008**, *28*, 17–24. [CrossRef]
75. Ng, M.S.Y.; Tung, J.-P.; Fraser, J.F. Platelet storage lesions: What more do we know now? *Transfus. Med. Rev.* **2018**, *32*, 144–154. [CrossRef] [PubMed]
76. Prudova, A.; Serrano, K.; Eckhard, U.; Fortelny, N.; Devine, D.V.; Overall, C.M. TAILS N-terminomics of human platelets reveals pervasive metalloproteinase-dependent proteolytic processing in storage. *Blood Am. Soc. Hematol.* **2014**, *124*, e49–e60. [CrossRef] [PubMed]
77. Thiele, T.; Braune, J.; Dhople, V.; Hammer, E.; Scharf, C.; Greinacher, A.; Völker, U.; Steil, L. Proteomic profile of platelets during reconstitution of platelet counts after apheresis. *Proteom. Clin. Appl.* **2016**, *10*, 831–838. [CrossRef]
78. Rijkers, M.; van den Eshof, B.L.; van der Meer, P.F.; van Alphen, F.P.; de Korte, D.; Leebaeek, F.W.; Meijer, A.B.; Voorberg, J.; Jansen, A.G. Monitoring storage induced changes in the platelet proteome employing lable free quantative mass spectrometry. *Sci. Rep.* **2017**, *7*, 11045. [CrossRef] [PubMed]
79. Wang, S.; Jiang, T.; Fan, Y.; Zhao, S. A proteomic approach reveals the variation in human platelet protein composition after storage at different temperatures. *Platelets* **2019**, *30*, 403–412. [CrossRef]
80. Wood, B.; Padula, M.P.; Marks, D.C.; Johnson, L. Refrigerated storage of platelets initiates changes in platelet surface marker expression and localization of intracellular proteins. *Transfusion* **2016**, *56*, 2548–2559. [CrossRef]
81. Schubert, P.; Culibrk, B.; Karwal, S.; Goodrich, R.P.; Devine, D.V. Protein translation occurs in platelet concentrates despite riboflavin/UV light pathogen inactivation treatment. *Proteom. Clin. Appl.* **2016**, *10*, 839–850. [CrossRef]
82. Sonego, G.; Abonnenc, M.; Crettaz, D.; Lion, N.; Tissot, J.-D.; Prudent, M. Irreversible oxidations of platelet proteins after riboflavin-UVB pathogen inactivation. *Transfus. Clin. Biol.* **2020**, *27*, 36–42. [CrossRef]
83. Hermida-Nogueira, L.; Barrachina, M.N.; Izquierdo, I.; García-Vence, M.; Lacerenza, S.; Bravo, S.; Castrillo, A.; García, Á. Proteomic analysis of extracellular vesicles derived from platelet concentrates treated with Mirasol® identifies biomarkers of platelet storage lesion. *J. Proteom.* **2020**, *210*, 103529. [CrossRef]
84. Greening, D.W.; Sparrow, R.L.; Simpson, R.J. Preparation of platelet concentrates. *Plasma Proteom. Methods Protoc.* **2011**, *728*, 267–278.
85. Wrzyszcz, A.; Urbaniak, J.; Sapa, A.; Woźniak, M. An efficient method for isolation of representative and contamination-free population of blood platelets for proteomic studies. *Platelets* **2017**, *28*, 43–53. [CrossRef]

96. Kim, T.; Chen, I.R.; Parker, B.L.; Humphrey, S.J.; Crossett, B.; Cordwell, S.J.; Yang, P.; Yang, J.Y.H. QCMAP: An Interactive Web-Tool for Performance Diagnosis and Prediction of LC-MS Systems. *Proteomics* **2019**, *19*, 1900068. [CrossRef] [PubMed]
97. Van Houtven, J.; Agten, A.; Boonen, K.; Baggerman, G.; Hooyberghs, J.; Laukens, K.; Valkenborg, D. Qcquan: A web tool for the automated assessment of protein expression and data quality of labeled mass spectrometry experiments. *J. Proteome Res.* **2019**, *18*, 2221–2227. [CrossRef] [PubMed]
98. Chiva, C.; Olivella, R.; Borras, E.; Espadas, G.; Pastor, O.; Sole, A.; Sabido, E. QCloud: A cloud-based quality control system for mass spectrometry-based proteomics laboratories. *PLoS ONE* **2018**, *13*, e0189209. [CrossRef] [PubMed]
99. Chen, C.; Hou, J.; Tanner, J.J.; Cheng, J. Bioinformatics methods for mass spectrometry-based proteomics data analysis. *Int. J. Mol. Sci.* **2020**, *21*, 2873. [CrossRef] [PubMed]
100. Solari, F.A.; Dell'Aica, M.; Sickmann, A.; Zahedi, R.P. Why phosphoproteomics is still a challenge. *Mol. Biosyst.* **2015**, *11*, 1487–1493. [CrossRef] [PubMed]
101. Swieringa, F.; Solari, F.A.; Pagel, O.; Beck, F.; Huang, J.; Feijge, M.A.; Jurk, K.; Körver-Keularts, I.M.; Mattheij, N.J.; Faber, J. Impaired iloprost-induced platelet inhibition and phosphoproteome changes in patients with confirmed pseudohypoparathyroidism type Ia, linked to genetic mutations in GNAS. *Sci. Rep.* **2020**, *10*, 11389. [CrossRef] [PubMed]
102. Looße, C.; Swieringa, F.; Heemskerk, J.W.; Sickmann, A.; Lorenz, C. Platelet proteomics: From discovery to diagnosis. *Expert. Rev. Proteom.* **2018**, *15*, 467–476. [CrossRef]
103. Chen, L.; Kashina, A. Post-translational Modifications of the Protein Termini. *Front. Cell. Dev. Biol.* **2021**, *9*, 719590. [CrossRef]
104. Martínez-Botía, P.; Villar, P.; Carbajo-Argüelles, G.; Jaiteh, Z.; Acebes-Huerta, A.; Gutiérrez, L. Proteomics-wise, how similar are mouse and human platelets? *Platelets* **2023**, *34*, 2220415. [CrossRef]
105. Monaco, G.; van Dam, S.; Casal Novo Ribeiro, J.L.; Larbi, A.; de Magalhães, J.P. A comparison of human and mouse gene co-expression networks reveals conservation and divergence at the tissue, pathway and disease levels. *BMC Evol. Biol.* **2015**, *15*, 259. [CrossRef]
106. Schmitt, A.; Guichard, J.; Massé, J.-M.; Debili, N.; Cramer, E.M. Of mice and men: Comparison of the ultrastructure of megakaryocytes and platelets. *Exp. Hematol.* **2001**, *29*, 1295–1302. [CrossRef]
107. Thijs, T.; Deckmyn, H.; Broos, K. Model systems of genetically modified platelets. *Blood Am. Soc. Hematol.* **2012**, *119*, 1634–1642. [CrossRef]
108. Jirouskova, M.; Shet, A.; Johnson, G.J. A guide to murine platelet structure, function, assays, and genetic alterations. *Thromb. Haemost.* **2007**, *5*, 661–669. [CrossRef] [PubMed]
109. Takemoto, A.; Miyata, K.; Fujita, N. Platelet-activating factor podoplanin: From discovery to drug development. *Cancer Metastasis Rev.* **2017**, *36*, 225–234. [CrossRef] [PubMed]
110. Herzog, B.H.; Fu, J.; Wilson, S.J.; Hess, P.R.; Sen, A.; McDaniel, J.M.; Pan, Y.; Sheng, M.; Yago, T.; Silasi-Mansat, R.; et al. Podoplanin maintains high endothelial venule integrity by interacting with platelet CLEC-2. *Nature* **2013**, *502*, 105–109. [CrossRef]
111. Mobarrez, F.; He, S.; Broijersen, A.; Wiklund, B.; Antovic, A.; Antovic, J.; Egberg, N.; Jorneskog, G.; Wallen, H. Atorvastatin reduces thrombin generation and expression of tissue factor, P-selectin and GPIIIa on platelet-derived microparticles in patients with peripheral arterial occlusive disease. *Thromb. Haemost.* **2011**, *106*, 344–352. [CrossRef] [PubMed]
112. Watanabe, N.; Kidokoro, M.; Tanaka, M.; Inoue, S.; Tsuji, T.; Akatuska, H.; Okada, C.; Iida, Y.; Okada, Y.; Suzuki, Y.; et al. Podoplanin is indispensable for cell motility and platelet-induced epithelial-to-mesenchymal transition-related gene expression in esophagus squamous carcinoma TE11A cells. *Cancer Cell Int.* **2020**, *20*, 263. [CrossRef]
113. Kato, Y.; Kaneko, M.K.; Kunita, A.; Ito, H.; Kameyama, A.; Ogasawara, S.; Matsuura, N.; Hasegawa, Y.; Suzuki-Inoue, K.; Inoue, O.; et al. Molecular analysis of the pathophysiological binding of the platelet aggregation-inducing factor podoplanin to the C-type lectin-like receptor CLEC-2. *Cancer Sci.* **2008**, *99*, 54–61. [CrossRef]
114. Suzuki-Inoue, K.; Kato, Y.; Inoue, O.; Kaneko, M.K.; Mishima, K.; Yatomi, Y.; Yamazaki, Y.; Narimatsu, H.; Ozaki, Y. Involvement of the snake toxin receptor CLEC-2, in podoplanin-mediated platelet activation, by cancer cells. *J. Biol. Chem.* **2007**, *282*, 25993–26001. [CrossRef]
115. Mach, F.; Schonbeck, U.; Libby, P. CD40 signaling in vascular cells: A key role in atherosclerosis? *Atherosclerosis* **1998**, *137*, 89–95. [CrossRef]
116. de Lemos, J.A.; Zirlik, A.; Schonbeck, U.; Varo, N.; Murphy, S.A.; Khera, A.; McGuire, D.K.; Stanek, G.; Lo, H.S.; Nuzzo, R.; et al. Associations between soluble CD40 ligand, atherosclerosis risk factors, and subclinical atherosclerosis: Results from the Dallas Heart Study. *Arterioscler. Thromb. Vasc. Biol.* **2005**, *25*, 2192–2196. [CrossRef] [PubMed]
117. Lacy, M.; Burger, C.; Shami, A.; Ahmadsei, M.; Winkels, H.; Nitz, K.; van Tiel, C.M.; Seijkens, T.T.P.; Kusters, P.J.H.; Karshovka, E.; et al. Cell-specific and divergent roles of the CD40L-CD40 axis in atherosclerotic vascular disease. *Nat. Commun.* **2021**, *12*, 3754. [CrossRef]
118. Andrae, J.; Gallini, R.; Betsholtz, C. Role of platelet-derived growth factors in physiology and medicine. *Genes Dev.* **2008**, *22*, 1276–1312. [CrossRef] [PubMed]
119. Schmahl, J.; Raymond, C.S.; Soriano, P. PDGF signaling specificity is mediated through multiple immediate early genes. *Nat. Genet.* **2007**, *39*, 52–60. [CrossRef]
120. Zeller, J.A.; Tschoepe, D.; Kessler, C. Circulating platelets show increased activation in patients with acute cerebral ischemia. *Thromb. Haemost.* **1999**, *81*, 373–377. [PubMed]

111. O'Connor, C.M.; Gurbel, P.A.; Serebruany, V.L. Usefulness of soluble and surface-bound P-selectin in detecting heightened platelet activity in patients with congestive heart failure. *Am. J. Cardiol.* **1999**, *83*, 1345–1349. [CrossRef]
112. Tschoepe, D.; Schultheiss, H.P.; Kolarov, P.; Schwippert, B.; Dannehl, K.; Nieuwenhuis, H.K.; Kehrel, B.; Strauer, B.; Gries, F.A. Platelet membrane activation markers are predictive for increased risk of acute ischemic events after PTCA. *Circulation* **1993**, *88*, 37–42. [CrossRef]
113. Blann, A.D.; Nadar, S.K.; Lip, G.Y. The adhesion molecule P-selectin and cardiovascular disease. *Eur. Heart J.* **2003**, *24*, 2166–2179. [CrossRef]
114. Bielinski, S.J.; Berardi, C.; Decker, P.A.; Kirsch, P.S.; Larson, N.B.; Pankow, J.S.; Sale, M.; de Andrade, M.; Sicotte, H.; Tang, W.; et al. P-selectin and subclinical and clinical atherosclerosis: The Multi-Ethnic Study of Atherosclerosis (MESA). *Atherosclerosis* **2015**, *240*, 3–9. [CrossRef] [PubMed]
115. Fullard, J.F. The role of the platelet glycoprotein IIb/IIIa in thrombosis and haemostasis. *Curr. Pharm. Des.* **2004**, *10*, 1567–1576. [CrossRef]
116. Lippi, G.; Montagnana, M.; Danese, E.; Favaloro, E.J.; Franchini, M. Glycoprotein IIb/IIIa inhibitors: An update on the mechanism of action and use of functional testing methods to assess antiplatelet efficacy. *Biomark. Med.* **2011**, *5*, 63–70. [CrossRef]
117. Schneider, D.J. Anti-platelet therapy: Glycoprotein IIb-IIIa antagonists. *Br. J. Clin. Pharmacol.* **2011**, *72*, 672–682. [CrossRef]
118. Pellitero, S.; Reverter, J.L.; Tassies, D.; Pizarro, E.; Monteagudo, J.; Salinas, I.; Aguilera, E.; Sanmarti, A.; Reverter, J.C. Polymorphisms in platelet glycoproteins Ia and IIIa are associated with arterial thrombosis and carotid atherosclerosis in type 2 diabetes. *Thromb. Haemost.* **2010**, *103*, 630–637. [CrossRef] [PubMed]
119. Befekadu, R.; Christiansen, K.; Larsson, A.; Grenegard, M. Increased plasma cathepsin S and trombospondin-1 in patients with acute ST-segment elevation myocardial infarction. *Cardiol. J.* **2019**, *26*, 385–393. [CrossRef]
120. van Almen, G.C.; Verhesen, W.; van Leeuwen, R.E.; van de Vrie, M.; Eurlings, C.; Schellings, M.W.; Swinnen, M.; Cleutjens, J.P.; van Zandvoort, M.A.; Heymans, S.; et al. MicroRNA-18 and microRNA-19 regulate CTGF and TSP-1 expression in age-related heart failure. *Aging Cell* **2011**, *10*, 769–779. [CrossRef] [PubMed]
121. Pereira, A.; Palma Dos Reis, R.; Rodrigues, R.; Sousa, A.C.; Gomes, S.; Borges, S.; Ornelas, I.; Freitas, A.I.; Guerra, G.; Henriques, E.; et al. Association of ADAMTS7 gene polymorphism with cardiovascular survival in coronary artery disease. *Physiol. Genom.* **2016**, *48*, 810–815. [CrossRef]
122. Bauer, R.C.; Tohyama, J.; Cui, J.; Cheng, L.; Yang, J.; Zhang, X.; Ou, K.; Paschos, G.K.; Zheng, X.L.; Parmacek, M.S.; et al. Knockout of Adamts7, a novel coronary artery disease locus in humans, reduces atherosclerosis in mice. *Circulation* **2015**, *131*, 1202–1213. [CrossRef]
123. Hofmann, B.; Adam, A.C.; Jacobs, K.; Riemer, M.; Erbs, C.; Bushnaq, H.; Simm, A.; Silber, R.E.; Santos, A.N. Advanced glycation end product associated skin autofluorescence: A mirror of vascular function? *Exp. Gerontol.* **2013**, *48*, 38–44. [CrossRef]
124. de Vos, L.C.; Lefrandt, J.D.; Dullaart, R.P.; Zeebregts, C.J.; Smit, A.J. Advanced glycation end products: An emerging biomarker for adverse outcome in patients with peripheral artery disease. *Atherosclerosis* **2016**, *254*, 291–299. [CrossRef]
125. Singh, V.P.; Bali, A.; Singh, N.; Jaggi, A.S. Advanced glycation end products and diabetic complications. *Korean J. Physiol. Pharmacol.* **2014**, *18*, 1–14. [CrossRef]
126. Thygesen, K.; Alpert, J.S.; Jaffe, A.S.; Chaitman, B.R.; Bax, J.J.; Morrow, D.A.; White, H.D.; Executive Group on behalf of the Joint European Society of Cardiology/American College of Cardiology/American Heart Association/World Heart Federation Task Force for the Universal Definition of Myocardial Infarction. Fourth Universal Definition of Myocardial Infarction (2018). *J. Am. Coll. Cardiol.* **2018**, *72*, 2231–2264. [CrossRef]
127. Samman Tahhan, A.; Sandesara, P.; Hayek, S.S.; Hammadah, M.; Alkhoder, A.; Kelli, H.M.; Topel, M.; O'Neal, W.T.; Ghasemzadeh, N.; Ko, Y.A.; et al. High-Sensitivity Troponin I Levels and Coronary Artery Disease Severity, Progression, and Long-Term Outcomes. *J. Am. Heart Assoc.* **2018**, *7*, e007914. [CrossRef] [PubMed]
128. Evans, J.D.W.; Dobbin, S.J.H.; Pettit, S.J.; Di Angelantonio, E.; Willeit, P. High-Sensitivity Cardiac Troponin and New-Onset Heart Failure: A Systematic Review and Meta-Analysis of 67,063 Patients With 4,165 Incident Heart Failure Events. *JACC Heart Fail.* **2018**, *6*, 187–197. [CrossRef] [PubMed]
129. Filion, K.B.; Agarwal, S.K.; Ballantyne, C.M.; Eberg, M.; Hoogeveen, R.C.; Huxley, R.R.; Loehr, L.R.; Nambi, V.; Soliman, E.Z.; Alonso, A. High-sensitivity cardiac troponin T and the risk of incident atrial fibrillation: The Atherosclerosis Risk in Communities (ARIC) study. *Am. Heart J.* **2015**, *169*, 31–38. [CrossRef] [PubMed]
130. Zethelius, B.; Berglund, L.; Sundstrom, J.; Ingelsson, E.; Basu, S.; Larsson, A.; Venge, P.; Arnlov, J. Use of multiple biomarkers to improve the prediction of death from cardiovascular causes. *N. Engl. J. Med.* **2008**, *358*, 2107–2116. [CrossRef]
131. Shin, D.S.; Kim, H.N.; Shin, K.D.; Yoon, Y.J.; Kim, S.J.; Han, D.C.; Kwon, B.M. Cryptotanshinone inhibits constitutive signal transducer and activator of transcription 3 function through blocking the dimerization in DU145 prostate cancer cells. *Cancer Res.* **2009**, *69*, 193–202. [CrossRef] [PubMed]
132. Oi, T.; Asanuma, K.; Matsumine, A.; Matsubara, T.; Nakamura, T.; Iino, T.; Asanuma, Y.; Goto, M.; Okuno, K.; Kakimoto, T.; et al. STAT3 inhibitor, cucurbitacin I, is a novel therapeutic agent for osteosarcoma. *Int. J. Oncol.* **2016**, *49*, 2275–2284. [CrossRef]
133. Pidgeon, G.P.; Barr, M.P.; Harmey, J.H.; Foley, D.A.; Bouchier-Hayes, D.J. Vascular endothelial growth factor (VEGF) upregulates BCL-2 and inhibits apoptosis in human and murine mammary adenocarcinoma cells. *Br. J. Cancer* **2001**, *85*, 273–278. [CrossRef] [PubMed]

34. Chung, J.; Bachelder, R.E.; Lipscomb, E.A.; Shaw, L.M.; Mercurio, A.M. Integrin (alpha 6 beta 4) regulation of eIF-4E activity and VEGF translation: A survival mechanism for carcinoma cells. *J. Cell Biol.* **2002**, *158*, 165–174. [CrossRef] [PubMed]
35. Shibuya, M. Vascular Endothelial Growth Factor (VEGF) and Its Receptor (VEGFR) Signaling in Angiogenesis: A Crucial Target for Anti- and Pro-Angiogenic Therapies. *Genes Cancer* **2011**, *2*, 1097–1105. [CrossRef] [PubMed]
36. McDonnell, T.; Wincup, C.; Buchholz, I.; Pericleous, C.; Giles, I.; Ripoll, V.; Cohen, H.; Delcea, M.; Rahman, A. The role of beta-2-glycoprotein I in health and disease associating structure with function: More than just APS. *Blood Rev.* **2020**, *39*, 100610. [CrossRef] [PubMed]
37. Maiolino, G.; Rossitto, G.; Caielli, P.; Bisogni, V.; Rossi, G.P.; Calo, L.A. The role of oxidized low-density lipoproteins in atherosclerosis: The myths and the facts. *Mediat. Inflamm.* **2013**, *2013*, 714653. [CrossRef] [PubMed]
38. Pitari, G.M.; Cotzia, P.; Ali, M.; Birbe, R.; Rizzo, W.; Bombonati, A.; Palazzo, J.; Solomides, C.; Shuber, A.P.; Sinicrope, F.A.; et al. Vasodilator-Stimulated Phosphoprotein Biomarkers Are Associated with Invasion and Metastasis in Colorectal Cancer. *Biomark. Cancer* **2018**, *10*, 1179299X18774551. [CrossRef]
39. Aratani, Y. Myeloperoxidase: Its role for host defense, inflammation, and neutrophil function. *Arch. Biochem. Biophys.* **2018**, *640*, 47–52. [CrossRef] [PubMed]
40. van der Veen, B.S.; de Winther, M.P.; Heeringa, P. Myeloperoxidase: Molecular mechanisms of action and their relevance to human health and disease. *Antioxid. Redox Signal* **2009**, *11*, 2899–2937. [CrossRef]
41. Arnhold, J. The Dual Role of Myeloperoxidase in Immune Response. *Int. J. Mol. Sci.* **2020**, *21*, 8057. [CrossRef]
42. Lipkova, J.; Parenica, J.; Duris, K.; Helanova, K.; Tomandl, J.; Kubkova, L.; Vasku, A.; Goldbergova Pavkova, M. Association of circulating levels of RANTES and -403G/A promoter polymorphism to acute heart failure after STEMI and to cardiogenic shock. *Clin. Exp. Med.* **2015**, *15*, 405–414. [CrossRef]
43. Appay, V.; Rowland-Jones, S.L. RANTES: A versatile and controversial chemokine. *Trends Immunol.* **2001**, *22*, 83–87. [CrossRef]
44. Ueba, T.; Nomura, S.; Inami, N.; Yokoi, T.; Inoue, T. Elevated RANTES level is associated with metabolic syndrome and correlated with activated platelets associated markers in healthy younger men. *Clin. Appl. Thromb. Hemost.* **2014**, *20*, 813–818. [CrossRef]
45. Amabile, N.; Rautou, P.E.; Tedgui, A.; Boulanger, C.M. Microparticles: Key protagonists in cardiovascular disorders. *Semin. Thromb. Hemost.* **2010**, *36*, 907–916. [CrossRef] [PubMed]
46. Margolis, J.; Kenrick, K.G. 2-dimensional resolution of plasma proteins by combination of polyacrylamide disc and gradient gel electrophoresis. *Nature* **1969**, *221*, 1056–1057. [CrossRef]
47. Tan, K.T.; Tayebjee, M.H.; Lynd, C.; Blann, A.D.; Lip, G.Y. Platelet microparticles and soluble P selectin in peripheral artery disease: Relationship to extent of disease and platelet activation markers. *Ann. Med.* **2005**, *37*, 61–66. [CrossRef] [PubMed]
48. Namba, M.; Tanaka, A.; Shimada, K.; Ozeki, Y.; Uehata, S.; Sakamoto, T.; Nishida, Y.; Nomura, S.; Yoshikawa, J. Circulating platelet-derived microparticles are associated with atherothrombotic events: A marker for vulnerable blood. *Arterioscler. Thromb. Vasc. Biol.* **2007**, *27*, 255–256. [CrossRef] [PubMed]
49. Badimon, L.; Suades, R.; Fuentes, E.; Palomo, I.; Padro, T. Role of Platelet-Derived Microvesicles as Crosstalk Mediators in Atherothrombosis and Future Pharmacology Targets: A Link between Inflammation, Atherosclerosis, and Thrombosis. *Front. Pharmacol.* **2016**, *7*, 293. [CrossRef]
50. Chiva-Blanch, G.; Suades, R.; Padro, T.; Vilahur, G.; Pena, E.; Ybarra, J.; Pou, J.M.; Badimon, L. Microparticle Shedding by Erythrocytes, Monocytes and Vascular Smooth Muscular Cells Is Reduced by Aspirin in Diabetic Patients. *Rev. Esp. Cardiol. Engl. Ed.* **2016**, *69*, 672–680. [CrossRef]
51. Getts, D.R.; Terry, R.L.; Getts, M.T.; Deffrasnes, C.; Muller, M.; van Vreden, C.; Ashhurst, T.M.; Chami, B.; McCarthy, D.; Wu, H.; et al. Therapeutic inflammatory monocyte modulation using immune-modifying microparticles. *Sci. Transl. Med.* **2014**, *6*, 219. [CrossRef]
52. Chiva-Blanch, G.; Crespo, J.; Suades, R.; Arderiu, G.; Padro, T.; Vilahur, G.; Cubedo, J.; Corella, D.; Salas-Salvado, J.; Aros, F.; et al. CD142+/CD61+, CD146+ and CD45+ microparticles predict cardiovascular events in high risk patients following a Mediterranean diet supplemented with nuts. *Thromb. Haemost.* **2016**, *116*, 103–114. [CrossRef] [PubMed]
53. Almog, N.; Henke, V.; Flores, L.; Hlatky, L.; Kung, A.L.; Wright, R.D.; Berger, R.; Hutchinson, L.; Naumov, G.N.; Bender, E.; et al. Prolonged dormancy of human liposarcoma is associated with impaired tumor angiogenesis. *FASEB J.* **2006**, *20*, 947–949. [CrossRef] [PubMed]
54. Naumov, G.N.; Bender, E.; Zurakowski, D.; Kang, S.Y.; Sampson, D.; Flynn, E.; Watnick, R.S.; Straume, O.; Akslen, L.A.; Folkman, J.; et al. A model of human tumor dormancy: An angiogenic switch from the nonangiogenic phenotype. *J. Natl. Cancer Inst.* **2006**, *98*, 316–325. [CrossRef] [PubMed]
55. Cervi, D.; Yip, T.T.; Bhattacharya, N.; Podust, V.N.; Peterson, J.; Abou-Slaybi, A.; Naumov, G.N.; Bender, E.; Almog, N.; Italiano, J.E., Jr.; et al. Platelet-associated PF-4 as a biomarker of early tumor growth. *Blood* **2008**, *111*, 1201–1207. [CrossRef] [PubMed]
56. Hansson, G.K. Inflammation, atherosclerosis, and coronary artery disease. *N. Engl. J. Med.* **2005**, *352*, 1685–1695. [CrossRef] [PubMed]
57. Ozawa, K.; Muller, M.A.; Varlamov, O.; Tavori, H.; Packwood, W.; Mueller, P.A.; Xie, A.; Ruggeri, Z.; Chung, D.; Lopez, J.A.; et al. Proteolysis of Von Willebrand Factor Influences Inflammatory Endothelial Activation and Vascular Compliance in Atherosclerosis. *JACC Basic Transl. Sci.* **2020**, *5*, 1017–1028. [CrossRef] [PubMed]

158. Takaya, H.; Namisaki, T.; Kitade, M.; Kaji, K.; Nakanishi, K.; Tsuji, Y.; Shimozato, N.; Moriya, K.; Seki, K.; Sawada, Y.; et al. VWF/ADAMTS13 ratio as a potential biomarker for early detection of hepatocellular carcinoma. *BMC Gastroenterol.* **2019**, *19*, 167. [CrossRef] [PubMed]
159. De Meyer, S.F.; Stoll, G.; Wagner, D.D.; Kleinschnitz, C. von Willebrand factor: An emerging target in stroke therapy. *Stroke* **2012**, *43*, 599–606. [CrossRef]
160. Qin, F.; Impeduglia, T.; Schaffer, P.; Dardik, H. Overexpression of von Willebrand factor is an independent risk factor for pathogenesis of intimal hyperplasia: Preliminary studies. *J. Vasc. Surg.* **2003**, *37*, 433–439. [CrossRef]
161. Chen, G.F.; Xu, T.H.; Yan, Y.; Zhou, Y.R.; Jiang, Y.; Melcher, K.; Xu, H.E. Amyloid beta: Structure, biology and structure-based therapeutic development. *Acta Pharmacol. Sin.* **2017**, *38*, 1205–1235. [CrossRef]
162. Perneczky, R.; Guo, L.H.; Kagerbauer, S.M.; Werle, L.; Kurz, A.; Martin, J.; Alexopoulos, P. Soluble amyloid precursor protein beta as blood-based biomarker of Alzheimer's disease. *Transl. Psychiatry* **2013**, *3*, 227. [CrossRef]
163. O'Brien, R.J.; Wong, P.C. Amyloid precursor protein processing and Alzheimer's disease. *Annu. Rev. Neurosci.* **2011**, *34*, 185–204. [CrossRef]
164. Mai, W.; Liao, Y. Targeting IL-1beta in the Treatment of Atherosclerosis. *Front. Immunol.* **2020**, *11*, 589654. [CrossRef] [PubMed]
165. Libby, P. Interleukin-1 Beta as a Target for Atherosclerosis Therapy: Biological Basis of CANTOS and Beyond. *J. Am. Coll. Cardiol.* **2017**, *70*, 2278–2289. [CrossRef] [PubMed]
166. Gonzalez, L.; Rivera, K.; Andia, M.E.; Martinez Rodriguez, G. The IL-1 Family and Its Role in Atherosclerosis. *Int. J. Mol. Sci.* **2022**, *24*, 17. [CrossRef] [PubMed]
167. Peiro, C.; Lorenzo, O.; Carraro, R.; Sanchez-Ferrer, C.F. IL-1beta Inhibition in Cardiovascular Complications Associated to Diabetes Mellitus. *Front. Pharmacol.* **2017**, *8*, 363. [CrossRef] [PubMed]
168. Shrestha, S.; Nazy, I.; Smith, J.W.; Kelton, J.G.; Arnold, D.M. Platelet autoantibodies in the bone marrow of patients with immune thrombocytopenia. *Blood Adv.* **2020**, *4*, 2962–2966. [CrossRef] [PubMed]
169. Zito, F.; Drummond, F.; Bujac, S.R.; Esnouf, M.P.; Morrissey, J.H.; Humphries, S.E.; Miller, G.J. Epidemiological and genetic associations of activated factor XII concentration with factor VII activity, fibrinopeptide A concentration, and risk of coronary heart disease in men. *Circulation* **2000**, *102*, 2058–2062. [CrossRef] [PubMed]
170. Miller, G.J.; Esnouf, M.P.; Burgess, A.I.; Cooper, J.A.; Mitchell, J.P. Risk of coronary heart disease and activation of factor XII in middle-aged men. *Arterioscler. Thromb. Vasc. Biol.* **1997**, *17*, 2103–2106. [CrossRef]
171. Ishii, K.; Oguchi, S.; Murata, M.; Mitsuyoshi, Y.; Takeshita, E.; Ito, D.; Tanahashi, N.; Fukuuchi, Y.; Oosumi, K.; Matsumoto, K.; et al. Activated factor XII levels are dependent on factor XII 46C/T genotypes and factor XII zymogen levels, and are associated with vascular risk factors in patients and healthy subjects. *Blood Coagul. Fibrinolysis* **2000**, *11*, 277–284.
172. Johansson, K.; Jansson, J.H.; Johansson, L.; Bylesjo, I.; Nilsson, T.K.; Eliasson, M.; Soderberg, S.; Lind, M. Factor XII as a Risk Marker for Hemorrhagic Stroke: A Prospective Cohort Study. *Cerebrovasc. Dis. Extra* **2017**, *7*, 84–94. [CrossRef] [PubMed]
173. Bonnez, Q.; Sakai, K.; Vanhoorelbeke, K. ADAMTS13 and Non-ADAMTS13 Biomarkers in Immune-Mediated Thrombotic Thrombocytopenic Purpura. *J. Clin. Med.* **2023**, *12*, 6169. [CrossRef] [PubMed]
174. Gupta, A.K.; Joshi, M.B.; Philippova, M.; Erne, P.; Hasler, P.; Hahn, S.; Resink, T.J. Activated endothelial cells induce neutrophil extracellular traps and are susceptible to NETosis-mediated cell death. *FEBS Lett.* **2010**, *584*, 3193–3197. [CrossRef] [PubMed]
175. Villanueva, E.; Yalavarthi, S.; Berthier, C.C.; Hodgin, J.B.; Khandpur, R.; Lin, A.M.; Rubin, C.J.; Zhao, W.; Olsen, S.H.; Klinker, M.; et al. Netting neutrophils induce endothelial damage, infiltrate tissues, and expose immunostimulatory molecules in systemic lupus erythematosus. *J. Immunol.* **2011**, *187*, 538–552. [CrossRef] [PubMed]
176. Bruschi, M.; Petretto, A.; Santucci, L.; Vaglio, A.; Pratesi, F.; Migliorini, P.; Bertelli, R.; Lavarello, C.; Bartolucci, M.; Candiano, G.; et al. Neutrophil Extracellular Traps protein composition is specific for patients with Lupus nephritis and includes methyl-oxidized alphaenolase (methionine sulfoxide 93). *Sci. Rep.* **2019**, *9*, 7934. [CrossRef] [PubMed]
177. Kaplan, M.J.; Radic, M. Neutrophil extracellular traps: Double-edged swords of innate immunity. *J. Immunol.* **2012**, *189*, 2689–2695. [CrossRef] [PubMed]
178. Ho, A.S.; Chen, C.H.; Cheng, C.C.; Wang, C.C.; Lin, H.C.; Luo, T.Y.; Lien, G.S.; Chang, J. Neutrophil elastase as a diagnostic marker and therapeutic target in colorectal cancers. *Oncotarget* **2014**, *5*, 473–480. [CrossRef] [PubMed]
179. Jia, W.; Luo, Q.; Wu, J.; Shi, Y.; Guan, Q. Neutrophil elastase as a potential biomarker related to the prognosis of gastric cancer and immune cell infiltration in the tumor immune microenvironment. *Sci. Rep.* **2023**, *13*, 13447. [CrossRef]
180. Taylor, S.; Dirir, O.; Zamanian, R.T.; Rabinovitch, M.; Thompson, A.A.R. The Role of Neutrophils and Neutrophil Elastase in Pulmonary Arterial Hypertension. *Front. Med.* **2018**, *5*, 217. [CrossRef]
181. Thalin, C.; Aguilera, K.; Hall, N.W.; Marunde, M.R.; Burg, J.M.; Rosell, A.; Daleskog, M.; Mansson, M.; Hisada, Y.; Meiners, M.J.; et al. Quantification of citrullinated histones: Development of an improved assay to reliably quantify nucleosomal H3Cit in human plasma. *J. Thromb. Haemost.* **2020**, *18*, 2732–2743. [CrossRef]
182. Mauracher, L.M.; Posch, F.; Martinod, K.; Grilz, E.; Daullary, T.; Hell, L.; Brostjan, C.; Zielinski, C.; Ay, C.; Wagner, D.D.; et al. Citrullinated histone H3, a biomarker of neutrophil extracellular trap formation, predicts the risk of venous thromboembolism in cancer patients. *J. Thromb. Haemost.* **2018**, *16*, 508–518. [CrossRef] [PubMed]
183. Heo, K.S.; Chang, E.; Le, N.T.; Cushman, H.; Yeh, E.T.; Fujiwara, K.; Abe, J. De-SUMOylation enzyme of sentrin/SUMO-specific protease 2 regulates disturbed flow-induced SUMOylation of ERK5 and p53 that leads to endothelial dysfunction and atherosclerosis. *Circ. Res.* **2013**, *112*, 911–923. [CrossRef] [PubMed]

84. Wilhelmsen, K.; Xu, F.; Farrar, K.; Tran, A.; Khakpour, S.; Sundar, S.; Prakash, A.; Wang, J.; Gray, N.S.; Hellman, J. Extracellular signal-regulated kinase 5 promotes acute cellular and systemic inflammation. *Sci. Signal* **2015**, *8*, 86. [CrossRef]
85. Kim, J.; Lee, Y.R.; Lee, C.H.; Choi, W.H.; Lee, C.K.; Kim, J.; Bae, Y.M.; Cho, S.; Kim, B. Mitogen-activated protein kinase contributes to elevated basal tone in aortic smooth muscle from hypertensive rats. *Eur. J. Pharmacol.* **2005**, *514*, 209–215. [CrossRef]
86. McLimans, K.E.; Willette, A.A. Alzheimer's Disease Neuroimaging Initiative: Autotaxin is Related to Metabolic Dysfunction and Predicts Alzheimer's Disease Outcomes. *J. Alzheimers Dis.* **2017**, *56*, 403–413. [CrossRef]
87. Araki, T.; Okumura, T.; Hiraiwa, H.; Mizutani, T.; Kimura, Y.; Kazama, S.; Shibata, N.; Oishi, H.; Kuwayama, T.; Kondo, T.; et al. Serum autotaxin as a novel prognostic marker in patients with non-ischaemic dilated cardiomyopathy. *ESC Heart Fail.* **2022**, *9*, 1304–1313. [CrossRef]
88. Linton, M.F.; Fazio, S. Cyclooxygenase products and atherosclerosis. *Drug Discov. Today Ther. Strateg.* **2008**, *5*, 25–36. [CrossRef] [PubMed]
89. Schonbeck, U.; Sukhova, G.K.; Graber, P.; Coulter, S.; Libby, P. Augmented expression of cyclooxygenase-2 in human atherosclerotic lesions. *Am. J. Pathol.* **1999**, *155*, 1281–1291. [CrossRef] [PubMed]

Disclaimer/Publisher's Note: The statements, opinions and data contained in all publications are solely those of the individual author(s) and contributor(s) and not of MDPI and/or the editor(s). MDPI and/or the editor(s) disclaim responsibility for any injury to people or property resulting from any ideas, methods, instructions or products referred to in the content.

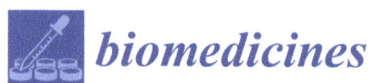

Review

New Approaches to the Management of Cardiovascular Risk Associated with Sleep Respiratory Disorders in Pediatric Patients

Esther Solano-Pérez [1,2,3], Carlota Coso [1,2,3], Sofía Romero-Peralta [1,2,3,4], María Castillo-García [1,2,3,4,5], Sonia López-Monzoni [1,3], Alfonso Ortigado [5,6,†] and Olga Mediano [1,2,3,5,*,†]

1. Sleep Unit, Pneumology Department, Hospital Universitario de Guadalajara, 19002 Guadalajara, Spain; 1399esther@gmail.com (E.S.-P.); carlootacs@gmail.com (C.C.); sofiamp10@hotmail.com (S.R.-P.); mariacastillogarcia37@gmail.com (M.C.-G.); sonialopezmonzoni@gmail.com (S.L.-M.)
2. Centro de Investigación Biomédica en Red de Enfermedades Respiratorias (CIBERES), 28029 Madrid, Spain
3. Instituto de Investigación Sanitaria de Castilla la Mancha (IDISCAM), 45071 Toledo, Spain
4. Sleep Research Institute, 28036 Madrid, Spain
5. Medicine Department, Universidad de Alcalá, 28805 Madrid, Spain; aortigado@secardiologia.es
6. Paediatric Department, Hospital Universitario de Guadalajara, 19002 Guadalajara, Spain
* Correspondence: olgamediano@hotmail.com
† These authors contributed equally to this work.

Abstract: Exposure to risk factors in youth can exacerbate the development of future cardiovascular disease (CVD). Obstructive sleep apnea (OSA), characterized by repetitive episodes of airway obstructions, could trigger said CVD acting as a modifiable risk factor. Measurements from echocardiography have shown impairments in the anatomy and function of the heart related to the severity of OSA. Therefore, the aim of this review was to propose a new clinical approach to the management of cardiovascular risk (CVR) in children based on treating OSA. The review includes studies assessing echocardiographic parameters for cardiac function and structure in pediatric OSA diagnosed using the apnea–hypopnea index (AHI) $\geq 1/h$ using polysomnography (PSG) and conducted within a year. Based on the reviewed evidence, in addition to PSG, echocardiography should be considered in OSA children in order to indicate the need for treatment and to reduce their future CVR. A follow-up echocardiography after treatment could be performed if impairments in the anatomy and function were found. Prioritizing parameters intimately connected to comorbidity could propel more effective patient-centered care. In conclusion, a reevaluation of pediatric OSA strategies should be considered, emphasizing comorbidity-related parameters in the cardiovascular field. Further studies are needed to assess this approach, potentially leading to enhanced protocols for more effective pediatric OSA treatment and CVR prevention.

Keywords: cardiovascular; echocardiography; sleep apnea; adenotonsillectomy; children

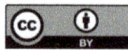

1. Introduction

1.1. Cardiovascular Disease in the Pediatric Population

Cardiovascular disease (CVD) is the main cause of death globally [1]. Although these adverse events are infrequent in children, the basis of these CVDs, atherosclerosis, may begin in childhood [2–4]. The exposure to risk factors and behaviors in youth can exacerbate its development. Hence, both addressing the social, economic, and environmental determinants of health to prevent the onset of risk factors (primordial prevention) and intervening to prevent risk factors from progressing into clinical diseases in adulthood (primary prevention) should be contemplated [2,5].

Focusing on primary prevention, some of these factors are related to life habits, while others are hereditary or the result of diseases [6]. The most common factors are excess body mass, high blood pressure (HBP), tobacco, low physical activity, and alterations in glucose and lipid metabolism [3–5,7]. Controlling said morbidities could decrease the atherosclerotic process and delay future cardiometabolic disease [8–10]. However, the importance of sleep as a possible trigger of CVD is often not considered despite the recent evidence highlighting its association [11,12]. It is imperative to consider the diagnosis and treatment of sleep disorders, even in the absence of clinically manifested CVD, as these may serve as potential contributors to them.

1.2. Sleep Disordered Breathing in the Pediatric Population

Sleep disturbances, and more concisely, sleep disordered breathing (SDB), are prevalent conditions in the pediatric population. SDB ranges from primary snoring (PS) to obstructive sleep apnea (OSA), being the prevalence of SDB of 10–17% and between 1 and 4% in OSA [13–15]. OSA is characterized by repetitive episodes of partial (hypopnea) or total (apnea) airway obstructions, driving immediate consequences that include changes in intrathoracic pressure, intermittent hypoxia, and sleep fragmentation [16]. The gold standard test to diagnose OSA is polysomnography (PSG), an objective sleep study that collects neurophysiological and cardiorespiratory variables, which is performed in-laboratory during the night. OSA in children is considered when the apnea–hypopnea index (AHI), a parameter obtained from the sleep study that collects the number of respiratory events per hour of sleep, is greater than 1–3 events per hour. Adenotonsillectomy (AT) is the first line and effective treatment in moderate-to-severe OSA patients (AHI $\geq$ 5) when adenotonsillar hypertrophy, the most-frequent cause in children, is also present [16,17].

1.3. OSA Treatment as a Modifiable Cardiovascular Risk Factor

OSA has particularly been related to adverse cardiovascular (CV) responses due to its associated immediate consequences [18], which result in the activation of the sympathetic nervous system, increased oxidative stress, and a proinflammatory and hypercoagulable state [19]. All these processes taking place in children with OSA have an impact on their CV sphere: alterations in hemodynamic and cardiac structure and function, increase in blood pressure (BP) levels with special impact during night, activation of the inflammatory cascade, and dysfunction of endothelium [20]. Therefore, treating OSA could reduce these intermediate mechanisms acting as a modifiable risk factor in the development of future CVD.

In the present review, CV risk (CVR) was evaluated through the alteration of both the anatomy and function of the heart, assessed using the ultrasound-based imaging technique (echocardiography). On the other hand, OSA was considered for the narrative review when AHI $\geq$ 1/h was identified from PSG performed in-laboratory. Performing an echocardiography as a complementary test to the PSG could help to identify children who have OSA and concomitant increased CVR. Therefore, the main aim of this review was to propose a new clinical management of CVR in children based on treating OSA as a potential modulator of this risk.

2. Material and Methods

For the narrative review, Table 1 contains reports including information about echocardiography and PSG within the pediatric population. The terms "echocardiography" and "obstructive sleep apnea" were used in PubMed and Web of Science to search for these articles. The reports had to meet the following criteria: (1) echocardiographic parameters evaluating cardiac function and anatomy; (2) OSA diagnosis using an AHI $\geq$ 1/h obtained from in-laboratory PSG; (3) realization of PSG and echocardiography within 1 year; (4) age below 18 years; (5) articles written in English from 2000 to the present. Exclusion criteria were as follows: (1) participants with comorbidities, neuromuscular disorders, or syndromic disorders; (2) systematic reviews and meta-analyses; (3) obese-only populations. Finally, after a careful evaluation of all the studies, 10 studies with adequate data meeting the criteria of the authors were integrated into the narrative synthesis.

3. Results and Discussion
3.1. Association between OSA and Echocardiography Parameters
3.1.1. The Impact of OSA on Cardiac Structure and Function

There is inconsistency in the evidence supporting an association between pediatric OSA and cardiac remodeling. As suggested by previous reviews [21,22], said controversy may be due to heterogeneity in their designs, comprising characteristics of participants (anthropometric variables and medical history), recruitment strategies, follow-up periods, OSA diagnosis and stratification, composition of control groups, echocardiographic parameters, and echocardiographic imaging methods.

OSA in children has been associated with cardiac alterations involving both left (LV) and right (RV) ventricles and pulmonary arteries. Said CV disturbances may be worsened as OSA severity increases but reverted with effective treatment. Related to LV structure impairments associated with OSA, Amin et al., 2002 and 2005 [23,24], found a statistically significant increase in the LV mass associated with OSA severity measured using the AHI, desaturation index (DI), and oxygen saturation (SpO_2). This hypertrophy improved after treatment. Similarly, Villa et al., 2011 [25], indicated that SDB children (OSA and PS), but not no-SDB participants, had a tendency for increased LV mass. Chan et al., 2009 [26], showed increased relative wall thickness (RWT) and interventricular septal thickness index to height (IVSI) in moderate-to-severe OSA children (AHI > 5/h) vs. mild OSA (AHI 1–5/h). These variables improved in OSA children adequately treated but not in persistent OSA. The same results have been recently published by Domany et al., 2021, in which OSA children (obstructive AHI—OAHI > 1/h) had increased LV mass worsened with OSA severity.

3.1.2. OSA Impact in Cardiac Function

Regarding LV function, the study by Amin et al., 2002 and 2005 [23,24], identified a decrease in LV diastolic function as E/A ratio, which measures flow velocities across the mitral valve, was diminished in PS (AHI < 1/h) and OSA (AHI $\geq$ 1/h) children. Comparing both groups, this dysfunction only improved in OSA but not in PS after treatment. Similar results were shown by Ugur et al., 2008 [27], in which OSA children (AHI > 2/h) presented diastolic dysfunction demonstrated by an increase in the mitral Em/Am ratio, with changes after AT. Similar results were reported by Chan et al., 2009 [26], demonstrating an alteration in diastolic function with E/e', a marker of LV filling pressure, which was elevated when the severity of OSA increased. Kaditis et al., 2010 [28], showed decreased LV systolic function in moderate-to-severe OSA (OAHI > 5/h) vs. PS (AHI $\leq$ 2/h) measured through lower LV ejection fraction (LVEF), defined by the volume ejected in systole in relation to the volume in the ventricle at the end of diastole, and LV shortening fraction (LVSF), a measure of LV contractility. In the study by Villa et al., 2011 [25], LV dysfunction was demonstrated through a diminished LVEF in OSA children (AHI $\geq$ 1/h) vs. PS (AHI < 1/h), decreased E/A ratio, and increased isovolumetric relaxation time (IVRT). Recently, Domany et al., 2021 [29], reported that, in OSA children (OAHI > 1/h), LV diastolic dysfunction worsened with OSA severity with improvements after AT, measured by a decrease in the E/e' ratio in the follow-up.

Regarding the association of the RV architecture and OSA, Amin et al., 2002 [23], indicated an association between the OSA and RV dimensions in children independent of BP and body mass, with RV abnormalities being more common in OSA patients (AHI $\geq$ 1/h) compared to PS (AHI < 1/h). In terms of RV function, Ugur et al., 2008 [27], observed RV diastolic dysfunction through lower tricuspid Em/Am values in the OSA group (AHI > 2/h), with a favorable change after AT, demonstrated by the elevation of this value in the surgery group. In the study by Chan et al., 2009 [26], many measurements of RV dysfunction were significantly different when OSA severity increased: greater RV systolic volume index (RVSVI), lower RV ejection fraction (RVEF), and right ventricular myocardial performance index (RVMPI). Also, an improvement in RVMPI values related to a significant reduction in the AHI was shown after treatment (surgery or nasal steroid therapy). These results were not effective in the group with persistent OSA. Goldbart et al., 2010 [30], found a strong association between the measurement of RV function, tricuspid regurgitation (TR), and OSA severity. Prior to AT, TR values were elevated in comparison to normal values for children, and these measurements normalized after surgery.

Finally, few studies have investigated the effect of OSA on pulmonary arterial pressure (PAP). Ugur et al., 2008 [27], communicated an increase in PAP in OSA children, with a decrease after treatment through surgery. Similarly, Tinano et al., 2022 [31], showed a reduction in pulmonary arterial systolic pressure (PASP) after AT.

However, although most of the studies reported alterations in the CV sphere, other studies have shown that these abnormalities in preoperative echocardiography were not directly associated with OSA severity. Also, these studies did not find a direct association between surgery and cardiac impairments. Kaditis et al., 2010 [28], could not find an association between diastolic function and cardiac structure in SDB. Goldbart et al., 2010 [30], did not find a correlation between the AHI and LV end-diastolic diameter, suggesting a stronger impact on RV than on LV in OSA children with an AHI $\geq 5/h$. Finally, Teplitzky et al., 2019 [32], showed no significant functional or structural cardiac impairments in a very severe OSA cohort (AHI $\geq 30/h$).

In summary, it has been shown that OSA could trigger cardiac alterations involving LV and RV, highlighting impairments in diastolic and systolic functions, increased mass, and higher PAP. These disturbances, in terms of architecture and function, were usually worsened as OSA severity increased, as measured using the AHI. In many studies, the impact of treatment was assessed, leading to an observation of a general improvement when children were adequately treated.

Therefore, it seems that OSA is an important risk factor in the CV sphere and that OSA treatment may be useful for the health of the heart in this population. The early identification and management of both cardiac issues and sleep disturbances might improve the overall health and quality of life of children, potentially reducing the risk of complications and improving long-term health outcomes.

Table 1. Summary of previous reports about the association of OSA diagnosis and treatment and CV consequences.

Study (Author, Year)	Type of Study	Number of Participants (Control/OSA)	Age (Years)	Sex (% Males)	OSA Classification	Mean Follow-Up	Other Characteristics	Main CV Outcomes
Tinano MM. et al., 2022 [31]	Retrospective case series study	-/15 (11 AT/ 4 non-AT)	<10 years	53.3%	OAHI ≥ 1/h Moderate OAHI ≥ 5 < 10/h Severe ≥ 10/h	18.7 months	Brodsky's grades 3–4 >75% adenoid hypertrophy AT indication	PASP decreased in all AT children (16.6%); The OAHI did not decrease in six AT children (55%) and three non-AT children (75%); Mean min SpO$_2$ increased in the AT children (from 87.5% to 90.2%); Clinical improvements were reported despite the persistence of altered OAHI in six children.
Domany KA. et al., 2021 [29]	Combined from 2 prospective longitudinal studies	174/199	5–13 years	59.3%	OAHI > 1/h	6–24 months	Hypertrophy of palatine tonsils who were scheduled for AT	At baseline, OSA children presented LV diastolic dysfunction and increased LV mass, which worsened as OSA severity increased. After AT, there was an improvement in diastolic dysfunction; no similar changes occurred in the controls. OAHI improved following AT, the E/e′ ratio decreased, and e′ increased.
Teplitzky T. et al., 2019 [32]	Case series, retrospective study	47	1–17 years	70.2%	Severe OSA: AHI ≥ 30/h	-	Echocardiographic evaluation within six months prior to AT	Severe OSA children who underwent echocardiographic screening prior to AT did not show significant functional or structural cardiac impairments. Thus, preoperative echocardiographic screening did not identify any abnormalities.

Table 1. *Cont.*

Study (Author, Year)	Type of Study	Number of Participants (Control/OSA)	Age (Years)	Sex (% Males)	OSA Classification	Mean Follow-Up	Other Characteristics	Main CV Outcomes
Villa MP. et al., 2011 [25]	Cross-sectional, observational study	21/18 PS/31 OSA	2–16 years	75.7%	PS: AHI < 1/h OSA: AHI ≥ 1/h	-	Echocardiographic examinations were performed in the morning following PSG	A tendency for increased LV mass between the control group and SDB (PS or OSA) was found but was not statistically significant. Significantly higher LVEF values were observed in OSA patients than in patients with PS. SDB patients compared with control subjects presented an alteration in the late phase of LV diastolic function: (1) increase in the A wave amplitude and a reduction in the E/A ratio, although this difference was statistically significant only in patients with PS. (2) statistically higher IVRT values.
Goldbart AD. et al., 2010 [30]	Prospective study	45/90	<3 years	70.4%	AHI ≥ 5/h	3 months	Echocardiography was performed on the morning of AT and 3 months later	The severity of the disease measured using AHI was strongly correlated with the measurements of RV function (TR). Also, TR values were abnormal, and these measurements were normalized before AT. However, no such correlations were seen with LVEDD (diastolic capacity of the heart), suggesting a stronger impact on the RV than on the LV in young children with OSA.
Kaditis AG. et al., 2010 [28]	Cross-sectional study	19/13 PS/14 OSA	2–12 years	52.2%	PS: OAHI ≤ 2/h Mild OSA: OAHI > 2 ≤ 5/h Moderate-to-severe OSA: OAHI > 5/h	-	Echocardiography was carried out the morning after completion of the sleep study;	The main finding was the lower LV systolic function in children with moderate-to-severe OSA compared to subjects with PS (LVEF and LVSF). Diastolic function and cardiac structure indices in the current study were not related to severity of SDB.

Table 1. Cont.

Study (Author, Year)	Type of Study	Number of Participants (Control/OSA)	Age (Years)	Sex (% Males)	OSA Classification	Mean Follow-Up	Other Characteristics	Main CV Outcomes
Chan JY. et al., 2009 [26]	Community-based study	35/66	6–13 years	73.3%	Mild OSA: AHI $\geq 1 \leq 5$/h Moderate-to-severe OSA: AHI > 5/h	6 months	36 OSA subjects had follow-up assessment: 8 had AT, 9 received nasal steroid therapy, and 19 refused any forms of treatment but agreed to have follow-up assessment	This study documented RV and LV dysfunction and remodeling: RVSVI, RVEF, RVMPI, and E/e' were significantly different between controls, mild OSA, and moderate-to-severe OSA. RWT and the IVSI were significantly higher in the moderate to severe group compared with the mild group. Only RVMPI, IVSI improved in children with effective treatment. After controlling for age, gender, and BMI z score, children with moderate to severe OSA had a 4.2-fold increased risk of abnormal LV geometry compared with the control group. The cardiac abnormalities improved when treatment for OSA was effective but not in the group with persistent OSA.
Ugur MB. et al., 2008 [27]	Prospective study	26 PS/29 OSA		52.7%	PS: AHI ≤ 2/h OSA: AHI > 2/h	6 months	Echocardiography was performed in the preoperative period and then was repeated in the 6th postoperative month in the OSA group and once in the control group. Adenoidectomy, tonsillectomy, or AT were carried out in 11, 10, and 8 patients, respectively	The results of TDI showed high PAP values in children with adenotonsillar hypertrophy and OSA. There was a remarkable decrease in PAP in the postoperative period. RV diastolic dysfunction was observed, with favorable change after AT, which was demonstrated by the increase in tricuspid Em and Em/Am values in the surgery group. Similarly, mitral Em/Am values increased after surgery, suggesting that LV dysfunction improved postoperatively.

Table 1. Cont.

Study (Author, Year)	Type of Study	Number of Participants (Control/OSA)	Age (Years)	Sex (% Males)	OSA Classification	Mean Follow-Up	Other Characteristics	Main CV Outcomes
Amin RS. et al., 2005 [24]	Prospective study	15/48	5–18 years	65.1%	PS: AHI < 1/h OSA: -Group 2: AHI ≥ 1 ≤ 5/h -Group 3: AHI > 5/h	1 year	PSG was repeated 8 weeks and 1 year after the initial evaluation; 10 adequately treated OSA children and 10 age- and gender-matched children with PS were recruited for a 1-year follow-up study. Children were managed with different treatments: AT, uvulopalatoplasty, and CPAP	A decrease in the LV diastolic function (decrease in the E/A ratio) was found across the 3 groups. It improved after treatment in the OSA group but not in children with PS. Negative correlation between OSA severity and LV diastolic function was independent of obesity, BP, and LV mass. Increased LV mass index was observed with increased severity of OSA, which improved after the disorder was adequately treated.
Amin RS. et al., 2002 [23]	Cross-sectional study	19 PS/28 OSA	2–18 years	63.8%	PS: AHI < 1/h OSA: AHI ≥ 1/h	-	-	Children with OSA had a statistically significant increased LV mass compared with children with PS. This was correlated with AHI, DI, and lowest SpO$_2$. The results of logistic regression (controlling for age, sex, and BMI) indicated that patients with OSA were more likely to have RV (6-fold) and LV (11-fold) abnormalities than patients with PS.

Abbreviation: OSA: obstructive sleep apnea; CV: cardiovascular; AT: adenotonsillectomy; OAHI: obstructive apnea-hypopnea index; PASP: pulmonary arterial systolic pressure; SpO$_2$: oxygen saturation; LV: left ventricle; AHI: apnea-hypopnea index; PS: primary snoring; PSG: polysomnography; SDB: sleep disordered breathing; LVEF: left ventricle ejection fraction; IVRT: isovolumetric relaxation time; RV: right ventricle; TR: tricuspid regurgitation; LVEDD: left ventricular end-diastolic diameter; LVSF: left ventricular shortening fraction; RVSVI: right ventricle systolic volume index; RVEF: right ventricle ejection fraction; RVMPI: right ventricular myocardial performance index; RWT: relative wall thickness; IVSI: interventricular septal thickness index to height; BMI: body mass index; TDI: tissue Doppler imaging; PAP: pulmonary arterial pressure; BP: blood pressure; CPAP: continuous positive airway pressure; DI: desaturation index.

3.2. Advantages of Performing an Echocardiography Complementary to Polysomnography

In this sense, performing an echocardiography in addition to the sleep study has several advantages. First, it is a short-term, non-invasive, and easy-to-perform technique compared to other procedures such as blood sample analysis used to obtain specific biomarkers described for evaluating cardiac function. Moreover, it is the most used technique in the study of heart disease due to its low cost and its wide availability [33].

Secondly, knowing that OSA has a negative impact on cardiac structure and function, it could be used to identify patients in whom treating OSA with AT could reverse these alterations [24,26,27,29–31].

Thirdly, it may help to better characterize OSA patients. Actually, OSA management is based on the AHI, which does not reflect the heterogeneity of the disease [34]. Selecting OSA patients undergoing surgery based on only the AHI could explain the different results found on AT, being the disease resolved in only 60–80% of children [35,36]. Unresolved OSA may not reverse the negative consequences promoted by OSA and could lead to neurocognitive deficits, behavioral changes, low academic performance, and low quality of life, among others [37]. Therefore, in addition to the AHI, new variables including echocardiographic parameters could be considered for better OSA management and define the phenotype of children undergoing AT. In this sense, the echocardiographic study could identify the group of patients in whom, regardless of its severity measured using the AHI, OSA is having an impact on their cardiac function and/or structure. Furthermore, these are potentially reversible changes which could reduce the development of short- and long-term adverse health outcomes. In the same way, follow-up echocardiography and PSG could help monitor the effectiveness of treatment for cardiac conditions and sleep disorders, enabling adjustments to be made when needed [38].

Fourthly, children are an ideal population to perform this technique since their risk factors can be modified before CVD is well established or advanced [20]. Additionally, first-line treatment in said population (AT) is effective in terms of compliance while in adults, first-line treatment, continuous positive airway pressure (CPAP), is conditioned by its adherence. Although the association between OSA and CVD is well known in adults, randomized clinical trials have failed to demonstrate the effect of CPAP in reducing major CV events [39–41]. The most sustained hypotheses are the low compliance of treatment and the inclusion of patients with CVD (secondary prevention) in said studies. Thus, selecting the pediatric population could clarify the response to the intervention of OSA in CVR without confounding factors or biases.

Finally, echocardiography is used to identify cardiac abnormalities that can lead to perioperative and postoperative complications in patients with severe OSA, as recommended by the American Thoracic Society (ATS) and American Heart Association (AHA) [42]. Therefore, performing an echocardiography for OSA children treated with AT could prevent said surgery-related difficulties due to cardiac impairments.

Otherwise, echocardiography has several limitations that need to be commented on. The main limitation is the need for qualified personnel who are essential for the realization and interpretation of the results obtained. Both PSG and echocardiography procedures could cause discomfort, particularly in children, which could lead to stress during the tests, potentially affecting the accuracy of the results. Another disadvantage could be the waiting time for both tests to be performed, which might lead to delays in surgery. Finally, echocardiography measures cardiac structure and function but no other important CV alterations such as elevated BP values, which have been related to future CVD in children [39,43].

3.3. Management Proposal for Children with CVR and OSA

Historically, the AHI has served as a primary marker guiding surgical indications for values ≥ 5 events per hour of sleep. Recent studies, however, have illuminated structural and functional cardiac abnormalities in children with AHI values below this threshold. Notably, these alterations appear to be potentially reversible with appropriate treatment. In this discourse, we advocate for a paradigm shift in the assessment of treatment indications, favoring a focus on preventing future comorbidities rather than relying solely on parameters that may not encapsulate the entire spectrum of the disease.

Furthermore, emerging data introduce novel parameters within the realm of OSA, which exhibit stronger associations with CV consequences more than the traditional AHI. Consequently, we propose that future clinical guidelines for the OSA definition in children and severity levels should be based on associated comorbidities and their potential ramifications. However, research exploring the genetic basis of OSA and its relationship with CV outcomes has uncovered candidate genes and pathways that may play crucial roles in both conditions. These genetic factors could influence not only the severity and susceptibility to OSA but also contribute to the development and progression of CV comorbidities associated with the disorder [44].

A transformative approach to diagnostic methods is suggested, directing efforts towards parameters more intricately linked to comorbidity. This would not only simplify diagnostic processes but also enhance their relevance in clinical decision-making. We posit that the diagnostic algorithm should incorporate assessments for organic damage, particularly CV impact. Compared to adults, the management of OSA in children faces two relevant problems: (1) the scientific knowledge in OSA and CVR association is less explored and slower in the child population; (2) the incorporation of the results into clinical practice is delayed. In order to mitigate these problems, strategic actions are relevant, including the following: developing research to transfer the knowledge to the pediatric population and the periodic updating of clinical guidelines based on scientific evidence.

Although guidelines published by ATS and AHA recommend performing preoperative echocardiography only on children with severe OSA [42], the reviewed studies have reported that children with SDB from PS to OSA may have cardiac abnormalities. Accordingly, children referred to the sleep unit for suspected SDB should undergo echocardiography in addition to the PSG, to adapt the treatment to the complete resolution of OSA and reduce their CVR. Additionally, a reevaluation of children after treatment may decide future readjustment when necessary, although it is not clear what the ideal follow-up period should be.

Beyond its role in diagnosis, echocardiography serves as a valuable tool for indicating the necessity of treatment and mitigating CVR. By employing echocardiographic parameters that intimately link to comorbidities, such as cardiac structure and function, clinicians can enhance their understanding of the diverse CV manifestations associated. This approach not only aids in treatment decision-making but also in more tailored and patient-centered care strategies. Furthermore, the integration of follow-up echocardiography post treatment, when necessary, provides an additional insight into the effectiveness of interventions, allowing for the continuous refinement of management strategies.

Implementing these modifications would fundamentally alter the current treatment management algorithm, allowing for the identification of patient cohorts deriving clear treatment benefits. This risk-based approach, departing from arbitrary measures, offers a more personalized framework for the management of pediatric OSA. The delay produced in the application of these advances involves the development and implementation of tailored educational programs for healthcare professionals. These programs could focus on disseminating the latest research findings to clinicians to make them well-informed about advancements in the field. Furthermore, fostering collaboration between researchers and healthcare practitioners (specialist and primary care practitioners) through interdisciplinary forums and conferences may enhance mutual understanding and facilitate the translation of research findings into clinical practice also in primary care levels.

As always, in the health management of children, promoting a supportive relationship, addressing parental concerns, promoting understanding, and obtaining informed consent are integral components of the diagnostic and treatment processes. By prioritizing these aspects, healthcare providers can enhance the quality of care and outcomes for pediatric patients.

Finally, the strengths and limitations of this review need to be commented on. The strengths of the study include a summarized broad spectrum of literature that provides a comprehensive overview of echocardiographic parameters in pediatric OSA. The inclusion of rigorous selection criteria, such as the strict age limit (under 18 years), standardized diagnostic criteria (PSG) for diagnosis and classification, and the temporal proximity between both methods, enhances the internal validity of our findings. Moreover, this population is of special interest as it offers insights into a critical developmental stage.

Within the limitations of the study, there is some controversy on the reported results, which may be due to the heterogeneity of the populations, composition of the control group that was predominantly PS children, different follow-up periods for reevaluation, and differences in echocardiographic performance. Additionally, the inclusion criteria for papers may have introduced selection bias, as only studies published in English were included, and those with participants presenting comorbidities or specific disorders were excluded. Additionally, there may be an underrepresentation of certain populations or recent advancements. These limitations should be considered when interpreting the results, and future research could address these constraints to understand the interplay between pediatric OSA and CV health.

4. Conclusions

In conclusion, we advocate for a comprehensive reevaluation of definitions, as well as diagnostic and management strategies, in pediatric OSA. By prioritizing parameters intimately connected to comorbidity and organic damage, we can propel the field towards a more effective, patient-centered care.

More studies with an adequate design are necessary to evaluate the possible implementation of this proposed management in the pediatric population. These studies may include a useful test for OSA diagnosis, and echocardiographic parameters should be considered for treatment indication according to its objective impact and reversibility. Therefore, it may prompt the development of novel protocols that could enhance the management of children's OSA treatment.

Author Contributions: Conceptualization, E.S.-P., C.C. and O.M.; methodology, E.S.-P., C.C. and O.M.; validation, E.S.-P., C.C. and O.M.; investigation, E.S.-P., C.C., S.R.-P., M.C.-G., S.L.-M., A.O. and O.M.; resources, O.M.; writing—original draft preparation, E.S.-P. and C.C.; writing—review and editing, O.M.; supervision, O.M.; funding acquisition, O.M. All authors have read and agreed to the published version of the manuscript.

Funding: This work was funded by the Instituto de Salud Carlos III (ISCIII: PI18/00565 and PI22/01653) and co-funded by the European Regional Development Fund (ERDF)/"A way to make Europe", the Spanish Respiratory Society (Sociedad Española de Neumología y Cirugía Torácica-SEPAR) (535-2018, 1073-2020 and 1425/2023), and an unconditional research grant from Menarini Laboratories and NEUMOMADRID (Sociedad Madrileña de Neumología y Cirugía Torácica).

Conflicts of Interest: The authors declare no conflicts of interest.

References

1. Cardiovascular Diseases. Available online: https://www.who.int/health-topics/cardiovascular-diseases (accessed on 22 December 2023).
2. De Ferranti, S.D.; Steinberger, J.; Ameduri, R.; Baker, A.; Gooding, H.; Kelly, A.S.; Mietus-Snyder, M.; Mitsnefes, M.M.; Peterson, A.L.; St-Pierre, J.; et al. Cardiovascular Risk Reduction in High-Risk Pediatric Patients: A Scientific Statement from the American Heart Association. *Circulation* **2019**, *139*, e603–e634. [CrossRef]
3. Raitakari, O.; Pahkala, K.; Magnussen, C.G. Prevention of Atherosclerosis from Childhood. *Nat. Rev. Cardiol.* **2022**, *19*, 543–554. [CrossRef] [PubMed]
4. Genovesi, S.; Giussani, M.; Orlando, A.; Battaglino, M.G.; Nava, E.; Parati, G. Prevention of Cardiovascular Diseases in Children and Adolescents. *High Blood Press. Cardiovasc. Prev.* **2019**, *26*, 191–197. [CrossRef]
5. Daniels, S.R.; Pratt, C.A.; Hayman, L.L. Reduction of Risk for Cardiovascular Disease in Children and Adolescents. *Circulation* **2011**, *124*, 1673–1686. [CrossRef] [PubMed]

Rada, D.A.G. Factores de Riesgo Cardiovascular en los Niños y los Adolescentes. In *Libro de la salud cardiovascular del Hospital Clínico San Carlos y la fundación BBVA*; Nerea S.A.: Bilbao, Spain, 2009; Chapter 2.

Candelino, M.; Tagi, V.M.; Chiarelli, F. Cardiovascular Risk in Children: A Burden for Future Generations. *Ital. J. Pediatr.* **2022**, *48*, 57. [CrossRef]

Chung, S.T.; Onuzuruike, A.U.; Magge, S.N. Cardiometabolic Risk in Obese Children. *Ann. N. Y. Acad. Sci.* **2018**, *1411*, 166–183. [CrossRef]

Cominato, L.; Franco, R.R.; Ybarra, M.; Frascino, A.V.; Steinmetz, L.; Ferraro, A.A.; Aivazoglou Carneiro, J.D.; Damiani, D. Obesity as a Thrombogenic and Cardiovascular Risk Factor in Children. *Horm. Res. Paediatr.* **2021**, *94*, 410–415. [CrossRef]

10. Drozdz, D.; Alvarez-Pitti, J.; Wójcik, M.; Borghi, C.; Gabbianelli, R.; Mazur, A.; Herceg-Čavrak, V.; Lopez-Valcarcel, B.G.; Brzeziński, M.; Lurbe, E.; et al. Obesity and Cardiometabolic Risk Factors: From Childhood to Adulthood. *Nutrients* **2021**, *13*, 4176. [CrossRef] [PubMed]

11. Wolk, R.; Gami, A.; Garciatouchard, A.; Somers, V. Sleep and Cardiovascular Disease. *Curr. Probl. Cardiol.* **2005**, *30*, 625–662. [CrossRef]

12. Cappuccio, F.P.; Miller, M.A. Sleep and Cardio-Metabolic Disease. *Curr. Cardiol. Rep.* **2017**, *19*, 110. [CrossRef]

13. Gokdemir, Y.; Civelek, E.; Cakir, B.; Demir, A.; Kocabas, C.N.; Ikizoglu, N.B.; Karakoc, F.; Karadag, B.; Ersu, R. Prevalence of Sleep-Disordered Breathing and Associated Risk Factors in Primary School Children in Urban and Rural Environments. *Sleep Breath.* **2021**, *25*, 915–922. [CrossRef] [PubMed]

14. Aroucha Lyra, M.C.; Aguiar, D.; Paiva, M.; Arnaud, M.; Filho, A.A.; Rosenblatt, A.; Thérèse Innes, N.P.; Heimer, M.V. Prevalence of Sleep-Disordered Breathing and Associations with Malocclusion in Children. *J. Clin. Sleep Med.* **2020**, *16*, 1007–1012. [CrossRef]

15. Williamson, A.A.; Johnson, T.J.; Tapia, I.E. Health Disparities in Pediatric Sleep-Disordered Breathing. *Paediatr. Respir. Rev.* **2023**, *45*, 2–7. [CrossRef] [PubMed]

16. Luz Alonso-Álvarez, M.; Canet, T.; Cubell-Alarco, M.; Estivill, E.; Fernández-Julián, E.; Gozal, D.; Jurado-Luque, M.J.; Lluch-Roselló, M.A.; Martínez-Pérez, F.; Merino-Andreu, M.; et al. Documento de consenso del síndrome de apneas-hipopneas durante el sueño en niños (versión completa). *Arch. de Bronconeumol.* **2011**, *47*, 2–18. [CrossRef]

17. Kaditis, A.G.; Gozal, D. Adenotonsillectomy: The Good, the Bad and the Unknown. *Curr. Opin. Pulm. Med.* **2022**, *28*, 537–542. [CrossRef] [PubMed]

18. Drager, L.F.; McEvoy, R.D.; Barbe, F.; Lorenzi-Filho, G.; Redline, S. Sleep Apnea and Cardiovascular Disease: Lessons from Recent Trials and Need for Team Science. *Circulation* **2017**, *136*, 1840–1850. [CrossRef] [PubMed]

19. Sánchez-de-la-Torre, M.; Campos-Rodriguez, F.; Barbé, F. Obstructive Sleep Apnoea and Cardiovascular Disease. *Lancet Respir. Med.* **2013**, *1*, 61–72. [CrossRef]

20. Castillo-García, M.; Solano-Pérez, E.; Coso, C.; Romero-Peralta, S.; García-Borreguero, D.; Izquierdo, J.L.; Mediano, O. Impact of Obstructive Sleep Apnea in Cardiovascular Risk in the Pediatric Population: A Systematic Review. *Sleep Med. Rev.* **2023**, *71*, 101818. [CrossRef]

21. Poupore, N.S.; Gudipudi, R.; Nguyen, S.A.; Pecha, P.P.; Pecha, T.J.; Carroll, W.W. Tissue Doppler Echocardiography in Children with OSA before and after Tonsillectomy and Adenoidectomy: A Systematic Review and Meta-Analysis. *Int. J. Pediatr. Otorhinolaryngol.* **2022**, *152*, 111002. [CrossRef]

22. Pettitt-Schieber, B.; Tey, C.S.; Nemeth, J.; Raol, N. Echocardiographic Findings in Children with Obstructive Sleep Apnea: A Systematic Review. *Int. J. Pediatr. Otorhinolaryngol.* **2021**, *145*, 110721. [CrossRef]

23. Amin, R.S.; Kimball, T.R.; Bean, J.A.; Jeffries, J.L.; Willging, J.P.; Cotton, R.T.; Witt, S.A.; Glascock, B.J.; Daniels, S.R. Left Ventricular Hypertrophy and Abnormal Ventricular Geometry in Children and Adolescents with Obstructive Sleep Apnea. *Am. J. Respir. Crit. Care Med.* **2002**, *165*, 1395–1399. [CrossRef]

24. Amin, R.S.; Kimball, T.R.; Kalra, M.; Jeffries, J.L.; Carroll, J.L.; Bean, J.A.; Witt, S.A.; Glascock, B.J.; Daniels, S.R. Left Ventricular Function in Children with Sleep-Disordered Breathing. *Am. J. Cardiol.* **2005**, *95*, 801–804. [CrossRef] [PubMed]

25. Villa, M.P.; Ianniello, F.; Tocci, G.; Evangelisti, M.; Miano, S.; Ferrucci, A.; Ciavarella, G.M.; Volpe, M. Early domanyCardiac Abnormalities and Increased C-Reactive Protein Levels in a Cohort of Children with Sleep Disordered Breathing. *Sleep Breath.* **2012**, *16*, 101–110. [CrossRef] [PubMed]

26. Chan, J.Y.S.; Li, A.M.; Au, C.-T.; Lo, A.F.C.; Ng, S.-K.; Abdullah, V.J.; Ho, C.; Yu, C.-M.; Fok, T.-F.; Wing, Y.-K. Cardiac Remodelling and Dysfunction in Children with Obstructive Sleep Apnoea: A Community Based Study. *Thorax* **2009**, *64*, 233–239. [CrossRef] [PubMed]

27. Ugur, M.B.; Dogan, S.M.; Sogut, A.; Uzun, L.; Cinar, F.; Altin, R.; Aydin, M. Effect of Adenoidectomy and/or Tonsillectomy on Cardiac Functions in Children with Obstructive Sleep Apnea. *ORL* **2008**, *70*, 202–208. [CrossRef] [PubMed]

28. Kaditis, A.G.; Alexopoulos, E.I.; Dalapascha, M.; Papageorgiou, K.; Kostadima, E.; Kaditis, D.G.; Gourgoulianis, K.; Zakynthinos, E. Cardiac Systolic Function in Greek Children with Obstructive Sleep-Disordered Breathing. *Sleep Med.* **2010**, *11*, 406–412. [CrossRef] [PubMed]

29. Domany, K.A.; Huang, G.; Hossain, M.M.; Schuler, C.L.; Somers, V.K.; Daniels, S.R.; Amin, R. Effect of Adenotonsillectomy on Cardiac Function in Children Age 5–13 Years with Obstructive Sleep Apnea. *Am. J. Cardiol.* **2021**, *141*, 120–126. [CrossRef] [PubMed]

30. Goldbart, A.D.; Levitas, A.; Greenberg-Dotan, S.; Ben Shimol, S.; Broides, A.; Puterman, M.; Tal, A. B-Type Natriuretic Peptide and Cardiovascular Function in Young Children with Obstructive Sleep Apnea. *Chest* **2010**, *138*, 528–535. [CrossRef] [PubMed]

31. Tinano, M.M.; Becker, H.M.G.; Franco, L.P.; Dos Anjos, C.P.G.; Ramos, V.M.; Nader, C.M.F.F.; Godinho, J.; De Párcia Gontijo, H.; Souki, B.Q. Morphofunctional Changes Following Adenotonsillectomy of Obstructive Sleep Apnea Children: A Case Series Analysis. *Prog. Orthod.* **2022**, *23*, 29. [CrossRef]
32. Teplitzky, T.B.; Pereira, K.D.; Isaiah, A. Echocardiographic Screening in Children with Very Severe Obstructive Sleep Apnea. *Int. J. Pediatr. Otorhinolaryngol.* **2019**, *126*, 109626. [CrossRef]
33. Chasco Ronda, J. El ecocardiograma. *Imagen Diagnóstica* **2010**, *1*, 14–18. [CrossRef]
34. Redline, S.; Azarbarzin, A.; Peker, Y. Obstructive Sleep Apnoea Heterogeneity and Cardiovascular Disease. *Nat. Rev. Cardiol.* **2023**, *20*, 560–573. [CrossRef] [PubMed]
35. Marcus, C.L.; Moore, R.H.; Rosen, C.L.; Giordani, B.; Garetz, S.L.; Taylor, H.G.; Mitchell, R.B.; Amin, R.; Katz, E.S.; Arens, R.; et al. A Randomized Trial of Adenotonsillectomy for Childhood Sleep Apnea. *N. Engl. J. Med.* **2013**, *368*, 2366–2376. [CrossRef] [PubMed]
36. Bhattacharjee, R.; Kheirandish-Gozal, L.; Spruyt, K.; Mitchell, R.B.; Promchiarak, J.; Simakajornboon, N.; Kaditis, A.G.; Splaingard, D.; Splaingard, M.; Brooks, L.J.; et al. Adenotonsillectomy Outcomes in Treatment of Obstructive Sleep Apnea in Children: A Multicenter Retrospective Study. *Am. J. Respir. Crit. Care Med.* **2010**, *182*, 676–683. [CrossRef] [PubMed]
37. Ersu, R.; Chen, M.L.; Ehsan, Z.; Ishman, S.L.; Redline, S.; Narang, I. Persistent Obstructive Sleep Apnoea in Children: Treatment Options and Management Considerations. *Lancet Respir. Med.* **2023**, *11*, 283–296. [CrossRef] [PubMed]
38. Solano-Pérez, E.; Coso, C.; Castillo-García, M.; Romero-Peralta, S.; Lopez-Monzoni, S.; Laviña, E.; Cano-Pumarega, I.; Sánchez-de-la-Torre, M.; García-Río, F.; Mediano, O. Diagnosis and Treatment of Sleep Apnea in Children: A Future Perspective Is Needed. *Biomedicines* **2023**, *11*, 1708. [CrossRef]
39. Yang, L.; Magnussen, C.G.; Yang, L.; Bovet, P.; Xi, B. Elevated Blood Pressure in Childhood or Adolescence and Cardiovascular Outcomes in Adulthood: A Systematic Review. *Hypertension* **2020**, *75*, 948–955. [CrossRef] [PubMed]
40. McEvoy, R.D.; Antic, N.A.; Heeley, E.; Luo, Y.; Ou, Q.; Zhang, X.; Mediano, O.; Chen, R.; Drager, L.F.; Liu, Z.; et al. CPAP for Prevention of Cardiovascular Events in Obstructive Sleep Apnea. *N. Engl. J. Med.* **2016**, *375*, 919–931. [CrossRef]
41. Sánchez-de-la-Torre, M.; Sánchez-de-la-Torre, A.; Bertran, S.; Abad, J.; Duran-Cantolla, J.; Cabriada, V.; Mediano, O.; Masdeu, M.J.; Alonso, M.L.; Masa, J.F.; et al. Effect of Obstructive Sleep Apnoea and Its Treatment with Continuous Positive Airway Pressure on the Prevalence of Cardiovascular Events in Patients with Acute Coronary Syndrome (ISAACC Study): A Randomised Controlled Trial. *Lancet Respir. Med.* **2020**, *8*, 359–367. [CrossRef]
42. Abman, S.H.; Hansmann, G.; Archer, S.L.; Ivy, D.D.; Adatia, I.; Chung, W.K.; Hanna, B.D.; Rosenzweig, E.B.; Raj, J.U.; Cornfield, D.; et al. Pediatric Pulmonary Hypertension: Guidelines from the American Heart Association and American Thoracic Society. *Circulation* **2015**, *132*, 2037–2099. [CrossRef]
43. Tirosh, A.; Afek, A.; Rudich, A.; Percik, R.; Gordon, B.; Ayalon, N.; Derazne, E.; Tzur, D.; Gershnabel, D.; Grossman, E.; et al. Progression of Normotensive Adolescents to Hypertensive Adults: A Study of 26 980 Teenagers. *Hypertension* **2010**, *56*, 203–209. [CrossRef] [PubMed]
44. Goodman, M.O.; Cade, B.E.; Shah, N.A.; Huang, T.; Dashti, H.S.; Saxena, R.; Rutter, M.K.; Libby, P.; Sofer, T.; Redline, S. Pathway-Specific Polygenic Risk Scores Identify Obstructive Sleep Apnea-Related Pathways Differentially Moderating Genetic Susceptibility to Coronary Artery Disease. *Circulation* **2022**, *15*, e003535. [CrossRef] [PubMed]

Disclaimer/Publisher's Note: The statements, opinions and data contained in all publications are solely those of the individual author(s) and contributor(s) and not of MDPI and/or the editor(s). MDPI and/or the editor(s) disclaim responsibility for any injury to people or property resulting from any ideas, methods, instructions or products referred to in the content.

MDPI AG
Grosspeteranlage 5
4052 Basel
Switzerland
Tel.: +41 61 683 77 34

Biomedicines Editorial Office
E-mail: biomedicines@mdpi.com
www.mdpi.com/journal/biomedicines

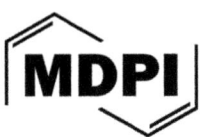

Disclaimer/Publisher's Note: The statements, opinions and data contained in all publications are solely those of the individual author(s) and contributor(s) and not of MDPI and/or the editor(s). MDPI and/or the editor(s) disclaim responsibility for any injury to people or property resulting from any ideas, methods, instructions or products referred to in the content.